# Neuromuscular *and* Electrodiagnostic Medicine Board Review

# Neuromuscular and Electrodiagnostic Medicine Board Review

**Thananan Thammongkolchai, MD**
Consultant Neurologist
Clinical Neurophysiology Unit, EMG Laboratory and Neuromuscular
Medicine Section
Division of Neurology, Department of Medicine
Ramathibodi Hospital, Mahidol University
Bangkok Thailand

**Pichet Termsarasab, MD**
Associate Professor and Consultant Neurologist
Division of Neurology, Department of Medicine
Ramathibodi Hospital, Mahidol University
Bangkok, Thailand

**Bashar Katirji, MD, FAAN**
Professor of Neurology
Case Western Reserve University School of Medicine
Director, Neuromuscular Center and EMG Laboratory
Department of Neurology
University Hospitals Cleveland Medical Center
Cleveland, Ohio, United States

**David C. Preston, MD, FAAN**
Professor of Neurology
Case Western Reserve University School of Medicine
Program Director, Neurology Residency
Vice Chairman, Department of Neurology
University Hospitals Cleveland Medical Center
Cleveland, Ohio, United States

ELSEVIER

Elsevier
1600 John F. Kennedy Blvd.
Ste 1800
Philadelphia, PA 19103-2899

---

**Notice**

Practitioners and researchers must always rely on their own experience and knowledge in evaluating and using any information, methods, compounds or experiments described herein. Because of rapid advances in the medical sciences, in particular, independent verification of diagnoses and drug dosages should be made. To the fullest extent of the law, no responsibility is assumed by Elsevier, authors, editors or contributors for any injury and/or damage to persons or property as a matter of products liability, negligence or otherwise, or from any use or operation of any methods, products, instructions, or ideas contained in the material herein.

---

**International Standard Book Number:** 9780323790758

*Content Strategist:* Mary Hegeler
*Content Development Specialists:* Shweta Pant, Ambika Kapoor
*Publishing Services Manager:* Shereen Jameel
*Project Manager:* Shereen Jameel
*Design Direction:* Amy Buxton

Printed in India

Last digit is the print number:   9  8  7  6  5  4  3  2  1

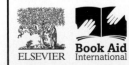

Working together
to grow libraries in
developing countries

www.elsevier.com • www.bookaid.org

*We dedicate this book to our families.*

*To my husband and beloved family, Suchin, Waraporn, Sopida, Apinya, and Bubble – TT*

*To my parents, Boonreun and Veerachai, and to Grandma Lung – PT*

*To my wife, Patricia, our children, Linda and Michael, and my mother, Malak – BK*

*To my wife, Barbara, and our daughters, Hannah and Abby – DCP*

# Preface

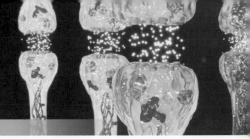

Why a board review book on neuromuscular and electrodiagnostic medicine?

First, an increasing number of neurology physicians and physical medicine and rehabilitation (PM&R) physicians are taking the initial and recertification board examinations, which involve knowledge (partial or complete), skills, and aptitude in neuromuscular medicine and electrodiagnostic medicine. These examinations include Neurology, Neuromuscular Medicine, and Clinical Neurophysiology under the American Board of Psychiatry and Neurology; PM&R and Neuromuscular Medicine under the American Board of Physical Medicine and Rehabilitation; and Electrodiagnostic Medicine under the American Board of Electrodiagnostic Medicine. While not intended to be a single comprehensive resource for all of neuromuscular and electrodiagnostic medicine, nor to replace classic textbooks, this book is a solid comprehensive review for physicians studying for those exams in tandem with other study tools and practices. We hope the book is also a useful resource for residents preparing for in-training examinations. In addition, practicing physicians can benefit from this text as a means to brush up on (or fill gaps in) knowledge that will improve their clinical practice.

Second, people have different learning styles, and this book is for the "question learners." Questions are thought provoking and invite active participation, as opposed to passive reading through long texts. We have included case vignettes, practical points, pitfalls, and important facts to remember. Reading and thinking through case vignettes that are based on real patients simulate and enhance the skill of clinical thinking when encountering patients.

The book is organized in twenty-one chapters. Chapters 1 and 2 review the applied anatomy and physiology of the peripheral nervous system. Chapters 3 through 8 review electrodiagnostic medicine. Chapters 9 through 11 discuss additional testing in neuromuscular disorders, including autonomic testing (and relevant clinical autonomic disorders), muscle and nerve biopsy, and neuromuscular ultrasound. Chapters 12 through 20 review clinical neuromuscular disorders, including disorders of motor neuron, nerve, neuromuscular junction, and muscle. Small fiber and autonomic neuropathies are reviewed again in Chapter 20. Chapter 21 covers the important topics of rehabilitation and ethics in neuromuscular disorders and electrodiagnostic medicine.

Each chapter has two parts: First, we list all questions – consecutively and without answers – so that readers can think through each question without any bias from knowing the answers. This is followed by the answer section where, for convenience, we repeat each question along with the answers (no need to flip back and forth between pages). We include a detailed Comments and Discussion section to provide not only the explanation for the correct and incorrect answers but also to expand on points in the topic(s) relevant to the question. The easy-to-read bulleted format makes these a "quick and dirty" review for the associated topics. Figures, video clips, and tracings (useful tools for visual learners) are incorporated throughout to simulate the actual board examination. We also include high-yield facts and mnemonics, which serve as a "candid" way to study (and are not typically found in formal textbooks). Suggested readings are listed neatly in one place at the end of each chapter. For deeper understanding and more comprehensive study of the subjects covered, we encourage closer review of the references and suggested readings.

Finally, our hope is that readers enjoy thinking through each of the questions posed and that they learn from the answers, ultimately leading to better patient care.

**Thananan Thammongkolchai, MD**
**Pichet Termsarasab, MD**
**Bashar Katirji, MD, FAAN**
**David C. Preston, MD, FAAN**

# Acknowledgments

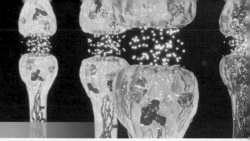

We thank our patients, residents, and fellows – and we are indebted to our mentors and colleagues. *For TT:* Bashar Katirji, MD, FAAN; David C. Preston, MD, FAAN; Barbara E. Shapiro, MD, PhD; Mark Cohen, MD; Supoch Tunlayadechanont, MD; Teeratorn Pulkes, MD, PhD. Ramathibodi EMG team, including Charungthai Dejthevaporn, MD, PhD; Kanlaya Kaokum, and Somlak Anwiset. *For PT:* Bashar Katirji, MD, FAAN; David C. Preston, MD, FAAN; Steven J. Frucht, MD; Paul E. Greene, MD; Tumtip Sangruchi, MD; Kanokwan Boonyapisit, MD; Kristina Simonyan, MD, PhD; Mark Cohen, MD; Xinglong Wang, PhD; Supoch Tunlayadechanont, MD; and Teeratorn Pulkes, MD, PhD. *For BK:* Asa J. Wilbourn, MD; Oscar Reinmuth, MD; Robert B. Daroff, MD. *For DCP;* Eric L. Logigian, MD; Martin A. Samuels, MD; John J. Kelly Jr., MD; Robert B. Daroff, MD.

We are grateful to Mark Cohen, MD, for providing many of the neuropathology figures and to Chat Iamsirikij, MD, for reviewing the physical medicine and rehabilitation questions in Chapter 21. We also thank the publishing team at Elsevier: Melanie Tucker, Mary Hegeler, Shweta Pant, Ambika Kapoor, Shereen Jameel, and Amy Buxton.

# Contents

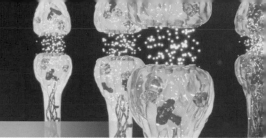

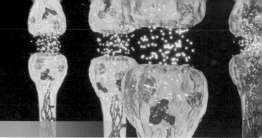

# CHAPTER 1

# Neuromuscular Applied Anatomy

## PART 1 | PRACTICE TEST

**Q1.** Which of the following is **TRUE** regarding the brachial plexus?
  A. There are three trunks: lateral, medial, and posterior.
  B. Each trunk divides into three divisions.
  C. All major upper extremity nerves originate from the trunks.
  D. The trunks are formed by the anterior rami of C5-T1.
  E. The cords form proximal to the level of the clavicle.

**Q2.** Which of the following muscles would be affected by a C5 radiculopathy but not an upper trunk lesion of the brachial plexus?
  A. Rhomboids
  B. Supraspinatus
  C. Infraspinatus
  D. Biceps
  E. Clavicular head of pectoralis major

**Q3.** Which of the following is **NOT** associated with an upper trunk lesion of the brachial plexus?
  A. Burner or stinger syndrome from contact sports
  B. Pancoast tumor
  C. Trauma
  D. Penetrating injury
  E. Obstetrical injury

**Q4.** Which of the following is **TRUE** regarding the cords of the brachial plexus?
  A. The posterior division of the lower trunk forms the medial cord.
  B. All three posterior divisions form the lateral cord.
  C. The upper trunk continues as the lateral cord.
  D. The anterior division of the upper trunk contributes to the lateral cord.
  E. The anterior divisions of the middle and lower trunks form the medial cord.

**Q5.** A 22-year-old man is referred to an electromyography (EMG) lab for evaluation of left arm weakness after a motorcycle accident 2 months ago. Needle examination of which of the following muscles would help differentiate an upper trunk from a lateral cord lesion of the brachial plexus?
  A. Brachialis
  B. Brachioradialis
  C. Rhomboids
  D. Supraspinatus
  E. Serratus anterior

**Q6.** Which of the following muscles is affected in a middle trunk but not in a posterior cord lesion of the brachial plexus?
  A. Teres minor
  B. Brachioradialis
  C. Triceps
  D. Pronator teres
  E. Abductor pollicis brevis

**Q7.** Which of the following muscles would be affected by a lower trunk lesion but not a medial cord lesion of the brachial plexus?
  A. Deltoid
  B. Extensor indicis proprius
  C. Abductor pollicis brevis
  D. Abductor digiti minimi
  E. Flexor digitorum profundus of the index finger

**Q8.** Which of the following muscles would be affected by a median nerve lesion in the forearm but not a carpal tunnel syndrome?
  A. Flexor carpi ulnaris
  B. Flexor carpi radialis
  C. Abductor pollicis longus
  D. Adductor pollicis
  E. Opponens pollicis

**Q9.** A 35-year-old man develops weakness of right thumb flexion at the interphalangeal joint. In addition, he cannot flex the index and middle fingers at the distal interphalangeal joints. However, the ring and little fingers are normal, and there is no sensory loss. What is the other muscle most likely to be affected?
A. Abductor pollicis brevis
B. Flexor carpi radialis
C. Flexor digitorum superficialis
D. Pronator teres
E. Pronator quadratus

**Q10.** A 44-year-old woman develops weakness of the right hand for 6 weeks. Electromyography (EMG) examination of which of the following muscles is useful to differentiate a median nerve lesion from a C8 nerve root lesion?
A. Abductor pollicis brevis
B. Opponens pollicis
C. Flexor pollicis longus
D. Flexor digitorum profundus of the index finger
E. Extensor indicis proprius

**Q11.** In a severe ulnar nerve lesion at Guyon's canal, which of the following clinical findings is **MOST LIKELY** to be **PRESENT**?
A. Intact sensation over the distal medial palm
B. Intact sensation over the medial side of the dorsum of the hand
C. Intact sensation over the little finger
D. Intact posture of the little and ring fingers
E. Normal abduction of the index finger

**Q12.** Which of the following upper extremity muscles has a dual nerve supply?
A. Flexor digitorum superficialis
B. Flexor pollicis brevis
C. Flexor pollicis longus
D. Opponens pollicis
E. Dorsal interossei

**Q13.** A patient presents with a wrist and finger drop. Which muscle would be affected by a radial neuropathy but not a posterior interosseous neuropathy?
A. Extensor digitorum indicis
B. Extensor digitorum communis
C. Extensor carpi ulnaris
D. Abductor pollicis longus
E. Brachioradialis

**Q14.** A 50-year-old man has weakness and atrophy of the left infraspinatus, but the left supraspinatus is normal. What is the most likely location of the lesion?
A. Suprascapular notch
B. Superior transverse scapular ligament
C. Anterior coracoscapular ligament
D. Spinoglenoid notch
E. Neck of the humerus

**Q15.** A woman presents with scapular winging as shown in the following photo. Which of the following muscles is most likely affected?

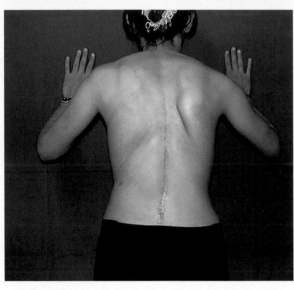

Ameri, E., Behtash, H. & Omidi-Kashani, F. *J Med Case Reports* **3**, 7366 (2009).

A. Trapezius
B. Rhomboids
C. Subscapularis
D. Serratus anterior
E. Teres minor

**Q16.** Which of the following muscles would be affected by a lumbosacral trunk but not a sciatic nerve lesion?
A. Iliacus
B. Tensor fascia latae
C. Adductor longus
D. Medial hamstrings
E. Short head of the biceps femoris

**Q17.** A 65-year-old man develops weakness of the right leg after he undergoes coronary angiography for evaluation of chest pain. Examination reveals weakness of right knee extension. Which of the following muscles would be affected by a lumbar plexus lesion but not a femoral nerve lesion?
A. Iliacus
B. Adductor longus
C. Gluteus medius
D. Quadriceps
E. Hamstrings

**Q18.** A 65-year-old man presents with weakness of the right leg after surgical repair of a right inguinal hernia. Examination demonstrates weakness of right knee extension. Which of the following skin areas of the right lower extremity is most likely to reveal sensory impairment?
A. Medial lower leg
B. Lateral lower leg
C. Dorsum of the foot
D. Lateral aspect of the foot
E. Sole

**Q19.** The tibial division of the sciatic nerve innervates the:
A. tibialis anterior.
B. adductor magnus.
C. peroneus longus.
D. peroneus brevis.
E. adductor longus.

**Q20.** A 23-year-old man presents with the left foot drop. To differentiate an L5 radiculopathy from a peroneal neuropathy, which of the following muscle testing would be useful?
A. Hip extension
B. Hip internal rotation
C. Knee extension
D. Knee flexion
E. Plantar flexion

**Q21.** A 45-year-old woman presents with right foot drop. Which of the following muscles on needle electromyography (EMG) would be affected by a sciatic nerve lesion but not a common fibular (peroneal) nerve lesion around the fibular neck?
A. Extensor hallucis longus
B. Peroneus longus
C. Short head of biceps femoris
D. Gluteus medius
E. Tensor fascia latae

**Q22.** Which of the following muscles is supplied by the superficial fibular (peroneal) nerve?
A. Tibialis anterior
B. Extensor hallucis longus
C. Extensor digitorum brevis
D. Peroneus brevis
E. Peroneus tertius

**Q23.** A 33-year-old woman presents with numbness of the lateral lower leg for one week. Which of the following diagnoses is **LEAST** likely?
A. L5 radiculopathy
B. Sciatic neuropathy
C. Common fibular (peroneal) neuropathy
D. Isolated superficial fibular (peroneal) neuropathy
E. Isolated deep fibular (peroneal) neuropathy

**Q24.** The sural communicating nerve:
A. is also known as the medial sural nerve.
B. is also known as the tibial communicating nerve.
C. originates from the common fibular (peroneal) nerve.
D. originates from the superficial fibular (peroneal) nerve.
E. originates from the deep fibular (peroneal) nerve.

**Q25.** Which matching between the muscle and the nerve root(s) is **CORRECT**?
A. Anconeus – C5
B. Pronator teres – C8
C. Flexor digitorum longus – L5 and S1
D. Extensor digitorum brevis – L4
E. Long head of biceps femoris – L3 and 4

**PART 2 | QUESTIONS WITH ANSWERS AND DISCUSSION**

**QUESTION 1.** Which of the following is **TRUE** regarding the brachial plexus?
A. There are three trunks: lateral, medial. and posterior.
B. Each trunk divides into three divisions.
C. All major upper extremity nerves originate from the trunks.
D. The trunks are formed by the anterior rami of C5-T1.
E. The cords form proximal to the level of the clavicle.

**ANSWER:** D. The trunks are formed by the anterior rami of C5-T1

**COMMENTS AND DISCUSSION**
- Brachial plexus anatomy (Fig. 1.1).
  - Most commonly formed by the anterior rami of the C5-T1 nerve roots
  - Passes between the anterior and middle scalene muscles to continue in the posterior triangle of the neck
  - Uncommon variations:
    - Prefixed brachial plexus has a more cephalic orientation; formed by the C4-C8 nerve roots
    - Postfixed brachial plexus has a more caudal orientation; formed by the C6-T2 nerve roots

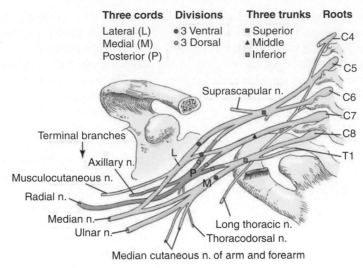

| Three cords | Divisions | Three trunks | Roots |
|---|---|---|---|

Three cords: Lateral (L), Medial (M), Posterior (P)
Divisions: 3 Ventral, 3 Dorsal
Three trunks: Superior, Middle, Inferior

**Fig. 1.1** Brachial plexus. From Nagelhout ES, Heiner JJ, Surname? JS Nurse Anesthesia. 7th ed. 2022.

- Classic structure:
  - Five anterior rami of the C5-T1 nerve roots
  - Three trunks: upper (superior), middle, lower (inferior)
  - Six divisions: one anterior and one posterior from each trunk
  - Three cords: lateral, medial, and posterior
- Location in relationship to the clavicle:
  - Above the clavicle (often referred to as supraclavicular plexus): anterior rami and trunks
  - Immediately behind the clavicle: divisions
  - Below the clavicle (often referred to as infraclavicular plexus): cords

**QUESTION 2.** Which of the following muscles would be affected by a C5 radiculopathy but not an upper trunk lesion of the brachial plexus?

A. Rhomboids
B. Supraspinatus
C. Infraspinatus
D. Biceps
E. Clavicular head of pectoralis major

**ANSWER:** A. Rhomboids

**COMMENTS AND DISCUSSION**

- Pre-plexus: Two nerves originate directly from the anterior rami of the nerve roots before the brachial plexus (Fig. 1.1):
  - Dorsal scapular nerve, supplying the rhomboid muscles (C4-5 fibers)
  - Long thoracic nerve, supplying the serratus anterior muscle (C5-6-7 fibers)
- Rhomboids are supplied by the dorsal scapular nerve, which is derived primarily from the C5 nerve root (and some C4) and arises before the formation of the upper trunk.
- Thus rhomboids are affected in a C5 radiculopathy but spared in an upper trunk lesion.

The table below demonstartes the correct innervation of these muscles (Tables 1.3 and 1.8).

| Muscle | Nerve | Cord | Trunk | Root |
|---|---|---|---|---|
| Rhomboids | Dorsal scapular | N/A | N/A | C4-5 |
| Supraspinatus | Suprascapular | N/A | Upper | C5-6 |
| Infraspinatus | Suprascapular | N/A | Upper | C5-6 |
| Biceps | Musculocutaneous | Lateral | Upper | C5-6 |
| Clavicular head of pectoralis major | Lateral pectoral | Lateral | Upper, middle | C5-7 |

**TABLE 1.1** High-yield key muscles in the upper extremity.

| Muscle | Nerve | Cord | Trunk | Myotome |
|---|---|---|---|---|
| Rhomboids | Dorsal scapular | - | - | C5 |
| Deltoid | Axillary | Posterior | U | C5,6 |
| Supraspinatus | Suprascapular | - | U | C5,6 |
| Infraspinatus | Suprascapular | - | U | C5,6 |
| Serratus anterior | Long thoracic | - | U, M | C5,6,7 |
| Biceps | Musculocutaneous | Lateral | U | C5,6 |
| Brachioradialis | Radial | Posterior | U | C**5**,6 |
| Triceps | Radial | Posterior | U, **M**, L | C6,**7**,8 |
| Pronator teres | Median | Lateral | U, M | C6,7 |
| Flexor carpi radialis | Median | Lateral | U, M | C6,7 |
| Flexor digitorum longus | Digits 2, 3 - AIN (Median) Digits 4, 5 - Ulnar | Lateral, **Medial** | M, L | C7,**8** |
| Flexor carpi ulnaris | Ulnar | Medial | L | C8,T1 |
| Flexor pollicis longus | AIN (Median) | Lateral, **Medial** | M, L | C7,**8** |
| Extensor digitorum communis | PIN (Radial) | Posterior | **M**, L | C7,**8** |
| Extensor indicis proprius | PIN (Radial) | Posterior | M, **L** | C7,**8** |
| First dorsal interossei | Ulnar | Medial | L | C8,**T1** |
| Abductor pollicis brevis | Median | Medial | L | **C8**,T1 |
| Abductor digiti minimi | Ulnar | Medial | L | C8,**T1** |

*U*, upper trunk; *M*, middle trunk; *L*, lower trunk of the brachial plexus; *AIN*, anterior interosseous nerve; *PIN*, posterior interosseous nerve

- Both the supraspinatus and infraspinatus are supplied by the suprascapular nerve, which has contributions from the C5 and C6 nerve roots and comes off the upper trunk of the brachial plexus (Table 1.1).
- Thus, the supraspinatus and infraspinatus are affected in both C5 radiculopathy and upper trunk lesions.
- Biceps is supplied by the musculocutaneous nerve, which has contributions from the C5 and C6 nerve roots. However, the musculocutaneous nerve is a branch of lateral cord and upper trunk. Thus, the biceps can be affected in both C5 radiculopathy and an upper trunk lesion.
- The pectoralis major is supplied by the lateral and medial pectoral nerves. The clavicular head of pectoralis major has contributions from C5 and C6 nerve roots, whereas the sternal head has contributions from C7, C8, and T1. The lateral pectoral nerve comes off the lateral cord, which supplies the clavicular head of the pectoralis major. Therefore, it can also be affected in both C5 radiculopathy and an upper trunk lesion.

**QUESTION 3.** Which of the following is **NOT** associated with an upper trunk lesion of the brachial plexus?
A. Burner or stinger syndrome from contact sports
B. Pancoast tumor
C. Trauma
D. Penetrating injury
E. Obstetrical injury

**ANSWER:** B. Pancoast tumor

**COMMENTS AND DISCUSSION**
- Three trunks of the brachial plexus (Fig. 1.1)
  ○ Upper (Superior) trunk
    - Formed by the anterior rami of the C5-6 nerve roots
    - Suprascapular nerve originates directly from the upper trunk
      - Supplies the supraspinatus and infraspinatus muscles
      - No cutaneous sensory fibers, but supplies deep pain fibers to the shoulder joint
    - Common etiologies of upper trunk plexopathy include:
      - Burner or stinger syndrome from contact sports
      - Midshaft clavicular fracture
      - Trauma (especially the head and shoulder striking the ground following motor vehicle or biking accidents)

- Penetrating injury
- Rucksack syndrome (wearing heavy backpack)
- Obstetrical injury (Erb-Duchenne palsy)
  - Middle trunk
    - Formed solely by the anterior ramus of the C7 nerve root
    - Isolated middle trunk plexopathies are very rare; when seen are usually caused by trauma
  - Lower (Inferior) trunk
    - Formed by the anterior rami of the C8-T1 nerve roots
    - Common etiologies of lower trunk plexopathy:
      - Pancoast tumor
      - Neurogenic thoracic outlet syndrome (TOS)
      - Metastatic disease
      - Post-median sternotomy
      - Traction from shoulder hyperextension (e.g., body dragged from pulling the arm)
      - Obstetrical injury: Dejerine-Klumpke palsy

 **KEY POINT**

**Upper trunk C5, C6**
**Middle trunk C7**
**Lower trunk C8, T1**

 **HIGH-YIELD FACT**

**L**ateral **A**nte**b**rachial **C**utaneous nerve (**LABC**) arises from the musculocutaneous nerve (C5-6 fibers). It can be affected in **upper trunk or lateral cord** lesions. It is a pure sensory nerve supplying the skin of the **lateral forearm**.
    **M**edial **A**nte**b**rachial **C**utaneous nerve (**MABC**) arises from the medial cord (C8-T1 fibers). It can be affected in **lower trunk or medial cord** lesions, especially in the true neurogenic thoracic outlet syndrome. It is a pure sensory nerve supplying the skin of the **medial forearm**.

 **KEY POINT**

**Upper trunk/lateral cord → abnormal LABC**
**Lower trunk/medial cord → abnormal MABC**

**QUESTION 4.** Which of the following is **TRUE** regarding the cords of the brachial plexus?
    A. The posterior division of the lower trunk forms the medial cord.
    B. All three posterior divisions form the lateral cord.
    C. The upper trunk continues as the lateral cord.
    D. The anterior division of the upper trunk contributes to the lateral cord.
    E. The anterior divisions of the middle and lower trunks form the medial cord.

**ANSWER:** D. The anterior division of the upper trunk contributes to the lateral cord.

**COMMENTS AND DISCUSSION**
- Divisions and derivation of the cords (Fig. 1.1)
  - Each trunk divides into one anterior and one posterior divisions
  - Thus there are six divisions total
    - Medial cord is derived from one division: anterior division of the lower trunk
    - Lateral cord is derived from two divisions: anterior divisions of the upper and middle trunks
    - Posterior cord is derived from three divisions: posterior divisions of the upper, middle, and lower trunks
- Major nerves originating from the cords
  - Nerves originating from the lateral cord:
    - Lateral pectoral nerve, supplying the pectoralis major

- Median nerve (also receives a contribution from the medial cord)
- Musculocutaneous nerve
  o Nerves originating from the medial cord:
    - Medial pectoral nerve, supplying the pectoralis major and minor
    - Medial brachial cutaneous nerve (MBC), supplying the lateral arm
    - Medial antebrachial cutaneous nerve (MABC), supplying the lateral forearm
    - Median nerve (also receives a contribution from the lateral cord)
    - Ulnar nerve
  o Nerves originating from the posterior cord:
    - Upper subscapular nerve, supplying the subscapularis
    - Lower subscapular nerve, supplying the subscapularis and teres major
    - Thoracodorsal nerve, supplying the latissimus dorsi
    - Axillary nerve, supplying the deltoid and teres minor
    - Radial nerve

## 🔑 KEY POINT

**Teres Major** → Lower subscapular nerve
**Teres Minor** → Axillary nerve

**QUESTION 5.** A 22-year-old man is referred to an electromyography (EMG) lab for evaluation of left arm weakness after a motorcycle accident 2 months ago. Needle examination of which of the following muscles would help differentiate an upper trunk from a lateral cord lesion of the brachial plexus?
 A. Brachialis
 B. Brachioradialis
 C. Rhomboids
 D. Supraspinatus
 E. Serratus anterior

**ANSWER:** B. Brachioradialis

**COMMENTS AND DISCUSSION**
The table below demonstartes the correct innervation of these muscles (Tables 1.3 and 1.8).

| Muscle | Nerve | Cord | Trunk | Root |
|---|---|---|---|---|
| Brachialis | Musculocutaneous | Lateral | Upper | C5-6 |
| Brachioradialis | Radial | Posterior | Upper | C5-6 |
| Rhomboids | Dorsal scapular | N/A | N/A | C4-5 |
| Supraspinatus | Suprascapular | N/A | Upper | C5-6 |
| Serratus anterior | Long thoracic | N/A | N/A | C5-6-7 |

- Brachioradialis is affected in an upper trunk, but not a lateral cord lesion. It is supplied by the radial nerve, which arises from the posterior cord (Table 1.1).
- The brachialis is affected in both upper trunk and lateral cord lesions; thus it is not useful in differentiating between these two locations.
- Neither rhomboids nor serratus anterior are affected in the upper trunk or lateral cord lesions (Table 1.1).

**QUESTION 6.** Which of the following muscles is affected in a middle trunk but not in a posterior cord lesion of the brachial plexus?
 A. Teres minor
 B. Brachioradialis
 C. Triceps
 D. Pronator teres
 E. Abductor pollicis brevis

**ANSWER:** D. Pronator teres

## COMMENTS AND DISCUSSION

The table below demonstartes the correct innervation of these muscles (Tables 1.3 and 1.8).

| Muscle | Nerve | Cord | Trunk | Root |
|--------|-------|------|-------|------|
| Teres minor | Axillary | Posterior | Upper | C5-6 |
| Brachioradialis | Radial | Posterior | Upper | C5-6 |
| Triceps | Radial | Posterior | Upper, middle, lower | C6-8 |
| Pronator teres | Median | Lateral | Upper, middle | C6-7 |
| Abductor pollicis brevis | Median | Medial | Lower | C8, T1 |

- C7-innervated non–radial-innervated muscles such as the pronator teres and the flexor carpi radialis would be affected in a middle trunk but spared in a posterior cord lesion (Table 1.1 and 1.2).
  - These C7-innervated muscles are supplied by the median nerve and lateral cord fibers.
- The teres minor and the brachioradialis (as well as the deltoid) would be affected in a posterior cord but not in a middle trunk lesion.
- The triceps would be affected in both middle trunk and posterior cord lesions (Table 1.1 and 1.2).
- The abductor pollicis brevis (supplied by the median nerve, medial cord, lower trunk) is not affected in either middle trunk or posterior cord lesion (Table 1.1).

**TABLE 1.2** High-yield upper extremity muscles that are useful for lesion localization.

| Key muscles | Impaired in: | Normal in: |
|-------------|--------------|------------|
| Deltoid/brachioradialis | C5-6 radiculopathy <br> Upper trunk plexopathy | Lateral cord plexopathy |
| Pronator teres/flexor carpi radialis | C6-7 radiculopathy | Posterior cord plexopathy |
| Extensor indicis proprius | C8 radiculopathy | Medial cord plexopathy |
| Triceps/anconeus | High radial neuropathy | Radial neuropathy at the spiral groove |
| | Posterior cord plexopathy <br> C7 radiculopathy | Posterior interosseous neuropathy |
| Extensor carpi radialis longus | Radial neuropathy at the spiral groove | Posterior interosseous neuropathy |
| Flexor carpi ulnaris/flexor digitorum profundus to digits 4-5 | Ulnar neuropathy at the elbow | Ulnar neuropathy at Guyon's canal |

**QUESTION 7.** Which of the following muscles would be affected by a lower trunk lesion but not a medial cord lesion of the brachial plexus?

- A. Deltoid
- B. Extensor indicis proprius
- C. Abductor pollicis brevis
- D. Abductor digiti minimi
- E. Flexor digitorum profundus of the index finger

**ANSWER:** B. Extensor indicis proprius

## COMMENTS AND DISCUSSION

The table below demonstartes the correct innervation of these muscles (Tables 1.3 and 1.8).

| Muscle | Nerve | Cord | Trunk | Root |
|--------|-------|------|-------|------|
| Deltoid | Axillary | Posterior | Upper, middle | C5-6 |
| Extensor indicis proprius | Radial | Posterior | Middle, lower | C7-8 |
| Abductor pollicis brevis | Median | Medial | Lower | C8-T1 |
| Abductor digiti minimi | Ulnar | Medial | Lower | C8-T1 |
| Flexor digitorum profundus of the index finger (and also of the middle finger) | Median | Medial | Lower | C8-T1 |

**TABLE 1.3** Major upper extremity nerves and supplied muscles.

| Nerves | Muscles | Cutaneous Sensory | Myotomes |
|---|---|---|---|
| Dorsal scapular | Rhomboids | None | C4, **5** |
| Long thoracic | Serratus anterior | None | C5,6,7 |
| Suprascapular | Supraspinatus | None | C**5**,6 |
|  | Infraspinatus |  | C**5**,6 |
| Medial pectoral | Pectoralis minor | None | C8,T1 |
|  | Sternocostal head of pectoralis major |  |  |
| Lateral pectoral | Clavicular head of pectoralis major | None | C5,6,7 |
| Musculocutaneous | Biceps |  | C5,6 |
|  | Brachialis |  |  |
|  | Coracobrachialis |  |  |
| Median | Forearm Group |  |  |
|  | Pronator teres |  | C6,7 |
|  | Flexor carpi radialis |  | C6,7 |
|  | Palmaris longus |  | C7,8 |
|  | Flexor digitorum superficialis |  | C8,T1 |
|  | Hand Group |  |  |
|  | Abductor pollicis brevis |  | **C8**,T1 |
|  | Opponens pollicis |  | C8,T1 |
|  | Flexor pollicis brevis (superficial head) |  | C8,T1 |
|  | Lumbricals (1st and 2nd) acting on digits 2 and 3 |  | C8,T1 |
| Anterior interosseus, branch of median | Flexor digitorum profundus to digits 2 and 3 | None | C7,8 |
|  | Flexor pollicis longus |  | C7,**8** |
|  | Pronator quadratus |  | C7,**8** |

*Continued*

**TABLE 1.3**  Major upper extremity nerves and supplied muscles—cont'd

| Nerves | Muscles | Cutaneous Sensory | Myotomes |
|---|---|---|---|
| Ulnar | Forearm Group | | |
| | Flexor carpi ulnaris | | C8,T1 |
| | Flexor digitorum profundus to digits 4 and 5 | | C8,T1 |
| | Hypothenar Group | | |
| | Abductor digiti minimi | | C8,T1 |
| | Flexor digiti minimi | | C8,T1 |
| | Opponens digiti minimi | | C8,T1 |
| | Palmaris brevis | | C8,T1 |
| | Dorsal (4) and palmar (3) interossei | | C8,T1 |
| | Lumbricals (3rd and 4th) acting on digits 4 and 5 | | C8,T1 |
| | Thenar Group | | |
| | Adductor pollicis | | C8,T1 |
| | Flexor pollicis brevis (deep head) | | C8,T1 |
| Axillary | Deltoid (anterior, middle, and posterior heads) | | C5,6 |
| | Teres Minor | | C5,6 |

**TABLE 1.3** Major upper extremity nerves and supplied muscles—cont'd

| Nerves | Muscles | Cutaneous Sensory | Myotomes |
|---|---|---|---|
| Radial | Proximal to the Spiral Groove | | |
| | Triceps (medial, lateral, and long heads) | | C6,**7**,8 |
| | Anconeus | | C6,**7**,8 |
| | Distal to the Spiral Groove | | |
| | Brachioradialis | | C**5**,6 |
| | Extensor carpi radialis (longus and brevis) | | C7,8 |
| | Supinator | | C6,7 |
| Posterior interosseous (PIN) from radial | Superficial Group | None | |
| | Extensor digitorum communis | | C7,8 |
| | Extensor digit minimi | | C7,8 |
| | Extensor carpi ulnaris | | C7,8 |
| | Deep Group | | |
| | Abductor pollicis longus | | C7,8 |
| | Extensor pollicis (longus and brevis) | | C7,8 |
| | Extensor indicis proprius | | C7,8 |

- Extensor indicis proprius (supplied by the radial nerve through posterior cord) is affected in a lower trunk but not in a medial cord lesion (Table 1.1 and 1.2).
- Therefore, this muscle is key in differentiating between a lower trunk and a medial cord lesion.
- The abductor pollicis brevis, the abductor digiti minimi, and the flexor digitorum profundus of the index finger are affected in both medial cord and lower trunk lesions (Table 1.1).
- The deltoid is not affected in either lower trunk or medial cord lesion (Table 1.1 and 1.2).

**QUESTION 8.** Which of the following muscles would be affected by a median nerve lesion in the forearm but not a carpal tunnel syndrome?
    A. Flexor carpi ulnaris
    B. Flexor carpi radialis
    C. Abductor pollicis longus
    D. Adductor pollicis
    E. Opponens pollicis

**ANSWER:** B. Flexor carpi radialis

**COMMENTS AND DISCUSSION**

- Flexor carpi radialis is affected in high median nerve lesions but not in carpal tunnel syndrome (Fig. 1.2 and Table 1.3).
- Pronator teres and flexor carpi radialis are also useful to differentiate between a high median nerve lesion and carpal tunnel syndrome (Table 1.2 and 1.3).
- Abductor pollicis longus is supplied by the radial nerve (Table 1.3).
- Opponens pollicis is affected in both high median nerve lesions and carpal tunnel syndrome (Table 1.3).
- Flexor carpi ulnaris and adductor pollicis are supplied by the ulnar nerve (Table 1.3).
- Common entrapment sites of major upper extremity peripheral nerves including the median nerve are shown in Table 1.4.

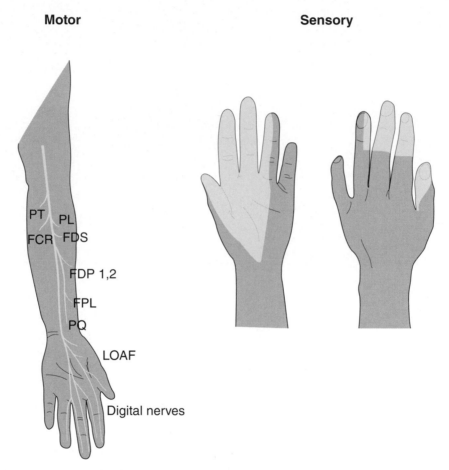

**Motor**　　　　　　　　　　　　　　**Sensory**

**Fig. 1.2**  Median nerve anatomy. Left: Motor branches of the median nerve; Right: Sensory areas innervated by the median nerve. *PT*, pronator teres; *FCR*, flexor carpi radialis; *PL*, palmaris longus; *FDS*, flexor digitorum superficialis; *FDP*, flexor digitorum profundus; *FPL*, flexor pollicis longus; *PQ*, pronator quadratus; *LOAF*, first and second Lumbricals, Opponens pollicis, Abductor pollicis brevis, Flexor pollicis brevis.

**TABLE 1.4**  Common entrapment sites of major upper extremity peripheral nerves.

| Nerves | Common entrapment sites |
|---|---|
| Median | • Carpal tunnel |
| Ulnar | • Ulnar groove at the elbow (between the medial epicodyle and the olecranon) |
| | • Cubital tunnel |
| | • Guyon canal at the wrist/palm |
| Radial | • Spiral groove at the mid-humerus |
| Posterior interosseous | • Between the two heads of the supinator muscle (arcade of Frohse) |

## ⊚ HIGH-YIELD FACT

**MUSCLES WITH DUAL NERVE SUPPLIES**

**Flexor digitorum profundus (FDP)**
Index and middle figures → median nerve
Ring and little fingers → ulnar nerve

**Flexor pollicis brevis (FPB)**
Superficial head → median nerve
Deep head → ulnar nerve

## MNEMONIC

**Hand muscles innervated by the median nerve: LOAF muscles**
**L**umbricals, 1st and 2nd
**O**pponens pollicis
**A**bductor pollicis brevis
**F**lexor pollicis brevis (superficial head)

**QUESTION 9.** A 35-year-old man develops weakness of right thumb flexion at the interphalangeal joint. In addition, he cannot flex the index and middle fingers at the distal interphalangeal joints. However, the ring and little fingers are normal, and there is no sensory loss. What is the other muscle most likely to be affected?
A. Abductor pollicis brevis
B. Flexor carpi radialis
C. Flexor digitorum superficialis
D. Pronator teres
E. Pronator quadratus

**ANSWER:** E. Pronator quadratus

## COMMENTS AND DISCUSSION

- Anterior interosseous nerve (AIN) (Table 1.3)
  - Relatively pure motor branch of the median nerve
  - No cutaneous sensory innervation, but it carries sensory fibers to the volar wrist joint capsule
  - Passes between the two heads of the pronator teres
  - Courses anterior along the interosseous membrane
  - Often affected in neuralgic amyotrophy
  - **"OK" sign** is seen in anterior interosseous neuropathy. Due to weakness of flexor pollicis longus (FPL) to the thumb and flexor digitorum profundus (FDP) to the index finger, a patient is unable to make an "OK" sign (Fig. 1.3 and see Fig. 14.7).

## ⊚ HIGH-YIELD FACT

**AIN supplies**
- Flexor digitorum profundus of index and middle fingers
- Flexor pollicis longus
- Pronator quadratus

- The clinical features described in the vignette are due to weakness of the FDP to the index and middle fingers, and the FPL. Therefore, the pronator quadratus is the only other muscle that is most likely affected. The AIN is a relatively pure motor nerve: there are only sensory branches that receive sensation from the joint capsule, but no sensory branch that receives sensation from the skin.

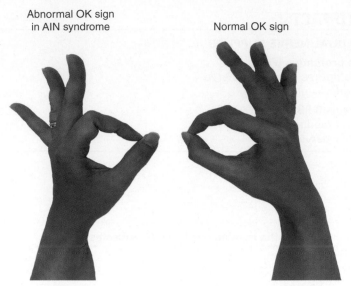

Abnormal OK sign
in AIN syndrome

Normal OK sign

**Fig. 1.3** "OK" sign in anterior interosseous neuropathy. This patient (right) has an anterior interosseus nerve (AIN) syndrome (aka Kiloh-Nevin syndrome) and cannot make an "OK" sign. The AIN supplies the flexor digitorum profundus (FDP) to the index and middle fingers, as well as flexor pollicis longus (FPL) and pronator quadratus (PQ).

**QUESTION 10.** A 44-year-old woman develops weakness of the right hand for 6 weeks. Electromyography (EMG) examination of which of the following muscles is useful to differentiate a median nerve lesion from a C8 nerve root lesion?
A. Abductor pollicis brevis
B. Opponens pollicis
C. Flexor pollicis longus
D. Flexor digitorum profundus of the index finger
E. Extensor indicis proprius

**ANSWER:** E. Extensor indicis proprius

**COMMENTS AND DISCUSSION**
- In order to differentiate between a median nerve lesion from a C8 nerve root lesion, one needs to examine a C8 non–median-innervated muscles such as those innervated by the ulnar or radial nerve (e.g., extensor indicis proprius) (Table 1.2 and 1.3).
- All other muscles in the question are supplied by the median nerve and the C8-T1 nerve roots, and thus are not useful for differentiating between a lesion in these two locations.

**QUESTION 11.** In a severe ulnar nerve lesion at Guyon's canal, which of the following clinical findings is **MOST LIKELY** to be **PRESENT**?
A. Intact sensation over the distal medial palm
B. Intact sensation over the medial side of the dorsum of the hand
C. Intact sensation over the little finger
D. Intact posture of the little and ring fingers
E. Normal abduction of the index finger

**ANSWER:** B. Intact sensation over the medial side of the dorsum of the hand

**COMMENTS AND DISCUSSION**
- The medial side of the dorsum of the hand is supplied by the dorsal ulnar cutaneous nerve (DUC), and is always spared in ulnar nerve lesions at the wrist (Guyon's canal) (Fig. 1.4).
- This nerve arises from the ulnar nerve, 6 to 8 cm proximal to the wrist. Sensation of the distal medial palm, digit 5, and the medial half of digit 4 is supplied by the ulnar sensory fibers.
- Clawing (not intact posture) of the little and ring fingers is likely to be seen in a severe ulnar nerve lesion at Guyon's canal (see Fig. 14.11). This occurs from weakness of the third and fourth lumbricals which are supplied by the ulnar nerve distal to Guyon's canal.
  - The normal action of the lumbricals is flexion of the metacarpophalangeal joints and extension of the interphalangeal joints.

**Motor**   **Sensory**

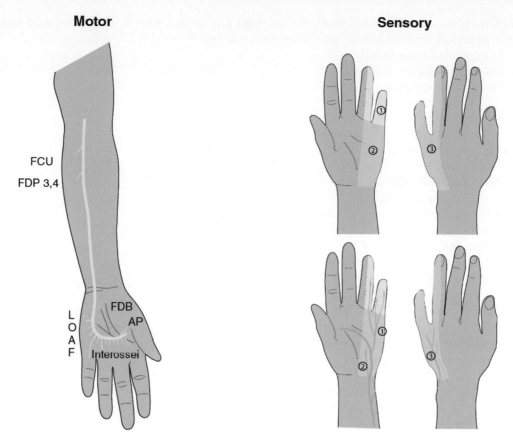

**Fig. 1.4** Ulnar nerve anatomy Left: Motor branches of the ulnar nerve. Right: Sensory areas supplied by the ulnar nerve. The ulnar sensory branches (lower panel) and their innervated skin areas (upper panel) are demonstrated. 1=Ulnar digital sensory branches. This is a part of superficial branch, and receives sensation from the volar surface of fourth (medial half) and fifth digits; 2=Palmar cutaneous branch. This arises 1-2 cm proximal to the wrist, and receives sensation from the ulnar side of the palm; 3=Dorsal ulnar cutaneous sensory branch. This arises more proximal to the wrist, and receives sensation from the ulnar side of the dorsal hand, fourth (medial half) and fifth digits.
*FCU*, flexor carpi ulnaris; *FDP*, flexor digitorum profundus; *LOAF*, thrid and fourth Lumbrical, Opponens digiti minimi, Abductor digiti minimi, Flexor digiti minimi; *FDB*, flexor digitorum brevis; *AP*, adductor pollicis.

- ○ Thus weakness of the lumbricals results in the opposite: extension of the metacarpophalangeal joints and flexion of the interphalangeal joints, which result in the clawed deformity.
- Abduction of the index finger is subserved by the first dorsal interossei, which is affected in all ulnar nerve lesions, including those at Guyon's canal.
- Ulnar nerve anatomy
  - ○ Innervates all intrinsic hand muscles, except the thenar muscles supplied by the median nerve and those supplied by the radial nerve
  - ○ Innervated muscles and common entrapment sites shown in Fig. 1.4 and Table 1.4.

**QUESTION 12.** Which of the following upper extremity muscles has a dual nerve supply?
   A. Flexor digitorum superficialis
   B. Flexor pollicis brevis
   C. Flexor pollicis longus
   D. Opponens pollicis
   E. Dorsal interossei

**ANSWER:** B. Flexor pollicis brevis

**COMMENTS AND DISCUSSION**
- Flexor pollicis brevis usually has double innervation.
- Most commonly, the superficial head is innervated by the recurrent branch of the median nerve, whereas the deep head is innervated by the deep branch of the ulnar nerve.
- The flexor digitorum superficialis and opponens pollicis are supplied by the median nerve.
- The flexor pollicis longus is supplied by the anterior interosseus nerve.
- All palmar and dorsal interossei are supplied by the ulnar nerve.

**QUESTION 13.** A patient presents with a wrist and finger drop. Which muscle would be affected by a radial neuropathy but not a posterior interosseous neuropathy?

A. Extensor digitorum indicis
B. Extensor digitorum communis
C. Extensor carpi ulnaris
D. Abductor pollicis longus
E. Brachioradialis

**ANSWER:** E. Brachioradialis

### COMMENTS AND DISCUSSION

- Radial nerve anatomy (Fig. 1.5)
  - In the upper arm, before the spinal groove, the radial nerve supplies:
    - Triceps
    - Anconeus
  - It then wraps around the spinal groove posteriorly to supply:
    - Brachioradialis
    - Extensor carpi radialis longus
  - It then divides into the superficial and deep branches.
  - The superficial branch is a primarily sensory branch that continues as the superficial radial nerve.
  - The deep branch is a primarily motor branch that initially supplies:
    - Extensor carpi radialis brevis
    - Supinator
  - The deep branch then runs through the tendinous arch between the two heads of the supinator muscle (arcade of Frohse), and becomes the posterior interosseous nerve
- Posterior interosseous nerve (PIN)
  - Relatively pure motor nerve with no cutaneous sensation but it carries sensory fibers to the dorsal wrist joint capsule
  - Courses posteriorly along the interosseous membrane

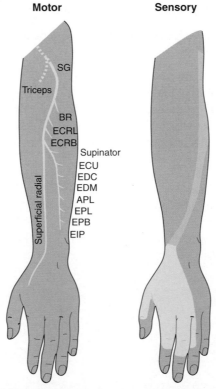

**Fig. 1.5** Radial nerve anatomy. Left: Motor branches of the radial nerve. Right: Sensory areas supplied by the radial nerve. The skin areas innervated by the superficial radial nerve (eggnog color) and by the posterior cutaneous nerve of forearm and arm (sepia color) are demonstrated.

*SG,* spiral groove; *BR,* brachioradialis; *ECRL,* extensor carpi radialis longus; *ECRB,* extensor carpi radial brevis; *ECU,* extensor carpi ulnaris; *EDC,* extensor digitorum communis; *EDM,* extensor digiti minimi; *APL,* abductor pollicis longus; *EPL,* extensor pollicis longus; *EPB,* extensor pollicis brevis; *EIP,* extensor indicis proprius.

- It innervates all remaining finger and wrist extensors
- Lesions affecting PIN result in finger drop and partial wrist drop. Wrist drop is partial and often associated with a radial deviation due to sparing of the extensor carpi radialis longus (ECRL)
- Preferably affected in neuralgic amyotrophy

## ◎ HIGH-YIELD FACT

**RADIAL NERVE**
**Branches before the spiral groove**
- Triceps
- Anconeus

**Branches after the spiral groove but before the posterior interosseus nerve (PIN)**
- Brachioradialis
- Extensor carpi radialis longus (ECRL)
- Extensor carpi radialis brevis (ECRB)

**QUESTION 14.** A 50-year-old man has weakness and atrophy of the left infraspinatus, but the left supraspinatus is normal. What is the most likely location of the lesion?
A. Suprascapular notch
B. Superior transverse scapular ligament
C. Anterior coracoscapular ligament
D. Spinoglenoid notch
E. Neck of the humerus

**ANSWER:** D. Spinoglenoid notch

### COMMENTS AND DISCUSSION
- The suprascapular nerve comes off the upper trunk of the brachial plexus and supplies both the supraspinatus and the infraspinatus (Fig. 1.1 and Table 1.3).
- It first supplies the supraspinatus after traveling through the suprascapular notch, and then innervates the infraspinatus after passing through the spinoglenoid notch.
- Thus, lesions, such as a ganglion cyst at the spinoglenoid notch, result in isolated weakness of the infraspinatus with sparing of the supraspinatus.
- A lesion of the suprascapular notch affects both the supraspinatus and the infraspinatus.
- The transverse scapular ligament connects the borders of the suprascapular notch.
- The anterior coracoscapular ligament attaches to the coracoid process and is inferior to the superior transverse scapular ligament.

**QUESTION 15.** A woman presents with scapular winging as shown in the following photo. Which of the following muscles is most likely affected?

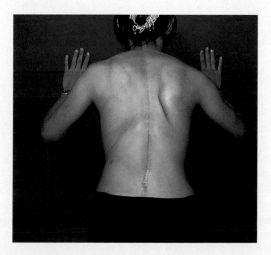

Ameri, E., Behtash, H. & Omidi-Kashani, F. Isolated long thoracic nerve paralysis - a rare complication of anterior spinal surgery: a case report. *J Med Case Reports* **3**, 7366 (2009).

    A. Trapezius
    B. Rhomboids
    C. Subscapularis
    D. Serratus anterior
    E. Teres minor

**ANSWER:** D. Serratus anterior

**COMMENTS AND DISCUSSION**

- Scapular winging (Table 1.5 and Fig. 1.6)
  - Muscle weakness results in an abnormally protruded scapula.
  - Medial scapular winging:
    - Weakness of serratus anterior
    - The serratus anterior weakness from involvement of the long thoracic nerve is classically seen in neuralgic amyotrophy and stretch injuries.
  - Lateral scapular winging:
    - Weakness of rhomboids or trapezius.
    - Weakness of trapezius also associated with a shoulder droop.
    - Rhomboids are rarely injured in isolation.
  - This patient has medial scapular winging, which is due to weakness of the serratus anterior from a long thoracic neuropathy.
  - Weakness of the subscapularis or the teres minor does not cause scapular winging.

**TABLE 1.5** Scapular winging.

|  | **Medial scapular winging** | **Lateral scapular winging** |
|---|---|---|
| **Definition** | • Elevation of the inferomedial corner of the scapula <br> • Medially protruded | • Dropping of the superomedial corner of the scapula <br> • Laterally protruded |
| **Weak muscle** | Serratus anterior | Trapezius or rhomboids |
| **Injured nerve** | Long thoracic | Spinal accessory (for trapezius) or dorsal scapular (for rhomboids) |
| **Aggravating maneuver** | Moving arms forward and pushing against resistance | Shoulder abduction |

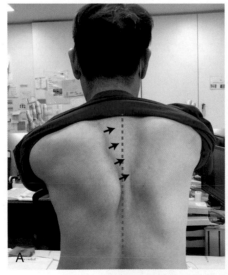
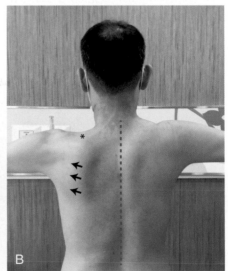

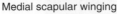

Medial scapular winging               Lateral scapular winging

**Fig. 1.6.** Scapular winging. Scapular winging is commonly divided into two catagories: medial (A) and lateral (B) scapular winging, according to movements of the scapula. The dotted line represents the midline. The arrows indicate the direction of scapular movements when moving the shoulder. If the scapula moves medially or towards the midline, it is called medial scapular winging (A). If the scapula moves laterally or away from the midline, it is called lateral scapular winging (B). A is a patient with neuralgic amyotrophy. B is a patient with spinal accessory neuropathy. The asterisk (*) indicate atrophy of the left trapezius muscle.

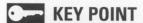 **KEY POINT**

**Muscles Stabilizing the Scapula**
- Serratus anterior
- Trapezius
- Rhomboids
- Levator scapulae

 **KEY POINT**

**Nerves preferably involved in neuralgic amyotrophy**
- Long thoracic
- Suprascapular
- Anterior interosseous

**Other nerves often involved in neuralgic amyotrophy**
- Phrenic
- Musculocutaneous
- Posterior interosseous

**QUESTION 16.** Which of the following muscles would be affected by a lumbosacral trunk but not a sciatic nerve lesion?
- A. Iliacus
- B. Tensor fascia latae
- C. Adductor longus
- D. Medial hamstrings
- E. Short head of the biceps femoris

**ANSWER:** B. Tensor fascia latae

**COMMENTS AND DISCUSSION**
The table below demonstartes the correct innervation of these muscles (Tables 1.3 and 1.8).

| Muscle | Nerve | Plexus | Root |
|---|---|---|---|
| Iliacus | Femoral | Lumbar (posterior division) | L2-4 |
| Tensor fascia latae | Superior gluteal | N/A | L4-5, S1 |
| Adductor longus | Obturator | Lumbar (anterior division) | L2-4 |
| Medial hamstrings | Sciatic | Lumbosacral | L4-5, S1 |
| Short head of the biceps femoris | Sciatic | Lumbosacral | **L5**, S1 |

- Tensor fascia latae is innervated by the superior gluteal nerve, which comes off the lumbosacral plexus before the formation of the sciatic nerve (Table 1.6 and 1.7). Thus, this muscle would be affected in the lumbosacral trunk lesion, but spared in the sciactic nerve lesion.
- The superior gluteal nerve also supplies the gluteus medius and minimus.
- The inferior gluteal nerve is another branch of the lumbosacral plexus and supplies the gluteus maximus.
- Both the medial hamstrings and the short head of the biceps femoris are supplied by the sciatic nerve, which arises from the lumbosacral plexus.
- The iliacus and the adductor longus are innervated by the femoral and obturator nerves, respectively (Table 1.8).
- Lumbar and lumbosacral plexus anatomy
  - Derived from the L1-S3 nerve roots
  - Divided into the lumbar plexus (L1-4) and the lumbosacral plexus (L4-S3)
    - Lumbar plexus
      - L2-3-4 nerve roots form the lumbar plexus which is divided into two divisions
      - Anterior division forms the obturator nerve

**TABLE 1.6** High-yield key muscles in the lower extremity.

| Muscles | Nerves | Plexus / division | Myotomes |
|---|---|---|---|
| Iliopsoas | Branches from L1,2,3 and femoral | - | **L1,2,**3 |
| Quadriceps | Femoral | Lumbar, posterior | L2,**3,**4 |
| Adductor longus, brevis and magnus, and gracilis | Obturator | Lumbar, anterior | L2,**3,**4 |
| Tibialis anterior | Deep peroneal | Lumbosacral | L4,5 |
| Tibialis posterior | Tibial | Lumbosacral | L5,S1 |
| Peroneus longus and brevis | Superficial peroneal | Lumbosacral | **L5,**S1 |
| Tensor fascia latae | Superior gluteal | Lumbosacral | L5,S1 |
| Gluteus medius | Superior gluteal | Lumbosacral | L5,S1 |
| Extensor hallucis longus | Deep peroneal | Lumbosacral | **L5** |
| Flexor digitorum longus | Tibial | Lumbosacral | L5,S1 |
| Gluteus maximus | Inferior gluteal | Lumbosacral | L5,**S1,**2 |
| Hamstring | Sciatic | Lumbosacral | |
| Medial hamstrings | | | **L5,**S1 |
| Lateral hamstrings | | | L5,**S1** |
| Gastrocnemius | Tibial | Lumbosacral | **S1,**2 |

**TABLE 1.7** High-yield lower extremity muscles that are useful for lesion localization.

| Key muscles | Impaired in: | Normal in: |
|---|---|---|
| Iliacus | Femoral neuropathy in the pelvis L2, 3, 4 radiculopathy Lumbar plexopathy | Femoral neuropathy at the inguinal ligament |
| Thigh adductors | L2, 3, 4 radiculopathy Lumbar plexopathy Obturator neuropathy | Femoral neuropathy |
| Tibialis posterior/flexor digitorum longus | L5 radiculopathy Sciatic neuropathy Tibial neuropathy | Common or deep peroneal neuropathy |
| Gluteus medius/tensor fascia latae | L5 radiculopathy Lumbosacral plexopathy | Peroneal neuropathy Sciatic neuropathy |
| Gluteus maximus | S1 radiculopathy Lumbosacral plexopathy | Tibial neuropathy Sciatic neuropathy |
| Short head biceps femoris | Sciatic neuropathy L5, S1 radiculopathy | Peroneal neuropathy at the fibular neck |

Adapted from Michael O'Brien. *Aids to the Examination of the Peripheral Nervous System*. 10th ed. Saunders; 2010.

- Posterior division forms the femoral nerve
- Other nerves:
  - Iliohypogastric (L1)
  - Ilioinguinal (L1)
  - Genitofemoral (L1, L2)
  - Lateral femoral cutaneous nerve (LFCN) (L2, L3) (aka lateral cutaneous nerve of the thigh)
- Lumbosacral plexus
  - Major nerve from the lumbosacral plexus is the sciatic nerve which is derived from L4-S3 fibers
  - Lumbosacral trunk receives contribution from the L5 and partial L4 nerve roots. This is often affected in "maternal obstetrical palsy".
  - Other nerves:
    - Superior gluteal (**L5**, S1) to the tensor fascia latae and gluteus medius and minimus muscles
    - Inferior gluteal (L5, **S1**) to the gluteus maximus muscle
    - Posterior cutaneous nerve of the thigh (S1, S2)
    - Pudendal (S2,3,4)

**TABLE 1.8** Nerves from lumbar and lumbosacral plexus and their supplied muscles.

| Nerves | Muscles | Sensory | Myotomes |
|---|---|---|---|
| Femoral | Iliacus | | L1,2,3 |
| | Quadriceps | | L2,3,4 |
| Obturator | Adductors | | L2,3,4 |
| Superior gluteal | Gluteus medius | None | L4,**5**,S1 |
| | Tensor fascia latae | | L4,**5**,S1 |
| Inferior gluteal | Gluteus maximus | None | L5, **S1**, S2 |
| Sciatic | Hamstrings | | L5,S1 |

*Continued*

**TABLE 1.8** Nerves from lumbar and lumbosacral plexus and their supplied muscles—cont'd

| Nerves | Muscles | Sensory | Myotomes |
|---|---|---|---|
| Tibial | Gastrocnemius | | S1,2 |
| | Soleus | | S1,2 |
| | Tibialis posterior | | L**5**, S1 |
| | Flexor digitorum longus | | **L5**, S1 |
| Peroneal (deep) | Tibialis anterior | | L4,**5** |
| | Extensor hallucis longus | | **L5** |
| | Extensor digitorum brevis | | **L5**, S1 |
| Peroneal (superficial) | Peroneus longus and brevis | | **L5** |
| Sural | None | | S1 |

Adapted from Michael O'Brien Aids to the Examination of the Peripheral Nervous System. Saunders; 2010. 10th ed.

## 🔑 KEY POINT

**Lateral Femoral Cutaneous Nerve (LFCN)**
- Meralgia paresthetica
- Numbness of anterolateral thigh without weakness
- Compression of LFCN occurs as it travels under the inguinal ligament

## MNEMONIC

| | | |
|---|---|---|
| **Gluteus medius** | Muscle locates higher | L5 predominant |
| **Gluteus maximus** | Muscle locates lower | S1 predominant |

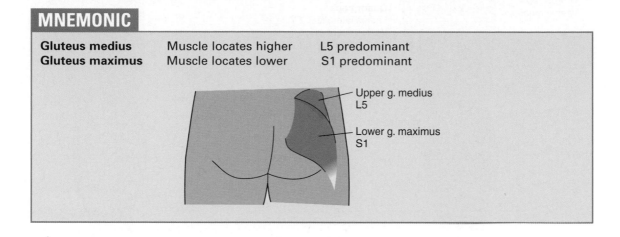

Upper g. medius L5

Lower g. maximus S1

**QUESTION 17.** A 65-year-old man develops weakness of the right leg after he undergoes coronary angiography for evaluation of chest pain. Examination reveals weakness of right knee extension. Which of the following muscles would be affected by a lumbar plexus lesion but not a femoral nerve lesion?
- A. Iliacus
- B. Adductor longus
- C. Gluteus medius
- D. Quadriceps
- E. Hamstrings

**ANSWER:** B. Adductor longus

### COMMENTS AND DISCUSSION

The table below demonstartes the correct innervation of these muscles (Tables 1.3 and 1.8).

| Muscle | Nerve | Plexus | Root |
|---|---|---|---|
| Iliacus | Femoral | Lumbar (posterior division) | L2-4 |
| Adductor longus | Obturator | Lumbar (anterior division) | L2-4 |
| Gluteus medius | Superior gluteal | N/A | L4-**5**, S1 |
| Quadriceps | Femoral | Lumbar (posterior division) | L2-4 |
| Medial hamstrings | Sciatic | Lumbosacral | L4-**5**, S1 |
| Lateral hamstrings (biceps femoris) | Sciatic | Lumbosacral | L5, **S1** |

- Both femoral and obturator nerves are derived from the lumbar plexus.
- The femoral nerve is formed from the posterior division, whereas the obturator is formed from the anterior division.
- Thus, to differentiate a lumbar plexus lesion from a femoral nerve lesion, one should examine the muscles innervated by the obturator nerve to assess involvement of the anterior division of the lumbar plexus.
- The thigh adductors are innervated by the obturator nerve.
- The iliacus and the quadriceps are innervated by the femoral nerve, which would be affected in both a femoral nerve lesion and a lumbar plexus lesion (Fig. 1.7).
- The gluteus medius and hamstrings would not be affected in either a femoral nerve or a lumbar plexus lesion.

**Motor**                                    **Sensory**

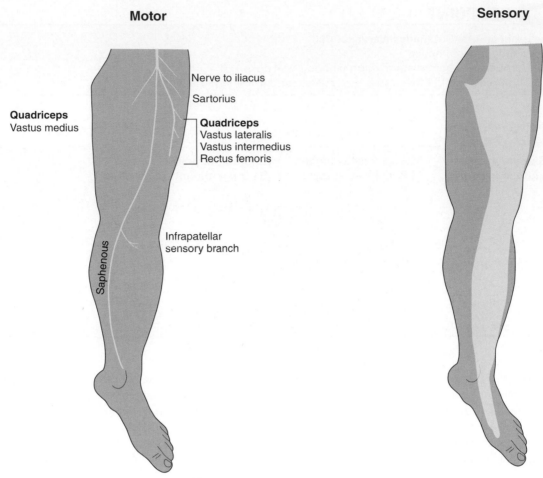

**Fig. 1.7** Anatomy of the femoral nerve.

**QUESTION 18.** A 65-year-old man presents with weakness of the right leg after surgical repair of a right inguinal hernia. Examination demonstrates weakness of right knee extension. Which of the following skin areas of the right lower extremity is most likely to reveal sensory impairment?
A. Medial lower leg
B. Lateral lower leg
C. Dorsum of the foot
D. Lateral aspect of the foot
E. Sole

**ANSWER:** A. Medial lower leg

**COMMENTS AND DISCUSSION**
- This patient most likely has femoral neuropathy after surgical repair of his inguinal hernia.
- Right knee extension is due to weakness of the quadriceps, which is supplied by the femoral nerve.
- The saphenous nerve is the terminal sensory branch of the femoral nerve that supplies sensation to the medial lower leg.
- Thus, when femoral neuropathy is suspected, testing sensation over the medial leg can be useful.
- In addition, the medial and intermediate cutaneous nerves of the thigh are sensory branches of the femoral nerve that supply sensation to the medial and anterior thigh.
- Sensation in the lateral leg, especially in the lower part, and in the dorsum of the foot (except the first web space) is supplied by the superficial fibular (peroneal) nerve (Table 1.8).
- The sural nerve supplies sensation to the lateral aspect of the foot, and is formed by branches of both the tibial and fibular (peroneal) nerves (Table 1.8).
- The sensation in the sole is supplied mainly by the medial and lateral plantar nerves, which are branches of the tibial nerve.

- Major lower extremity nerves
  - Femoral nerve (Fig. 1.7)
    - The largest branch of the lumbar plexus; arises from the posterior division
    - Innervates the psoas and iliacus (iliopsoas) first, and then runs under the inguinal ligament to supply muscles in the anterior thigh including quadriceps, sartorius, and pectineus

 **HIGH-YIELD FACT**

**Femoral N.**
From **posterior** division, but supplies **anterior** thigh muscles (e.g., quadriceps)
**Obturator N.**
From **anterior** division, but supplies more **posterior** thigh muscles (e.g., thigh adductors)

 **KEY POINT**

The infrapatellar sensory branch of the femoral nerve may be entrapped at the pes arserine bursa, or may be injured during knee surgeries

  - Obturator nerve (Fig. 1.8)
    - From the anterior division of the lumbar plexus
    - Supplies adductor muscles of the thigh

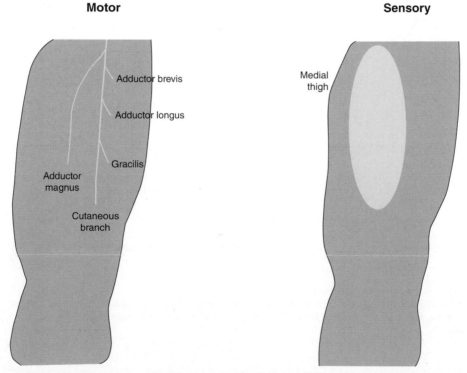

**Motor**

**Sensory**

Adductor brevis

Adductor longus

Gracilis

Adductor magnus

Cutaneous branch

Medial thigh

Fig. 1.8 Anatomy of the obturator nerve.

**QUESTION 19.** The tibial division of the sciatic nerve innervates the:
  A. tibialis anterior.
  B. adductor magnus.
  C. peroneus longus.
  D. peroneus brevis.
  E. adductor longus.

**ANSWER:** B. adductor magnus.

## COMMENTS AND DISCUSSION

- In the thigh, the tibial division of the sciatic nerve co-innervates the adductor magnus with the obturator nerve.
- It also innervates most hamstring muscles except for the short head of biceps femoris muscle that is innervated by the fibular (peroneal) division of the sciatic nerve.
- The obturator nerve innervates the adductor longus (Fig. 1.8).
- The peroneal (fibular) nerve innervates the tibialis anterior, peroneus longus, and peroneus brevis (Fig. 1.9).
- Sciatic nerve (Fig. 1.9)
  - The largest branch of the lumbosacral plexus
  - Consists of two main bundles: tibial (lateral) and common peroneal (medial)
  - Supplies all hamstrings and part of lateral adductor magnus
  - Divides into two branches at the popliteal fossa: tibial and common peroneal (fibular) nerves

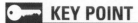 **KEY POINT**

This book uses **"peroneal"** nerve, which is also recently renamed as the **"fibular"** nerve.

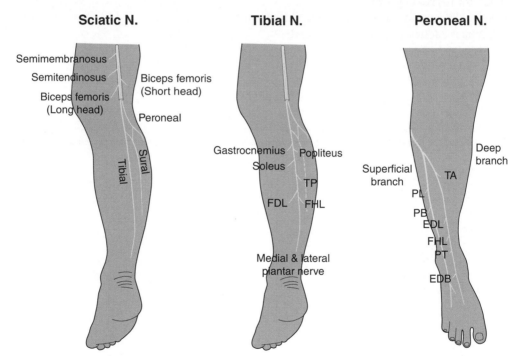

**Fig. 1.9** Sciatic, tibial, and peroneal nerve anatomy.
*TP*, tibialis posterior; *FDL*, flexor digitorum longus; *FHL*; flexor hallucis longus; *TA*, tibialis anterior; *PL*, peroneus longus; *PB*, peroneus brevis; *EDL*, extensor digitorum longus; *FHL*, flexor hallucis longus; *PT*, peroneus tertius; *EDB*, extensor digitorum brevis.

**QUESTION 20.** A 23-year-old man presents with left foot drop. To differentiate an L5 radiculopathy from a peroneal neuropathy, which of the following muscle testing would be useful?
A. Hip extension
B. Hip internal rotation
C. Knee extension
D. Knee flexion
E. Plantar flexion

**ANSWER:** B. Hip internal rotation

## COMMENTS AND DISCUSSION

The table below demonstartes the correct innervation of these muscles (Tables 1.3 and 1.8).

| Muscle action | Muscle | Nerve | Root |
|---|---|---|---|
| Hip extension | Gluteus maximus | Inferior gluteal | L5, **S1**, S2 |
| Hip internal rotation/abduction | Tensor fascia latae | Superior gluteal | L4, **L5**, S1 |
| Knee extension | Quadriceps | Femoral | L2-4 |
| Knee flexion | Hamstrings | Sciatic | L5-S1 |
| Plantar flexion | Gastrocsoleus | Sciatic | S1 |

- To differentiate an L5 radiculopathy from a peroneal neuropathy, testing of the non-peroneal L5-innervated muscles would be useful (Table 1.6).
- Tensor fascia latae is an L5 muscle innervated by the superior gluteal nerve (Table 1.7).
  - Its action includes internal rotation and abduction of the hip.
- Another muscle that is very useful is the tibialis posterior, which is a tibial L5-innervated muscle.
  - Its action is ankle inversion (Table 1.7).
- Hip extension is primarily an action of the gluteus maximus muscle, supplied by the inferior gluteal nerve and principally innervated by the S1 nerve root (Table 1.8).
- Knee flexion and plantar flexion are actions of the sciatic nerve and the tibial nerves, respectively, both supplied predominantly by the S1 nerve root (Table 1.6).
- Knee extension is an action of the quadriceps, which are supplied by the femoral nerve and the L2-4 nerve roots (Table 1.6).
- Common (fibular) peroneal nerve (Fig. 1.9 and Table 1.8)
  - Divides into superficial and deep branches, as well as articular branch
    - Superficial branch
      - Supplies ankle evertors which include the peroneus longus and brevis
      - Supplies sensation to the dorsum of the foot and the lateral calf (Fig. 1.10)

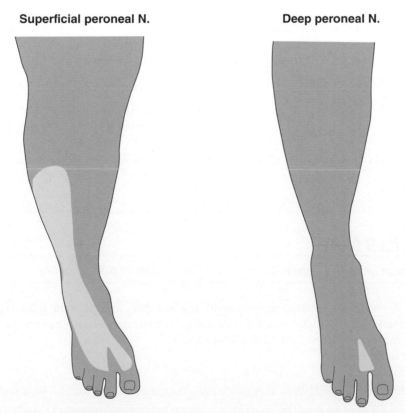

**Superficial peroneal N.**            **Deep peroneal N.**

**Fig. 1.10** Sensory areas innervated by the superficial and deep peroneal nerves.

- Deep branch
  - Supplies ankle dorsiflexors including the tibialis anterior, extensor digitorum longus and brevis, extensor hallucis longus, and peroneus tertius (also an ankle evertor)
  - Supplies sensation to the web space between the first and second toes (Fig. 1.10)
- Articular branch
  - Supplies the proximal tibiofibular joint

 **KEY POINT**

**Short head of biceps femoris** is the **only muscle** supplied by the **peroneal division** of the sciatic nerve

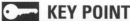 **HIGH-YIELD FACT**

**Ankle Evertors**
**Primary**
- Peroneus longus (superficial peroneal)
- Peroneus brevis (superficial peroneal)

**Secondary**
- Peroneus tertius (deep peroneal)
- Extensor digitorum longus (deep peroneal)

- Tibial nerve (Fig. 1.9)
  - Main motor nerve to the posterior compartment of the calf and most intrinsic foot muscles
  - Supplies muscles involved in ankle inversion and ankle and toe plantar flexion (Table 1.8)
  - Gives off the sural nerve, a pure sensory nerve that innervates the skin of the posterior calf and lateral foot and toes.
  - Terminal branches: medial and lateral plantar nerves and calcaneal nerves, which supplies sensation to the sole of the foot (Table 1.8) and is affected in tarsal tunnel syndrome (Table 1.9)

**TABLE 1.9** Common entrapment sites of lower extremity nerves.

| Nerves | Common entrapment sites |
|---|---|
| Lateral femoral cutaneous nerve of thigh (LFCN) | • Inguinal ligament (close to anterior superior iliac spine) |
| Femoral | • Within the psoas muscle (hematoma)<br>• Inguinal ligament (especially in the lithotomy position) |
| Obturator | • Isolated entrapment is unlikely<br>• Within pelvis (hematoma) |
| Sciatic | • Hip/buttock area (hip or buttock surgery) |
| Common peroneal | • Fibular neck |
| Tibial | • Tarsal tunnel |

 **HIGH-YIELD FACT**

**Baxter's (inferior calcaneal) nerve** is a first branch of the lateral plantar nerve.

**QUESTION 21.** A 45-year-old woman presents with right foot drop. Which of the following muscles on needle electromyography (EMG) would be affected by a sicatic nerve lesion but not a common fibular (peroneal) nerve lesion around the fibular neck?
A. Extensor hallucis longus
B. Peroneus longus
C. Short head of biceps femoris
D. Gluteus medius
E. Tensor fascia latae

**ANSWER:** C. Short head of biceps femoris

**COMMENTS AND DISCUSSION**

The table below demonstartes the correct innervation of these muscles (Tables 1.3 and 1.8).

| Muscle | Nerve | Root |
|--------|-------|------|
| Extensor hallucis longus | Peroneal | L5 |
| Peroneus longus | Peroneal | L5 |
| Short head of biceps femoris | Sciatic (peroneal division) | L5, S1 |
| Gluteus medius | Superior gluteal | L4, **5**, S1 |
| Tensor fascia latae | Superior gluteal | L4, **5**, S1 |

- The short head of biceps femoris is the only muscle innervated by the peroneal division of the sciatic nerve.
- Therefore, this muscle is very useful on electromyography (EMG) to differentiate common peroneal nerve lesions (e.g., at the fibular neck) from sciatic nerve lesions and L5 radiculopathies (Table 1.7).
- Examining the medial hamstring muscles (i.e., semimembranosus and semitendinosus) can also be useful but is clinically difficult due to strong medial hamstring muscles (Table 1.6).
- The extensor hallucis longus and peroneus longus are affected in both the common peroneal nerve and sciatic nerve lesions (Fig. 1.9 and Table 1.8).
- The gluteus medius and tensor fascia latae are both innervated by the superior gluteal nerve, and thus are not affected in either common peroneal nerve or sciatic nerve lesions (Table 1.6 and 1.8).

**QUESTION 22.** Which of the following muscles is supplied by the superficial fibular (peroneal) nerve?
- A. Tibialis anterior
- B. Extensor hallucis longus
- C. Extensor digitorum brevis
- D. Peroneus brevis
- E. Peroneus tertius

**ANSWER:** D. Peroneus brevis

**COMMENTS AND DISCUSSION**
- The superficial peroneal nerve is mainly a sensory nerve that supplies the lower lateral leg and dorsum of the foot (Fig. 1.10).
- It also innervates ankle evertors including the peroneus longus and peroneus brevis (Fig. 1.9 and Table 1.8).
- The only ankle evertor that is supplied by the deep peroneal nerve is the peroneus tertius (Fig. 1.9)
- The deep peroneal nerve is mainly a motor nerve that supplies the tibialis anterior, extensor hallucis longus, and extensor digitorum brevis (Table 1.8).
- It also supplies sensation to a small area of skin in the web space between the first and second toes (Fig. 1.10).

**QUESTION 23.** A 33-year-old woman presents with numbness of the lateral lower leg for one week. Which of the following diagnoses is **LEAST** likely?
- A. L5 radiculopathy
- B. Sciatic neuropathy
- C. Common fibular (peroneal) neuropathy
- D. Isolated superficial fibular (peroneal) neuropathy
- E. Isolated deep fibular (peroneal) neuropathy

**ANSWER:** E. Isolated deep fibular (peroneal) neuropathy

**COMMENTS AND DISCUSSION**
- The area of skin over the lower lateral lower leg is innervated by the L5 nerve root and the superficial peroneal nerve (Fig. 1.10 and Table 1.8).

- Because the superficial peroneal nerve is a branch from the sciatic nerve (peroneal division) and the common peroneal nerve, lesions in these locations may also result in numbness in this area.
- The deep peroneal nerve supplies sensation only to the web space between the first and second toes (Fig. 1.10).
- Thus an isolated deep peroneal neuropathy would not result in numbness of the lower lateral lower leg.

**QUESTION 24.** The sural communicating nerve:
- A. is also known as the medial sural nerve.
- B. is also known as the tibial communicating nerve.
- C. originates from the common fibular (peroneal) nerve.
- D. originates from the superficial fibular (peroneal) nerve.
- E. originates from the deep fibular (peroneal) nerve.

**ANSWER:** C. originates from the common fibular (peroneal) nerve.

**COMMENTS AND DISCUSSION**
- The sural nerve supplies sensation to the posterior calf and lateral foot (Table 1.8).
- The sural nerve is a pure sensory nerve with fibers from S1 root mostly.
- The sural nerve arises from the tibial nerve in the popliteal fossa, and is known as the medial sural nerve.
- In addition, a lateral sural nerve arises from the proximal common peroneal nerve in the popliteal fossa and travels down the posterior calf.
- In about 80% of individuals, lateral sural nerve has a branch (the sural communicating nerve) that joins the medial sural nerve in the lower calf.

 **KEY POINT**

> In elderly patients or patients with foot edema, sural sensory nerve action potentials (SNAPs) can be low or absent.

**QUESTION 25.** Which matching between the muscle and the nerve root(s) is **CORRECT**?
- A. Anconeus – C5
- B. Pronator teres – C8
- C. Flexor digitorum longus – L5 and S1
- D. Extensor digitorum brevis – L4
- E. Long head of biceps femoris – L3 and L4

**ANSWER:** C. Flexor digitorum longus – L5 and S1

**COMMENTS AND DISCUSSION**
The table below demonstrates the correct innervation of these muscles (Table 1.3 and 1.8)

| Muscle | Nerve | Root |
| --- | --- | --- |
| Anconeus | Radial | C6-8 (mainly C7) |
| Pronator teres | Median | C6-7 |
| Flexor digitorum longus | Tibial | L5, S1 (mainly L5) |
| Extensor digitorum brevis | Peroneal (deep) | L5, S1 |
| Long head of biceps femoris | Sciatic (tibial division) | L5, S1 |

**MNEMONIC**

> **L5 in**cludes ankle **in**version deficit.

- **Clues for lesion localization**
  - Clues for root lesion
    - Sensory impairment in dermatomal distribution
    - Motor impairment in myotomal distribution
  - Clues for individual nerve lesion
    - Sensory and/or motor impairment in peripheral nerve distribution
  - Clues for plexus lesion
    - Sensory and/or motor impairment in combined distribution of different nerves in the same trunk, cord, or part of the plexus

## SUGGESTED READINGS

Preston DC, Shapiro BE. *Electromyography and neuromuscular disorders: Clinical-electrophysiologic-ultrasound Correlations.* 4th ed. Philadelphia: Elsevier; 2021.

O'Brien Michael, On behalf of the Guarantor of Brain. *Aids to the Examination of the Peripheral Nervous System.* 6th ed. Philadelphia: Elsevier; 2022.

Katirji B, Kaminski HJ, Ruff RL, eds. *Neuromuscular disorders in Clinical Practice.* 2nd ed. New York: Springer; 2014.

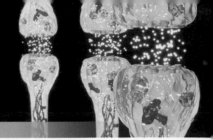

# CHAPTER 2

# Basic Science of Neuromuscular Disorders

## PART 1 | PRACTICE TEST

**Q1.** Which statement is **TRUE** regarding nerve action potentials?
A. Resting membrane potential is approximately +70 millivolts (mV).
B. During depolarization, sodium influxes occurs through the $Na^+/K^+$ ATPase pump.
C. Identical action potential occurs when the membrane potential rises above the resting potential.
D. During repolarization, potassium influx results in more positive membrane potentials.
E. Inactivation of sodium channels during repolarization results in a refractory period.

**Q2.** During depolarization of an axon:
A. sodium channels open.
B. sodium channels close.
C. potassium channels open.
D. potassium channels close.
E. calcium channels open.

**Q3.** Which of the following results in **slower** conduction velocity of the nerve?
A. Increased diameter of axon
B. Increased myelin thickness
C. Decreased temperature
D. Decreased number of nodes of Ranvier
E. Decreased number of calcium channels

**Q4.** The function of $Na^+/K^+$ ATPase is to move:
A. 2 $Na^+$ out of the cell and 3 $K^+$ in.
B. 3 $Na^+$ out of the cell and 2 $K^+$ in.
C. 2 $Na^+$ into the cell and 3 $K^+$ out.
D. 3 $Na^+$ into the cell and 2 $K^+$ out.
E. 3 $Na^+$ out of the cell and 3 $K^+$ in.

**Q5.** Which sensory receptor perceives deep pressure sensation?
A. Pacinian corpuscle
B. Meissner corpuscle
C. Merkel disc
D. Ruffini ending
E. Free nerve ending

**Q6.** Which statement is **CORRECT**?
A. C fibers are myelinated fibers that perceive vibration sensation.
B. The fastest sensory fiber is the Ia fiber originating from muscle spindles.
C. Deep pressure is conducted through unmyelinated fibers.
D. Large fibers represent motor nerves, and small fibers represent sensory nerves.
E. Sympathetic nerve contains myelinated, fast-conducting fibers.

**Q7.** A 33-year-old man had an accident while skiing; he fell with his right leg hitting a rock. He developed a right foot drop and numbness over his right lateral calf and the dorsum of his right foot. In addition, he had moderate pain over the right knee region. On examination, right ankle dorsiflexion and eversion power was 2/5, but plantar flexion and inversion were preserved. The results of electromyography (EMG) performed 15 days later are shown in the following table. Which statement is **CORRECT**?
A. This patient has neurapraxia of the right common peroneal nerve.
B. The prognosis in this case is poor.
C. There are injuries to the myelin sheath, endoneurium, perineurium, and epineurium.
D. The supporting structures are also involved.
E. This patient has a 3rd grade nerve injury, according to Sunderland classification.

Table for Question 7

| Nerve stimulated | Stimulating site | Amplitude (mV) | | Distal latency (ms) | | Conduction velocity (m/s) | |
|---|---|---|---|---|---|---|---|
| | | Pt | NL | Pt | NL | Pt | NL |
| R Superficial peroneal (s) | Leg | 10 | ≥6 | 2.4 | ≤4.4 | 42 | ≥40 |
| R Sural (s) | Calf | 18 | ≥6 | 3.2 | ≤4.4 | 48 | ≥40 |
| R Peroneal (m, EDB) | Ankle | 4.5 | ≥2.6 | 4.5 | ≤6.5 | | ≥44 |
| | Below fibular head | 3.5 | | | | 48 | |
| | Knee | 0.8 | | | | 30 | |
| R Peroneal (m, TA) | Below fibular head | 4.5 | ≥3.0 | 2.6 | ≤6.7 | | ≥44 |
| | Knee | 0.4 | | | | 22 | |
| R Tibial (m, AH) | Ankle | 10 | ≥5.3 | 4.4 | ≤6.1 | | ≥41 |
| | Popliteal fossa | 8 | | | | 46 | |

*AH*, abductor hallucis; *EDB*, extensor digitorum brevis; *m*, motor; *m/s*, meters per second; *ms*, millisecond; *mV*, millivolt; *NL*, normal; *Pt*, patient; *R*, right; *s*, sensory; *TA*, tibialis, anterior.

Q8. When the nerve action potential reaches the presynaptic nerve terminal, there is:
A. opening of sodium channels.
B. opening of potassium channels.
C. opening of calcium channels.
D. opening of acetylcholine receptors.
E. opening of ryanodine receptors-1.

Q9. Presynaptic vesicular acetylcholine (ACh) quanta distribute into three separate stores: primary, secondary, and tertiary. When the latter is needed, which protein plays an important role in transporting these tertiary ACh quanta from the cell body to the presynaptic bouton?
A. Rapsyn
B. SNAP-25
C. Kinesin
D. Dynein
E. Actinin

Q10. What is the main function of SNARE protein in the presynaptic nerve terminal in relation to acetylcholine?
A. Packaging into vesicles
B. Delivery of vesicles from the cell body to the nerve terminal
C. Fusion of vesicles to the presynaptic membrane
D. Breakdown of molecules
E. Clustering of receptors

Q11. Which statement is TRUE regarding the neuromuscular junction?
A. The postsynaptic acetylcholine receptor is a voltage-gated channel.
B. When acetylcholine receptors are activated, endplate potentials are generated.
C. Endplate potentials always open $Ca^{2+}$ channels in the sarcoplasmic reticulum.
D. Choline acetyltransferase metabolizes acetylcholine at the synaptic cleft.
E. Acetyl coenzyme A (acetyl-CoA) is transported back to the presynaptic terminal by the acetyl-CoA transporter.

Q12. Which of the following is FALSE regarding the muscle-specific kinase (MuSK) protein?
A. MuSK increases the rate of acetylcholine receptor opening.
B. MuSK has a role in the clustering and anchoring of acetylcholine receptors.
C. MuSK has a role in the formation of neuromuscular junctions.
D. MuSK enhances the transcription of genes that encode synaptic proteins.
E. The activation of MuSK requires agrin-induced LRP4 binding and recruitment of DOK-7.

Q13. Which statement is TRUE regarding ryanodine receptor-1 (RYR1)?
A. It resides on the sarcoplasmic reticulum membrane.
B. It is a part of T-tubule.
C. Activation of this receptor causes $Na^+$ influx via the postsynaptic muscle membrane.
D. It inhibits dihydropyridine receptor.
E. It promotes clustering of acetylcholine receptors.

Q14. What is the function of calcium ($Ca^{2+}$) in excitation-contraction coupling?
A. Binding to troponin C, resulting in movements of tropomyosin
B. Dissociation of the actin-myosin complex
C. Returning of the myosin head to resting conformation
D. Changing the conformation of myosin heads, resulting in a power stroke
E. Releasing adenosine diphosphate (ADP) from myosin

Q15. Which statement is TRUE regarding excitation-contraction coupling and the cross-bridge cycle?
A. $Ca^{2+}$ required in this process is mainly from the extracellular space.
B. $Ca^{2+}$ required in this process enters the intracellular space via acetylcholine receptors.
C. ATP is required for the release of the myosin head from actin after the power stroke.
D. Titin stabilizes the sarcolemma membrane and actin.
E. In rigor mortis, actin-myosin cross-bridges separate due to a lack of ATP.

**Q16.** During muscle contraction, which part of the sarcomere has a constant length?
A. A-band
B. H-band
C. I-band
D. Area between two M-lines
E. Area between two Z-lines

**Q17.** Which of the following is a property of a type 1 muscle fiber, compared to a type 2 fiber?
A. Faster twitching
B. Higher fatigue rate
C. Higher intensity of contraction
D. Fewer mitochondria
E. Associated with smaller motor neurons

**Q18.** What neurotransmitter is released from most postganglionic sympathetic neurons?
A. Acetylcholine (binding to muscarinic receptors)
B. Acetylcholine (binding to nicotinic receptors)
C. Glutamate
D. γ-Aminobutyric acid (GABA)
E. Norepinephrine

## PART 2 | QUESTIONS WITH ANSWERS AND DISCUSSION

**QUESTION 1.** Which statement is **TRUE** regarding nerve action potentials?
A. Resting membrane potential is approximately +70 millivolts (mV).
B. During depolarization, sodium influx occurs through the $Na^+/K^+$ ATPase pump.
C. Identical action potential occurs when the membrane potential rises above the resting potential.
D. During repolarization, potassium influx results in more positive membrane potentials.
E. Inactivation of sodium channels during repolarization results in a refractory period.

**ANSWER:** E. Inactivation of sodium channels during repolarization results in a refractory period.

### COMMENTS AND DISCUSSION
- Nerve action potential (Fig. 2.1)
  - Resting nerve membrane potential: $-70$ mV (inside as compared to outside)
  - Potassium is located primarily within the cell, and sodium is located mostly outside.
  - "All or none" principle: When the membrane potential depolarizes above threshold, an action potential occurs ("all"); if the depolarization does not reach threshold, no action potential occurs ("none").
  - The action potential then propagates down the nerve.
  - During depolarization: $Na^+$ influx occurs through voltage-gated $Na^+$ channels.
  - During repolarization: inactivation of the $Na^+$ channels occurs followed by $K^+$ efflux, resulting in a more negative membrane potential.
  - Inactivation of $Na^+$ channels during repolarization results in a refractory period.
    - Absolute refractory period: no action potential can be generated.
    - Relative refractory period: later, action potential can be generated but the threshold is increased.
  - $Na^+/K^+$ ATPase (pump) then re-establishes the concentration gradient by pumping 3 $Na^+$ out for every 2 $K^+$ pumped in.

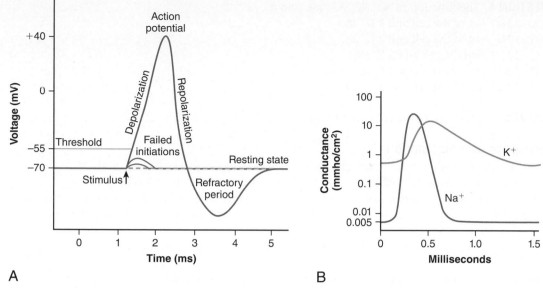

Fig. 2.1 Action potentials. From A: https://commons.wikimedia.org/wiki/File:Action_potential.svg under the Creative Commons Attribution-Share Alike 3.0 Unported license. B; adjusted from Hall, J. E. (2016). Guyton and hall textbook of medical physiology. 13th ed. Philadelphia, PA: Elsevier:67.

**QUESTION 2.** During depolarization of an axon:
  A. sodium channels open.
  B. sodium channels close.
  C. potassium channels open.
  D. potassium channels close.
  E. calcium channels open.

**ANSWER:** A. sodium channels open

**COMMENTS AND DISCUSSION**
- During depolarization, sodium channels open. (Fig. 2.1B)
- Entrance of sodium into the cell results in a more-positive membrane potential relative to baseline.
- Potassium channels remain unchanged (remain closed) during the depolarization phase.

**QUESTION 3.** Which of the following results in **slower** conduction velocity of the nerve?
  A. Increased diameter of axon
  B. Increased myelin thickness
  C. Decreased temperature
  D. Decreased number of nodes of Ranvier
  E. Decreased number of calcium channels

**ANSWER:** C. Decreased temperature

**COMMENTS AND DISCUSSION**
- Low temperature slows nerve conduction velocity by prolonging the inactivation of sodium channels, resulting in longer depolarization times.
- Nerve axons with larger diameters and thicker myelin sheaths have faster conduction velocities.
- Fewer nodes of Ranvier result in longer internodal distances for saltatory conduction, which in turn leads to faster nerve conduction velocity.
- Decreased numbers of calcium channels would not affect the conduction velocity.

**QUESTION 4.** The function of Na$^+$/K$^+$ ATPase is to move:
A. 2 Na$^+$ out of the cell and 3 K$^+$ in.
B. 3 Na$^+$ out of the cell and 2 K$^+$ in.
C. 2 Na$^+$ into the cell and 3 K$^+$ out.
D. 3 Na$^+$ into the cell and 2 K$^+$ out.
E. 3 Na$^+$ out of the cell and 3 K$^+$ in.

**ANSWER:** B. 3 Na$^+$ out of the cell and 2 K$^+$ in.

**COMMENTS AND DISCUSSION**
- During depolarization, Na$^+$ influx into the cell occurs along its concentration gradient.
- During repolarization, K$^+$ efflux out of the cell occurs along its electrochemical gradient.
- To maintain the electrochemical gradient (i.e., higher concentration of Na$^+$ extracellularly and higher concentration of K$^+$ intracellularly), active transport of 3 Na$^+$ out of the cell in exchange for 2 K$^+$ into the cell occurs.
- This process requires ATP and is therefore referred to as primary active transport.

**QUESTION 5.** Which sensory receptor perceives deep pressure sensation?
A. Pacinian corpuscle
B. Meissner corpuscle
C. Merkel disc
D. Ruffini ending
E. Free nerve ending

**ANSWER:** A. Pacinian corpuscle

**COMMENTS AND DISCUSSION**
- Sensory receptors (Fig. 2.2 and Table 2.1)
  ○ Are distributed in different layers of the skin and convey various sensory modalities to nerve fibers
  ○ Three main types of sensory receptors in the skin include:
    - Mechanoreceptors (detecting touch, mechanical compression, or stretching)
    - Thermoreceptors (detecting hot or cold temperature)
    - Nociceptors (detecting pain)

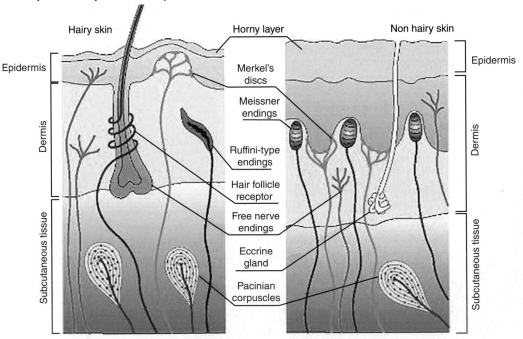

**Fig. 2.2** Sensory receptors in skin layers. Adapted from https://www.pediagenosis.com/2018/07/sensory-receptors.html

**TABLE 2.1** Sensory receptors, function, and related nerve fibers.

| Sensory receptor | Location | Received modality | Related nerve fiber group |
|---|---|---|---|
| Pacinian corpuscles | Dermis/hypodermis (deep) | Vibration, pressure | Aα, Aβ |
| Meissner corpuscles | Superficial dermis at dermal papillae | Point discrimination, touch, flutter | Aα, Aβ |
| Merkel discs | Basal epidermis | Light touch/pressure | Aα, Aβ |
| Ruffini endings (corpuscles) | Superficial dermis | Skin stretch | Aα, Aβ |
| Thermoreceptors | Dermis | Hot/cold temperature | Aδ, C |
| Free nerve endings | Dermis | Pain | Aδ, C |

- Pacinian corpuscles, Meissner corpuscles, Merkel disc, and Ruffini endings are mechanoreceptors.
- Free nerve endings are nociceptors.
- Pacinian corpuscles and Meissner corpuscles both have corpuscular structures but Pacinian corpuscles are lamellated (like onions).
- Pacinian corpuscles are located deep in the hypodermis and thus mediate vibration and deep pressure.
- Ruffini endings are sensitive to skin stretching.
- Free nerve endings terminate in the dermis; therefore skin injuries to dermal layers (e.g., second-degree burns) result in pain.

## MNEMONICS

Pacinian corpuscles are located deep in the hypodermis, and mediate deep pressure and vibration.

**QUESTION 6.** Which statement is **CORRECT**?
A. C fibers are myelinated fibers that perceive vibration sensation.
B. The fastest sensory fiber is the Ia fiber originating from muscle spindles.
C. Deep pressure is conducted through unmyelinated fibers.
D. Large fibers represent motor nerves, and small fibers represent sensory nerves.
E. Sympathetic nerve contains myelinated, fast-conducting fibers.

**ANSWER:** B. The fastest sensory fiber is the Ia fiber originating from muscle spindles.

**COMMENTS AND DISCUSSION**
- There are two commonly used nerve fiber classification systems (Fig. 2.3 and Table 2.2):
  - Erlanger-Gasser classification for motor, sensory, and autonomic nerves. This system divides nerve fibers, from large to small diameter, into Aα, Aβ, Aγ, Aδ, B, and C fibers.
  - Lloyd classification for **sensory** fibers only; divides fibers from large to small diameters: I, II, III, and IV fibers.
    - Nerve fibers with larger diameters have faster conduction velocities.
    - Ia fibers have the largest diameters, and hence are the fastest sensory fibers.
    - The Ia fibers receive sensation from muscle spindles.
  - Large fibers (i.e., types A and B) include both motor and sensory (Ia, Ib, and III) fibers.
  - Myelinated fibers have faster conduction velocities than unmyelinated fibers.
  - C fibers (type IV fibers) are the only fiber type that is unmyelinated; these fibers have the smallest diameters, and accordingly the slowest conduction velocities.
  - C fibers mediate slow pain, warm and cold temperature, and crude touch, as well as postganglionic sympathetic fibers.
  - "Small" sensory fibers include Aδ and C fibers, which mediate pain and temperature.
  - "Large" sensory fibers include Aα and Aβ, which receive vibration and proprioception.
    - Deep pressure is received by Pacinian corpuscles, which then conduct through Aα and Aβ fibers; these are myelinated and have large diameters.

## ◎ HIGH-YIELD FACT

Aδ and C fibers convey pain sensation. Impairment of Aδ and C fibers results in small fiber neuropathies.

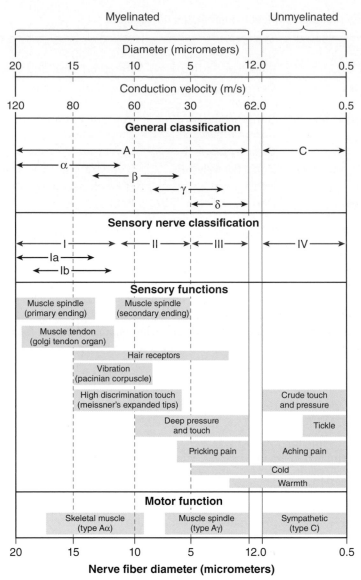

**Fig. 2.3** Nerve fiber classifications and function. From Hall, JE. and Hall ME. Sensory receptor, neuronal circuits for processing information. In: *Guyton and Hall Textbook of Medical Physiology*. 14th ed. Philadelphia PA: Elsevier;2020;7:587–598.

**TABLE 2.2** Comparison of first and second nerve classifications and function.

| First nerve classification[a] | Function | Second nerve classification (only sensory) |
| --- | --- | --- |
| Aα | Somatic motor | - |
| | Sensory (proprioception) | Ia (from muscle spindle) |
| | | Ib (from Golgi tendon organ) |
| Aβ | Sensory (vibration, proprioception from muscle spindle only, light touch) | II (from muscle spindle only) |
| Aγ | Motor to muscle spindle | - |
| Aδ | Fast pain and cold temperature | III |
| B | Preganglionic autonomic | - |
| C[b] | Slow pain, warm and cold temperature, crude touch | IV |
| | Postganglionic sympathetic (autonomic) | - |

[a]The upper ones have larger diameters and faster conduction velocities.
[b]C fibers are unmyelinated; all other types are myelinated.

**QUESTION 7.** A 33-year-old man had an accident while skiing; he fell with his right leg hitting a rock. He developed a right foot drop and numbness over his right lateral calf and the dorsum of his right foot. In addition, he had moderate pain over the right knee region. On examination, right ankle dorsiflexion and eversion power was 2/5, but plantar flexion and inversion were preserved. The results of electromyography (EMG) performed 15 days later are shown in the following table. Which statement is **CORRECT**?

| Nerve stimulated | Stimulating site | Amplitude (mV) | | Distal latency (ms) | | Conduction velocity (m/s) | |
|---|---|---|---|---|---|---|---|
| | | Pt | NL | Pt | NL | Pt | NL |
| R Superficial peroneal (s) | Leg | 10 | ≥6 | 2.4 | ≤4.4 | 42 | ≥40 |
| R Sural (s) | Calf | 18 | ≥6 | 3.2 | ≤4.4 | 48 | ≥40 |
| R Peroneal (m, EDB) | Ankle | 4.5 | ≥2.6 | 4.5 | ≤6.5 | | ≥44 |
| | Below fibular head | 3.5 | | | | 48 | |
| | Knee | 0.8 | | | | 30 | |
| R Peroneal (m, TA) | Below fibular head | 4.5 | ≥3.0 | 2.6 | ≤6.7 | | ≥44 |
| | Knee | 0.4 | | | | 22 | |
| R Tibial (m, AH) | Ankle | 10 | ≥5.3 | 4.4 | ≤6.1 | | ≥41 |
| | Popliteal fossa | 8 | | | | 46 | |

*AH,* abductor hallucis; *EDB,* extensor digitorum brevis; *m,* motor; *m/s,* meters per second; *ms,* millisecond; *mV,* millivolt; *NL,* normal; *Pt,* patient; *R,* right; *s,* sensory; *TA,* tibialis.

A. This patient has neurapraxia of the right common peroneal nerve.
B. The prognosis in this case is poor.
C. There are injuries to the myelin sheath, endoneurium, perineurium, and epineurium.
D. The supporting structures are also involved.
E. This patient has a 3rd grade nerve injury, according to Sunderland classification.

**ANSWER:** A. This patient has neurapraxia of the right common peroneal nerve.

**COMMENTS AND DISCUSSION**
- Two main classification systems for **nerve injuries**: Seddon and Sunderland (Fig. 2.4, Table 2.3 and see Fig. 14.1)
  - Seddon classification (from mild to severe):
    - Neurapraxia
    - Axonotmesis
    - Neurotmesis
  - Sunderland classification (from mild to severe): 1st to 5th degrees
    - 1st degree
    - 2nd degree
    - 3rd degree
    - 4th degree
    - 5th degree
  - Neurapraxia or 1st-degree injury:
    - Only myelin sheath disruption
    - Conduction block (due to demyelination) on electrodiagnostic studies
    - Good recovery
  - Recovery is poorer if there is disruption of axon and/or supporting structures (e.g., endoneurium, perineurium, and epineurium). Neurotmesis has poorest prognosis, and typically requires surgical repair.

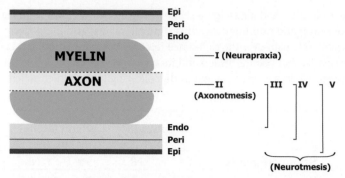

**Fig. 2.4** Diagram of structures involved in each degree of nerve injury based on Sunderland (in Roman numbers) and Seddon (in parentheses) classifications. *Endo*, endoneurium; *Epi*, epineurium; *Peri*, perineurium.

**TABLE 2.3** Seddon and Sunderland classifications of nerve injury. The injured structures, electrodiagnostic findings and prognosis are shown for each degree of nerve injuries.

| Seddon classification | Sunderland classification (grade) | Myelin sheath | Axon | Supporting structures | EDx | Recovery |
|---|---|---|---|---|---|---|
| Neurapraxia | 1st | ✗ | ✓ | ✓ | Conduction block; velocity focal slowing | Best |
| Axonotmesis | 2nd | ✗ | ✗ | ✓ | Axonal features | Good |
| Neurotmesis | 3rd | ✗ | ✗ | ✗ Endoneurium | Axonal features | Fair |
| | 4th | ✗ | ✗ | ✗ Endoneurium + perineurium | Axonal features | Poor |
| | 5th | ✗ | ✗ | ✗ Endoneurium + perineurium + epineurium | Axonal features | Worst |

*X*, injured; *✓*, intact; *EDx*, electrodiagnosis.

**QUESTION 8.** When the nerve action potential reaches the presynaptic nerve terminal, there is:
   A. opening of sodium channels.
   B. opening of potassium channels.
   C. opening of calcium channels.
   D. opening of acetylcholine receptors.
   E. opening of ryanodine receptors-1.

**ANSWER:** C. opening of calcium channels

 **HIGH-YIELD FACT**

In neurapraxia, only the myelin sheath is injured. Electrodiagnosis shows conduction block with or without conduction velocity slowing, and the recovery is good.

**COMMENTS AND DISCUSSION**
- Physiology of the neuromuscular junction (Fig. 2.5)
   - The neuromuscular junction (NMJ) comprises the presynaptic nerve terminal, synaptic cleft, and postsynaptic membrane of the muscle.
      - Presynaptic nerve terminal
         - Action potentials (depolarization) travel down the motor axon.
         - Depolarization results in opening of the P/Q type voltage-gated calcium channels, resulting in calcium entering the presynaptic terminal.
         - After calcium influx, synaptic vesicles containing acetylcholine (ACh) link to synaptic membrane by intertwining of SNARE proteins are SNAP REceptors (Soluble Nsf [*N*-ethylmaleimide sensitive factor] Attachment Protein REceptors).

- ACh is produced from acetyl-CoA (from Krebs cycle in mitochondria) and choline that enters the presynaptic nerve terminal from the synaptic cleft via the choline transporter.
- ACh is then stored within presynaptic vesicles.
- SNARE proteins at the vesicular membrane (v-SNARE) intertwine with those at the synaptic membranes.
  - Synaptobrevin and synaptotagmin are located at the vesicular membrane
  - Syntaxin and SNAP-25 are located at the synaptic membrane
  - After intertwining of SNARE proteins, synaptic vesicles fuse with synaptic membrane and release ACh.

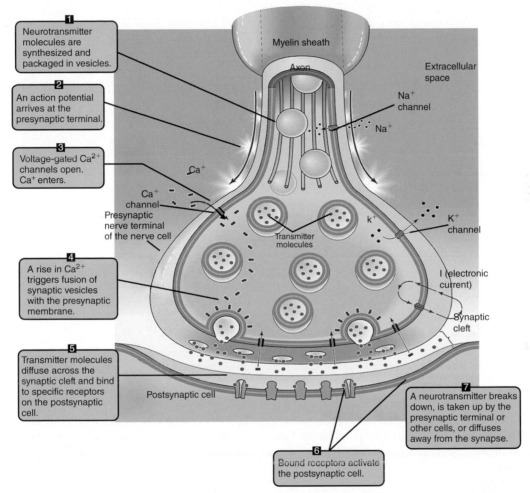

**Fig. 2.5** Physiology of the neuromuscular junction. From Boron WF, Boulpaep EL. *Medical Physiology*. 2nd ed. Philadelphia, PA: Elsevier; 2012.

- Synaptic cleft
  - ACh diffuses across the synaptic cleft.
  - ACh binds to ligand-gated nicotinic acetylcholine receptor (nAChR) at the postsynaptic site.
  - ACh is metabolized by the enzyme cholinesterase (ChE) to acetate and choline; the latter will then be transported back to presynaptic nerve terminal via the choline transporter.
- Postsynaptic membrane
  - ACh binds to ligand-gated nAChR resulting in endplate potentials (EPPs).
  - Summation of EPPs above threshold results in depolarization of voltage-gated sodium channels. Action potentials travel along the postsynaptic membrane to the T-tubules.
  - The T-tubule is the invagination or cleft of postsynaptic membrane.
  - One sarcoplasmic reticulum (SR) is located on each side of a T-tubule.
  - T-tubule + 2 SR on both sides = triad
  - SR stores $Ca^{2+}$ inside.

- Depolarization of the T-tubule membrane leads to linkage of the dihydropyridine receptor (DHPR) on the T-tubule membrane to ryanodine receptor-1 (RYR1) on the SR membrane, resulting in calcium release from SR.
- $Ca^{2+}$ then binds to troponin C, which subsequently activates excitation-contraction coupling.
- Other important proteins at postsynaptic site (Fig. 2.6)
    - Muscle-specific kinase (MuSK) is a tyrosine kinase important for clustering and anchoring of AChRs at the NMJ.
    - Agrin is important in the development of the NMJ.
    - LRP4: agrin binds LRP4, which then activates MuSK.
    - Rapsyn has a role in clustering of AChR.

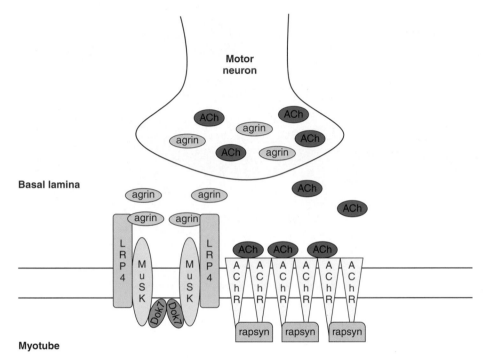

**Fig. 2.6** Important proteins in clustering of acethycholine receptors (AChR) in the postsynaptic membrane. From Hubbard SR, Gnanasambandan K. Structure and activation of MuSK, a receptor tyrosine kinase central to neuromuscular junction formation. *Biochim Biophys Acta.* 2012;1834(10):2166–2169.

**QUESTION 9.** Presynaptic vesicular acetylcholine (ACh) quanta distribute into three separate stores: primary, secondary, and tertiary. When the latter is needed, which protein plays an important role in transporting these tertiary ACh quanta from the cell body to the presynaptic bulb?
A. Rapsyn
B. SNAP-25
C. Kinesin
D. Dynein
E. Actinin

**ANSWER:** C. Kinesin

**COMMENTS AND DISCUSSION**
- Axonal or axoplasmic transport is a process that ships organelles and other chemical substances from one end of the axon to the other.
- There were two types of axonal transport:
    - Anterograde (away from the cell body)
    - Retrograde (toward the cell body)
- These processes are run by specific proteins that navigate microtubules. These proteins move vesicles and organelles along microtubule filaments.
    - Anterograde transport requires kinesin.
    - Retrograde transport requires dynein.

- To deliver tertiary ACh quanta from the cell body to the neuromuscular junction, anterograde transport occurs, and this process requires kinesin.
- Rapsyn is located at the postsynaptic membrane (muscle) and has a role in clustering of postsynaptic nicotinic ACh receptors.
- SNAP-25 is one of the SNARE proteins (in addition to synaptobrevin and synaptotagmin, among others) located at the vesicular membrane within presynaptic nerve terminals, and it has a role in fusion of the vesicular membrane and plasma membrane before release of neurotransmitter from the presynaptic site.
- Actinin, a microfilament protein that is a part of muscle fiber, binds to actin.

**QUESTION 10.** What is the main function of SNARE protein in the presynaptic nerve terminal in relation to acetylcholine?
  A. Packaging into vesicles
  B. Delivery of vesicles from the cell body to the nerve terminal
  C. Fusion of vesicles into the presynaptic membrane
  D. Breakdown of molecules
  E. Clustering of receptors

**ANSWER:** C. Fusion of vesicles to the presynaptic membrane

**COMMENTS AND DISCUSSION**
- SNARE proteins play an important role in exocytosis of synaptic vesicular ACh. After $Ca^{2+}$ influx into the presynaptic nerve terminals, synaptobrevin and synaptotagmin at the vesicular membranes attach to SNAP-25 and syntaxin at the synaptic membrane, to form the SNARE complex, resulting in fusion of the vesicular and synaptic membranes. ACh can then be released into the synaptic cleft.
- Packaging of ACh into presynaptic vesicles requires vesicular ACh transporters.
- Delivery of ACh from the cell body to the presynaptic nerve terminal requires kinesin.
- ACh that remains in the synaptic cleft after release will then be metabolized by acetylcholinesterase into choline and acetate.
- Rapsyn has a role in clustering of ACh receptors at the postsynaptic site.

**QUESTION 11.** Which statement is **TRUE** regarding the neuromuscular junction?
  A. The postsynaptic acetylcholine receptor is a voltage-gated channel.
  B. When acetylcholine receptors are activated, endplate potentials are generated.
  C. Endplate potentials always open $Ca^{2+}$ channels in the sarcoplasmic reticulum.
  D. Choline acetyltransferase metabolizes acetylcholine at the synaptic cleft.
  E. Acetyl coenzyme A (acetyl-CoA) is transported back to the presynaptic terminal by the acetyl-CoA transporter.

**ANSWER:** B. When acetylcholine receptors are activated, endplate potentials are generated.

**COMMENTS AND DISCUSSION**
- Within the presynaptic nerve terminal, acetylcholine (ACh) is produced from acetyl-CoA and choline by a choline acetyltransferase enzyme.
- After the release from the presynaptic nerve terminal into the synaptic cleft, ACh attaches to the postsynaptic ACh receptor, a ligand-gated (not voltage-gated) nicotinic acetylcholine receptor (nAChR).
- The remaining ACh in the synaptic cleft is metabolized by cholinesterase into choline and acetate.
- Choline is then transported back to the presynaptic terminal via the choline transporter.
- Acetyl-CoA is synthesized from pyruvate within the presynaptic nerve terminal, not from the synaptic cleft.
- When nAChRs are activated, endplate potentials (EPPs) are generated. Summation of EPPs that reach threshold then result in $Na^+$ influx via voltage-gated $Na^+$ channel and muscle depolarization. Depolarization along the sarcolemmal membrane then spreads to the T-tubule, where the sarcoplasmic reticulum resides on both sides of the membrane invagination.
- For $Ca^{2+}$ to be released from the sarcoplasmic reticulum, EPPs need to be summated to reach the depolarization threshold.

**QUESTION 12.** Which of the following is **FALSE** regarding the muscle-specific kinase (MuSK) protein?
   A. MuSK increases the rate of acetylcholine receptor opening.
   B. MuSK has a role in the clustering and anchoring of acetylcholine receptors.
   C. MuSK has a role in the formation of neuromuscular junctions.
   D. MuSK enhances the transcription of genes that encode synaptic proteins.
   E. The activation of MuSK requires agrin-induced LRP4 binding and recruitment of DOK-7.

**ANSWER:** B. MuSK has a role in the clustering and anchoring of acetylcholine receptors.

**COMMENTS AND DISCUSSION**
- MuSK is a tyrosine kinase protein that has an important role in the formation of the neuromuscular junctions, clustering and anchoring acetylcholine receptors, enhancing transcription of genes encoding synaptic proteins, as well as stimulation of presynaptic differentiation.
- MuSK does not have role in increasing or decreasing the rate of acetylcholine receptor opening.
- Activation of MuSK requires agrin-induced low-density lipoprotein-related protein 4 (LRP4) binding and also recruitment of the downstream of tyrosine kinase 7 (DOK-7) protein (See Fig. 2.6).
- Mutations of the genes encoding for MuSK, agrin, LRP4, and DOK-7 can result in congenital myasthenic syndromes.

**QUESTION 13.** Which statement is **TRUE** regarding ryanodine receptor-1 (RYR1)?
   A. It resides on the sarcoplasmic reticulum membrane.
   B. It is a part of T-tubule.
   C. Activation of this receptor causes $Na^+$ influx via the postsynaptic muscle membrane.
   D. It inhibits dihydropyridine receptor.
   E. It promotes clustering of acetylcholine receptors.

**ANSWER:** A. It resides on the sarcoplasmic reticulum membrane.

**COMMENTS AND DISCUSSION**
- Ryanodine receptor-1 (RYR1) is located on the sarcoplasmic reticulum (SR) membrane (Fig. 2.7).
- When action potentials travel along the sarcolemmal membrane and reach the T-tubule, which is the invagination of the postsynaptic membrane, dihydropyridine receptors (DHPRs) residing on the T-tubule membrane are activated and linked to RYR1.
- This results in the release of $Ca^{2+}$ from the SR, which is required for excitation-contraction coupling.
- RYR1 does not inhibit DHPR, and it does not have a role in clustering of acetylcholine receptors.
- One T-tubule, together with two SR membranes on both sides of it, is called "triad." RYR1 is on the SR membrane, and thus a part of the triad. However, RYR1 is not a part of T-tubule.

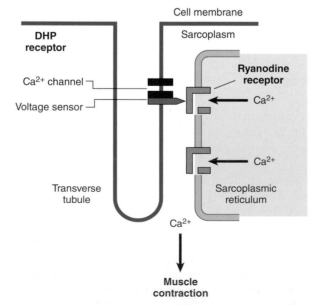

**Fig. 2.7** $Ca^{2+}$ and receptors for excitation-contraction coupling. From Pascual JM, Brady ST. Disorders of muscle excitability. In: Brady ST, Siegel GJ, Albers RW, et al., eds. *Basic Neurochemistry: Principles of Molecular, Cellular, and Medical Neurobiology.* 8th ed. Amsterdam: Academic Press; 2012.

**QUESTION 14.** What is the function of calcium ($Ca^{2+}$) in excitation-contraction coupling?
  A. Binding to troponin C, resulting in movements of tropomyosin
  B. Dissociation of the actin-myosin complex
  C. Returning of the myosin head to resting conformation
  D. Changing the conformation of myosin heads, resulting in a power stroke
  E. Releasing adenosine diphosphate (ADP) from myosin

**ANSWER:** A. Binding to troponin C, resulting in movements of tropomyosin

**COMMENTS AND DISCUSSION**
- Physiology of muscle
  - The sarcomere is located within the sarcolemma.
    - One sarcomere = a unit between two Z-lines (Fig. 2.8).
    - During muscle contraction, the A-band does not change, whereas the H- and I-bands are shorter.

 **HIGH-YIELD FACT**

During muscle contraction, the A-band is constant.

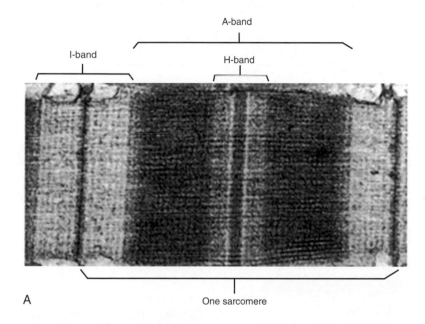

A — One sarcomere

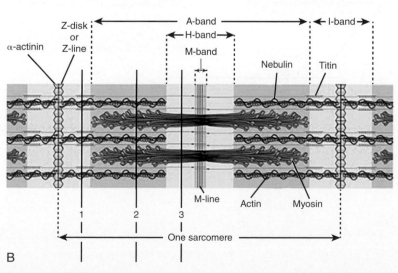

B

**Fig. 2.8** Structure of sarcomere. (A) Electron micrograph revealing the structure of sarcomere. (B) Comparative model representing the key components and architecture of the sarcomere. From Boron WF, Boulpaep EL. *Medical Physiology.* 2nd ed. Philadelphia, PA: Elsevier; 2012.

- Cross-bridge cycle (Fig. 2.9)
  - $Ca^{2+}$ binds to troponin C, resulting in movement of tropomyosin, which in turn exposes the myosin-binding site on actin (thin filament).
  - During the cross-bridge cycle, myosin (thick filament) binds to actin and slides the thin filament in the direction close to the M-line.
  - The release of phosphate leads to a conformational change of myosin heads and the power stroke.
  - Dissociation of the actin-myosin complex occurs after the binding of ATP to the myosin head.
  - Hydrolysis of ATP (to ADP and inorganic phosphate) allows the myosin head to return to its resting conformation.
  - Subsequently, a new cross-bridge between actin and myosin can be formed.
  - To terminate muscle contraction (relax), $Ca^{2+}$ is sequestered back into SR, and some $Ca^{2+}$ moves out through the sarcolemma. Once $Ca^{2+}$ is released from troponin C, tropomyosin returns to cover the myosin-binding site on actin, preventing the cross-bridge cycle

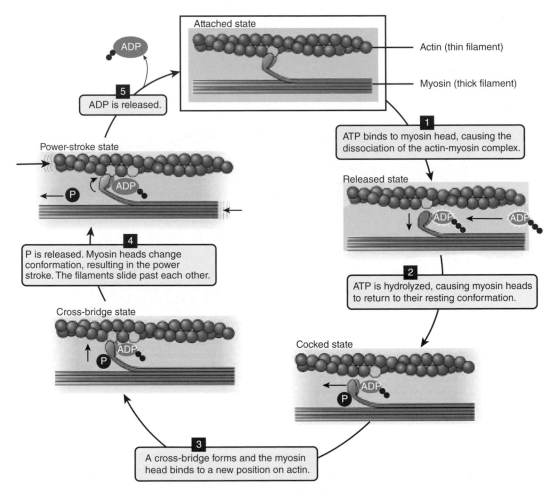

**Fig. 2.9** The cross-bridge cycle in skeletal muscle. From Boron WF, Boulpaep EL. *Medical Physiology.* 2nd ed. Philadelphia, PA: Elsevier; 2012.

**QUESTION 15.** Which statement is **TRUE** regarding excitation-contraction coupling and the cross-bridge cycle?

A. $Ca^{2+}$ required in this process is mainly from the extracellular space.

B. $Ca^{2+}$ required in this process enters the intracellular space via acetylcholine receptors.

C. ATP is required for the release of the myosin head from actin after the power stroke.

D. Titin stabilizes the sarcolemma membrane and actin.

E. In rigor mortis, actin-myosin cross-bridges separate due to a lack of ATP.

**ANSWER:** C. ATP is required for the release of the myosin head from actin after the power stroke.

**COMMENTS AND DISCUSSION**

- To initiate the cross-bridge cycle, $Ca^{2+}$ needs to bind troponin C to expose the myosin-binding site on actin.
- The source of this $Ca^{2+}$ is the sarcoplasmic reticulum (SR), which releases $Ca^{2+}$ via the ryanodine receptor (RYR) (Fig. 2.10), not the acetylcholine receptor.
- During the cross-bridge cycle, ATP is required to detach the myosin head from the actin filament.
- In states where muscle lacks ATP, such as death, the myosin head cannot detach from the actin filament. This results in failure of muscle to relax, as seen in rigor mortis after death.
- Titin is the largest known human protein. It is located between the myosin thick filament and the Z-disc and has a major role in stabilization of the thick filaments in the sarcomere.

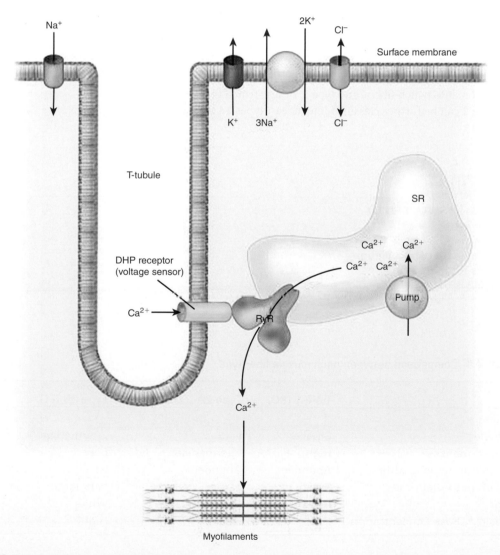

**Fig. 2.10** Excitation-contraction coupling of skeletal muscle. From Jurkat-Rott K, Lehmann-Horn F. Muscle channelopathies and critical points in functional and genetic studies. *J Clin Invest.* 2005;115(8):2000–2009.

**QUESTION 16.** During muscle contraction, which part of the sarcomere has a constant length?
  A. A-band
  B. H-band
  C. I-band
  D. Area between two M-lines
  E. Area between two Z-lines

**ANSWER:** A. A-band

**COMMENTS AND DISCUSSION**
- During muscle contraction, the A-band is constant. An A-band contains a single, thick (myosin) filament (Fig. 2.8B).
- The H-band and I-band become shorter during muscle contraction.
- The area between two Z-lines is one sarcomere, which is shorter during muscle contraction.
- The area between two M-lines (D) is also shorter during muscle contraction.

**QUESTION 17.** Which of the following is a property of a type 1 muscle fiber, compared to a type 2 fiber?
  A. Faster twitching
  B. Higher fatigue rate
  C. Higher intensity of contraction
  D. Fewer mitochondria
  E. Associated with smaller motor neurons

**ANSWER:** E. Associated with smaller motor neurons

**COMMENTS AND DISCUSSION**
- Muscle fiber types are classified by myosin ATPase histochemical reactions into two main categories: type 1, or slow-twitch fibers, and type 2, or fast-twitch fibers (Table 2.4).
  ○ Type 2 can be further classified into at least types 2A and 2B.

---

**MNEMONIC**

Type 1 fiber: **SLOW RED OX**
  **Slow**-twitch
  **Red** fiber
  **Ox**idative phosphorylation
Type 1 is for marathon.
  Type 2 is for sprinting.

---

**TABLE 2.4** Comparison between each muscle fiber type.

|  | Type 1 (SO) | Type 2A (FOG) | Type 2B (FG) |
|---|---|---|---|
| **Structure** | | | |
| Diameter | Smaller | Largest | Intermediate |
| Capillary density | High | Intermediate | Low |
| Amount of mitochondria | Abundant | Abundant | Less |
| Size of motor neurons | Small | Large | Very large |
| Color | Red | Red/pink | White |
| Myosin ATPase concentration | Low | High | High |

**TABLE 2.4**  Comparison between each muscle fiber type—cont'd

|  | Type 1 (SO) | Type 2A (FOG) | Type 2B (FG) |
| --- | --- | --- | --- |
| **Metabolism** | | | |
| Oxidative capacity | High | High | Low |
| Glycolytic capacity | Low | High | High |
| Major storage fuel | Triglycerides | Creatine phosphate, glycogen | Creatine phosphate, glycogen |
| **Mechanical property** | | | |
| Contraction speed | Slow twitch | Fast twitch | Fast twitch |
| Resistance to fatigue | High | Intermediate | Low |
| Power produced | Low | Medium | High |

*SO*, slow oxidative; *FOG*, fast oxidative glycolytic; *FG*, fast glycolytic.

**QUESTION 18.**  What neurotransmitter is released from most postganglionic sympathetic neurons?
  A. Acetylcholine (binding to muscarinic receptors)
  B. Acetylcholine (binding to nicotinic receptors)
  C. Glutamate
  D. γ-Aminobutyric acid (GABA)
  E. Norepinephrine

**ANSWER:** E. Norepinephrine

**COMMENTS AND DISCUSSION**
- The autonomic nervous system is divided into three main categories:
  - Parasympathetic
  - Sympathetic
  - Enteric nervous system
- Parasympathetic nervous system (see Fig. 9.1)
  - Preganglionic neurons are located in the brain stem (e.g., dorsal motor nucleus of vagus nerve) and sacral parasympathetic nucleus at levels S2 through S4 spinal segments, and thus called "craniosacral outflow."
  - Second-order neurons are located at or near target organs (e.g., cardiac or bladder wall).
  - Neurotransmitters: acetylcholine (ACh) for preganglionic AND postganglionic neurons (binding to muscarinic receptors at target organs) (Fig. 2.11)
- Sympathetic nervous system (see Fig. 9.1)
  - Preganglionic neurons are located in the lateral gray horns at spinal levels T1 through L3, and thus called "thoracolumbar outflow."
  - Second-order neurons are usually located far from target organs (e.g., in cervical ganglia or adrenal glands)
  - Neurotransmitters: ACh for preganglionic neurons, and mostly norepinephrine (NE) for postganglionic neurons (binding to adrenergic receptors at target organs) (Fig. 2.11)
    - Exception: postganglionic parasympathetic neurons to the sweat glands use ACh as a neurotransmitter, which then binds to muscarinic receptors at sweat glands.

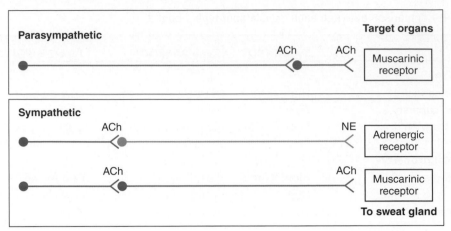

**Fig. 2.11** Pre-/post-synaptic nerve fibers and neurotransmitters in parasympathetic and sympathetic systems.

## SUGGESTED READINGS

Bate-Smith EC, Bendall JR. Rigor mortis and adenosine-triphosphate. *J Physiol.* 1947;106(2):177-185.

Boron WF, Boulpaep EL. *Medical Physiology: A Cellular and Molecular Approach.* Updated 3rd ed. Elsevier; 2016.

Hall JE. *Guyton and Hall Textbook of Medical Physiology.* 13th ed. Elsevier; 2016.

Palfreyman MT, Jorgensen EM. Chapter 3: roles of SNARE proteins in synaptic vesicle fusion. In: Wang Z, ed. *Molecular Mechanism of Neurotransmitter Release.* Humana Press; 2008.

Preston DC, Shapiro BE. *Electromyography and Neuromuscular Disorders: Clinical-electrophysiologic-ultrasound Correlations.* 4th ed. Elsevier; 2021.

Sleigh JN, Rossor AM, Fellows AD, et al. Axonal transport and neurological disease. *Nat Rev Neurol.* 2019;15:691-703.

Dubowitz V, Sewry CA, Oldfors A. *Muscle Biopsy: A Practical Approach.* 5th ed. Elsevier; 2021.

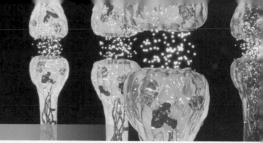

# CHAPTER 3

# Electrodiagnostic Medicine I: Nerve Conduction Studies

## PART 1 | PRACTICE TEST

**Q1.** Which type of nerve fibers are recorded on routine nerve conduction studies (NCSs)?
A. Large myelinated fibers
B. Unmyelinated fibers
C. Type B fibers
D. Type C fibers
E. All fiber types

**Q2.** Which of the following statements is **TRUE**?
A. Only signals from the active recording electrode (G1) are amplified.
B. Current from the reference electrode (G2) is added to the active electrode (G1) before being amplified.
C. The signal of interest is magnified from differential amplification.
D. High electrode impedance is recommended for nerve conduction studies (NCSs).
E. Common mode rejection results in poor resolution of the signal of interest.

**Q3.** Which statement is **TRUE** regarding a needle electrode for near-nerve stimulation, compared to a surface electrode?
A. Lower cost
B. More stimulus artifact
C. More stimulating current required
D. More stimulus spread
E. Able to access nerves in deeper locations

**Q4.** Which is **TRUE** of motor nerve conduction studies?
A. Muscle-belly montage is used.
B. Supramaximal stimulation is necessary only at the distal stimulation site.
C. Amplitudes are typically in the μV (microvolt) range.
D. Conduction velocity can be calculated by using the data from one stimulation site.
E. Motor studies are more affected by electrical noise than sensory studies.

**Q5.** Which is **TRUE** regarding sensory nerve conduction studies?
A. They typically require higher stimulation currents than motor studies.
B. The orthodromic method results in higher amplitude responses than the antidromic method.
C. Amplitudes are typically in the μV (microvolt) range.
D. Conduction velocity can be calculated only from two stimulation sites.
E. The high-frequency filter is typically set higher than the one for motor studies.

**Q6.** An electromyography (EMG) equipment converts biological data to digital waveforms. An adequate sampling frequency is required to avoid:
A. common-mode rejection.
B. high signal-to-noise ratio.
C. stimulus artifact.
D. aliasing.
E. collision.

**Q7.** When a median motor conduction study is performed, the waveform at the proximal stimulation appears to have a higher amplitude than the one at the distal stimulation site. Which of the following is most likely?
A. Cold temperature
B. Co-stimulation at the proximal site
C. Co-stimulation at the distal site
D. Conduction block
E. Temporal dispersion

**Q8.** Which statement is **CORRECT** regarding onset and peak latencies?
A. Both are standard measurements for compound muscle action potentials (CMAPs) and sensory nerve action potentials (SNAPs).
B. Marking for onset latency is more precise than peak latency for sensory studies.
C. Peak latency reflects the fastest sensory fibers.
D. Onset latency is used for calculation of nerve conduction velocity.
E. Peak latency is often obscured by electrical noise.

**Q9.** You observe your technologist performing an ulnar motor study and note that he/she places the cathode of the stimulator proximal to an anode. What would you expect from the recording?
A. Unable to get a response at all
B. Increased amplitude
C. Prolonged latency
D. Increased duration
E. Slowed motor conduction velocity

**Q10.** When performing a median sensory study recording the index finger by using the antidromic technique, ring electrodes are placed with a separation between G1 and G2 of 2 cm instead of 4 cm. Which of the following findings would be expected?
A. Shorter distal latency from shorter separation
B. Longer distal latency from subtracting out more of the G2 recording
C. Smaller amplitude from subtracting out more of the G2 recording
D. Higher amplitude due to summation of the G1 and G2 signals
E. No difference between 2-cm or 4-cm separation of G1 and G2 electrodes

**Q11.** Which of the following electrodiagnostic findings is **NOT** a principal feature of demyelination on motor nerve conduction studies?
A. Prolonged distal latency
B. Reduced amplitude
C. Slowed conduction velocity
D. Conduction block
E. Temporal dispersion

**Q12.** After a complete peroneal nerve transection at the fibular neck, a nerve conduction study is performed 4 days after the injury. Which of the following findings is expected?
A. Both the compound muscle action potential (CMAP) and sensory nerve action potential (SNAP) are absent.
B. Only the CMAP is absent but the SNAP is preserved.
C. Only the SNAP is absent but the CMAP is preserved.
D. CMAP amplitude is reduced but the SNAP is normal.
E. SNAP amplitude is slightly reduced but the CMAP is normal.

**Q13.** A 34-year-old woman is referred to an electromyography (EMG) lab for evaluation of numbness and pain in the right hand in the morning. A median sensory study stimulating at the wrist (WR), antecubital fossa (AF), and the axilla (AX) is recorded and shown in the figure. Which statement is **CORRECT** regarding the findings in this patient?
A. This study demonstrates normal temporal dispersion as commonly seen in sensory studies.
B. On the distal stimulation, the high amplitude is due to muscle artifact.
C. Smaller responses at proximal stimulation sites are suggestive of cold temperature.
D. Conduction block from focal demyelination is present in this sensory study.
E. There is a change in the waveform morphology, consistent with pathological temporal dispersion.

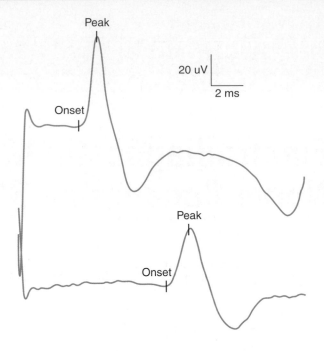

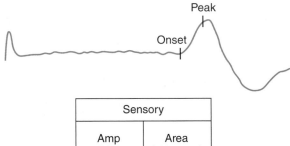

| Sensory | | |
|---|---|---|
| | Amp (uV) | Area (uV × ms) |
| WR | 36.2 | 10.9 |
| AF | 27.5 | 8.5 |
| AX | 13 | 4.7 |

From Preston DC, Shapiro BE. *Electromyography and Neuromuscular Disorders: Clinical-electrophysiologic-ultrasound Correlations.* 4th ed. Elsevier; 2021.

**Q14.** A nerve conduction study is performed in a patient with a hand temperature of 29°C. A compound muscle action potential (CMAP) from median nerve stimulation at the wrist shows an amplitude of 6 mV, a distal latency of 4.6 ms, and a proximal conduction velocity of 46 m/s. Since the desired temperature is 32°C, which statement is **CORRECT**?
A. She has median neuropathy at the wrist.
B. The measurements need to be adjusted for height.
C. The amplitude adjusted for the temperature is 9 mV.
D. The distal latency adjusted for the temperature is 5.2 ms.
E. The conduction velocity adjusted for the temperature is 52 m/s.

**Q15.** While performing a nerve conduction study you observe this waveform on the monitor. Which of the following is **LEAST** useful in troubleshooting this problem?

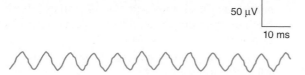

From Preston DC, Shapiro BE. *Electromyography and Neuromuscular Disorders: Clinical-electrophysiologic-ultrasound Correlations.* 4th ed. Elsevier; 2021.

   A. Checking that all electrodes and wires are intact
   B. Using a coaxial cable
   C. Proper skin preparation with alcohol
   D. Securing G1 and G2 firmly to skin
   E. Removing ground electrode, as only G2 (reference electrode) is needed

**Q16.** Which of the following is the consequence of changing the low-frequency filter from 10 Hz to 1 Hz?
   A. Shortened latency
   B. Decreased amplitude
   C. Increased amplitude
   D. Decreased duration
   E. Increased duration

**Q17.** Waveform A is a normal baseline waveform. Which situation can change waveform A to waveform B?

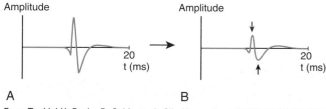

From Tankisi H, Burke D, Cui L, et al. *Clin Neurophysiol.* 2020;131(1):243-258.

   A. Cooling the recording limb
   B. Changing to antidromic technique
   C. Lowering the low frequency filter
   D. Lowering the high-frequency filter
   E. Reducing the impedance mismatch

**Q18.** Which statement is **CORRECT** regarding this sensory recording?

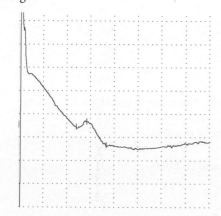

   A. Supramaximal stimulation is not achieved.
   B. The ground is placed between G1 and the stimulator.
   C. There is volume conduction artifact from the stimulator.
   D. The baseline contains high-frequency noise.
   E. The low-frequency filter is too low.

**Q19.** Which of the following is **FALSE** regarding the very proximal stimulation such as at Erb's point?
   A. It requires high current intensity for stimulation.
   B. Co-stimulation is common.
   C. Conduction velocity between axilla and Erb's point is as accurate as at more distal sites.
   D. Waveform morphology may be different than that of distal stimulation.
   E. It may be difficult to obtain supramaximal in obese subjects.

**Q20.** Which statement is **CORRECT** regarding the Martin-Gruber anastomosis (MGA)?
   A. It is a form of median neuropathy at the wrist.
   B. In MGA, the ulnar nerve gives a branch supplying a median innervated muscle (e.g., abductor pollicis brevis).
   C. The most common innervated muscle in an MGA is the flexor carpi ulnaris.
   D. The first dorsal interossei may receive fibers from the radial nerve.
   E. MGA needs to be considered when encountering a conduction block pattern of the ulnar nerve in the forearm segment.

**Q21.** When performing a peroneal (fibular) motor study recording the extensor digitorum brevis (EDB) muscle, you observe larger responses from stimulation below the fibular head and at the popliteal fossa, compared to the one obtained from stimulation at the ankle, as shown in the following figure. What is the next best action?

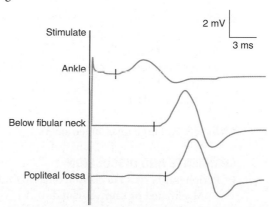

From Preston DC, Shapiro BE. *Electromyography and Neuromuscular Disorders: Clinical-electrophysiologic-ultrasound Correlations.* 4th ed. Elsevier; 2021.

   A. Warm the knee and restimulate.
   B. Increase the current intensity below the fibular head and at the popliteal fossa.
   C. Decrease the current intensity at the ankle.
   D. Record an additional response by stimulating behind the lateral malleolus and recording the EDB.
   E. Try to perform peroneal motor study recording the tibialis anterior (TA) instead.

**Q22.** Which of the following electrodiagnostic findings is seen in a patient who has both a median neuropathy at the wrist and a Martin-Gruber anastomosis (MGA)?
A. Motor response with an initially positive dip when stimulating at the wrist
B. Factitiously fast conduction velocity at the forearm segment
C. Normal distal latency but slowed proximal conduction velocity
D. Prolonged distal latency and slowed proximal conduction velocity
E. Conduction block between the wrist and antecubital fossa

**Q23.** Which of the following is consistent with a Riche-Cannieu anastomosis?
A. Reversed Martin-Gruber anastomosis
B. Communication between median and radial nerves in the palm
C. All-median hand
D. All-ulnar hand
E. All-radial hand

**Q24.** When performing an ulnar motor study, the amplitude at the wrist is much higher than that when stimulating the below-elbow site. Which of the following can result in this pattern?
A. Co-stimulation at the wrist
B. Submaximal stimulation at the below-elbow site
C. Martin-Gruber anastomosis
D. Conduction block in the forearm
E. All of the above

**Q25.** Which is **TRUE** regarding physiologic factors that can affect nerve conduction studies?
A. Increased height is associated with faster nerves.
B. Cold limb temperatures are associated with small-amplitude sensory nerve action potentials (SNAPs).
C. Limb position does not influence calculated conduction velocities.
D. Age can affect both amplitude and conduction velocity.
E. All of the above.

**Q26.** Which is **TRUE** regarding motor and sensory nerve conduction studies after a nerve injury?
A. The most common pattern seen is axonal loss.
B. Demyelination is more prominent in lower extremity nerves.
C. Motor nerves are preferentially affected.
D. Demyelination is always present if the conduction velocity is lower than the lower limit of normal.
E. All of the above.

---

## PART 2 | QUESTIONS WITH ANSWERS AND DISCUSSION

**QUESTION 1.** Which type of nerve fibers are recorded on routine nerve conduction studies (NCSs)?
A. Large myelinated fibers
B. Unmyelinated fibers
C. Type B fibers
D. Type C fibers
E. All fiber types

**ANSWER:** A. Large myelinated fibers

**COMMENTS AND DISCUSSION**
- Peripheral nerves are classified based on the following attributes:
  - Myelinated or unmyelinated
  - Somatic or autonomic
  - Motor (efferent) or sensory (afferent)
  - Diameter
- Direct relationship between fiber diameter and conduction velocity: the larger the diameter, the faster the conduction velocity.
- *Only the large, myelinated fibers are measured in clinical NCSs.* These fibers are:
  - Somatic motor efferents to muscle (A fibers)
  - Muscle afferents from muscle spindles and Golgi tendons (Ia and Ib fibers)
    - These fibers are recorded only during mixed NCSs
  - Cutaneous afferents from skin and hair (Aβ fibers)

- *Small myelinated (Aδ, B) and unmyelinated (C) fibers are not recorded with standard nerve conduction techniques.* These fibers include:
  - Preganglionic autonomic efferents (B fibers)
  - Postganglionic autonomic efferents (C fibers)
  - Somatic pain and temperature sensations (Aδ and C fibers)

**QUESTION 2.** Which of the following statements is **TRUE**?
  A. Only signals from the active recording electrode (G1) are amplified.
  B. Current from the reference electrode (G2) is added to the active electrode (G1) before being amplified.
  C. The signal of interest is magnified from differential amplification.
  D. High electrode impedance is recommended for nerve conduction studies (NCSs).
  E. Common mode rejection results in poor resolution of the signal of interest.

**ANSWER:** C. The signal of interest is magnified from differential amplification.

**COMMENTS AND DISCUSSION**
- All electrodiagnostic data are derived from waveforms recording a potential difference (i.e., voltage difference) between two electrodes.
- Recording electrodes
  - Active electrode, black in color (known as G1)
  - Reference electrode, red in color (known as G2) (The "G" is derived from "Grid," when electrodes were formerly attached to different grids in an oscilloscope)
  - Ground, green in color, used to suppress stray electrical noise
- Amplification
  - Biological signals range from microvolts ($\mu$V) to millivolts (mV)
  - Biological signals needed to be amplified prior to analysis
  - Differential amplification
    - Two identical amplifiers are used; the first amplifier receives the signal from the active electrode (G1) and the second amplifier receives an inverted signal from the reference electrode (G2).
    - Amplified signals from two amplifiers are summated (G1+(−G2)), which is called *difference-mode signal.*
    - In contrast, when the same signal is present on both electrodes, these potentials cancel each other out, known as *common-mode rejection.*
    - The active electrode carries a signal of interest but also electrical noise. If the reference electrode carries similar electrical noise, the electrical noise will be subtracted out by differential amplification, leaving the signal of interest.
    - Differential amplification improves the signal-to-noise ratio as electrical noise is cancelled out and only the signal of interest remains.
  - Input impedance
    - Recording electrode impedance must be very low to prevent the loss of signal between its source and the amplifier.
    - However, the amplifier impedance must be very high so that the signal remains unchanged at the amplifier input.

**QUESTION 3.** Which statement is **TRUE** regarding a needle electrode for near-nerve stimulation, compared to a surface electrode?
  A. Lower cost
  B. More stimulus artifact
  C. More stimulating current required
  D. More stimulus spread
  E. Able to access nerves in deeper locations

**ANSWER:** E. Able to access nerves in deeper locations

**COMMENTS AND DISCUSSION**

- Near-nerve stimulation using a monopolar needle as the cathode and a surface recording as the anode can be used on some occasions.
- Because near-nerve stimulation is placed closer to the nerve, less current is used.
- There is less stimulus artifact and less stimulus spreading compared to surface stimulation.
- Because a needle is used, the cost is higher than surface stimulation.
- Needle stimulation can access nerves in deeper locations that surface stimulators cannot reach (e.g., nerve roots).
- Likewise, needles can be used as recording electrodes in place of surface electrodes, with similar advantages and disadvantages.

**QUESTION 4.** Which is **TRUE** of motor nerve conduction studies?
    A. Muscle-belly montage is used.
    B. Supramaximal stimulation is necessary only at the distal stimulation site.
    C. Amplitudes are typically in the μV (microvolt) range.
    D. Conduction velocity can be calculated by using the data from one stimulation site.
    E. Motor studies are more affected by electrical noise than sensory studies.

**ANSWER:** A. Muscle-belly montage is used.

**COMMENTS AND DISCUSSION**

- Nerve is depolarized under the stimulator resulting in an action potential that runs down the nerve to the neuromuscular junction (NMJ). The electrical signal is then converted to the chemical signal crossing the NMJ resulting in depolarization of multiple muscle fibers and muscle fiber action potentials (Fig. 3.1).
- The recording electrodes are placed by using the belly-tendon montage technique (Fig. 3.2).
- CMAP (compound muscle action potential):
  - Summation of all underlying single muscle fiber action potentials
  - Typically, a biphasic potential with an initial negativity
  - The CMAP distal latency reflects the conduction time of the motor nerve from the stimulator to the NMJ, time across the NMJ, and then muscle fiber depolarization time.

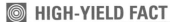 **HIGH-YIELD FACT**

If CMAP appears with an initial positivity or downward deflection, it means either
1. G1 is **NOT** placed over the belly (i.e., motor point) of the tested muscle **OR**
2. there are additional responses from adjacent muscles (**co-stimulation**).

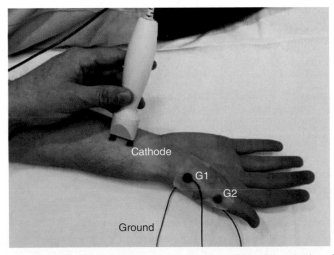

**Fig. 3.1** Motor nerve conduction study. The depolarization occurs under the cathode of the stimulator. The cathode should be facing the active recording electrode (G1). From Preston DC, Shapiro BE. Electromyography and Neuromuscular Disorders: Clinical-electrophysiologic-ultrasound Correlations. 4th ed. Elsevier; 2021;3:24.

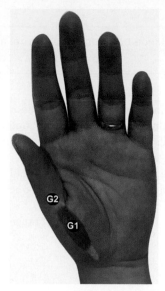

**Fig. 3.2** Belly-tendon technique for motor studies. The figure illustrates the recording electrode (G1), which is placed over the muscle belly, and the reference electrode (G2), which is placed over the tendon. This "belly-tendon" montage is used for motor studies.

- Amplitudes of motor responses are usually in the range of millivolts (mV).
- Less affected by artifacts and electrical noise due to larger responses (mV), as opposed to sensory and mixed responses (μV)
- Onset latency is measured for CMAP.
- Motor conduction velocity (Fig. 3.1)
  - Stimulation of two sites along a nerve is needed to calculate a conduction velocity across this nerve segment. This method would eliminate the distal nerve conduction time, the NMJ time, and the muscle fiber depolarization time.
  - Conduction velocity is calculated by measuring the distance between proximal and distal sites, and dividing it by the difference between the proximal and distal latencies (Fig. 3.3).
  - It is essential that supramaximal stimulation is achieved at all sites to ensure that all fibers, including the fastest fibers, have been stimulated.

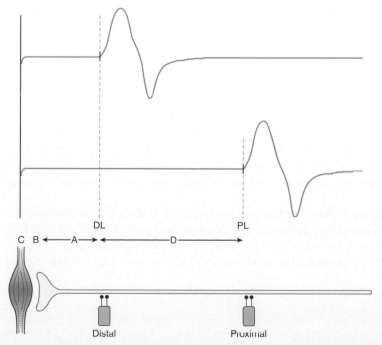

**Fig. 3.3** Conduction velocity (CV). CV represents speed of depolarization along the motor nerve but only in the segment between the proximal and distal stimulating sites. The formula for calculation is shown below. From Preston DC, Shapiro BE. *Electromyography and Neuromuscular Disorders: Clinical-electrophysiologic-ultrasound Correlations.* 4th ed. Elsevier; 2021;3:25.

## ◎ HIGH-YIELD FACT

$$\text{Conduction velocity} = \frac{\text{Distance between the proximal and distal stimulation site}}{\text{Proximal latency} - \text{distal latency}}$$

**QUESTION 5.** Which is **TRUE** regarding sensory nerve conduction studies?
  A. They typically require higher stimulation currents than motor studies.
  B. The orthodromic method results in higher amplitude responses than the antidromic method.
  C. Amplitudes are typically in the μV (microvolt) range.
  D. Conduction velocity can be calculated only from two stimulation sites.
  E. The high-frequency filter is typically set higher than the one for motor studies.

**ANSWER:** C. Amplitudes are typically in the μV (microvolt) range.

## COMMENTS AND DISCUSSION

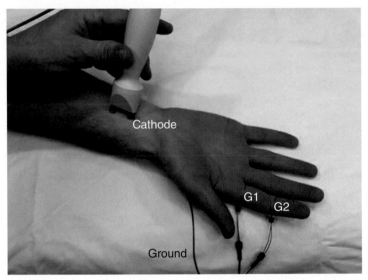

**Fig. 3.4** Sensory nerve conduction study. The depolarization occurs under the cathode of the stimulator. The cathode should be facing the active recording electrode (G1). G1 and G2 should be 2.5 to 4 cm apart, which prevents simultaneous depolarization of the nerve under both electrodes and reducing the amplitude of the response. From Preston DC, Shapiro BE. *Electromyography and Neuromuscular Disorders: Clinical-electrophysiologic-ultrasound Correlations.* 4th ed. Elsevier; 2021;3:26.

- Sensory nerve conduction studies require lower stimulation threshold compared to motor studies.
- Sensory conduction velocity can be calculated with one stimulation site, as there is no need for subtraction of neuromuscular junction (NMJ) and muscle conduction time, in contrast to motor nerve conduction studies.
- SNAP can be either biphasic or triphasic, and typically in the μV (microvolt) range.
- Because SNAPs have short durations, they are composed predominantly of high frequencies, which can more easily be obscured by high-frequency noises. Thus the high-frequency filter setting is typically lower for sensory as compared to motor studies (2 kHz versus 10 kHz, respectively) (Table 3.1).

**TABLE 3.1** Typical filter settings for motor and sensory conduction studies

| Conduction study | Low-frequency filter setting | High-frequency filter setting |
|---|---|---|
| Motor | 10 Hz | 10 kHz |
| Sensory | 20 Hz | 2 kHz |

## ◎ HIGH-YIELD FACT

Reduced low-frequency filter → Increased duration of the potentials
Reduced high frequency filter → Reduced amplitude of the potentials

- Two techniques can be used for sensory studies: orthodromic and antidromic (Table 3.2)
  - Orthodromic recording obtains sensory potentials that conduct in the physiologic direction from distal to proximal.
    - Recording electrodes are placed proximally over the nerve; stimulating electrodes are placed distally over the nerve.
    - In orthodromic recording, it may be challenging to obtain abnormal small sensory responses.
    - This recording technique is performed primarily for median and ulnar sensory nerve potentials.
  - Antidromic technique is the reverse of orthodromic.
    - Recording electrodes are placed distally over the nerve (e.g., ring electrodes on the fingers); stimulator is placed over the proximal nerve (Fig. 3.4).

**TABLE 3.2** Orthodromic versus antidromic sensory studies

| Orthodromic | Antidromic |
|---|---|
| Same direction as physiologic conduction | Opposite direction to physiologic conduction |
| Stimulate only sensory nerve/fibers | Depending on the nerve, stimulation may occur for motor in addition to sensory fibers |
| Response unlikely to be contaminated from nearby volume conduction potentials | Higher likelihood of response to be contaminated by nearby volume conduction potentials from muscle |
| Recording through more tissue (e.g., at wrist) results in some attenuation of the signal | Recording closer to the nerve (e.g., at finger) results in less attenuation of the signal |
| Smaller amplitude | Larger amplitude |
| May be more painful to stimulate | Easier to stimulate |
| More subject to noise and artifacts due to smaller sesnory nerve action potnetial (SNAP) | Subject to muscle artifacts due to co-stimulation of motor fibers |
| More difficult to mark latency due to smaller SNAP | Easier to mark latency due to larger SNAP |

**QUESTION 6.** An electromyography (EMG) equipment converts biological data to digital waveforms. An adequate sampling frequency is required to avoid:
  A. common-mode rejection.
  B. high signal-to-noise ratio.
  C. stimulus artifact.
  D. aliasing.
  E. collision.

**ANSWER:** D. aliasing.

### COMMENTS AND DISCUSSION
- The EMG machine needs to convert analog biological signals to digital data.
- The sampling rate must be adequate to avoid error.
- Aliasing is an error resulting when the sampling frequency is less than twice the highest frequency of the signal of interest (Fig. 3.5).

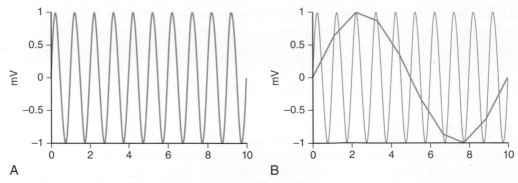

**Fig. 3.5 Aliasing.** Aliasing occurs when the sampling frequency is lower than twice the highest frequency of the signal of interest. In panel A, the signal of interest has frequency of 1 Hz. However, in panel B, the sampling of that waveform is set frequency of 0.9 Hz. The output signal does not correctly reproduce the original signal. Indeed, the output waveform has an apparent frequency of 0.1 Hz. This effect caused by insufficient sampling is called "Aliasing." From Tankisi H, Burke D, Cui L, et al. Standards of instrumentation of EMG. Clin Neurophysiol. 2020 Jan;131(1):243-258.

- Common mode rejection refers to the use of a differential amplifier that rejects common electrical noise between recording and reference electrodes, leaving only the signal of interest. This results in an improved signal-to-noise ratio.
- Stimulus artifact is caused by volume conduction from the stimulator through tissue, which is then picked up by the recording electrodes.
- Collision is an advanced technique using two stimulators to eliminate unavoidable co-stimulation of a nearby nerve. For example, when stimulating the median nerve in the axilla, it is not possible to avoid co-stimulating the ulnar nerve. Collision can eliminate the ulnar nerve response in this case.

### 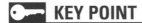 KEY POINT

**To Avoid Aliasing**
Minimum sampling frequency of a waveform must be at least twice the highest frequency component in the waveform. This is known as the Nyquist sampling theorem.

**QUESTION 7.** When a median motor conduction study is performed, the waveform at the proximal stimulation appears to have a higher amplitude than the one at the distal stimulation site. Which of the following is most likely?
A. Cold temperature
B. Co-stimulation at the proximal site
C. Co-stimulation at the distal site
D. Conduction block
E. Temporal dispersion

**ANSWER:** B. Co-stimulation at the proximal site

### COMMENTS AND DISCUSSION
- Waveforms recorded from a distal stimulation normally have the same or slightly larger amplitude than those recorded from proximal stimulation sites.
- For proximal stimulation sites, longer distances result in more physiologic temporal dispersion and phase cancellation, and thus similar or slightly decreased amplitudes compared to the distal stimulation (Fig. 3.6)
  - Nerve fibers in normal peripheral nerve have a range of conduction velocities. Some conduct faster, others are slower, and most are in the middle. As a result, responses from individual nerve fibers arrive at their destination at slightly different times. This results in normal *temporal dispersion*.
  - The conduction distances along faster nerve fibers separate more from those along slower fibers when travelling through longer distances. Thus normal temporal dispersion occurs in both compound muscle action potential (CMAP) and sensory nerve action potential (SNAP) when proximal sites are stimulated.

- However, normal temporal dispersion is more prominent for SNAPs than CMAPs, as individual sensory fiber action potentials have much shorter unit durations than those of muscle fiber action potentials (1–2 ms versus 5–6 ms). Thus temporal dispersion of 1 ms results in sensory fiber action potentials being much more out of phase than muscle fiber action potentials. If negative and positive phases overlap, *phase cancellation* occurs (Fig. 3.6).

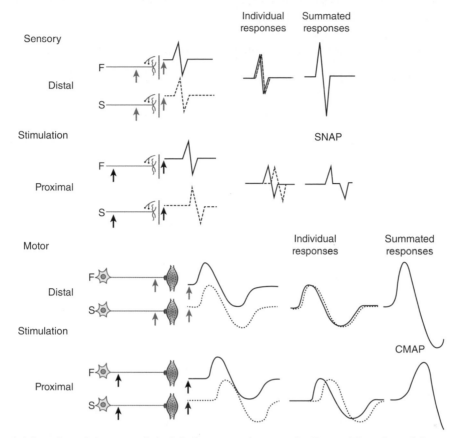

**Fig. 3.6** Temporal dispersion and phase cancellation in both sensory and motor studies. Temporal dispersion and phase cancellation are normal physiologic factors seen in both motor and sensory waveforms, which are more pronounced by longer distances. Sensory nerve action potentials (SNAPs) have more phase cancellation, since the responses are much shorter. In contrast, compound muscle action potentials (CMAPs) have less phase cancellation as the same amount of temporal dispersion results in much less overlap of positive and negative phases. From Preston DC, Shapiro BE. *Electromyography and Neuromuscular Disorders: Clinical-electrophysiologic-ultrasound Correlations.* 4th ed. Elsevier; 2021;3:31. From Kimura J, Machida M, Ishida T, et al. Relationship between size of compound sensory or muscle action potentials, and length of nerve segment. *Neurology* 1986;36:647, with permission of Little, Brown and Company.

- Temporal dispersion and phase cancellation results in reduction of the amplitude.
- In the case of a higher amplitude from proximal stimulation, the most common cause is a technical error from co-stimulation proximally: the stimulation at the proximal site is too strong, causing co-stimulation through adjacent soft tissues to nearby nerves. The recorded waveform would contain the signal of interest plus additional signals from nearby muscles that are depolarized from the co-stimulated nerves.
- Co-stimulation at the distal site would evoke a higher distal CMAP amplitude. This would not result in a higher proximal CMAP amplitude.
- Cold temperature:
  - Results in delayed inactivation of sodium channels and a longer depolarization time.
  - The longer depolarization time results in a slower conduction velocity.
  - As more sodium moves into cells, amplitudes are also larger and durations are longer.
  - Effects from cold temperature usually occur more prominently in distal sites, since proximal sites are closer to the body core.

## ◎ HIGH-YIELD FACT

For every 1°C drop in temperature → CV slows by 1 m/s
→ DL prolongs by 0.2 ms

**QUESTION 8.** Which statement is **CORRECT** regarding onset and peak latencies?
- A. Both are standard measurements for compound muscle action potentials (CMAPs) and sensory nerve action potentials (SNAPs).
- B. Marking for onset latency is more precise than peak latency for sensory studies.
- C. Peak latency reflects the fastest sensory fibers.
- D. Onset latency is used for calculation of nerve conduction velocity.
- E. Peak latency is often obscured by electrical noise.

**ANSWER:** D. Onset latency is used for calculation of nerve conduction velocity.

### COMMENTS AND DISCUSSION

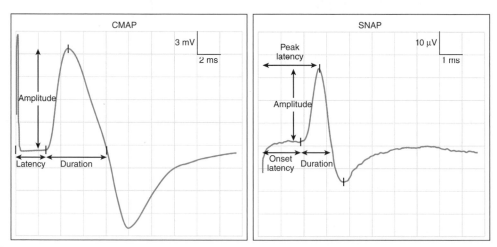

**Fig. 3.7** Standard measurements for motor and sensory waveforms. Compound muscle action potential (CMAP) waveform is biphasic, with an initial negativity when the G1 active electrode is correctly placed over the motor point. Parameters for CMAP include latency (only onset latency for CMAP), amplitude, duration, and area. Sensory nerve action potential (SNAP) waveforms can be either biphasic or triphasic. Parameters for SNAP include onset and peak latencies, amplitude, and duration. Amplitude and area reflect the number of muscle fibers (for motor studies) or nerve fibers (for sensory studies) that depolarize. Amplitude is conventionally used to assess the number of nerve fibers present. However, area may be more accurate for assessing conduction block of motor fibers. Distal latency reflects the conduction time of the fastest nerve fibers from the stimulation to the recording site. Duration reflects synchrony (time variation) between the fast and slow muscle or nerve fibers. Nerve conduction velocity reflects the speed of depolarization of the fastest axons. From Preston DC, Shapiro BE. *Electromyography and Neuromuscular Disorders: Clinical-electrophysiologic-ultrasound Correlations.* 4th ed. Elsevier; 2021;3:24.

- In sensory studies, SNAP latency can be measured by using either peak or onset latency (Fig. 3.7).
  - Peak latency
    - Advantages:
      - Excellent interrater reliability
      - Easy to perform
      - Minimal effect from electrical noise and technical factors
    - Disadvantages:
      - It cannot be used to calculate a conduction velocity.
      - A set distance must be used, as normal values are based on a set distance.
  - Onset latency
    - Measured as the time from the stimulus to the initial negative (upward) deflection for a biphasic waveform.
    - Measured as the time from the stimulus to the initial positive (downward) for a triphasic waveform.
    - Advantages:
      - Reflects the true fastest sensory fiber
      - Can be used to calculate a true conduction velocity
      - Does not require a set distance
    - Disadvantages:
      - More affected by technical factors, especially stimulus artifact and electrical noise
      - Unless there is an abrupt onset, poorer interrater reliability

- Smaller waveforms (e.g., orthodromic recordings) become even more difficult to measure accurately.
- May be more difficult to measure (Fig. 3.8)

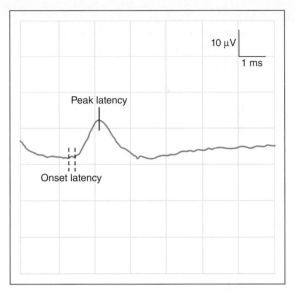

**Fig. 3.8** Marking for onset and peak latencies. Unless the onset deflection of the sensory nerve action potential (SNAP) is abrupt, it is difficult to precisely mark the onset latency. In contrast, the point for peak latency is easily marked with little inter-examiner variability. From Preston DC, Shapiro BE. *Electromyography and Neuromuscular Disorders: Clinical-electrophysiologic-ultrasound Correlations.* 4th ed. Elsevier; 2021;3:27.

**QUESTION 9.**   You observe your technologist performing an ulnar motor study and note that he/she places the cathode of the stimulator proximal to an anode. What would you expect from the recording?
  A. Unable to get a response at all
  B. Increased amplitude
  C. Prolonged latency
  D. Increased duration
  E. Slowed motor conduction velocity

**ANSWER:** C. Prolonged latency

**COMMENTS AND DISCUSSION**
- A standard nerve stimulator has two prongs: current flows from the cathode (source of negative charges) to the anode (positive)
- Depolarization occurs under the cathode
- Theoretically, if the anode is placed distally, anodal block occurs. Anodal block is a local block caused by membrane hyperpolarization under the anode, which then inhibits propagation of the action potential running from the cathode. However, this phenomenon is reported in animal studies only—not in humans.
- In clinical practice, there is a separation of the cathode and anode by 2–3 cm. The proximal cathode is still able to depolarize and induces propagation through the nerve. With the cathode and anode reversed, the distance between the cathode and recording electrodes is longer. Thus a measured distance of 10 cm is actually 12–13 cm. All latency measurements including distal latency are then slightly prolonged.

**QUESTION 10.** When performing a median sensory study recording the index finger by using the antidromic technique, ring electrodes are placed with a separation between G1 and G2 of 2 cm instead of 4 cm. Which of the following findings would be expected?
  A. Shorter distal latency from shorter separation
  B. Longer distal latency from subtracting out more of the G2 recording
  C. Smaller amplitude from subtracting out more of the G2 recording
  D. Higher amplitude due to summation of the G1 and G2 signals
  E. No difference between 2-cm or 4-cm separation of G1 and G2 electrodes

**ANSWER:** C. Smaller amplitude from subtracting out more of the G2 recording

## COMMENTS AND DISCUSSION

- Sensory nerve action potentials (SNAPs) are recorded from skin overlying the cutaneous sensory nerves.
- Inter-electrode distance should be 2.5 to 4 cm.
- This separation is to ensure that the peak of recording potential passes through the G1 electrode before the initial of the potential reaching G2 electrode. The reason is to avoid amplitude subtraction of potential from G2 from G1 electrode. There is no effect on latency. (Fig. 3.9)

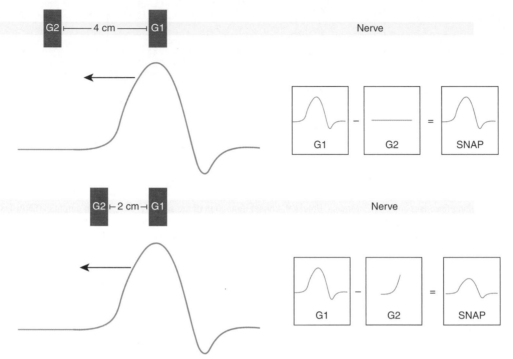

**Fig. 3.9** Significance of inter-electrode distance in sensory nerve studies. Upper trace shows recording electrode (G1) and reference electrode (G2) placed over the sensory nerve with an inter-electrode distance of 4 cm. The sensory potential travels from G1 to G2. When the negative peak of the potential passes G1, the initial deflection of the potential has not yet arrived at G2. Therefore, the subtracted sensory nerve action potential (SNAP) is equal or close to the true potential. The lower tracing shows G1 and G2 with an inter-electrode distance of 2 cm. When the potential negative peak has passed G1, the initial deflection of the potential has arrived at G2. Therefore, the subtracted SNAP has a smaller amplitude, compared to the upper tracing.

**QUESTION 11.** Which of the following electrodiagnostic findings is **NOT** a principal feature of demyelination on motor nerve conduction studies?
- A. Prolonged distal latency
- B. Reduced amplitude
- C. Slowed conduction velocity
- D. Conduction block
- E. Temporal dispersion

**ANSWER:** B. Reduced amplitude

## COMMENTS AND DISCUSSION

- The myelin sheath acts as an insulator, resulting in saltatory conduction along the nodes of Ranvier.
- Injuries to the myelin sheath (i.e., demyelination) lead to slow conduction, when if severe, result in conduction failure or block.
- Electrodiagnostic features of demyelination include primarily:
  - Prolonged distal latency (longer than 130% of the upper normal limit)
  - Slowed conduction velocity (slower than 75% of the lower normal limit)
  - Conduction block for conduction failure
  - Pathological temporal dispersion
- Reduction in amplitude most often reflects axonal loss. However, reduced amplitudes do occur in demyelination if conduction block is present, and if the stimulation is proximal to the block.

**QUESTION 12.** After a complete peroneal nerve transection at the fibular neck, a nerve conduction study is performed 4 days after the injury. Which of the following findings is expected?
- A. Both the compound muscle action potential (CMAP) and sensory nerve action potential (SNAP) are absent.
- B. Only the CMAP is absent but the SNAP is preserved.
- C. Only the SNAP is absent but the CMAP is preserved.
- D. CMAP amplitude is reduced but the SNAP is normal.
- E. SNAP amplitude is slightly reduced but the CMAP is normal.

**ANSWER:** D. CMAP amplitude is reduced but the SNAP is normal.

**COMMENTS AND DISCUSSION**
- After a complete nerve transection, Wallerian degeneration of the axons distal to the lesion ensues.
- CMAP and SNAP remain normal in the first 2 days.
- The CMAP amplitude begins to drop on day 3 due to first neuromuscular junction failure, and reaches the nadir around day 5–6.
- The SNAP amplitude begins to drop on day 5 (later than the CMAP) and reaches the nadir on day 10–11.
- In the case when the nerve conduction study is performed on day 4, CMAP amplitude already decreases but has not reached the nadir (reduced but not absent), whereas SNAP amplitude has not begun to decrease (still normal).

**QUESTION 13.** A 34-year-old woman is referred to an electromyography (EMG) lab for evaluation of numbness and pain in the right hand in the morning. A median sensory study stimulating at the wrist (WR), antecubital fossa (AF), and the axilla (AX) is recorded and shown in the figure. Which statement is **CORRECT** regarding the findings in this patient?

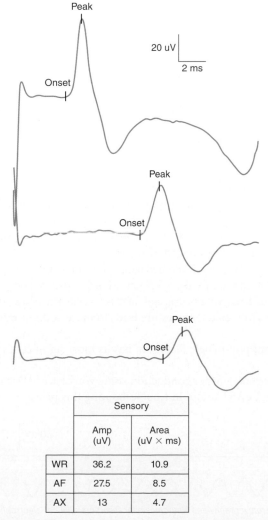

| | Sensory | |
| --- | --- | --- |
| | Amp (uV) | Area (uV × ms) |
| WR | 36.2 | 10.9 |
| AF | 27.5 | 8.5 |
| AX | 13 | 4.7 |

From Preston DC, Shapiro BE. *Electromyography and Neuromuscular Disorders: Clinical-electrophysiologic-ultrasound Correlations.* 4th ed. Elsevier; 2021;3:30.

A. This study demonstrates normal temporal dispersion as commonly seen in sensory studies.
B. On the distal stimulation, the high amplitude is due to muscle artifact.
C. Smaller responses at proximal stimulation sites are suggestive of cold temperature.
D. Conduction block from focal demyelination is present in this sensory study.
E. There is a change in the waveform morphology, consistent with pathological temporal dispersion.

**ANSWER:** A. This study demonstrates normal temporal dispersion as commonly seen in sensory studies.

## COMMENTS AND DISCUSSION
- When the proximal site is stimulated for sensory studies, the responses have longer durations with markedly reduced amplitudes and areas as compared to distal responses due to the combination of normal temporal dispersion and phase cancellation. This is a normal physiologic finding.
- Temporal dispersion and phase cancellation are also present in motor studies but are much less prominent. Larger amplitudes and longer durations of the compound muscle action potential (CMAP) result in less phase cancellation between responses from fast- and slow-conducting fibers.
- Cold temperature results in higher sensory nerve action potential (SNAP) amplitudes which are more evident with distal stimulation sites, as distal limbs are often cooler. Duration also prolongs with cooler temperature, which is not present in this study.
- Decrease of area at proximal stimulation, compared to distal stimulation, of more than 50% is diagnostic of a conduction block, which is a feature of focal demyelination. However, this criterion is only for motor studies. In sensory studies, physiologic temporal dispersion and phase cancellation are prominent in normal nerves. Thus, conduction block is typically not evaluated from sensory studies.
- In this figure, the change in waveform morphology proximally represents normal temporal dispersion.

**QUESTION 14.** A nerve conduction study is performed on a patient with a hand temperature of 29°C. A compound muscle action potential (CMAP) from median nerve stimulation at the wrist shows an amplitude of 6 mV, a distal latency of 4.6 ms, and a conduction velocity of 46 m/s. Since the desired temperature is 32°C, which statement is **CORRECT**?
A. She has median neuropathy at the wrist.
B. The measurements need to be adjusted for height.
C. The amplitude adjusted for the temperature is 9 mV.
D. The distal latency adjusted for the temperature is 5.2 ms.
E. The conduction velocity adjusted for the temperature is 52 m/s.

**ANSWER:** E. The conduction velocity adjusted for the temperature is 52 m/s.

## COMMENTS AND DISCUSSION
- Temperature is one of the most important physiological factors affecting nerve conduction study data.
- Cooler temperature results in delayed inactivation of sodium channels, and thus slow nerve conduction velocities.
- For every 1°C drop in temperature, conduction velocity (CV) decreases by 1.5–2.5 m/s (average is 2 m/s), and distal latency (DL) is prolonged by 0.2 ms.
- In this case, the temperature is 3°C from the desired temperature of 32°C. CV adjusted for the temperature is $(3 \times 2.0) + 46 = 52$ m/s. DL adjusted for the temperature is $4.6 - (0.2 \times 3) = 4.0$ m/s. Thus after adjustment for the temperature, the distal latency is normal, and there is no evidence of median neuropathy at the wrist.
- Prolonged depolarization from cold temperature leads to more sodium influx into cells, and higher amplitudes.
- Height is also an important physiologic factor but has its most significant impact on late responses.

**QUESTION 15.** While performing a nerve conduction study you observe this waveform on the monitor. Which of the following is **LEAST** useful in troubleshooting this problem?

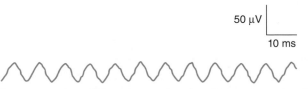

50 μV

10 ms

From Preston DC, Shapiro BE. *Electromyography and Neuromuscular Disorders: Clinical-electrophysiologic-ultrasound Correlations.* 4th ed. Elsevier; 2021;8:81.

A. Checking that all electrodes and wires are intact
B. Using a coaxial cable
C. Proper skin preparation with alcohol
D. Securing G1 and G2 firmly to skin
E. Removing ground electrode, as only G2 (reference electrode) is needed

**ANSWER:** E. Removing ground electrode as only G2 (reference electrode) is needed

## COMMENTS AND DISCUSSION

- This waveform demonstrates a 60-Hz artifact, which is a common non-physiologic artifact.
- 60-Hz interference is derived from lights, electric outlet, and heaters, among other sources of electrical noise.
- If there is impedance mismatch between G1 and G2, the electrical artifact will be different among the two electrodes and will not be subtracted out by a differential amplifier.
- To reduce and minimize 60-Hz artifact, impedance mismatch can be decreased by the following measures:
    - Ensuring all electrode and wires are intact
    - Using a coaxial cable
    - Proper skin preparation with alcohol
    - Using adequate electrode jelly or conducting cream
    - Securing G1 and G2 firmly to skin
    - Placing ground between the stimulator and G1
- G2 (aka. the reference electrode) and the ground are not the same. The ground has a lower potential and less resistance compared to G2. The ground can help remove any stray currents that result in electrical artifact.

**QUESTION 16.** Which of the following is the consequence of changing the low-frequency filter from 10 Hz to 1 Hz?
A. Shortened latency
B. Decreased amplitude
C. Increased amplitude
D. Decreased duration
E. Increased duration

**ANSWER:** E. Increased duration

## COMMENTS AND DISCUSSION

- Changing filter settings impacts waveforms.
- Filters aim to exclude unwanted signals with frequencies above (high-frequency filter) and below (low-frequency filter) their settings and leave the signal of interest relatively unchanged.
- However, filters also impact the signal of interest.
- If the low-frequency filter setting is reduced, more low-frequency waveforms will pass through. Therefore, the **duration** of the signal will be increased slightly. If the high-frequency filter setting is higher, more high-frequency signals will pass through. Therefore, the **amplitude** of the signal will slightly increase.

### MNEMONIC

- Think of "duration" as a "low-frequency" component and "amplitude" as a "high-frequency" component
- Thus more "low-frequency" component → increased duration and more "high-frequency" component → increased amplitude

**QUESTION 17.** Waveform A is a normal baseline waveform. Which situation can change waveform A to waveform B?

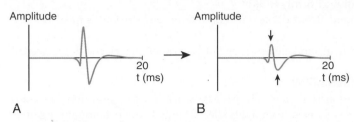

From Tankisi H, Burke D, Cui L, et al. *Clin Neurophysiol.* 2020 Jan;131(1):243-258.

A. Cooling the recording limb
B. Changing to antidromic technique
C. Lowering the low-frequency filter
D. Lowering the high-frequency filter
E. Reducing the impedance mismatch

**ANSWER:** D. Lowering the high-frequency filter

## COMMENTS AND DISCUSSION

- Waveform B has a lower amplitude signal compared to waveform A. This is the consequence of reducing the high-frequency filter (Fig. 3.10).
- When the high-frequency filter is lowered, less high-frequency waveforms will pass through. Therefore, the amplitude of the signal will be reduced.

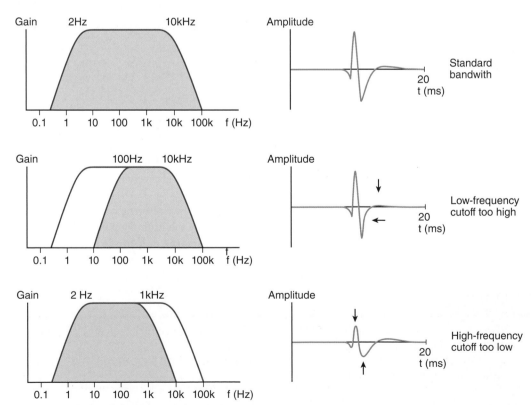

**Fig. 3.10** Changing filter parameters affects the waveform. The upper panel represents a usual standard waveform when applying typical low- and high-frequency filter settings. In the middle panel, when the low-frequency filter is higher (increased), more low-frequency waveforms are filtered, which results in decreased duration of the waveform. In the lower panel, the high-frequency filter is lowered, high-frequency waveforms are filtered out, which results in decreased amplitude of the waveform. C. Bischoff, A. Fuglsang-Fredriksen, L. Vendelbo, A. Sumner Standards of instrumentation of EMG. The international federation of clinical neurophysiology Electroencephalogr *Clin Neurophysiol Suppl,* 52 (1999), pp. 199-211.

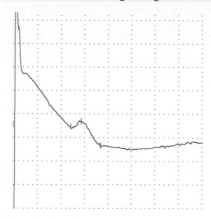

A. Supramaximal stimulation is not achieved.
B. The ground is placed between G1 and the stimulator.
C. There is volume conduction artifact from the stimulator.
D. The baseline contains high-frequency noise.
E. The low-frequency filter is too low.

**ANSWER:** C. There is volume conduction artifact from the stimulator.

## COMMENTS AND DISCUSSION

- The baseline of this tracing is not flat, obscuring the true onset latency of this sensory nerve action potential (SNAP), causing a falsely delayed distal latency.
- This baseline artifact results from stimulus artifact where a volume conducted potential from the stimulator is transmitted through tissue to the recording electrode.
- Stimulus artifact can interfere with take-off point amplitude, and other measurements, especially for sensory potentials.
- To reduce stimulus artifact:
  - Increase the distance between the stimulator and recording electrodes if possible.
  - Ensure the stimulator is optimally placed over the nerve so less stimulus intensity is needed to obtain supramaximal stimulation.
  - Place the ground between the stimulator and G1.
  - Use a coaxial cable.
  - Rotate the anode slightly while keeping the cathode position unchanged. For example (Fig. 3.11), the black waveform with the flat initial baseline was obtained by rotating the anode, compared to the original waveform (in gray).

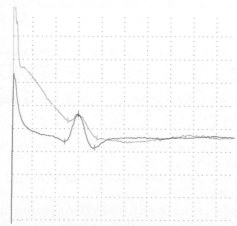

**Fig. 3.11** Stimulus artifact can affect the baseline of the recording potentials (potential in gray), resulting in falsely delayed distal latency. To reduce the artifact, moving the anode around while fixing the cathode can improve the baseline (potential in blue).

- If low-frequency filter is lowered, the duration of the waveform will be increased but will not create this type of artifact.

**QUESTION 19.** Which of the following is **FALSE** regarding the very proximal stimulation such as at Erb's point?
   A. It requires high current intensity for stimulation.
   B. Co-stimulation is common.
   C. Conduction velocity between axilla and Erb's point is as accurate as at more distal sites.
   D. Waveform morphology may be different than that of distal stimulation.
   E. It may be difficult to obtain supramaximal in obese subjects.

**ANSWER:** C. Conduction velocity between axilla and Erb's point is as accurate as more distal sites.

**COMMENTS AND DISCUSSION**
- Nerve conduction studies are routinely performed in the distal parts of the body, since nerves are more superficial and can easily be stimulated.
- Stimulation at very proximal sites such as the axilla or Erb's point can be technically challenging due to the following:
  - Due to the deep location, it can be difficult to obtain supramaximal stimulation, especially in obese subjects.
  - Much higher current intensity is needed to be able to stimulate nerves, which may cause more discomfort and pain.
  - At proximal sites, nerves from the plexus or multiple nerves run close to each other. This almost always results in co-stimulation. Waveform morphology is useful to help determine if co-stimulation has occurred. With co-stimulation, the morphology would be different from those waveforms from more distal stimulation of the studied nerve.
  - The distance measurement can be inaccurate due to the anatomy, which can affect the conduction velocity calculation. Thus conduction velocity at these proximal sites may be less accurate.

**QUESTION 20.** Which statement is **CORRECT** regarding the Martin-Gruber anastomosis (MGA)?
   A. It is a form of median neuropathy at the wrist.
   B. In MGA, the ulnar nerve gives a branch supplying a median innervated muscle (e.g., abductor pollicis brevis).
   C. The most common innervated muscle in an MGA is the flexor carpi ulnaris.
   D. The first dorsal interossei may receive fibers from the radial nerve.
   E. MGA needs to be considered when encountering a conduction block pattern of the ulnar nerve in the forearm segment.

**ANSWER:** E. MGA needs to be considered when encountering a conduction block pattern of the ulnar nerve in the forearm segment.

**COMMENTS AND DISCUSSION**
- Martin-Gruber anastomosis (MGA) is the most common anomalous innervation in the upper extremity, found in 15%–30% of individuals presenting to electromyography (EMG) laboratories.
- It is a crossover of median nerve motor fibers to the ulnar nerve in the forearm segment (not ulnar to median) (See Fig. 8.1).
- The median nerve fibers that cross over may supply ulnar-innervated hand muscles: hypothenar muscles (abductor digiti minimi), first dorsal interossei, thenar muscles (adductor pollicis), or a combination of these.
- The most common innervation is to the first dorsal interossei muscle. Proximal ulnar muscles (e.g., the flexor carpi ulnaris) are not involved.
- When to suspect MGA?
  - Most common: apparent conduction block of the ulnar nerve in the forearm segment, which is an uncommon location for an entrapment (See Fig. 8.1)
  - Apparent conduction block of ulnar study between below-elbow and above-elbow site (when an MGA is located between cubital tunnel and groove)
  - Increased compound muscle action potential (CMAP) amplitude at a proximal site on a median motor study (when an MGA innervates the thenar muscles)
- MGA is not a form of median neuropathy at the wrist.
- MGA has no innervation from the radial nerve.

**QUESTION 21.** When performing a peroneal (fibular) motor study recording the extensor digitorum brevis (EDB) muscle, you observe larger responses from stimulation below the fibular head and at the popliteal fossa, compared to the one obtained from stimulation at the ankle, as shown in the following figure. What is the next best action?

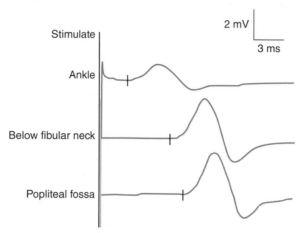

From Preston DC, Shapiro BE. *Electromyography and Neuromuscular Disorders: Clinical-electrophysiologic-ultrasound Correlations.* 4th ed. Elsevier;7, 24.

A. Warm the knee and restimulate.
B. Increase the current intensity below the fibular head and at the popliteal fossa.
C. Decrease the current intensity at the ankle.
D. Record an additional response by stimulating behind the lateral malleolus and recording the EDB.
E. Try to perform peroneal motor study recording the tibialis anterior (TA) instead.

**ANSWER:** D. Record an additional response by stimulating behind the lateral malleolus and recording the EDB.

### COMMENTS AND DISCUSSION

- The figure in this question demonstrates a peroneal motor study showing a smaller compound muscle action potential (CMAP) from stimulation at the ankle, but larger potentials from stimulation at more proximal sites. There are three main possibilities in this case:
  - Co-stimulation at proximal sites. However, co-stimulation of the peroneal nerve usually occurs when stimulating at the popliteal fossa, since peroneal and tibial nerves run close to each other. Co-stimulation rarely occurs when stimulating at the fibular head, where the peroneal nerve is not close to the tibial nerve. Nevertheless, if co-stimulation is suspected (e.g., when the waveform morphology is different from those obtained from the distal sites), decreasing (not increasing) the current intensity may be tried.
  - Submaximal stimulation at the ankle. When this is suspected, increasing current intensity at the ankle until reaching supramaximal stimulation should be undertaken. However, co-stimulation when using higher intensity should be cautioned.
  - The presence of an accessory peroneal nerve, a normal anatomic variation, where the EDB muscle receives additional supply from both the superficial peroneal nerve and the deep peroneal nerve. To confirm this anatomic variation, stimulating behind the lateral malleolus will produce an additional response with an amplitude approximately equal to the difference in amplitudes observed between below the fibular neck and the ankle (Fig. 3.12).
- Warming the proximal sites or performing a peroneal motor study recording the tibialis anterior muscle would not be helpful.

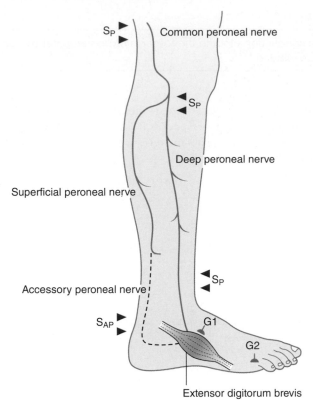

**Fig. 3.12** Accessory peroneal nerve. Normally, the extensor digitorum brevis is supplied by the deep peroneal nerve. When the accessory peroneal nerve which is a normal variation is present, the superficial peroneal nerve continues as a branch passing posterior to the lateral malleolus to supply the lateral extensor digitorum brevis. This branch is called the accessory peroneal nerve. From Preston DC, Shapiro BE. *Electromyography and Neuromuscular Disorders: Clinical-electrophysiologic-ultrasound Correlations.* 4th ed. Elsevier; 2021;7:73.

## ◎ HIGH-YIELD FACT

Causes of larger CMAP amplitude at proximal stimulation sites on peroneal motor studies recording the EDB
- Submaximal stimulation at ankle (distal) site
- Co-stimulation of the tibial nerve at the fibular neck/knee (proximal) site
- Accessory peroneal nerve

**QUESTION 22.** Which of the following electrodiagnostic findings is seen in a patient who has both a median neuropathy at the wrist and a Martin-Gruber anastomosis (MGA)?
A. Motor response with an initially positive dip when stimulating at the wrist
B. Factitiously fast conduction velocity at the forearm segment
C. Normal distal latency but slowed proximal conduction velocity
D. Prolonged distal latency and slowed proximal conduction velocity
E. Conduction block between the wrist and antecubital fossa

**ANSWER:** B. Factitiously fast conduction velocity at the forearm segment

## COMMENTS AND DISCUSSION
- Both MGA and median neuropathy at the wrist are common and can co-exist. Median neuropathy at the wrist slows the distal latency of the median nerve across the wrist. MGA is a crossover of median motor fibers to the ulnar nerve in the forearm segment.
- When median neuropathy at the wrist and MGA co-exist, the median motor study stimulating at the wrist shows the usual recording of a prolonged median motor distal latency. However,

when the forearm is stimulated, the crossover fibers travel to the ulnar nerve without slowing at the wrist. When these fibers terminate in the ulnar thenar muscles, the following findings are encountered (Fig. 3.13):

- Notably faster calculated conduction velocity of the median nerve in the forearm segment. Note that conduction velocity in the forearm segment is calculated from the distal latency, which is prolonged in this case, and the proximal latency, which is relatively "normal" due to crossover fibers that are not slowed the wrist.
- Positive dip or deflection of the median response when stimulating at the antecubital fossa. The median fibers which cross over arrive first at the hand as they are not slowed at the carpal tunnel. When they depolarize a muscle in or close to the thenar eminence, a positive deflection is picked up by the median recording electrodes.

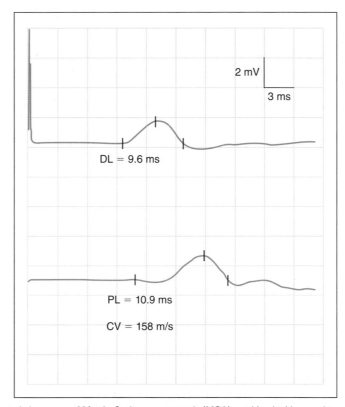

Fig. 3.13 Median motor study in a case of Martin-Gruber anastomosis (MGA) combined with carpal tunnel syndrome. The upper trace is a response from wrist stimulation. Prolonged distal latency is seen from carpal tunnel syndrome. The lower trace is a response from antecubital fossa stimulation. The positive dip represents a motor response from volume conduction of ulnar innervated muscles that is supplied by median nerve fibers from MGA. Since crossover median nerve fibers travelling to the ulnar nerve via the MGA bypass the carpal tunnel, calculated conduction velocity (CV) of the median nerve is spuriously fast. From Preston DC, Shapiro BE. *Electromyography and Neuromuscular Disorders: Clinical-electrophysiologic-ultrasound Correlations.* 4th ed. Elsevier; 2021;7:72.

◎ **HIGH-YIELD FACT**

When encountering a positive dip at a proximal stimulation site during a median motor study that is not present at the distal site, especially with an unusually fast conduction velocity, the combination of MGA and CTS should always be considered.

**QUESTION 23.** Which of the following is consistent with a Riche-Cannieu anastomosis?
A. Reversed Martin-Gruber anastomosis
B. Communication between median and radial nerves in the palm
C. All-median hand
D. All-ulnar hand
E. All-radial hand

**ANSWER:** D. All-ulnar hand

**COMMENTS AND DISCUSSION**
- Riche-Cannieu anastomosis is a very rare anomalous innervation in which there is a connection between the median and ulnar nerves in the palm.
- It is an anastomosis of the deep palmar branch of the ulnar and median nerves.
- It results in muscles usually innervated by the median nerve to be partially or completely/innervated by the ulnar nerve.
- May result in an "all-ulnar hand."
- When to suspect Riche-Cannieu anastomosis?
    o Compound muscle action potential (CMAP) of the median nerve has markedly reduced amplitude or absent; yet thenar muscle bulk and strength are normal. Thenar muscles usually innervated by the median nerve are supplied by the ulnar nerve. Thus when the median nerve is stimulated at the wrist there is no response when recording the thenar muscles.
    o Median-innervated thenar muscles are unexpectedly involved when the clinical presentation is ulnar neuropathy (caution—this pattern can also be seen in the medial cord, lower trunk, and C8 to T1 lesions)

**QUESTION 24.** When performing an ulnar motor study, the amplitude at the wrist is much higher than that when stimulating the below-elbow site. Which of the following can result in this pattern?
A. Co-stimulation at the wrist
B. Submaximal stimulation at the below-elbow site
C. Martin-Gruber anastomosis
D. Conduction block in the forearm
E. All of the above

**ANSWER:** E. All of the above

**COMMENTS AND DISCUSSION**
- A much lower motor amplitude at a proximal stimulation site as compared to the distal stimulation site usually indicates a conduction block. However, this pattern can also be seen with (Fig. 3.14):
    o Anomalous innervation, especially in the forearm segment when performing an ulnar motor study in a patient with an MGA
    o Submaximal stimulation at the proximal site
    o Co-stimulation of adjacent nerves at the distal site
        • Co-stimulation often occurs in the following circumstances:
            • If a very high current is used to stimulate or the stimulator is not optimally placed over the nerve.
            • At anatomic locations where nerves are very close to each other (e.g., median and ulnar nerves at the axilla or Erb's point)
            • If the response is small and unexpected, there is a natural tendency to increase the current further to try to make the response "more normal."
        • Actions to avoid co-stimulation of adjacent nerves:
            • Start low and go slow with the stimulating current
            • Ensure that the stimulator is optimally placed over the nerve
            • Observe waveform morphology. If there is co-stimulation, the morphology may change abruptly as current is increased.

- Observe the motor twitch. If there is co-stimulation, there will be twitching of muscles beyond the muscle intended to stimulate
- If unavoidable, collision studies may be used to distinguish and separate components from two different nerve pathways.

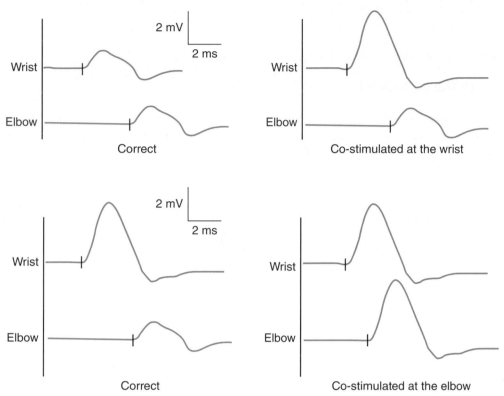

**Fig. 3.14** Co-stimulation and conduction block. Upper trace shows co-stimulation at the wrist resulting in a "pseudo-conduction block." The lower trace shows co-stimulation at the elbow resulting in a falsely large proximal response, and the true conduction block is missed. From Preston DC, Shapiro BE. *Electromyography and Neuromuscular Disorders: Clinical-electrophysiologic-ultrasound Correlations*. 4th ed. Elsevier; 2021;8:89.

## ◎ HIGH YIELD FACT

Co-stimulation at distal site can result in falsely large distal amplitude, and be misinterpreted as conduction block.

- Conversely, a higher amplitude proximally on a motor study can occur with:
  - Submaximal stimulation distally
  - Co-stimulation proximally
  - The presence of an anomalous innervation, especially an accessory peroneal nerve routine during routine peroneal motor studies.

## ☞ KEY POINT

Causes of a larger recording response from proximal stimulation
- Submaximal stimulation at distal site
- Co-stimulation of adjacent nerve at proximal site
- Anomalous innervation (e.g., accessroy peroneal nerve)

**QUESTION 25.** Which is **TRUE** regarding physiologic factors that can affect nerve conduction studies?
A. Increased height is associated with faster nerves.
B. Cold limb temperatures are associated with small-amplitude sensory nerve action potentials (SNAPs).
C. Limb position does not influence calculated conduction velocities.
D. Age can affect both amplitude and conduction velocity.
E. All of the above.

**ANSWER:** D. Age can affect both amplitude and conduction velocity.

**COMMENTS AND DISCUSSION**
- Age
  - Normal reference values for nerve conduction studies (NCS) are usually applied for subjects with ages between 10-60 years. Amplitudes are small in pediatric population, and then increase to adult values during adolescence. Amplitudes, especially those of sensory nerve action potentials (SNAPs), slowly decrease in the sixth decade.
  - Conduction velocity (CV) is greater in myelinated nerves due to saltatory conduction of action potentials requiring less total nerve length to depolarize.
    - Accordingly, CV correlates with the degree of myelination (i.e., CV is faster in well-myelinated nerves relative to poorly myelinated ones).
    - Myelination occur in utero and infancy and is not completed until age 3–5 years. Thus infants and children younger than 3–5 years of age normally have slower conduction velocities (Fig. 3.15).
    - In aging, there is a normal loss of motor and sensory neurons, resulting in decreased conduction velocity of nerves, simply by loss of some of the faster axons.
    - In adults 60 years and older, CV decreases 0.5–4.0 m/s per decade.

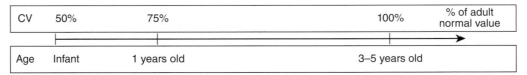

**Fig. 3.15** Age and conduction velocity. The *arrow* represents changes in the conduction velocity across the ages, from the infantile period. In the newborn, myelination is not fully completed; normal conduction velocity for this age is only 50% of the adult normal value. Conduction velocity increases to 75% of the adult normal value in the first year of age, and is the same as adults (100% of adult normal value) by the age of 3–5 years.

### ◎ HIGH-YIELD FACT

Peroneal CMAP (recording EDB) and sural SNAP can be low or absent in the elderly.

- Height
  - In tall subjects
    - The nerve length is longer, and there is more tapering of the nerves as they run distally.
    - Because nerve diameter is proportional to conduction velocity, more tapered nerves result in slower CV and longer distal latencies.
    - Latencies in late responses (F-waves and H-reflexes) are more prolonged due to longer nerve lengths in taller individuals.
- Temperature
  - Cool temperatures result in higher SNAP amplitude due to delayed inactivation and more sodium entering the nerve fiber.
- Limb position and measurement
  - In some nerves, proper limb position is required for accurate measurement, which then affects the calculated CV.
  - This is especially true for the ulnar nerve, where the distance measured in the elbow-bent position more correctly reproduces the actual nerve distance than in the elbow-straight position.
    - Some measurements are unavoidably inaccurate (e.g., radial nerve study below and above the groove of the humerus and the median and ulnar nerves between the axilla and Erb's point).

> ## 🔑 KEY POINT
>
> For an ulnar nerve study at the elbow, the nerve is slack when the arm is extended. Nerve conduction studies should be performed with the arm flexed at the elbow (at least 90 degrees) for accurate measurement.

**QUESTION 26.** Which is **TRUE** regarding motor and sensory nerve conduction studies after a nerve injury?
 A. The most common pattern seen is axonal loss.
 B. Demyelination is more prominent in lower extremity nerves.
 C. Motor nerves are preferentially affected.
 D. Demyelination is always present if the conduction velocity is lower than the lower limit of normal.
 E. All of the above.

**ANSWER:** A. The most common pattern seen is axonal loss.

## COMMENTS AND DISCUSSION

- Neurogenic lesions can be divided into axonal loss and demyelination (Table 3.3).
  - Axonal loss
    - The most common pattern seen on routine nerve conduction study (NCS)
    - Reduced amplitude is the primary abnormality due to loss of axons.
    - In axonal loss, latency and conduction velocity are usually normal but can be slightly slow if the fastest-conducting axons are lost.
  - Demyelination
    - Conduction velocity and distal latency are markedly slowed.
    - With sufficient demyelination, conduction block occurs.
    - Common features of demyelinating lesions on NCSs
      - Slowed conduction velocity (<75% of the lower normal limit)
      - Prolonged distal latency (>130% of the upper normal limit)
    - Features of acquired demyelination
      - Conduction block (unequivocal if area decrease is >50% for motor studies, probable for most decreases in amplitude >20% during routine motor studies)
      - Pathological temporal dispersion (proximal/distal CMAP duration ratio >1.15)

**TABLE 3.3** Effects on the potentials from axonal loss and demyelination

| Type of nerve injury | Amplitude | Latency | Conduction velocity |
|---|---|---|---|
| Axonal loss | ↓↓↓ | NL/↑ | NL/↓ |
| Demyelination | NL/↓ | ↑↑↑ | ↓↓↓ |

*Nl*: normal, ↓; slightly decreased, ↓↓↓; markedly decreased, ↑; slightly prolonged, ↑↑↑; markedly prolonged

## SUGGESTED READINGS

Dumitru D, Zwarts MJ. Instrumentation. In: Dumitru D, Amato A, Zwarts MJ, eds. *Electrodiagnostic Medicine.* 2nd ed. Philadelphia: Hanley & Belfus; 2002.

Kimura J. *Electrodiagnosis in Diseases of Nerve and Muscle, Principles and Practice.* 4th ed. New York: Oxford University Press; 2013.

Preston DC, Shapiro BE. *Electromyography and Neuromuscular Disorders: Clinical-electrophysiologic-ultrasound Correlations.* 4th ed. Philadelphia, PA: Elsevier; 2021.

Chen S, Andary M, Buschbacher R, et al. Electrodiagnostic reference values for upper and lower limb nerve conduction studies in adult populations. *Muscle Nerve.* 2016;54(3):371-377. doi:10.1002/mus.25203. 27238640.

Ryan CS, Conlee EM, Sharma R, et al. Nerve conduction normal values for electrodiagnosis in pediatric patients. *Muscle Nerve.* 2019;60(2):155-160. doi:10.1002/mus.26499.31032944.

Katirji B. *Electromyography in Clinical Practice.* 3rd ed. New York, NY: Oxford University Press; 2018.

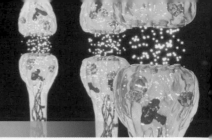

# CHAPTER 4

# Electrodiagnostic Medicine II: Needle Electromyography

## PART 1 | PRACTICE TEST

**Q1.** Which of the following is **FALSE** regarding the needle electromyography (EMG) examination?
A. The needle electrode is placed through the skin and subcutaneous tissue into the muscle to be sampled.
B. The needle is intramuscular.
C. The needle is intracellular.
D. The recording potentials are all voltages.
E. Each muscle is assessed for insertional activity, spontaneous activity, and voluntary activity.

**Q2.** You are invited to perform needle electromyography (EMG) in the off-campus lab. Only monopolar needles are available, whereas you normally use concentric needles in your lab. Which of the following would you expect on a needle EMG study when using a monopolar needle, compared to a concentric needle?
A. Less background noise
B. Smaller amplitudes of motor unit action potentials (MUAPs)
C. Longer duration of MUAPs
D. Reduced recruitment
E. No expected difference

**Q3.** Which of the following is **CORRECT** regarding electromyography (EMG) needles?
A. The monopolar needle has the exposed needle tip as a recording electrode.
B. The monopolar needle contains a fine insulated wire at the tip.
C. The concentric needle has a Teflon-coated shaft as a reference electrode.
D. The concentric needle has a larger area of recording compared to the monopolar needle.
E. The concentric needle needs a separated surface reference electrode.

**Q4.** Which of the following is **CORRECT** regarding insertional activity?
A. Insertional activity reflects the presence and vitality of the muscle.
B. Normal insertional activity has a duration greater than 300 ms.
C. Normal insertional activity can be seen in an actively denervating muscle.
D. Increased insertional activity is seen in a fibrotic muscle.
E. Decreased insertional activity is seen in inflammatory myopathy.

**Q5.** Which of the following is **FALSE** regarding spontaneous activity?
A. Muscle is normally quiet at rest when being recorded.
B. Any electrical activity occurring at rest is known as spontaneous activity.
C. All spontaneous activity is abnormal.
D. The source generator of the waveform can be determined by assessing the morphology of the spontaneous waveform.
E. Sound on the loudspeaker can help the electromyographer identify the type of spontaneous activity.

**Q6.** Which of the following is the waveform in the video?
A. Endplate noise
B. Fibrillation potentials
C. Normal insertional activity
D. Complex repetitive discharges
E. Cramp potentials

**Q7.** You perform the needle electromyography (EMG) in the right first dorsal interosseous muscle and encounter the waveform shown in the video. Which of the following is **CORRECT**?
A. The patient is likely experiencing pain.
B. There is evidence of active denervation.
C. The patient is not relaxing the tested muscle.
D. This waveform is classic for benign fasciculation syndrome.
E. This patient has a C8 radiculopathy.

**Q8.** Fibrillation potentials can be seen in which of the following?
A. Myositis
B. Botulism
C. Diabetic neuropathy
D. Amyotrophic lateral sclerosis (ALS)
E. All of the above

**Q9.** Which of the following is the waveform in the video?
A. Endplate spikes
B. Positive sharp waves
C. Fasciculations
D. Myokymic discharges
E. Motor unit action potentials

**Q10.** Positive sharp waves are most likely seen in which of the following conditions?
A. Benign fasciculation syndrome
B. Carpal tunnel syndrome
C. Guillain-Barré syndrome on day 2 from the onset of symptoms
D. Remote poliomyelitis
E. Multiple sclerosis

**Q11.** A 20-year-old woman presents with ascending numbness with proximal muscle weakness. You suspect Guillain-Barré syndrome. How long after the onset would you expect to visualize evidence of active denervation on needle electromyography (EMG)?
A. Immediately
B. 3 hours
C. 24 hours
D. 3 days
E. 21 days

**Q12.** Which of the following represents the activity seen in the video?
A. Endplate noise
B. Myotonic discharges
C. Complex repetitive discharges
D. Myokymic discharges
E. Cramp potentials

**Q13.** A 35-year-old man presents with generalized weakness. Needle electromyography (EMG) of the abductor pollicis brevis muscle demonstrates the activity as shown in the video. What is the **MOST LIKELY** diagnosis?
A. Carpal tunnel syndrome
B. C8 radiculopathy
C. Radiation plexitis
D. Myotonic dystrophy
E. Hypocalcemic tetany

**Q14.** Which of the following is the activity recorded in the video?
A. Endplate noise
B. Myotonic discharges
C. Complex repetitive discharges
D. Myokymic discharges
E. Cramp potentials

**Q15.** Which of the following represents the waveform seen in this video?
A. Endplate spikes
B. Fibrillations
C. Fasciculations
D. Myokymic discharges
E. Voluntary motor units

**Q16.** Which of the following is classically associated with tetany?
A. Positive sharp waves
B. Fibrillations
C. Doublets
D. Cramp discharges
E. Voluntary motor unit

**Q17.** Which of the following is demonstrated in this video?
A. Endplate noise
B. Myotonic discharges
C. Doublets
D. Myokymic discharges
E. Neuromyotonia

**Q18.** A 36-year-old woman is referred to the electromyography (EMG) lab for further workup of facial twitching. She has no known underlying past medical history except for only one episode of transient band-like numbness in her chest 6 months ago. Needle EMG is performed in the mentalis, and there is an activity as demonstrated in the video. What is the next best step of investigation?
A. EMG of the upper and lower extremities
B. Visual-evoked potentials
C. Computed tomography (CT) of the brain without contrast
D. Magnetic resonance imaging (MRI) of the brain with gadolinium
E. Electroencephalography (EEG)

**Q19.** A 55-year-old man presents with an inability to lift the right arm and numbness in the right thumb for 2 months. Examination reveals atrophy and weakness of the deltoid, biceps, and brachioradialis muscles. You perform electromyography (EMG), and found that these muscles demonstrates the activity as in the following figure. Which of the following clinical scenarios is **MOST LIKELY** associated with her condition?

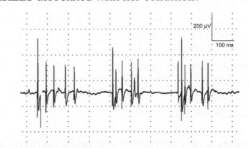

A. Guillain-Barré syndrome 5 years ago—in complete remission
B. Nasopharyngeal carcinoma status post radiation
C. Tongue atrophy with diffuse fasciculations in all extremities
D. Family history of muscle weakness
E. Progressive weakness of bilateral quadriceps muscles

**Q20.** Which of the following is associated with cramp potentials?
A. Any neuropathic condition
B. Can occur with exercise
C. Endocrine disorders
D. Metabolic disorders
E. All of the above

**Q21.** Which of the following is characteristic of neuromyotonia?
A. Waxing and waning of frequency
B. Initial frequencies up to 50 Hz
C. Waning of amplitude
D. Frequently seen as a benign phenomenon
E. Generated from a muscle fiber

**Q22.** Which of the following spontaneous discharges originate from a muscle fiber?
A. Endplate spikes
B. Fasciculations
C. Myotonic discharges
D. Myokymic discharges
E. Cramp potentials

**Q23.** Which of the following waveforms originates from the motor axon?
A. Endplate noise
B. Fibrillations
C. Fasciculations
D. Myotonic discharges
E. Complex repetitive discharges

**Q24.** When assessing voluntary activity during needle electromyography (EMG), which motor unit action potentials (MUAPs) are recruited first?
A. Small MUAPs; type I fibers
B. Small MUAPs; type II fibers
C. Large MUAPs; type I fibers
D. Large MUAPs; type II fibers
E. MUAPs closest to the needle

**Q25.** Which of the following motor unit action potential (MUAP) parameter is used to indicate the acceptable proximity of the tip of the recording needle electrode to the motor unit being studied?
A. Amplitude
B. Major spike rise time
C. Duration
D. Amplitude
E. Number of phases

**Q26.** Voluntary motor unit action potentials (MUAPs) are assessed routinely for all the following **EXCEPT**?
A. Amplitude
B. Phases
C. Duration
D. Jitter
E. Recruitment

**Q27.** A 65-year-old man presents for evaluation of right leg weakness. When the patient is asked to contract one of the weak muscles during needle electromyography (EMG) testing, you find motor unit action potentials (MUAPs) as shown in the following figure. What is the most likely time course of the weakness in this patient?

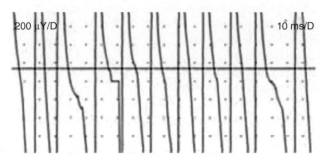

200 µY/D        10 ms/D

From Preston DC, Shapiro BE. Electromyography and Neuromuscular Disorders: Clinical-electrophysiologic-ultrasound Correlations. Philadelphia, PA: Elsevier; 2020:240. 4th ed.

A. 1 hour
B. 1 day
C. 1 week
D. 1 month
E. 1 year

**Q28.** Which of the following is **NOT** expected in a subacute (e.g., 4-week) axonal loss lesion?
A. Reduced compound muscle action potential (CMAP) amplitude
B. Reduced sensory nerve action potential (SNAP) amplitude
C. Fibrillation potentials
D. Large motor unit action potentials (MUAPs)
E. Reduced recruitment

**Q29.** In a case of pure focal demyelination of a peripheral nerve containing motor and sensory fibers, which of the following is expected?
A. Reduced compound muscle action potential (CMAP) amplitude distal to the lesion
B. Reduced sensory nerve action potential (SNAP) amplitude distal to the lesion
C. Fibrillation potentials in muscles supplied by the nerve, provided 4 weeks has passed
D. Large motor unit action potentials (MUAPs)
E. Reduced recruitment, if conduction block is present

**Q30.** In a case of a subacute inflammatory myopathy, which of the following is expected?
A. Fibrillation potentials
B. Reduced compound muscle action potential (CMAP) amplitude
C. Reduced sensory nerve action potential (SNAP) amplitude
D. Reduced recruitment of small, short, polyphasic motor unit action potentials (MUAPs)
E. Large MUAPs

## PART 2 | QUESTIONS WITH ANSWERS AND DISCUSSION

**QUESTION 1.** Which of the following is **FALSE** regarding the needle electromyography (EMG) examination?
A. The needle electrode is placed through the skin and subcutaneous tissue into the muscle to be sampled.
B. The needle is intramuscular.
C. The needle is intracellular.
D. The recording potentials are all voltages.
E. Each muscle is assessed for insertional activity, spontaneous activity, and voluntary activity.

**ANSWER:** C. The needle is intracellular.

### COMMENTS AND DISCUSSION
- The second part of the standard electrodiagnostic study, which follows the nerve conduction study, is the needle EMG examination.
- A needle electrode is placed through the skin and subcutaneous tissue into the muscle to be sampled.
- The needle is intramuscular but extracellular to the muscle fibers (i.e., the needle is much larger than individual muscle fibers).
- Similar to all data recorded in nerve conduction studies (NCS) and EMG, the waveforms sampled on needle EMG are all voltages (i.e., electrical potential differences between two electrodes).
- Each muscle is assessed for insertional, spontaneous, and voluntary activity.
- Practical steps for needle EMG
  - Formulate a differential diagnosis, based on the history, exam, and NCS findings.
  - Decide on which muscles are key to differentiate between possible anatomical locations or diagnoses.
  - Evaluate changes (both spontaneous and voluntary activity) in each muscle for:
    - Pattern of abnormal muscles, which often localizes the lesion (e.g., to an individual nerve, or nerve root)
    - The degree of abnormalities, which helps determine the severity
    - Many findings are time dependent and accordingly help determine the time course.
    - Useful information about the prognosis can be gained.

**QUESTION 2.** You are invited to perform needle electromyography (EMG) in the off-campus lab. Only monopolar needles are available, whereas you normally use concentric needles in your lab. Which of the following would you expect on a needle EMG study when using a monopolar needle, compared to a concentric needle?
A. Less background noise
B. Smaller amplitudes of motor unit action potentials (MUAPs)
C. Longer duration of MUAPs
D. Reduced recruitment
E. No expected difference

**ANSWER:** C. Longer duration of MUAPs

### COMMENTS AND DISCUSSION
- Monopolar and concentric needles are the two most common types of needles used for EMG in clinical practice.
- The recording area of the monopolar needle has a spherical configuration around the needle tip, whereas that of the concentric needle is a teardrop configuration from the bevel side of the needle.
- Thus, the monopolar needle can record a larger area and more muscle fibers resulting in a slightly longer duration and slightly higher amplitude MUAPs, compared to those recorded from the concentric needle (Fig. 4.1 and Table 4.1). Recruitment is not different between monopolar and concentric needles.
- The monopolar needle requires an additional surface reference electrode (G2), which is relatively far from the recording electrode (G1), whereas for the concentric needle, the shaft of the needle itself serves as the reference electrode (G2). Thus the distance between the recording electrode (G1) and the reference electrode (G2) is much longer when using the monopolar needle; this results in more background noise, compared to the concentric needle. Thus, the reference electrode (G2) should be placed as close as possible to the monopolar recording electrode (G1) site of insertion into the muscle in order to reduce the background noise.

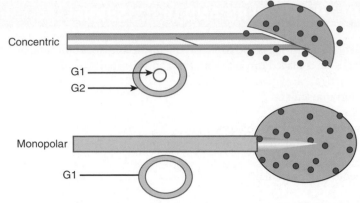

**Fig. 4.1 Concentric versus monopolar needles.** The concentric needle *(top)* is a bare, hollow needle with a fine insulated wire inside the core. At the tip, the beveled shape exposes the insulated wire inside (which is G1), surrounded by cannula (which is G2). With the concentric needle, G1 and G2 are next to each other. The recording area has hemispherical or teardrop shape. A separate G2 electrode is not required. The monopolar needle *(bottom)* is a stainless-steel core needle. The shaft is coated with Teflon. The needle tip is the recording electrode (G1). The recording area surrounding the tip has spherical shape. A separate surface reference electrode (G2) is required and should be placed close to the site of needle insertion into the muscle to reduce background noise. From Daube, JR, Rubin DI. Needle electromyography. *Muscle Nerve.* 2020;39:244–270.

**TABLE 4.1** The differences between monopolar and concentric needles.

|  | Monopolar needle | Concentric needle |
|---|---|---|
| Material | Stainless steel as a core electrode with a Teflon-coated shaft with a bare needle point | A bare, hollow needle with a small, insulated wire within the center |
| Active electrode | Tip of the needle | Tip of the small, insulated wire at its termination at the bevel of the needle |
| Reference electrode | Separated surface electrode close to the needle electrode | Shaft of the needle |
| Recording area | Spherical area around the needle tip | Hemispherical (teardrop-shaped) area around the bevel |
| Recorded MUAPs | Slightly longer duration and larger amplitude compared to MUAPs from concentric needle due to its larger recording area | Slightly shorter duration and smaller amplitude than monopolar needles |

*MUAP*, motor unit action potential.

**QUESTION 3.** Which of the following is **CORRECT** regarding electromyography (EMG) needles?
  A. The monopolar needle has the exposed needle tip as a recording electrode.
  B. The monopolar needle contains a fine insulated wire at the tip.
  C. The concentric needle has a Teflon-coated shaft as a reference electrode.
  D. The concentric needle has a larger area of recording compared to the monopolar needle.
  E. The concentric needle needs a separated surface reference electrode.

**ANSWER:** A. The monopolar needle has the exposed needle tip as a recording electrode.

**COMMENTS AND DISCUSSION**
- The monopolar needle is stainless steel coated with Teflon. Only the exposed needle tip serves as an active (recording) electrode (Fig. 4.1 and Table 4.1).
- A monopolar needle requires a separate surface reference electrode placed close to the needle.

- A concentric needle has a bare hollow needle with a very small, insulated wire running through the center of the needle.
- For a concentric needle, the beveled tip of the inner wire serves as an active electrode, and the shaft of the needle serves as a reference electrode.
- The recording area of the monopolar needle has a spherical configuration around the exposed tip, which is larger than the teardrop configuration from the beveled tip of the concentric needle (Fig. 4.1).

**QUESTION 4.** Which of the following is **CORRECT** regarding insertional activity?
A. Insertional activity reflects the presence and vitality of the muscle.
B. Normal insertional activity has a duration greater than 300 ms.
C. Normal insertional activity can be seen in an actively denervating muscle.
D. Increased insertional activity is seen in a fibrotic muscle.
E. Decreased insertional activity is seen in inflammatory myopathy.

**ANSWER:** A. Insertional activity reflects the presence and vitality of the muscle.

**COMMENTS AND DISCUSSION**
- Insertional activity
  - When the needle is placed in the muscle and moved slightly, nearby muscle fibers are mechanically deformed, depolarize, and fire briefly. This brief burst of muscle fiber firing is known as normal insertional activity.
  - Normal insertional activity lasts no longer than 200 to 300 ms.
  - Duration greater than 300 ms is considered as an increased insertional activity.
  - This reflects the presence and vitality of the muscle.
  - Increased insertional activity is seen in irritable muscle fibers from either neurogenic or myopathic conditions.
  - Decreased insertional activity is seen in end-stage fibrotic muscle fibers.
  - The presence of insertional activity is helpful in confirming that the needle is in muscle (as opposed to fat or connective tissue).

**QUESTION 5.** Which of the following is **FALSE** regarding spontaneous activity?
A. Muscle is normally quiet at rest when being recorded.
B. Any electrical activity occurring at rest when the patient is not contracting their muscle is known as spontaneous activity.
C. All spontaneous activity is abnormal.
D. The source generator of the waveform can be determined by assessing the morphology of the spontaneous waveform.
E. Sound on the loudspeaker can help the electromyographer identify the type of spontaneous activity.

**ANSWER:** C. All spontaneous activity is abnormal.

**COMMENTS AND DISCUSSION**
- Normally, muscle is quiet when recording at rest.
- There are many types of spontaneous activity (Table 4.2), which can be differentiated based on their:
  - Morphology, which indicates the source or generator
  - Stability
  - Firing characteristics, both rate and pattern
  - Sound of the discharges
- Most, but not all, spontaneous activity is abnormal. The exceptions are potentials generated at or near the muscle endplate: endplate noise and endplate spikes.
- Thus, not all spontaneous activity is abnormal.

**TABLE 4.2**  Spontaneous activity.

| Potential | Morphology | Stability | Firing rate | Firing pattern | Sound on speaker |
|---|---|---|---|---|---|
| **Normal spontaneous activity** | | | | | |
| *Originating from the NMJ* | | | | | |
| Endplate noise | Small, monophasic negative potentials | Stable | 20–40 Hz | Irregular | Seashell or hiss |
| *Originating from the terminal axon* | | | | | |
| Endplate spikes | Small, short, diphasic potentials with an initial negative (upward) deflection | Stable | 5–50 Hz | Irregular | Sputtering, fat in the frying pan |
| **Abnormal spontaneous activity** | | | | | |
| *Originating from muscle fiber* | | | | | |
| Fibrillation potentials | Small, short triphasic potentials with an initial positive (downward) deflection | Stable | 0.5–10 Hz | Regular | Rain on a tin roof |
| Positive sharp waves | Initial brief positive followed by a long, tailing negative | Stable | 0.5–10 Hz | Regular | Regular "pop – pop – pop" |
| Myotonic discharges | Either a brief spike or a positive wave morphology | Waxing/waning amplitude | 20–150 Hz | Waxing and waning | Revving engine |

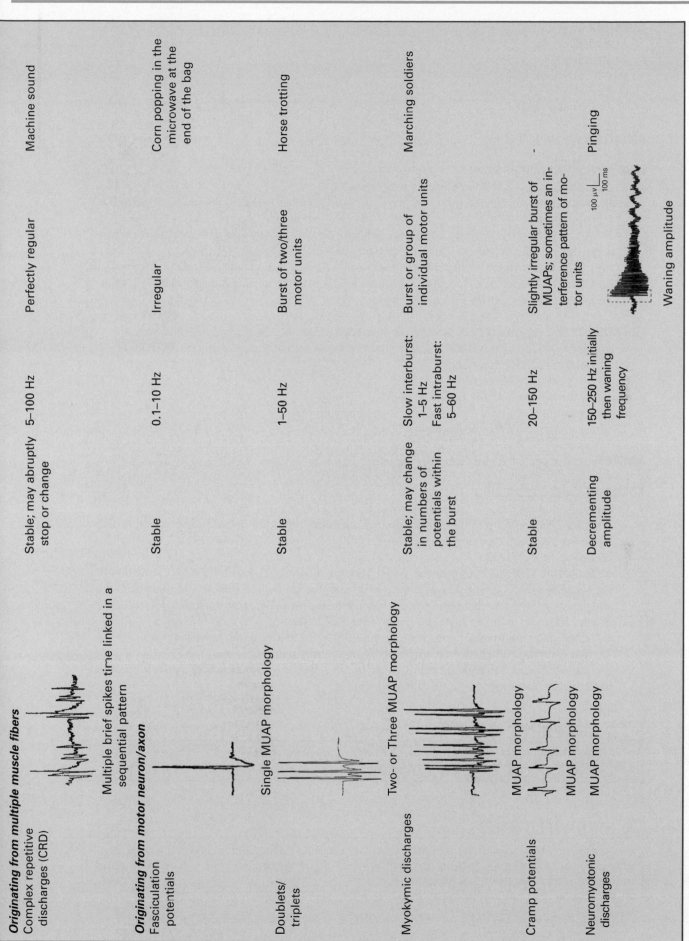

| | | Stability | Frequency | Firing Pattern | Sound |
|---|---|---|---|---|---|
| **_Originating from multiple muscle fibers_** | | | | | |
| Complex repetitive discharges (CRD) | Multiple brief spikes time linked in a sequential pattern | Stable; may abruptly stop or change | 5–100 Hz | Perfectly regular | Machine sound |
| **_Originating from motor neuron/axon_** | | | | | |
| Fasciculation potentials | Single MUAP morphology | Stable | 0.1–10 Hz | Irregular | Corn popping in the microwave at the end of the bag |
| Doublets/triplets | Two- or Three MUAP morphology | Stable | 1–50 Hz | Burst of two/three motor units | Horse trotting |
| Myokymic discharges | MUAP morphology | Stable; may change in numbers of potentials within the burst | Slow interburst: 1–5 Hz Fast intraburst: 5–60 Hz | Burst or group of individual motor units | Marching soldiers |
| Cramp potentials | MUAP morphology | Stable | 20–150 Hz | Slightly irregular burst of MUAPs; sometimes an interference pattern of motor units | - |
| Neuromyotonic discharges | MUAP morphology | Decrementing amplitude | 150–250 Hz initially then waning frequency | Waning amplitude | Pinging |

100 μV
100 ms

Adapted from Preston DC, Shapiro BE. _Electromyography and Neuromuscular Disorders._ 4th ed. Philadelphia, PA: Elsevier; 2020.

**QUESTION 6.** Which of the following is the waveform in the video?
- A. Endplate noise
- B. Fibrillations
- C. Normal insertional activity
- D. Complex repetitive discharges
- E. Cramp potentials

**ANSWER:** A. Endplate noise

**COMMENTS AND DISCUSSION**

- The waveform in the video demonstrates endplate noise
  - Endplate noise is generated from miniature endplate potentials (MEPPs) at the neuromuscular junction (NMJ).
  - MEPPs are potentials generated, at the postsynaptic membrane, by spontaneous release of normal acetylcholine quanta (vesicles) from the presynaptic membrane.
  - MEPPs do not reach the depolarization threshold of the muscle action potential and fail to propagate.
  - Endplate noise represents a background sound, louder than the normal quiet baseline.
  - Endplate noise sounds like a seashell or hiss.

**QUESTION 7.** You perform the needle electromyography (EMG) in the right first dorsal interosseous muscle and encounter the waveform shown in the video. Which of the following is **CORRECT**?
- A. The patient is likely experiencing pain.
- B. There is evidence of active denervation.
- C. The patient is not relaxing the tested muscle.
- D. This waveform is classic for benign fasciculation syndrome.
- E. This patient has a C8 radiculopathy.

**ANSWER:** A. The patient is likely experiencing pain.

**COMMENTS AND DISCUSSION**

- The waveform in the video is an endplate spike, a normal finding (Fig. 4.2 and Table 4.2).
  - Endplate spikes result from the depolarization of a terminal axon twig caused by mechanical irritation by the needle, which then propagates across the NMJ to the muscle fiber, resulting in a muscle fiber action potential (MFAP).
  - Potentials are brief spikes (typically 3–5 ms), with an initial negative deflection (denoting that the depolarization is occurring very near the needle, and that the depolarization runs away from the endplate down the muscle fiber; there is never a time the depolarization is running toward the needle electrode; therefore there is never a positive deflection).
  - Endplate spikes are irregular and create a sound similar to sputtering fat in a frying pan.
  - There is no association between endplate spikes and unrelaxed muscle.
  - Endplate spikes are a normal spontaneous activity, thus they are not a feature of active denervation, benign fasciculation syndrome, or radiculopathy.

 **KEY POINT**

Endplate noise and endplate spikes both originate close to each other (NMJ and terminal axon twig, respectively); therefore these two are often present at the same time.

 **HIGH-YIELD FACT**

When the electromyographer encounters endplate noise and/or endplate spikes, the patient may experience deep pain because the needle location is close to the nerve. The needle should then be moved away from that location.

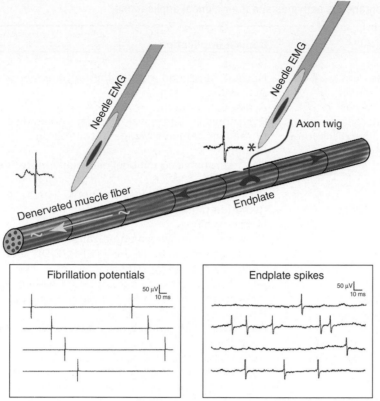

**Fig. 4.2 Endplate spikes versus fibrillation potentials.** Endplate spikes and fibrillation potentials are two similar potentials that can often be confused by electromyographers. It is crucial to differentiate between them, given different origins and implications. Endplate spikes originate from a depolarization of an axon twig, leading to an axonal twig action potential, which then travels across the neuromuscular junction (NMJ) to the muscle fiber and results in a muscle fiber action potential (MFAP). As the depolarization moves away from the needle electrode *(blue arrows)*, the initial deflection is negative or upward. Endplate spikes are irregular. In contrast, fibrillation potentials indicate active denervation. Because the potentials move towards the needle electrode *(yellow arrow)*, the initial deflection is positive or downward. The fibrillation potentials are regular. Adapted from Preston DC, Shapiro BE. *Electromyography and Neuromuscular Disorders.* 4th ed. Philadelphia, PA: Elsevier; 2020.

**QUESTION 8.** Fibrillation potentials can be seen in which of the following?
- A. Myositis
- B. Botulism
- C. Diabetic neuropathy
- D. Amyotrophic lateral sclerosis (ALS)
- E. All of the above

**ANSWER:** E. All of the above

**COMMENTS AND DISCUSSION**
- Fibrillation potentials (Fig. 4.2 and Table 4.2)
  - Origin: denervated muscle fiber depolarizes spontaneously, resulting in an abnormal muscle fiber action potential (MFAP)
  - Morphology: short duration, triphasic with an initial positive deflection
  - Stability: stable
  - Firing characteristic: regular with a frequency of 0.5–10 Hz
  - Sound: rain on a tin roof
  - Clinical application: they represent active or ongoing denervation (the muscle fiber has been disconnected from its nerve supply) (Table 4.3).
    - Classically this is seen in any neuropathic condition associated with axonal loss, including mononeuropathy, polyneuropathy, radiculopathy, and motor neuron disorders.
    - However, fibrillations also occur in some myopathies, especially inflammatory, necrotic, and some toxic myopathies.

**TABLE 4.3** Spontaneous activities and their clinical applications.

| Potentials | Clinical implication |
|---|---|
| Endplate noise | Normal |
| Endplate spikes | Normal; needle tip irritates the terminal nerve twig |
| Fibrillation potentials | Active denervation |
| Positive sharp waves | Active denervation |
| Myotonic discharges | Dystrophic and non-dystrophic myotonic disorders |
| Complex repetitive discharges | Chronic neurogenic/myopathic conditions |
| Fasciculation potentials | Benign |
| | Any neurogenic conditions, especially motor neuron diseases |
| Doublets/triplets | Hypocalcemic tetany |
| | Conditions similar to fasciculations |
| Myokymic discharges | Radiation plexopathy/neuropathy |
| | Pontine lesions |
| | Timber rattle snake envenomization |
| | Demyelinating neuropathies (GBS, CIDP, radiculopathy, entrapment neuropathy) |
| | Anti–VGKC-associated peripheral nerve hyperexcitability disorders (autoimmune and paraneoplastic) |
| Cramp potentials | Benign |
| | Associated with neurogenic, endocrinologic, or metabolic conditions |
| Neuromyotonic discharges | Anti–VGKC-associated peripheral nerve hyperexcitability disorders (autoimmune and paraneoplastic) |
| | Extremely chronic motor neuron disorders |

CIDP, chronic inflammatory demyelinating polyneuropathy; GBS, Guillain-Barré syndrome; VGKC, voltage-gated potassium channel.

- In addition, if transmission through the NMJ is severely blocked resulting in disconnection between the muscle fiber and its nerve supply, fibrillations can develop. This often occurs in botulism and, rarely, in myasthenia gravis.

## 🔑 KEY POINT

Due to its brief spike morphology, fibrillations can be confused with endplate spikes. Fibrillations are a sign of active denervation, whereas endplate spikes are a normal finding. To differentiate these, note the following factors (Fig. 4.2):
1. Initial deflection: positive (downward) in fibrillations versus negative (upward) in endplate spikes
2. Firing pattern: regular in fibrillations versus irregular in endplate spikes

**QUESTION 9.** Which of the following is the waveform in the video?
- A. Endplate spikes
- B. Positive sharp waves
- C. Fasciculations
- D. Myokymic discharges
- E. Motor unit action potentials

**ANSWER:** B. Positive sharp waves

### COMMENTS AND DISCUSSION
- Positive sharp waves (Table 4.2)
  - Origin: same as fibrillation potentials which originate from denervated muscle fiber that depolarizes spontaneously, resulting in an abnormal motor fiber action potential (MFAP). The difference is that, in positive sharp waves, the needle mechanically deforms the denervated muscle fiber, thereby preventing propagation of the action potential beyond this area.

- Morphology: initial brief positive deflection, followed by a long duration negative tail, biphasic
- Stability: stable
- Firing characteristic: regular with frequency of 0.5–10 Hz
- Sound: "pop – pop – pop"
- Clinical implication: they represent an active denervation, similar to fibrillation potentials (Table 4.3)
- Thus fibrillation potentials and positive sharp waves represent the same process: the spontaneous discharge of an denervated muscle fiber. Indeed, by moving the needle slightly, one can often change the morphology of the discharge from a fibrillation to a positive wave and vice versa.

**QUESTION 10.** Positive sharp waves are most likely seen in which of the following conditions?
A. Benign fasciculation syndrome
B. Carpal tunnel syndrome
C. Guillain-Barré syndrome on day 2 from the onset of symptoms
D. Remote poliomyelitis
E. Multiple sclerosis

**ANSWER:** B. Carpal tunnel syndrome

**COMMENTS AND DISCUSSION**
- Positive sharp waves are abnormal spontaneous activity.
- Similar to fibrillation potentials, they represent active denervation when the nerve is physically or functionally disconnected from the muscle.
- Positive sharp waves are seen in various neurogenic disorders involving anterior horn cells, nerve root, plexus, peripheral nerve, as well as some myopathies such as inflammatory myopathies and some severe neuromuscular junction disorders such as botulism.
- Among all choices, carpal tunnel syndrome is most likely to show positive sharp waves.
- In benign fasciculation syndrome, there is no active denervation and, therefore, positive sharp waves are not an expected finding.
- It takes at least 2–4 weeks for fibrillation potentials or positive sharp waves to appear, depending on the distance between the site of nerve injury and the tested muscle (i.e., it takes shorter time if the site of nerve injury is near the tested muscle). Immediately after a nerve injury, fibrillation potentials and positive sharp waves have not had sufficient time to develop. Two days after the onset of Guillain-Barré syndrome is too early to detect active denervating features.
- In very chronic neurogenic conditions lasting more than 6–12 months, fibrillation potentials and positive sharp waves become increasingly diminutive and disappear. Remote poliomyelitis is chronic, and active denervating features are not expected or are much less likely.
- Evidence of active (peripheral) denervation is generally not expected in central demyelination such as multiple sclerosis.

**QUESTION 11.** A 20-year-old woman presents with ascending numbness with proximal muscle weakness. You suspect Guillain-Barré syndrome. How long after the onset would you expect to visualize evidence of active denervation on needle electromyography (EMG)?
A. Immediately
B. 3 hours
C. 24 hours
D. 3 days
E. 21 days

**ANSWER:** E. 21 days

**COMMENTS AND DISCUSSION**
- In Guillain-Barré syndrome, the primary pathology is demyelination, but there is also often secondary axonal loss. The latter results in active denervation.
- However, the evidence of active denervation on needle electromyography (EMG) including fibrillation potentials and positive sharp waves takes time to appear, usually 10–14 days in the muscles closest to the site of nerve injury.
- It may take 3–4 weeks to appear in the distant muscles.

**QUESTION 12.** Which of the following represents the activity seen in the video?
   A. Endplate noise
   B. Myotonic discharges
   C. Complex repetitive discharges
   D. Myokymic discharges
   E. Cramp potentials

**ANSWER:** B. Myotonic discharges

**COMMENTS AND DISCUSSION**
- Myotonic discharges
  - Origin: single muscle fiber depolarization (same as fibrillation potentials and positive sharp waves)
  - Morphology: brief spike or positive wave (same as fibrillation potentials and positive sharp waves)
  - Stability: waxing and waning of amplitude
  - Firing characteristic: waxing and waning
  - Sound: a revving engine
  - Clinical implication: classically seen in the three major myotonic disorders including myotonic dystrophy, myotonia congenita, and paramyotonia congenita. In addition, it is classically seen in some toxic myopathies (e.g., statin-induced myopathy) and some inherited myopathies (particularly affecting the paraspinal and proximal muscles in cases of adult-onset acid maltase deficiency) (Table 4.4).

**TABLE 4.4** Location of myokymic discharges with associated conditions.

| Location of myokymia | Conditions |
| --- | --- |
| Face | Guillain-Barré syndrome |
| | Multiple sclerosis |
| | Pontine tumors |
| Limbs | Radiation injury (especially brachial plexopathy) |
| | Guillain-Barré syndrome |
| | Radiculopathy |
| | Nerve entrapments |
| Generalized | Timber rattle snake envenomization |
| | CIDP |

*CIDP*, Chronic inflammatory demyelinating polyneuropathy.

**QUESTION 13.** A 35-year-old man presents with generalized weakness. Needle electromyography (EMG) of the abductor pollicis brevis muscle demonstrates the activity as shown in the video. What is the **MOST LIKELY** diagnosis?
   A. Carpal tunnel syndrome
   B. C8 radiculopathy
   C. Radiation plexitis
   D. Myotonic dystrophy
   E. Hypocalcemic tetany

**ANSWER:** D. Myotonic dystrophy

**COMMENTS AND DISCUSSION**
- The waveform in this video demonstrates myotonic discharges, which originate from a single muscle fiber (Table 4.2). Myotonic discharges have either a brief spike or positive wave morphology similar to denervating potentials. In contrast, there is waxing and waning of the amplitude and frequency. This results in the sound of a revving engine. Myotonic discharges are unique and seen only in a few disorders.
- In carpal tunnel syndrome and C8 radiculopathy, active denervating features such as fibrillation potentials or positive sharp waves may be seen. In radiation plexitis, myokymic discharges are the pathognomonic finding (Table 4.4). In hypocalcemic tetany, doublets are the classic finding on needle EMG.

**QUESTION 14.** Which of the following is the activity recorded in the video?
  A. Endplate noise
  B. Myotonic discharges
  C. Complex repetitive discharges
  D. Myokymic discharges
  E. Cramp potentials

**ANSWER:** C. Complex repetitive discharges

**COMMENTS AND DISCUSSION**
- Complex repetitive discharges (CRDs) (Fig. 4.3 and Table 4.2)
  - Origin: depolarization from a denervated muscle fiber that initiates a circuit via ephaptic transmission to adjacent denervated muscle fibers (ephaptic referring to conduction from membrane to membrane without a synapse), and subsequently transmits back to the original fiber.
  - Morphology: a sequential group of repeating brief spikes that are perfectly time-linked to each other.
  - Stability: most are stable; however, they may change, start, or stop abruptly as additional loops or circuits drop in and out.
  - Firing frequency: due to a loop circuit, the rhythm of CRD is perfectly regular. Similar to their morphology, their frequency may change abruptly or stop abruptly.
  - Sound: a machine
  - Clinical implication: these occur in chronic conditions including chronic neuropathies and myopathies.
  - Pathological correlations
    - CRDs correlate with grouped atrophy in neurogenic conditions.
    - CRDs correlate with a group of necrotic muscle fibers, muscle fiber splitting, or inflammation in myopathic disorders.

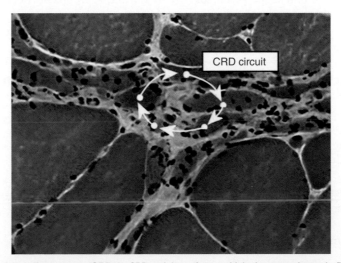

**Fig. 4.3  Complex repetitive discharges (CRDs).** CRDs originate from multiple denervated muscle fibers that lay adjacent to each other. This circus loop is facilitated by ephaptic transmission, which can spread to adjacent loops or dead-end circuits, resulting in abrupt changes. CRDs can also stop abruptly if one fiber in the circuit fails to maintain depolarization. These potentials indicate chronicity, which may be attributable to neurogenic or myopathic conditions. From Preston DC, Shapiro BE. *Electromyography and Neuromuscular Disorders.* 4th ed. Philadelphia, PA: Elsevier; 2020.

**QUESTION 15.** Which of the following represents the waveform seen in this video?
  A. Endplate spikes
  B. Fibrillations
  C. Fasciculations
  D. Myokymic discharges
  E. Voluntary motor units

**ANSWER:** C. Fasciculations

### COMMENTS AND DISCUSSION

- Fasciculation potentials (Table 4.2)
  - Origin: single motor unit/motor neuron or its axon
  - Morphology: similar to normal single motor unit action potentials (MUAPs), and may display complex and abnormal MUAP if there is an underlying pathology (e.g., in amyotrophic lateral sclerosis [ALS]). Typically, normal MUAPs have a duration of 5–15 msec, an amplitude up to 2 mV, and 2, 3, or 4 phases.
  - Stability: tend to be stable
  - Firing frequency: usually less than 1–2 Hz, which is too slow for voluntary motor units (that typically begin firing at 4–5 Hz); irregular firing pattern
  - Sound: popcorn popping in the microwave at the beginning or end of the bag
  - Clinical implication: can be seen as a benign and normal phenomenon (benign fasciculation syndrome) or in any neuropathic conditions, although they are classically associated with ALS and other motor neuron disorders (Table 4.3)

**QUESTION 16.** Which discharge is classically associated with tetany?
- A. Positive sharp waves
- B. Fibrillations
- C. Doublets
- D. Cramp discharges
- E. Voluntary motor units

**ANSWER:** C. Doublets

### COMMENTS AND DISCUSSION

- Doublets/triplets/multiplets (Table 4.2)
  - Origin: motor unit/motor neuron or its axon
  - Morphology: motor unit action potentials (MUAPs) firing in groups of two, three, or a few
  - Stability: tend to be stable
  - Firing frequency: a slightly irregular burst of two or three potentials, sometimes more, with a variable firing frequency ranging from 1–50 Hz
  - Sound: horse trotting
  - Clinical implication: classically present in tetany from hypocalcemia; in addition, can be seen in other conditions that are similar to those associated with fasciculations (Table 4.3)

**QUESTION 17.** Which of the following is demonstrated in this video?
- A. Endplate noise
- B. Myotonic discharges
- C. Doublets
- D. Myokymic discharges
- E. Neuromyotonia

**ANSWER:** D. Myokymic discharges

### COMMENTS AND DISCUSSION

- Myokymic discharges (Table 4.2)
  - Origin: motor unit/motor neuron or its axon
  - Morphology: motor unit action potentials (MUAPs; same as fasciculations) firing in groups, or bursts
  - Stability: usually stable
  - Firing pattern and rate: firing in burst. Interburst frequency is slow, typically 1–2 Hz, but intraburst frequency is much faster, in the range of 5–60 Hz.
  - Sound: marching soldiers
  - Clinical implication: classically seen in radiation-induced nerve injury (e.g., plexopathy or neuropathy); can be found in other conditions (Table 4.4).

**QUESTION 18.** A 36-year-old woman is referred to the electromyography (EMG) lab for further workup of facial twitching. She has no known underlying past medical history except for only one episode of transient band-like numbness in her chest 6 months ago. Needle EMG is performed in the mentalis, and there is an activity as demonstrated in the video. What is the next best step of investigation?

A. EMG of the upper and lower extremities
B. Visual-evoked potentials
C. Computed tomography (CT) of the brain without contrast
D. Magnetic resonance imaging (MRI) of the brain with gadolinium
E. Electroencephalography (EEG)

**ANSWER:** D. Magnetic resonance imaging (MRI) of the brain with gadolinium

**COMMENTS AND DISCUSSION**

- The video demonstrates myokymic discharges. Myokymic discharges are a well-known finding in radiation plexopathy or neuropathy, but can also be present in other conditions.
- This patient has facial twitching with myokymic discharges on EMG in the mentalis muscle.
- Facial myokymia is suggestive of lesions affecting the fascicles of the facial nerve as they exit the facial nucleus, first in the pons and then outside of the brain stem into the face.
- Facial myokymia is classically seen with pontine tumors (e.g., glioma), multiple sclerosis, and Guillain-Barré syndrome (Table 4.4).
- Given the previous episode of transient band-like numbness in her chest, multiple sclerosis is the most likely diagnosis. The next best step of investigation in this case is MRI of the brain with gadolinium to look for demyelinating lesion within the pons and other coexisting (previous or silent) demyelinating lesions.

**QUESTION 19.** A 55-year-old man presents with an inability to lift the right arm and numbness in the right thumb for 2 months. Examination reveals atrophy and weakness of the deltoid, biceps, and brachioradialis muscles. You perform electromyography (EMG), and found that these muscles demonstrate the activity shown in the following figure. Which of the following clinical scenarios is most likely associated with her condition?

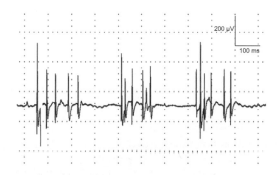

A. Guillain-Barré syndrome 5 years ago—in complete remission
B. Nasopharyngeal carcinoma status post radiation
C. Tongue atrophy with diffuse fasciculations in all extremities
D. Family history of muscle weakness
E. Progressive weakness of bilateral quadriceps muscles

**ANSWER:** B. Nasopharyngeal carcinoma status post radiation

**COMMENTS AND DISCUSSION**

- This figure demonstrates grouped repetitive discharges of the motor unit action potentials (MUAPs) or grouped fasciculations, compatible with myokymic discharges.
- Myokymic discharges are classically seen in radiation plexopathy/neuropathy, and less commonly in other conditions such as multiple sclerosis, pontine glioma, and Guillain-Barré syndrome, among others (Table 4.4).
- History of Guillain-Barré syndrome 5 years ago, but in complete remission now, is unlikely to show myokymic discharges. Also, this focal finding is unlikely to be due to a genealized neurogenic disorder.

**QUESTION 20.** Which of the following is associated with cramp potentials?
A. Any neuropathic condition
B. Can occur with exercise
C. Endocrine disorders
D. Metabolic disorders
E. All of the above

**ANSWER:** E. All of the above

### COMMENTS AND DISCUSSION
- Cramp potentials (Table 4.2)
  ○ Origin: motor unit/motor neuron or its axon
  ○ Morphology: motor unit action potential (MUAP)
  ○ Stability: tend to be stable
  ○ Firing frequency: irregularly high frequencies (40–75 Hz)
  ○ Clinical implication: can be seen in normal conditions (e.g., nocturnal or post-exercise cramps), or associated with any neuropathic conditions (non-specific). Additionally, they can also be seen in some electrolyte and metabolic disturbances (Table 4.3).

 **HIGH-YIELD FACT**

"Cramps" in metabolic myopathies (e.g., McArdle's disease) are not actually cramp potentials. The painful, involuntary contraction of muscle in a metabolic muscle disease is known as a contracture which is electrically silent on needle EMG.

**QUESTION 21.** Which of the following is characteristic of neuromyotonia?
A. Waxing and waning of frequency
B. Initial frequencies up to 50 Hz
C. Waning of amplitude
D. Frequently seen as a benign phenomenon
E. Generated from a muscle fiber

**ANSWER:** C. Waning of amplitude

### COMMENTS AND DISCUSSION
- Neuromyotonic discharges
  ○ Origin: motor unit/motor neuron or its axon
  ○ Morphology: motor unit action potential (MUAP)
  ○ Stability: unstable decrements (wanes) to a lower amplitude
  ○ Firing frequency: up to 250 Hz initially (highest frequency of all activities) and then decreases (wanes) in frequency
  ○ Sound: pinging sound
  ○ Clinical implication: neuromyotonic discharges have a limited number of differential diagnoses. They can be seen in an autoimmune/paraneoplastic peripheral nerve hyperexcitability syndrome caused by anti–voltage-gated potassium channel (VGKC) complex antibodies including Isaacs and Morvan syndromes. Additionally, they are observed in rare inherited disorders or extremely chronic motor neuron disorders (e.g., adult-onset spinal muscular atrophy) (Table 4.3).

**QUESTION 22.** Which of the following spontaneous discharges originates from a muscle fiber?
A. Endplate spikes
B. Fasciculations
C. Myotonic discharges
D. Myokymic discharges
E. Cramp potentials

**ANSWER:** C. Myotonic discharges

## COMMENTS AND DISCUSSION

- Spontaneous activity can originate from four main locations:
  - Muscle fiber
  - Neuromuscular junction
  - Axon twig
  - Motor neuron/its axon.
- Spontaneous activity that originates from a single muscle fiber include fibrillation potentials, positive sharp waves, and myotonic discharges.
- Complex repetitive discharges originate from multiple muscle fibers.
- Endplate spikes are normal spontaneous activity originating from an axon twig.
- Fasciculations, myokymic discharges, neuromyotonic discharges and cramp potentials originate from a motor neuron or its axon.

**QUESTION 23.** Which of the following waveforms originates from a motor axon?
- A. Endplate noise
- B. Fibrillations
- C. Fasciculations
- D. Myotonic discharges
- E. Complex repetitive discharges

**ANSWER:** C. Fasciculations

## COMMENTS AND DISCUSSION

- Fasciculations, myokymic discharges, cramp potentials, and neuromyotonia originate from motor neuron or its axon.
- Endplate noise is a normal spontaneous activity originating from the neuromuscular junction. It represents miniature endplate potentials (MEPPs).
- Fibrillations and myotonic discharges originate from a single muscle fiber.
- Complex repetitive discharges originate from multiple muscle fibers.

**QUESTION 24.** When assessing voluntary activity during needle electromyography (EMG), which motor unit action potentials (MUAPs) are recruited first?
- A. Small MUAPs; type I fibers
- B. Small MUAPs; type II fibers
- C. Large MUAPs; type I fibers
- D. Large MUAPs; type II fibers
- E. MUAPs closest to the needle

**ANSWER:** A. Small MUAPs type I fibers

## COMMENTS AND DISCUSSION

- Voluntary activity is the second part of the needle EMG examination, where the subject voluntarily contracts the tested muscle and MUAPs are analyzed.
- Several properties of MUAPs follow Henneman's "size principle": small motor units are recruited first, and large motor units are recruited last.
  - There is a wide range of normal motor unit sizes, from small to large.
  - Motor units with different sizes have different depolarization thresholds.
  - Size of the motor neuron positively correlates with:
    - size of the axon
    - thickness of the myelin sheath
    - conduction velocity (CV) of the axon
    - depolarization threshold
    - ratio of type II and type I muscle fibers.
  - Smaller motor neurons have smaller axons with thinner myelin and slower conduction velocities. They innervate type I fibers and have lower depolarization thresholds. Thus they are recruited first.
  - Larger motor neurons have larger axons with thicker myelin and the fastest conduction velocities. They innervate type II fibers and have high depolarization thresholds. Thus they are recruited last.

**HIGH-YIELD FACT**

**Small** motor neurons have smaller axons, which have thinner myelin sheaths, slower CVs, and lower thresholds to depolarize and innervate type I or slow-twitch muscle fibers. Due to their **low threshold,** these small motor neurons and units are **recruited first.**

**Large** motor neurons have larger axons, which have thicker myelin sheaths, faster CVs, and higher thresholds to depolarize and innervate type II or fast-twitch muscle fibers. Due to their **high threshold,** the largest motor neurons and units are recruited last during **maximum contraction.**

 **HIGH-YIELD FACT**

During routine EMG assessment of voluntary activity, the smaller MUAPs from motor neurons innervating type I muscle fibers are prominently present and analyzed.

**QUESTION 25.** Which of the following motor unit action potential (MUAP) parameter is used to indicate the acceptable proximity of the tip of the recording needle electrode to the motor unit being studied?
A. Amplitude
B. Major spike rise time
C. Duration
D. Amplitude
E. Number of phases

**ANSWER:** B. Major spike rise time

**COMMENTS AND DISCUSSION**
- Basics of motor unit action potentials (MUAPs)
  - Recorded MUAPs represent the summation of the extracellular muscle fiber action potentials within a motor unit, which is 1/10 to 1/100 of the actual transmembrane potentials.
  - MUAPs are analyzed to determine the following:
    - Morphology
    - Stability
    - Firing pattern
  - MUAP analysis should be performed when the electromyography (EMG) needle is close to the motor unit, which can be confirmed by:
    - The major spike of the MUAP having a short rise time (<500 μs)
    - The MUAPs sound sharp on the loudspeaker

**QUESTION 26.** Voluntary motor unit action potentials (MUAPs) are assessed routinely for all the following **EXCEPT?**
A. Amplitude
B. Phases
C. Duration
D. Jitter
E. Recruitment

**ANSWER:** D. Jitter

**COMMENTS AND DISCUSSION**
- MUAPs are analyzed routinely for their morphology (duration, amplitude, and phases), stability, and firing characteristic. Jitter is not typically used to assess MUAPs, but rather to evaluate the stability of the neuromuscular junction (NMJ).
  - Morphology (Fig. 4.4)
    - Duration
      - Best parameter that reflects the numbers of muscle fibers within a motor unit
      - Normal duration is 5–15 ms

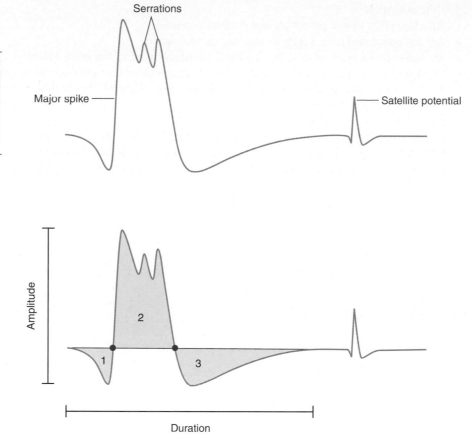

**Fig. 4.4 Motor unit action potential (MUAP) morphology and parameters.** Duration is measured from the point when the potential leaves the baseline to the point when it returns to the baseline. Amplitude is measured from the point of the most downward deflection to the point of the most upward deflection. Phases are measured by counting the points where the waveform crosses baseline and adding 1. The waveform in this figure has three phases. Serrations refer to changes in direction that do not cross the baseline, and these are not counted as additional phases. Satellite potentials are small spikes, following the major waveform with a fixed duration. The satellite potential is a muscle fiber action potential (MFAP) from collateral spouting, representing ongoing reinnervation. From Preston DC, Shapiro BE. *Electromyography and Neuromuscular Disorders*. 4th ed. Philadelphia, PA: Elsevier; 2020;15:248.

- Measured from the initial deflection from baseline to the final return
- Most reliable parameter of MUAP size
- Amplitude
  - Reflects primarily the muscle fibers that are closest to the EMG needle
  - Normal amplitude ranges between 100 μV to 2 mV, depending on the muscle
  - Measured from peak to peak
  - Not as a reliable parameter for assessing the size of MUAP size as compared to duration, since amplitude can be affected by several factors, such as the distance between the needle and the motor unit, the number and diameter of muscle fibers in the motor unit, and the degree of synchronization in the firing of muscle fibers.
- Phases
  - Reflects synchrony of muscle fibers (i.e., are muscle fibers within the MUAP firing more or less at the same time?)
  - Number of phases can be calculated by counting the number of baseline crossings and adding 1.
  - Normal MUAPs have two to four phases.
  - Polyphasia is nonspecific and can be seen in 5%–10% of most normal muscles. It can be increased in both neurogenic and myopathic conditions.
- Serrations
  - Also known as turns
  - Similar meaning to that of polyphasia (less-synchronous firing of muscle fibers in an MUAP), but the change in direction does not cross the baseline, unlike polyphasia where it does

- Satellite potentials
  - Also known as linked potentials and parasite potentials
  - Are abnormal and reflect early or ongoing reinnervation
  - Recognized as a brief spike(s) that trail and are time-linked to the main MUAP
  - Represent action potentials of muscle fiber(s) reinnervated by newly formed collateral axonal sprouts of the intact motor units. Because the collateral fiber is new and immature, and mostly unmyelinated, the conduction velocity is slow, resulting in the reinnervated muscle fiber(s) firing later than the main MUAP.
  - Often unstable because the NMJ on the reinnervated muscle fiber is also new and immature. When the sprouts become larger and more myelinated over time, the satellite potentials move closer to the main MUAPs, and eventually are incorporated into the main MUAP as a new phase.

 **KEY POINTS**

> **Duration** best reflects the **Number** of muscle fibers within a motor unit. The sound correlates with **pitch** (long durations are dull and thuddy, short durations are crisp and static-like).
>
> **Amplitude** best reflects the number of the **Nearby** muscle fibers within a motor unit. The sound correlates with **volume**.
>
> **Phases** reflects the **Synchrony** of the muscle fibers firing within a motor unit. Increased polyphasia has a sharp clicking sound.

◎ **HIGH-YIELD FACT**

> Among all parameters of the MUAP morphology, duration is the most reliable in assessement of the MUAP size.

- Stability
  - MUAPs are normally stable and have consistent morphology from one potential to another. This occurs because all muscle fibers under the same motor unit fire every time because of the safety factor of the NMJ (i.e., there are always sufficient quanta released to ensure that threshold is reached).
  - MUAPs that are unstable (change in morphology from one potential to another) means there are unstable NMJs.
  - Unstable NMJs are seen in:
    - primary NMJ disorders (e.g., myasthenia gravis).
    - any denervating process with early reinnervation (and new immature NMJ junctions). Although this is most often seen in neuropathic disorders, it is also seen as a secondary phenomenon in myopathies with segmental denervation of muscle (i.e., inflammatory, necrotic, and some toxic myopathies).
- Firing pattern
  - The most challenging aspect of the needle exam for the electromyographer
  - Normal motor units fire semi-rhythmically (almost, but not quite regular).
  - Under voluntary control, normal motor units begin firing at a frequency of 4–5 Hz.
  - Because the goal of motor unit firing is to create force, there are two ways to increase force:
    - Recruitment: there is firing of more motor units.
    - Activation: The motor units fire at a faster rate.

- Normally both recruitment and activation occur as more force is needed.
  - An increase in the number of MUAPs results in firing of more muscle fibers and generation of greater force.

 **HIGH-YIELD FACT**

| | | |
|---|---|---|
| Activation | = | ability to increase the firing rate |
| Recruitment | = | ability to increase the number of motor units |

- Firing MUAPs at a faster rate results in increased overlap and cross-bridging of actin and myosin within individual myofibrils, leading to generation of greater force.
- When a patient is first asked to contract the muscle:
  - Small MUAPs (type I muscle fibers) fire first at a rate of 4–5 Hz.
  - Voluntary motor unit cannot fire slower than 4-5 Hz.
  - As more force is required, this first MUAP fires faster. Once it reaches a rate of 10 Hz, the second MUAP is recruited. Once the second MUAP fires at a rate of 15 Hz, the third MUAP is recruited.
  - Maximum firing frequency of most muscles is 30–50 Hz.
- In neurogenic conditions where MUAPs are lost, an increased firing rate of the remaining MUAPs is required to compensate for the loss of force generation, resulting in a higher ratio of firing frequency per the number of MUAP). This is known as reduced recruitment.
- In myopathic conditions, there is normally no loss of motor units, but rather a loss of muscle fibers within a motor unit. Thus myopathic MUAPs have decreased number of muscle fibers firing in a motor unit. When a myopathic MUAP fires, it generates less force, requiring a larger number of motor units to fire simulatneously to generate an equivalent amount of force.
- Recruitment ratio does not change: at each firing frequency, the numbers of motor units recruited are still appropriate (5:1 ratio).
- Compared to the normal muscle, more motor units are recruited to generate the same force.
  - This is referred to as "early recruitment," meaning an inappropriately large number of MUAPs are needed to fire to generate a small amount of force.
- Decreased or poor activation is different from reduced recruitment.
  - When activation is poor, there is reduced firing frequency. However, the recruitment ratio remains normal (5:1).
  - Decreased activation is due to a central process, which includes:
    - Structural disorders of the brain or spinal cord
    - Functional weakness
    - Pain
    - Poor cooperation
    - Malingering

 **HIGH-YIELD FACT**

The ratio of firing frequency to the number of motor units firing is ~5:1.

- Interference pattern
  - Assessed while the subject is fully contracting the tested muscle
  - Complete interference pattern is when a large number of MUAPs fire simultaneously, resulting in the entire screen being filled and individual MUAPs being indistinguishable.
  - An incomplete interference pattern can be due to reduced recruitment or decreased activation (Fig. 4.5).

100 μV

80 ms

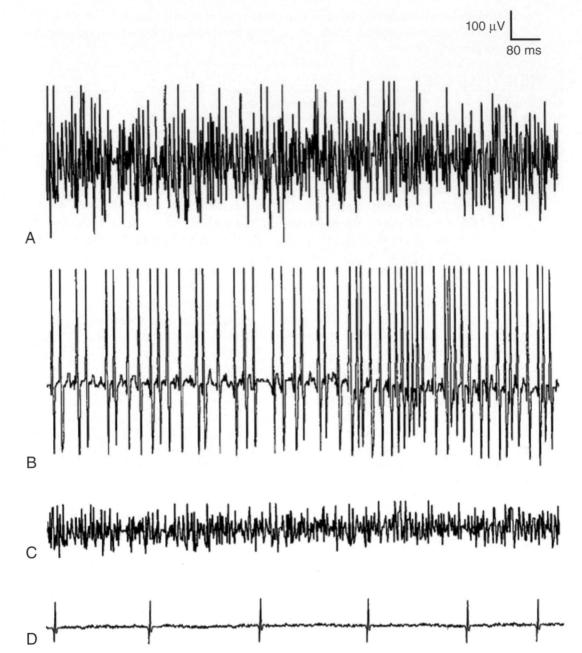

**Fig. 4.5 Interference patterns in different conditions.** The interference pattern is assessed when the tested muscle is fully contracted. A. Normal interference pattern. There are a combination of multiple motor unit action potentials (MUAPs) that cannot be distinguished individually. B. Incomplete interference pattern in neurogenic conditions. Only a single, large MUAP is recruited firing at high frequency, known as "the picket fence" pattern. C. Interference pattern in myopathy. Interference is complete; however, MUAPs appear small and polyphasic, due to the need for many MUAPs to fire to generate even a small amount of force. D. Incomplete interference pattern due to poor activation. A single, normal MUAP fires at a low frequency. This is found in individuals with central disorders, pain, or poor cooperation. From Preston DC, Shapiro BE. *Electromyography and Neuromuscular Disorders*. 4th ed. Philadelphia, PA: Elsevier; 2020;15:253.

**QUESTION 27.** A 65-year-old man presents for evaluation of right leg weakness. When the patient is asked to contract one of the weak muscles during needle electromyography (EMG) testing, you find motor unit action potentials (MUAPs), as shown in the following figure. What is the most likely time course of the weakness in this patient?

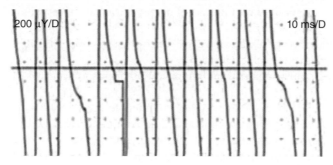

200 μV/D                                                                              10 ms/D

From Preston DC, Shapiro BE. Electromyography and Neuromuscular Disorders: Clinical-electrophysiologic-ultrasound Correlations. 4th ed. Philadelphia, PA: Elsevier; 2020:240.

 A. 1 hour
 B. 1 day
 C. 1 week
 D. 1 month
 E. 1 year

**ANSWER:** E. 1 year

**COMMENTS AND DISCUSSION**
- This figure demonstrates one MUAP with a very long duration and very large amplitude (exceeding the screen) (Table 4.5).
- The MUAPs recorded in this screen have the same morphology indicating generation from the same motor unit.
- The firing frequency is 50 Hz (10 MUAPs in 200 ms; therefore there are 50 MUAPs in 1000 ms or 1 s).
- If recruitment is normal, we would expect to see 10 different motor units. However, there is only one single motor unit in this recording.
- The recruitment is markedly reduced recruitment, indicative of chronic reinnervation.
- Large amplitude MUAPs represent chronicity, approximately more than 6 months.
- In hyperacute denervation, there is no change in motor unit morphology, but recruitment is reduced.
- In subacute denervation, the morphology of motor unit can be normal or show evidence of ongoing/immature reinnervation, including polyphasic and satellite potentials, and later, longer and higher MUAPs.

**TABLE 4.5** Parameters and sound in neurogenic and myopathic motor unit action potentials (MUAPs).

| Pathology | Duration | Pitch | Amplitude | Volume |
|---|---|---|---|---|
| Neurogenic MUAPs | Long | Dull and thuddy | Large | Loud |
| Myopathic MUAPs | Short | Crisp and static-like | Small | Soft |

**QUESTION 28.** Which of the following is **NOT** expected in a subacute (e.g., 4-week) axonal loss lesion?
 A. Reduced compound muscle action potential (CMAP) amplitude
 B. Reduced sensory nerve action potential (SNAP) amplitude
 C. Fibrillation potentials
 D. Large motor unit action potentials (MUAPs)
 E. Reduced recruitment

**ANSWER:** D. Large MUAPs

**COMMENTS AND DISCUSSION**

- Axonal pathology
  - Wallerian degeneration occurs from day 3 through day 11, initially affecting motor nerves before sensory nerves, resulting in reduced CMAP and SNAP amplitudes.
  - Spontaneous activity (fibrillation potentials and positive sharp waves) occurs 2–4 weeks after injury, depending on the distance between the site of nerve injury and the tested muscles. Muscles closer to the site of injury denervate first.
  - MUAP typically morphology remains normal in the early stages of nerve injury, and only the recruitment pattern is abnormally reduced.
  - MUAP morphology only changes when reinnervation begins to occur which can take several weeks to months.
    - Nascent and satellite units are signs of early reinnervation.
    - Reinnervation results in long duration and large-amplitude MUAPs, often accompanied by prominent polyphasia particularly in the initial stages (Table 4.6).
  - When reinnervation is complete, denervation potentials (i.e., fibrillation potentials and positive sharp waves) disappear, leaving only large and long MUAPs with reduced recruitment.

**TABLE 4.6** Motor unit action potential (MUAP) morphology in typical chronic neurogenic and myopathic conditions.

| Parameter | Neurogenic (chronic) | Myopathic |
|-----------|----------------------|-----------|
| Duration | Long | Short |
| Amplitude | Large | Small |
| Phases | Polyphasic (with early or ongoing reinnervation) Normal (chronic reinnervation) | Polyphasic |
| Recruitment | Reduced | Early |
| Activation | Normal | Normal |

 **HIGH-YIELD FACT**

Signs of active denervation (fibrillation potentials and positive sharp waves) appear 2-4 weeks after injury.

 **HIGH-YIELD FACT**

The **earliest MUAP finding** on needle EMG in neurogenic conditions is **reduced recruitment**.

**QUESTION 29.** In a case of pure focal demyelination of a peripheral nerve containing motor and sensory fibers, which of the following is expected?
- A. Reduced compound muscle action potential (CMAP) amplitude recording distal to the lesion
- B. Reduced sensory nerve action potential (SNAP) amplitude recording distal to the lesion
- C. Fibrillation potentials in muscles supplied by the nerve, provided 4 weeks has passed
- D. Large motor unit action potentials (MUAPs)
- E. Reduced recruitment, if conduction block is present

**ANSWER:** E. Reduced recruitment, if conduction block is present

**COMMENTS AND DISCUSSION**

- In pure demyelination
  - No abnormal spontaneous activity is seen, since only the myelin sheath is affected, and the underlying axon remains normal.
  - CMAP and SNAP amplitudes are normal when stimulating distal to the lesion, but reduced when stimulating above the lesion, provided a conduction block is present.

- ◦ MUAP morphology is normal, as there is no denervation or reinnervation.
- ◦ With conduction slowing alone, recruitment remains normal.
- ◦ With conduction block, recruitment is reduced.
  - • However, in clinical practice, there is often some secondary axonal loss after demyelination.
  - • Pure demyelination without axonal loss is uncommon.

 **HIGH-YIELD FACT**

In pure demyelination, only reduced recruitment pattern is seen on needle EMG provided conduction block is present.

**QUESTION 30.** In a case of a subacute inflammatory myopathy, which of the following is expected?
- A. Fibrillation potentials
- B. Reduced compound muscle action potential (CMAP) amplitude
- C. Reduced sensory nerve action potential (SNAP) amplitude
- D. Reduced recruitment of small, short, polyphasic motor unit action potentials (MUAPs)
- E. Large MUAPs

**ANSWER:** A. Fibrillation potentials

**COMMENTS AND DISCUSSION**
- • Myopathic abnormalities
  - ◦ SNAPs are always normal in isolated myopathies.
  - ◦ CMAP amplitudes are generally normal, as myopathies often affect proximal muscles, and it is the distal muscles that are assessed in routine motor conduction studies (n.b., in a distal myopathy or severe generalized myopathy, CMAP amplitudes will be reduced).
  - ◦ The number of functioning muscle fibers within a motor unit decreases but the number of motor units remains normal.
  - ◦ Due to the loss of muscle fibers, MUAPs are smaller in size, characterized by shorter duration and smaller amplitude (Table 4.6).
  - ◦ Recruitment is normal, or early in terms of the number of MUAPs needed to generate a small amount of force.
    - • Early recruitment can only be identified by the electromyographer performing the test, since it requires knowledge of the amount of force generated the patient during muscle contraction.
    - • Early recruitment cannot be assessed through the ratio of firing frequency and motor units displayed on the computer screen.
  - ◦ Fibrillation potentials usually indicate a neuropathic process, but can also be seen in several myopathic disorders, especially those that are inflammatory, necrotic, dystrophic, or toxic.

 **HIGH-YIELD FACT**

In myopathic changes, early recruitment is seen, **NOT** increased recruitment, since the number of motor units is constant.

**FURTHER READINGS**

1. Preston DC, Shapiro BE. *Electromyography and Neuromuscular Disorders.* Philadelphia, PA: Elsevier. 2020.4th ed..
2. Katirji B Electromyography in Clinical Practice. Oxford University Press; 2018. 3th ed..
3. Rubin DI. Needle electromyography: basic concepts and patterns of abnormalities. Neurol Clin. 2012 May;30(2): 429–456.
4. Daube JR, Rubin DI. Needle electromyography. Muscle Nerve. 2009 Feb;39(2):244-70.

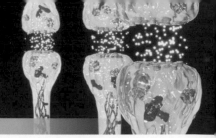

# CHAPTER 5

# Electrodiagnostic Medicine III: Late Responses

## PART 1 | PRACTICE TEST

**Q1.** Which of the following statements is **CORRECT** regarding F responses?
A. The afferent pathway is sensory nerve; the efferent pathway is motor nerve
B. The afferent pathway is sensory nerve; the efferent pathway is sensory nerve
C. The afferent pathway is motor nerve; the efferent pathway is sensory nerve
D. The afferent pathway is motor nerve; the efferent pathway is motor nerve

**Q2.** Abnormal F responses are most useful in which of the following condition?
A. Pathognomonic finding of polyneuropathy
B. Early active denervation
C. Reinnervation
D. Guillain-Barré syndrome
E. Radiculopathy

**Q3.** In normal individuals, F response can be impersistent or absent in which of the following nerves?
A. Median
B. Ulnar
C. Radial
D. Peroneal
E. Tibial

**Q4.** Which of the following statements is **CORRECT** regarding the F response?
A. F estimate is normally shorter than the shortest recorded F-wave latency.
B. F response is a true reflex arc.
C. F response originates from backfiring of motor neurons in the spinal cord through the sensory nerve.
D. F response can be performed in any motor nerve.
E. F response is absent in individuals with absent ankle jerks.

**Q5.** Which of the following factors **MOST LIKELY** affects F-wave latency?
A. Gender
B. Height
C. Weight
D. Ethnicity
E. Muscle mass

**Q6.** Which of the following F wave measurements is most commonly used in clinical practice?
A. Maximal F-wave amplitude
B. Average F-wave duration
C. Minimal F-wave latency
D. Maximal area
E. Mean F-wave latency

**Q7.** Which of the following statements is **CORRECT** regarding the H reflex?
A. It can be acquired only from the tibial nerve.
B. It is best evoked with long stimulus duration (1 ms).
C. It is best obtained with supramaximal stimulation.
D. It is not a true reflex arc.
E. Afferent pathway travels through the motor nerve.

**Q8.** Submaximal stimulation is used in which of the following studies?
A. Motor study
B. Sensory study
C. F response study
D. H-reflex study

**Q9.** Which of the following findings is common in polyneuropathy?
A. Normal F response in the tibial nerve
B. Minimal tibial F-wave latency shorter than F estimate
C. Absent A wave in the tibial nerve
D. M wave preceding H wave
E. Absent H reflex

**Q10.** In the figure below, what is the waveform B?

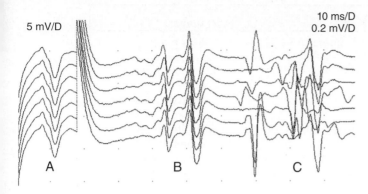

5 mV/D

10 ms/D
0.2 mV/D

A          B          C

From Katirji B. *Electromyography in Clinical Practice*. 3rd ed. Oxford University Press; 2018.

A. M wave
B. F wave
C. A wave
D. H wave
E. None of above

**Q11.** You perform a median F response study on a patient with numbness of the left thumb and index fingers for 2 weeks. You find A waves. Which of the following statements is **CORRECT**?
A. A wave is normally present in a median study.
B. This finding is consistent with the 2-week history.
C. A-wave latency measurement is required to determine the abnormality.
D. A wave merely indicates pathology in the left median nerve.
E. This patient has Guillain-Barré syndrome.

**Q12.** Which of the following statements is **CORRECT** regarding late responses?
A. H reflex can be performed only in the tibial nerve.
B. Minimal F-wave latency must be normal in median neuropathy at the wrist.
C. In C5 radiculopathy, median minimal F-wave latency is abnormal.
D. A wave is considered a normal finding if seen on ulnar motor study.
E. Submaximal stimulation is required when performing H-reflex study.

## PART 2 | QUESTIONS WITH ANSWERS AND DISCUSSION

**QUESTION 1.** Which of the following statements is **CORRECT** regarding F responses?
A. The afferent pathway is sensory nerve; the efferent pathway is motor nerve
B. The afferent pathway is sensory nerve; the efferent pathway is sensory nerve
C. The afferent pathway is motor nerve; the efferent pathway is sensory nerve
D. The afferent pathway is motor nerve; the efferent pathway is motor nerve

**ANSWER:** D. The afferent pathway is motor nerve; the efferent pathway is motor nerve

### COMMENTS AND DISCUSSION
- There are three late responses commonly seen in the limbs in clinical practice: F response, H reflex, and A wave (Table 5.1).
- Nerve conduction routinely studies the distal part of peripheral nervous system.
- Due to technical difficulty on stimulating proximal portion of peripheral nerve, plexus, and nerve root, late responses are potentially useful for assessment of very proximal lesions.
- F responses (Table 5.1)
  - Late response of the motor nerve
  - "F" is derived from "foot," when the response was first noticed from intrinsic foot muscles.
  - Pure motor response, seen only in motor nerve conduction study.
  - An electrical impulse from stimulation at the distal motor nerve travels both orthodromically (to the muscle) and antidromically (toward the anterior horn cells). When the antidromic volley arrives at the anterior horn cells, 1%–5% of the anterior horn cells backfire and the electrical impulse then travels down the same motor nerve to the neuromuscular junction and muscle, resulting in a small motor response (F response), which occurs after the motor response (M response).
  - F responses involve motor nerve in both afferent and efferent pathways.
  - If the stimulation point is moved more proximally, the motor latency (M wave or compound muscle action potential [CMAP]) becomes longer, but the F-response latency becomes shorter, reflecting its path is first antidromic.
  - F responses are generated from a different subgroup of 1%–5% of all motor neurons with each stimulus. Thus, there are slight differences in morphology and latency between successive F-wave recordings.
  - Normal values are based on at least 10 stimulations performed to increase the likelihood that some of the fastest motor axons are also included.

**TABLE 5.1**  Three major late responses: F response, H reflex, and A wave

|  | F Response | H reflex | A wave |
|---|---|---|---|
| **Afferent** | Motor axon | Ia sensory fibers (muscle spindle) | Motor axon |
| **Efferent** | Same motor axon as afferent | Motor axon | Motor axon that sprouts from the main motor axon |
| **Synapse** | No | Yes | No |
| **Mechanism** | Backfiring of motor neurons | Sensorimotor reflex loop | Sprouting of motor axons during reinnervation |
| **Nerves studied** | All motor nerves | Tibial-soleus (occasionally performed in median-FCR, femoral-quadriceps) | All motor nerves |
| **Dromicity (from the stimulus)** | Antidromic | Orthodromic | Antidromic |
| **Stimulation** | Supramaximal | Submaximal, long-duration pulse (1 ms) | Submaximal (may go away with supramaximal) |
| **Configuration** | Usually polyphasic Amplitude 1%–5% of CMAP morphology that varies with each simulation | Triphasic and stable Latency may shorten when H amplitude is growing. Present first with low-intensity stimulations, and larger with increased intensity. When M wave present, H wave becomes smaller. When M wave reaches its maximum, H wave decreases and then disappears. | Uniform and stable Same latency of all A waves When superimposed on all tracings, all A waves are perfectly on top of each other |
| **Measurements** | Minimal latency Chronodispersion Persistency | Minimal latency H/M ratio | Present or absent |
| **Major clinical utilities** | Early Guillain-Barré syndrome Polyneuropathy Internal control (entrapment neuropathy) | Early polyneuropathy S1 radiculopathy Early Guillain-Barré syndrome Tibial and sciatic neuropathy, sacral plexopathy | If present, indicative of reinnervation Early Guillain-Barré syndrome |

Adapted from Preston DC, Shapiro BE. *Electromyography and Neuromuscular Disorders: Clinical-electrophysiologic-ultrasound Correlations.* 4th ed. Elsevier; 2021:41; and Katirji B. *Electromyography in Clinical Practice.* 3rd ed. Oxford University Press; 2018:40.

- F response is *not* a true reflex (as there is no synapse).
- Most useful in assessing the integrity of the proximal nerve, plexus, and nerve root when routine motor conduction study is normal
- Measurements of F responses include the minimal (i.e., shortest) latency, persistency, and chronodispersion.
- The most commonly used parameter is minimal (i.e., shortest) latency.
- Performing the F-wave study (Fig. 5.1)
  - Setup is similar to that for motor nerve study.
  - The sweep and sensitivity require adjustment from that used in regular motor studies since F-wave amplitude is very small compared to the CMAP and has a much longer latency.
  - Sensitivity is decreased from 2–5 mV to 200–500 μV.
  - Sweep can be adjusted to 5–10 ms for the arm and 10–20 ms for the leg.
  - Ten stimulations are given with the rate less than 0.5 Hz (one stimulation every 2 s), to avoid collision from the previous stimulation and reduce pain.
  - If the F response is absent at rest, Jendrassik maneuver (e.g., making a fist or clenching teeth during each stimulation) may elicit the response. However, do not perform the Jendrassik maneuver unless the responses are absent or impersistent, as it can paradoxically make normal F responses more difficult to elicit.

**HIGH-YIELD FACT**

The F response is a response from a subpopulation of motor neurons (i.e., anterior horn cells) that backfires from the antidromic impulses, running down to the same motor axon; therefore, it is a pure motor response.

◎ **HIGH-YIELD FACT**

The F response is generated by only 1%–5% of all motor neurons or motor units, and a different 1%–5% are recorded each time.

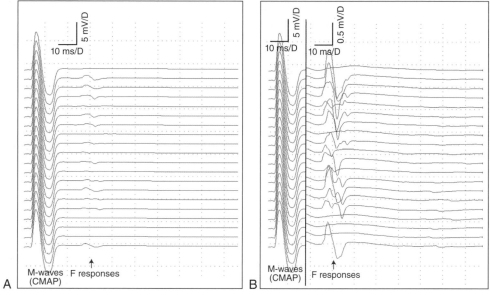

**Fig. 5.1 Setup for F responses is similar to when acquiring motor responses, but appropriate screen setting is required to enhance F response visualization.** (A) Median F responses following motor responses (M responses, compound muscle action potential [CMAP]) with a sweep of 5 mV/division (D) and 10 ms/D. F responses are much smaller than M waves and are easily missed. (B) Appropriate setting for the same median F responses as waveform A. The split screen with different sweeps is used to enhance F responses. On the left side of the screen, gain and sweep setting are 5 mV/D and 10 ms/D. On the right side, gain and sweep setting are changed to 0.5 mV/D and 10 ms/D. Note that F-response morphology and latency change from stimulation to stimulation.

**QUESTION 2.** Abnormal F responses are most useful in which of the following condition?
  A. Pathognomonic finding of polyneuropathy
  B. Early active denervation
  C. Reinnervation
  D. Guillain-Barré syndrome
  E. Radiculopathy

**ANSWER:** D. Guillain-Barré syndrome

**COMMENTS AND DISCUSSION**
- F responses are useful in the diagnosis of early Guillain-Barré syndrome (GBS), where they are often the first abnormality seen (Table 5.2). Otherwise, motor nerve conduction findings are often normal in GBS during the first few days.
- When the distal conductions are normal, F responses are useful to detect proximal lesions including the nerve roots. However, because all muscles are supplied by two or more myotomes, it is very unusual to see F-wave abnormalities with a single root lesion. In multiple root lesions (i.e., polyradiculopathy), F responses may be abnormal when recording from a muscle supplied by those nerve roots as occurs in early GBS (as GBS often starts as a polyradiculopathy).
- F responses are also useful for confirming abnormalities on motor studies. For example, in polyneuropathy, the F response should be abnormal if the motor study is abnormal, and likewise for distal entrapment neuropathies. However, the diagnosis of polyneuropathy and entrapment neuropathy should NOT be made solely from abnormal F responses.

**TABLE 5.2** Utility and caveats of F response in clinical practice

| Utility | Caveats |
|---|---|
| Helpful in early Guillain-Barré syndrome (GBS) when other parameters on nerve conduction studies (NCS) have not yet become abnormal<br>Serves as a good internal control for polyneuropathy and distal entrapment neuropathy | Nonspecific and nonlocalizable<br>Abnormal F response occurs when there is pathology in any segments of the motor nerve<br>Persistency is different on each nerve<br>May be absent in sedated subject<br>Painful procedure and less well tolerated compared to routine NCS, since at least 10 consecutive stimulations are required |

- F responses are not a sign of active denervation or reinnervation.
- F-wave measurements
  - Shortest or minimal F-response latency (Fig. 5.2).
    - Most commonly used parameter in clinical practice
    - Represents the fastest fibers
    - Normally, minimal F-response latency is 32 ms in the upper extremity and 56 ms in the lower extremity.
  - Persistence
    - Defined by the number of F waves recorded per the total number of stimuli (calculated as a percentage).
    - Approximately 50% in most nerves
    - Can be 0% (absent) in the normal peroneal nerve
    - Usually 100% or close to it in the normal tibial nerve
    - Caveat: F-response may be absent in asleep or sedated subjects.
  - F-wave chronodispersion
    - Chronodispersion is the difference between minimal and maximal F-response latency.
    - Normal values are 4 ms in the upper extremity and 6 ms in the lower extremity.

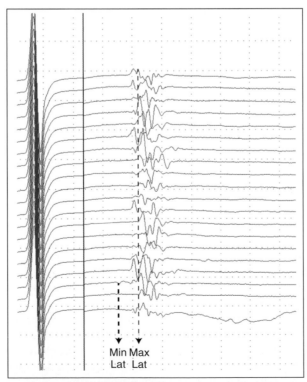

Min Max
Lat Lat

**Fig. 5.2 Minimal and maximal F response latencies.** F responses are obtained from at least 10 stimulations. In the figure, 20 stimulations are given on the tibial nerve. F responses are present with a persistence of 100%. Latency of the F response that is earliest, is marked as minimal F-response latency. Latency of the F-response that is latest is marked as maximal F-response latency. These two values are used in calculation of chronodispersion.

## ◎ HIGH-YIELD FACT

Prolonged, impersistent or absent F responses **are often the earliest electrodiagnostic finding in GBS.**

- F estimate (Fig. 5.3)
  - ○ Calculation of estimated F-response latency is based on the estimated length of the entire nerve (reflecting height and limb length), conduction velocity, and distal latency (Fig. 5.3).
  - ○ If the recorded minimum F-response latency is greater than the F estimate, this reflects that prolonged F response latency is due to a delay in the proximal segment, and cannot simply be due to the patient's height, conduction velocity, or distal latency. Indeed, in normal subjects, the minimum F-response latency is usually shorter than the F estimate.

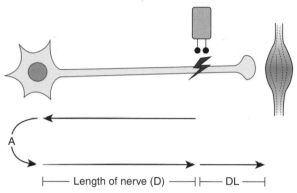

**Fig. 5.3 F estimate calculation.** Distance (*D*) is the length of nerve from this stimulation site to estimated anterior horn cell. Because the impulse for the F travels through the nerve twice, *D* has to be multiplied by 2. *A* is a turn-around time at the anterior horn cells, which has been determined experimentally to be ~1.0 ms., and *DL* is a distal latency from motor conduction study. For the upper extremity F responses, the length of the nerve can be approximated by measuring from the C7 spinous process to the stimulation site at the wrist for the median and ulnar nerves. For the peroneal and tibial nerves, the length can be approximated by measuring from the xiphoid process to the stimulation sites. F estimate can be calculated by using the formula below.

---

**F estimate = (2D/CV) × 10 + 1 ms + DL**

D, Length of the nerve (centimeter); CV, conduction velocity (millimeter/second); 10, conversion to milliseconds; 1 millisecond, turn-around time at anterior horn cells; DL, distal latency (millisecond).

---

**QUESTION 3.** In normal individuals, F response can be impersistent or absent in which of the following nerves?
- A. Median
- B. Ulnar
- C. Radial
- D. Peroneal
- E. Tibial

**ANSWER:** D. Peroneal

### COMMENTS AND DISCUSSION
- Peroneal F responses can be normally impersistent or absent.
- Persistence in other nerves such as the median and ulnar nerves is usually above 50%.
- Persistence in the tibial nerve is very high, typically 80%–100%.

## ◎ HIGH-YIELD FACT

F responses in the peroneal nerve can be absent in normal subjects.

**QUESTION 4.** Which of the following statements is **CORRECT** regarding the F response?
  A.  F estimate is normally shorter than the shortest recorded F-wave latency.
  B.  F response is a true reflex arc.
  C.  F response originates from backfiring of motor neurons in the spinal cord through the sensory nerve.
  D.  F response can be performed in any motor nerve.
  E.  F response is absent in individuals with absent ankle jerks.

**ANSWER:** D. F response can be performed in any motor nerve.

**COMMENTS AND DISCUSSION**
  •  F response is generated from an antidromic impulse from motor nerve stimulation back to anterior horn cells, which then backfires through the same motor nerve.
  •  Given no synapse, F response is not a true reflex arc.
  •  F response can be performed in any motor nerve.
  •  The shortest or minimal F-wave latency is the parameter commonly used, and usually shorter than the F estimate. This is because, in calculation of the F estimate, the measured conduction velocity in the distal limb (elbow to wrist; knee to ankle), which is often slower than that in the proximal limb, is used. The conduction velocity in the proximal part of the nerve is usually faster, due to the larger diameter of the nerve and warmer temperature.
  •  H reflex correlates with clinical examination of the ankle reflex, and is often absent (but not always) in an individual with absent ankle jerk. However, F response examines the integrity of the motor nerve, not the entire reflex arc, and does not always correlate with the ankle jerk.

**QUESTION 5.** Which of the following factors **MOST LIKELY** affects F-wave latency?
  A.  Gender
  B.  Height
  C.  Weight
  D.  Ethnicity
  E.  Muscle mass

**ANSWER:** B. Height

**COMMENTS AND DISCUSSION**
  •  Height correlates with leg and arm length, which influences the F-wave latency. The longer arm or leg length reflects the longer nerve and longer traveling distance for an electrical impulse in the generation of F responses.
  •  Gender, weight, ethnicity, and muscle mass do not affect F-wave latency.

**QUESTION 6.** Which of the following F wave measurements is most commonly used in clinical practice?
  A.  Maximal F-wave amplitude
  B.  Average F-wave duration
  C.  Minimal F-wave latency
  D.  Maximal area
  E.  Mean F-wave latency

**ANSWER:** C. Minimal F latency

**COMMENTS AND DISCUSSION**
  •  The most commonly used parameter for F responses is the minimal F-wave latency, which reflects the fastest nerve fiber.
  •  Other useful F-wave parameters include F-response persistence and F-wave chronodispersion.
  •  F-wave amplitude, duration, and area are usually not used; neither is mean F-wave latency.

**HIGH-YIELD FACT**

When CMAP is absent or has low amplitude, the F response cannot be elicited and should not be tested.

 **HIGH-YIELD FACT**

Abnormal F responses are **nonspecific**, and can reflect slowing in **any segment of the nerve**. DO **NOT** overdiagnose radiculopathy or plexopathy, based on abnormal F response only.

**QUESTION 7.** Which of the following statements is **CORRECT** regarding the H reflex?
   A. It can be acquired only from the tibial nerve.
   B. It is best evoked with long stimulus duration (1 ms).
   C. It is best obtained with supramaximal stimulation.
   D. It is not a true reflex arc.
   E. Afferent pathway travels through the motor nerve.

**ANSWER:** B. It is best evoked with long stimulus duration (1 ms).

**COMMENTS AND DISCUSSION**
- H reflex (Table 5.1)
  - "H" comes from Paul **H**offmann, the first person recognizing this reflex.
  - In contrast to the F response, the H is a true reflex, with an afferent sensory pathway (Ia sensory fiber), a synapse, and an efferent motor pathway.

 **HIGH-YIELD FACT**

| H-reflex circuit | Afferent: | **Ia sensory fibers** |
|---|---|---|
| | Efferent: | **motor fibers** |

- In contrast to motor, sensory, and F responses, in which supramaximal stimulation is used, the H reflex is obtained with *submaximal stimulation* and a long pulse stimulus duration (1 ms).
  - With submaximal sitmulation and a long pulse stimulus duration, the Ia sensory afferent fibers are more selectively stimulated (Fig. 5.4).
  - As the current is slowly increased, the H reflex will be larger.
  - As the current is increased further, the motor fibers will also be stimulated.
    - This results in an M response.
    - Then, the amplitude of H reflex starts to drop, due to collision effect from antidromic impulses from motor fibers.
    - At supramaximal stimulation, the M response is maximal, and the H reflex disappears and is often replaced by the F response.
- The H reflex is tested in only some, not all, peripheral nerves, unlike the F response.
- It is most commonly performed in the tibial nerve recording the gastroc-soleus in adults.
- Occasionally H reflex can be obtained from the median nerve recording the flexor carpi radialis (FCR) and the femoral nerve recording the quadriceps.
- Tibial H reflex correlates with the ankle jerk on clinical examination. If the ankle jerk can be elicited on the clinical examination, the tibial H reflex must be present.
- However, if the ankle jerk cannot be elicited, tibial H reflex can sometimes still be obtained on electrophysiologic studies.

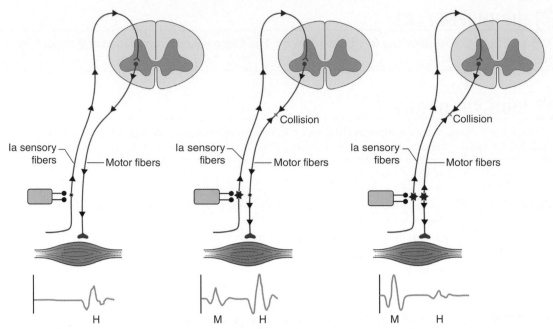

**Fig. 5.4 H reflex circuitry.** H reflex represents a complete reflex arc. The afferent pathway is Ia sensory fibers, and the efferent pathway is motor fibers. With low-intensity stimulation *(left)*, Ia sensory fibers are selectively stimulated, while motor fibers are not. Therefore, only the H reflex is present. When the intensity of the stimulation increases *(middle)*, the motor fibers are partially stimulated, in addition to the Ia sensory fibers. M wave is now present, but has a low amplitude due to submaximal stimulation. H reflex is still present, but there is some collision effect from the antidromic motor volley that travels proximally. When supramaximal stimulation is reached *(right)*, both sensory and motor fibers are stimulated. M wave has a maximal amplitude, whereas H reflex is very small or absent from greater collision effect. From Preston DC, Shapiro BE. *Electromyography and Neuromuscular Disorders: Clinical-electrophysiologic-ultrasound Correlations*. 4th ed. Elsevier; 2021:47.

## ◎ HIGH-YIELD FACT

The H reflex is best acquired with **submaximal stimulation.**

- Common measurements for the H reflex
  - Shortest H latency
    - Normal values depend on the leg length and the height of the patient (Fig. 5.5).
    - The contralateral side (performing at similar length or location) can also be used as an internal normal reference.
  - H/M ratio
    - Ratio of the maximal H amplitude divided by the maximal M amplitude
    - Reflects anterior horn cell excitability
    - Normal H/M ratio is ≤50%
    - H/M ratio is usually increased in upper motor neuron lesions.
- Obtaining H reflex
  - Duration of the stimulation pulse needs to be adjusted to 1 ms.
  - Stimulate tibial nerve in the popliteal fossa.
  - Record gastrocnemius (~2 fingerbreadths below mid-calf).
  - Start with low intensity until the H reflex appears; then stimulate on a rastered trace.
  - Slowly increase the stimulation intensity until the H reflex reaches its maximum.

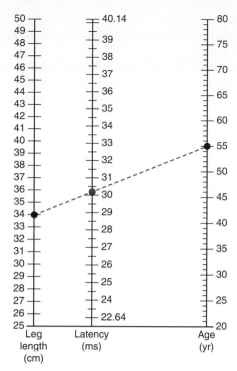

**Fig. 5.5 Shortest H latency normal values.** H latency normal values based on subject's leg length and age. Adapted with permission from Braddom, R.I., Johnson, E.W., 1974. Standardization of the H-reflex and diagnostic use in S1 radiculopathy. *Arch Phys Med Rehabil* 55, 161.

- ○ When the stimulation intensity is at the adequate level, the M response starts to appear.
- ○ When the amplitude of the M response is increasing with the higher stimulus intensity, the H reflex becomes smaller.
- ○ When the M response is maximum, H reflex becomes smaller and disappears.

**QUESTION 8.** Submaximal stimulation is used in which of the following studies?
A. Motor study
B. Sensory study
C. F response study
D. H-reflex study

**ANSWER:** D. H-reflex study

**COMMENTS AND DISCUSSION**
- H reflex is the only study in which submaximal stimulation is purposedly used.
- Submaximal stimulation along with a long stimulus pulse can selectively stimulate the Ia sensory afferent fibers (the sensory afferent limb of the H reflex).
- All other studies are performed with supramaximal stimulation to ensure that all fibers have been stimulated.

**QUESTION 9.** Which of the following findings are common in polyneuropathy?
A. Normal F response in the tibial nerve
B. Minimal tibial F-wave latency shorter than F estimate
C. Absent A wave in the tibial nerve
D. M wave preceding H wave
E. Absent H reflex

**ANSWER:** E. Absent H reflex

**COMMENTS AND DISCUSSION**

- In polyneuropathy, F responses in the lower extremities are often abnormal, prolonged, impersistent, or absent.
- Similarly, H reflex is also expected to be abnormal. Indeed, the two most important clinical utilities of the H reflex are for detecting S1 radiculopathy and early polyneuropathy.
- In normal nerves, minimal F-wave latency should be shorter than F estimate.
- A waves can be present in polyneuropathy, but are infrequently encountered in the EMG lab.
- On H reflex study, the M response normally appears before the H reflex.

**QUESTION 10.** In the figure below, what is the waveform B?

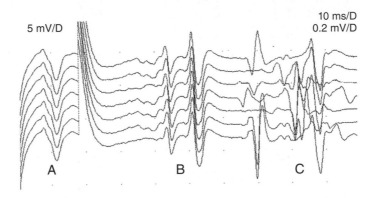

From Katirji B. *Electromyography in Clinical Practice.* 3rd ed. Oxford University Press; 2018.

A. M wave
B. F wave
C. A wave
D. H wave
E. None of above

**ANSWER:** C. A wave

**COMMENTS AND DISCUSSION**

- Waveform A: M wave. Waveform is the largest and appears first.
- Waveform B: A waves. Note the waveforms are stable and all responses look identical.
- Waveform C: F waves. Note that F responses have variable morphology and latency.
- Axon reflex A wave) (Table 5.1).
  - Not a true reflex
  - Present occasionally during the F-wave recording
  - Appears after the M waves but before the F waves
  - Has a uniform morphology with the same latency
  - All A waves can perfectly be superimposed on each other, **unlike** F responses.
  - A wave originates from an antidromic impulse that travels up an axon to a branching point, and then travels down orthodromically to the muscle fibers reinnervated by that axon sprout. Reinnervation by sprouting of the axon results in the proximal axonal branching (Fig. 5.6).
  - A wave represents evidence of reinnervation, but can also be visualized in early Guillain-Barré syndrome within several days from the onset due to resulting from ephaptic transmission between demyelinated axons.

**MNEMONICS**

**MAF: M** wave first, then the **A** wave, then the **F** responses

**MNEMONIC**

All **A** waves are the s**A**me, but **F** responses are di**FF**erent.

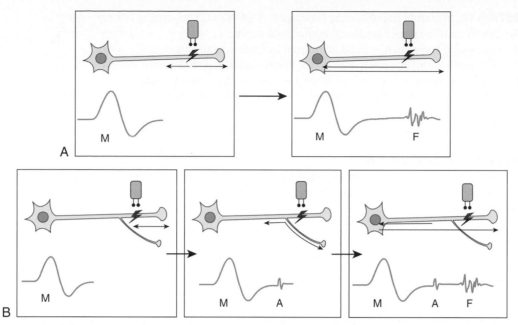

**Fig. 5.6 Pathway of M and F waves in normal nerve compared to M, A, and F waves in a reinnervated nerve.** (A) When the distal site of the normal nerve is stimulated, the impulse runs both orthodromically and antidromically. The orthodromic impulse arrives at the neuromuscular junction (NMJ), and activates the muscle, resulting in an M-wave. The antidromic impulse takes more time to travel up to the anterior horn cell, which then backfires and send the electrical activity along the nerve to the NMJ and the muscle, resulting in an F-wave. (B) When the distal site of the nerve with reinnervation (the axon sprout with a smaller diameter shown), the impulse also travels both orthodromically and antidromically. The orthodromic impulse arrives first due to the shorter distance and activates the muscle, resulting in an M wave. The antidromic impulse travels toward the anterior horn cell and also along the reinnervating axon that sprouts from the main nerve proximal to the stimulation site. The impulse travels along the sprouting branch and activates the reinnervated muscle fibers, resulting in an A wave. The other antidromic impulse reaches the anterior horn cell, which then backfires the electrical activity to the NMJ and the muscle, resulting in an F wave. Adapted from Preston DC, Shapiro BE. *Electromyography and Neuromuscular Disorders: Clinical-electrophysiologic-ultrasound Correlations.* 4th ed. Elsevier; 2021.

**QUESTION 11.** You perform a median F response study on a patient with numbness of the left thumb and index fingers for 2 weeks. You find A waves. Which of the following statements is **CORRECT**?
  A. A wave is normally present in a median study.
  B. This finding is consistent with the 2-week history.
  C. A-wave latency measurement is required to determine the abnormality.
  D. A wave merely indicates pathology in the left median nerve.
  E. This patient has Guillain-Barré syndrome.

**ANSWER:** D. A wave merely indicates pathology in the left median nerve.

**COMMENTS AND DISCUSSION**
• This patient has numbness in the left median nerve distribution.
• The presence of A waves in the median study is abnormal and likely denotes reinnervation.
• Reinnervation follows denervation, and typically takes many weeks to months. Thus the patient likely has an underlying subclinical pathology for much longer than 2 weeks.
• A-wave latency is not used to indicate abnormalities; only its presence is sufficient.
• Although A waves are common in Guillain-Barré syndrome, isolated numbness in the left median distribution and presence of A wave in one median study is not consistent with the diagnosis of Guillain-Barré syndrome.

**QUESTION 12.** Which of the following statements is **CORRECT** regarding late responses?
A. H reflex can be performed only in the tibial nerve.
B. Minimal F-wave latency must be normal in median neuropathy at the wrist.
C. In C5 radiculopathy, median minimal F-wave latency is abnormal.
D. A wave is considered a normal finding if seen on ulnar motor study.
E. Submaximal stimulation is required when performing H-reflex study.

**ANSWER:** E. Submaximal stimulation is required when performing H-reflex study.

### COMMENTS AND DISCUSSION

- H reflex is obtained with the submaximal stimulation. When the stimulation intensity is higher, motor response (M wave) becomes larger, and H reflex becomes smaller and eventually disappears at supramaximal stimulation.
- H reflex can be performed in nerves other than the tibial nerve such as the median nerve (recording the flexor carpi radialis).
- In median neuropathy at the wrist, minimal F-wave latency (stimulating the median nerve and recording the abductor pollicis brevis muscle) can be abnormal, since an electrical impulse also travels through the abnormal segment.
- On the median motor study, the recording electrode is on the abductor pollicis brevis muscle, which is supplied by the C8 and T1 nerve roots, not the C5. In C5 radiculopathy, median minimal F-wave latency should be normal.
- A waves originate from sprouting axons, and thus indicate reinnervation. The presence of A waves on the ulnar motor study is considered abnormal. Rarely, A waves can be seen in the tibial motor nerve in the absence of any pathology for unclear reasons.

 **HIGH-YIELD FACT**

A wave is usually seen in reinnervated nerve.

### SUGGESTED READINGS

Bischoff C. Neurography: Late responses. *Muscle Nerve.* 2002;25:S59–S65.

Fisher MA. H reflex and F waves. Fundamentals, normal and abnormal patterns. *Neurol Clin N Am.* 2002:20; 339–360.

Katirji B, ed. *Electromyography in Clinical Practice.* 3rd ed. New York, NY: Oxford University Press; 2018.

Kornhuber ME, Bischoff C, Mentrup H, Conrad B. Multiple A Waves in Guillain-Barre Syndrome. *Muscle Nerve.* 1999;22:394–399.

Preston DC, Shapiro BE, eds. *Electromyography and Neuromuscular Disorders: Clinical-electrophysiologic-ultrasound Correlations.* 4th ed. Elsevier; 2021.

Rowen J, Meriggioli MN. Electrodiagnostic significance of supramaximally stimulated A-waves. *Muscle Nerve.* 2000;23:1117–1120.

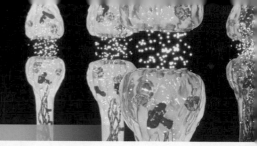

# CHAPTER 6

# Electrodiagnostic Medicine IV: Interpretation

**Q1.** Which of the following statements is **CORRECT** regarding electromyography (EMG) interpretation?
- A. EMG study should be performed without clinical information to avoid bias.
- B. Axonal loss can be identified on nerve conduction studies.
- C. Demyelinating features are mainly identified on needle EMG.
- D. EMG study is not useful in determining the prognosis of the condition.
- E. Nerve conduction study can often be performed in isolation without needle EMG.

**Q2.** Which of the following electrophysiologic findings indicate demyelination?
- A. Prolonged distal motor latency, 150% of the upper normal limit
- B. Slowed conduction velocity, 90% of the lower normal limit
- C. Reduced distal and proximal compound muscle action potential (CMAP) amplitudes, 25% of the lower normal limit
- D. A 15% drop in CMAP amplitude at the proximal stimulation site, compared to distal stimulation
- E. Temporal dispersion on sensory studies when stimulating at a proximal site

**Q3.** Demyelinating features on nerve conduction studies may be seen in which of the following conditions?
- A. Diabetic polyneuropathy
- B. Charcot-Marie-Tooth type 2
- C. Cisplatin-induced polyneuropathy
- D. Mononeuritis multiplex
- E. Multifocal motor neuropathy

**Q4.** A 30-year-old woman presents with gait imbalance for 5 years. On examination, there is pes cavus bilaterally, as well as areflexia. You suspect Charcot-Marie-Tooth type 1. Which of the following features is **NOT** expected on the nerve conduction study of this patient?
- A. Prolonged distal motor latencies of all studied nerves
- B. Slowed conduction velocities at all sites within the 10–20 m/s range
- C. Absent sensory nerve action potentials (SNAPs) in the lower extremities
- D. Conduction block on the median motor study
- E. Absent H-reflexes

**Q5.** A 45-year-old woman presents with progressive proximal muscle weakness. In addition, she has had numbness and paresthesia in both feet and all fingers for 3 months. On examination, she has weakness, Medical Research Council (MRC) grade 3 in the proximal lower extremities and grade 4 in the proximal upper extremities. Hyperesthesia is noted in all toes and fingers. Reflexes are all absent. Nerve conduction study demonstrates the finding in the tracing below. What is the **MOST LIKELY** diagnosis?

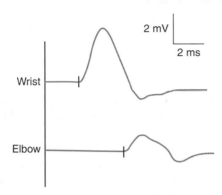

From Preston DC, Shapiro BE. *Electromyography and Neuromuscular Disorders: Clinical-electrophysiologic-ultrasound Correlations*. 4th ed. Philadelphia: Elsevier; 2020:89.

A. Charcot-Marie-Tooth type 1
B. Acute motor axonal neuropathy
C. Chronic inflammatory demyelinating polyneuropathy
D. Hypothyroidism
E. Vasculitic neuropathy

**Q6.** Which of the following statements is **CORRECT** regarding the median motor study below?

| Nerve-recording | Stimulating site | Latency (ms) | Amplitude (mV) | Conduction velocity (m/s) |
|---|---|---|---|---|
| Median-APB | Wrist | 4.4 | 1.2 | |
| | Elbow | | 1.0 | 45 |

*APB,* abductor pollicis brevis

A. There is a significantly prolonged distal latency, which indicates demyelination.
B. Reduction in the amplitude indicates axonal degeneration.
C. The decrease in amplitudes between the distal and proximal sites represents conduction block.
D. Conduction velocity is slowed within the demyelinating range.
E. This is a normal nerve conduction study.

**Q7.** A 19-year-old man presents with right wrist drop that he noticed upon awakening. He attended a party last night. You suspect Saturday night palsy. What is the earliest time after the onset for nerve conduction studies to determine the prognosis of wrist drop?
A. Day 1
B. Day 3
C. Day 7
D. Day 14
E. Day 21

**Q8.** Which of the following patients carries the **BEST** prognosis?
A. Mr. A presents with right foot drop. Nerve conduction study (NCS) on day 30 shows reduced amplitudes of right peroneal compound muscle action potential (CMAP).
B. Mr. B presents with weakness of the right intrinsic hand muscles. NCS on day 21 shows focal slowing of the right ulnar motor conduction velocity across the elbow.
C. Mr. C develops weakness of the left leg. Needle electromyography (EMG) reveals fibrillation potentials in the left tensor fascia latae with markedly reduced recruitment.
D. Mr. D presents with left wrist drop for 4 weeks. Needle EMG reveals fibrillation potentials with inability to activate any motor unit action potentials (MUAPs) in the extensor digitorum communis.
E. Mr. E presents with weakness of the right arm and leg for 6 weeks. He has known atrial fibrillation but is not on anticoagulation. Needle EMG reveals decreased activation but normal recruitment of muscles in the right arm.

**Q9.** Which of the following statements is **CORRECT** regarding Wallerian degeneration?
A. It occurs in both demyelination and axonal loss.
B. It occurs in retrograde fashion from the site of the injury to the neuronal cell body.
C. It takes ~5 days to complete.
D. Sensory fibers degenerate first due to their smaller size.
E. It indicates poorer prognosis compared to an isolated loss of the myelin sheath.

**Q10.** Distal compound muscle action potential (CMAP) amplitude is most likely normal in which of the following conditions?
A. Submaximal stimulation
B. Stimulator slipping off from the studied nerve
C. Distal demyelinating conduction block
D. Proximal demyelinating conduction block
E. Axonal loss

**Q11.** A 68-year-old man has difficulty lifting the right arm above his head for the past 3 months. In addition, he has a tingling sensation from the right shoulder down to the thumb. Examination reveals weakness of the right deltoid and biceps, Medical Research Council (MRC) grade 4. Sensory exam reveals decreased pinprick sensation in the right C5 through C6 distribution. Reflexes are 1+ in the right biceps and brachioradialis and 2+ in the other sites. You suspect right C5-6 radiculopathy. Which of the following findings is expected on the nerve conduction study?
A. Reduced median compound muscle action potential (CMAP) amplitude
B. Reduced ulnar CMAP amplitude
C. Reduced median sensory nerve action potential (SNAP) amplitude recording index finger
D. Reduced ulnar SNAP amplitude recording little finger
E. None of the above

**Q12.** A 25-year-old man presents with right wrist drop upon awakening for 1 day. He went to a party last night. He reports numbness and tingling over the dorsum of the right hand. You suspect right radial neuropathy at the spiral groove. Nerve conduction study performed on the same day demonstrates normal radial compound muscle action potential (CMAP) amplitude with stimulation at the elbow and below the spiral groove, but a reduced CMAP amplitude with stimulation above the spiral groove. Which of the following statements is **CORRECT**?
A. Reduced CMAP amplitude proximally represents axonal loss.
B. Conduction block over the spiral groove represents focal demyelination.
C. Martin-Gruber anastomosis at the forearm segment is suspected.
D. Co-stimulation at the proximal site causes pseudo-conduction block.
E. The pathology cannot be determined with certainty due to the time course.

**Q13.** A 68-year-old man is referred for an evaluation of bilateral leg weakness for 3 months. Recently, when walking for a long distance, he has to stop because of pain radiating from the back to the anterior thighs. The pain is relieved after bending or sitting. Examination reveals decreased tone in both legs. Motor exam shows intact strength of the lower extremities with normal sensation. Reflexes are 1+ in bilateral knees and 2+ elsewhere. Which of the following electrodiagnostic findings is **MOST LIKELY** seen in this patient?
A. Reduced tibial motor compound muscle action potential (CMAP) amplitudes
B. Absent superficial peroneal sensory neuron action potentials (SNAPs)
C. Active denervation in vastus medialis
D. Large motor unit action potentials (MUAPs) in the iliacus
E. Normal or equivocal study

**Q14.** A 26-year-old woman is referred for an evaluation of numbness and weakness of the right hand for 3 months. Nerve conduction study shows a markedly prolonged distal latency of a normal amplitude right median compound muscle action potential (CMAP) with an absent right median sensory nerve action potential (SNAP). Needle electromyography (EMG) of the right abductor pollicis brevis muscle shows normal spontaneous activity and normal motor unit action potential (MUAP) morphology, but markedly reduced recruitment. Which of the following statements is **CORRECT**?
A. The study needs to be repeated in the next 4 weeks when active denervation appears.
B. The reinnervation process is complete, so only reduced recruitment is seen.
C. This patient has a pure demyelinating lesion.
D. Reduced recruitment represents poor cooperation.
E. This study is inadequate for interpretation.

**Q15.** A 24-year-old man presents with right arm weakness and numbness from a traumatic brachial plexopathy. On nerve conduction study (NCS), all the sensory nerve action potentials (SNAPs) in the upper extremity are absent; the motor studies show reduced amplitudes with normal latencies and conduction velocities. On needle electromyography (EMG), there are fibrillations and positive sharp waves in all muscles. Motor unit action potential (MUAP) morphology is normal, but the recruitment is moderately decreased in all weak muscles. How old is the lesion?
A. Hyperacute (<1 week)
B. Acute (2–3 weeks)
C. Subacute (3–5 weeks)
D. Subacute to chronic (>6 weeks)
E. Very chronic (>2 years)

**Q16.** A 67-year-old man presented with weakness of his right ankle and toe dorsiflexion along with foot eversion weakness 3 weeks ago. In addition, he noted numbness on the top of his right foot. Yesterday, he developed weakness of his left-hand grip along with numbness of the ring and little fingers. How would you characterize this pattern of abnormalities?
A. Mononeuropathy
B. Polyneuropathy
C. Multiple mononeuropathies
D. Polyradiculopathy
E. Pure motor neuropathy

## PART 2 | QUESTIONS WITH ANSWERS AND DISCUSSION

**QUESTION 1.** Which of the following statements is **CORRECT** regarding electromyography (EMG) interpretation?
A. EMG study should be performed without clinical information to avoid bias.
B. Axonal loss can be identified on nerve conduction studies.
C. Demyelinating features are mainly identified on needle EMG.
D. EMG study is not useful in determining the prognosis of the condition.
E. Nerve conduction study can often be performed in isolation without needle EMG.

**ANSWER:** B. Axonal loss can be identified on nerve conduction studies.

### COMMENTS AND DISCUSSION
- Interpretation requires understanding of the pattern of pathological changes (i.e., demyelinating versus axonal process). The steps of EMG interpretation include:
  - List the differential diagnoses based on history and examination.
  - Identify nerve pathology patterns from nerve conduction study (demyelination versus axonal process).
  - Define the possible localization from the nerve conduction studies and muscle abnormalities on needle EMG.
  - Determine the pathological pattern whether it is normal, neurogenic, or myopathic from motor unit action potential (MUAP) morphology and the recruitment pattern on needle EMG.
  - Determine the time course based on nerve conduction study findings and spontaneous activity and MUAP morphology on needle EMG.
  - Identify any unique spontaneous activities (e.g., myotonia or myokymia)

 **KEY POINT**

For complete interpretation, EMG study requires both the nerve conduction study and needle EMG. Neither the nerve conduction study nor needle EMG should be routinely performed in isolation.

- EMG study is an extension of clinical history and examination; therefore, EMG should not be performed blinded.
- On nerve conduction studies, demyelination or axonal loss can be identified.
- Demyelinating features such as focal slowing, conduction block, or temporal dispersion are mainly identified on nerve conduction studies, not needle EMG.
- Needle EMG can determine neurogenic or myopathic changes, the degree of active denervation, and the degree of neurogenic loss. The latter two have implications in determination of prognosis.

**KEY POINT**

The most common abnormality seen in EMG labs is "neurogenic changes."

- Nerve conduction study can determine whether the process is demyelination or axonal loss; the first portends better prognosis.
- Therefore, both nerve conduction study and needle EMG are useful in prognostication.
- Because nerve conduction study and needle EMG provide different information, neither should be performed in isolation.

**QUESTION 2.** Which of the following electrophysiologic findings indicate demyelination?
A. Prolonged distal motor latency, 150% of the upper normal limit
B. Slowed conduction velocity, 90% of the lower normal limit
C. Reduced distal and proximal compound muscle action potential (CMAP) amplitudes, 25% of the lower normal limit
D. A 15% drop in CMAP amplitude at the proximal stimulation site, compared to distal stimulation
E. Temporal dispersion on sensory studies when stimulating at a proximal site

**ANSWER:** A. Prolonged distal motor latency, 150% of the upper normal limit

**COMMENTS AND DISCUSSION**
- Demyelination
  - Myelin sheath is crucial for saltatory conduction and faster conduction velocity.
  - Electrodiagnostic features of primary demyelination include (Fig. 6.1):
    - Prolonged distal latency, longer than 130% of the upper normal limit
    - Slowed conduction velocity, slower than 75% of the lower normal limit
    - Conduction block (only in acquired demyelination) with a drop of amplitude and area >50%
    - Temporal dispersion, duration of the proximal motor response >115% of the distal motor response (i.e., proximal/distal CMAP duration ratio >1.15)
      - All normal nerves have some physiological temporal dispersion and phase cancellation.
      - Normal motor nerves may show an increase in duration up to 15% at the proximal stimulation site when compared to the distal site (i.e., the proximal duration up to 115% of the distal duration), which can result in a decrease in proximal amplitude up to 20% compared to the distal site.
      - However, physiological temporal dispersion and phase cancellation are more pronounced for sensory nerve conduction studies, due to the much shorter durations of sensory fiber action potentials (which form the SNAP) as compared to muscle fiber action potentials (which form the CMAP). Even a slight amount of temporal dispersion in sensory studies can cause overlap of the positive and negative phases of single sensory fiber action potentials and subsequent phase cancellation, leading to a significant drop in amplitude between distal and proximal stimulation sites.
    - Amplitudes are variable in demyelination.
      - Sensory amplitude may be normal but is most often reduced or absent.
        - If there is a conduction block, the amplitudes from stimulation proximal to the block will be reduced.
        - Pathologic temporal dispersion and phase cancellation occur due to conduction slowing, leading to smaller or absent amplitudes, even in the absence of conduction block.
      - Motor amplitude may be normal or reduced.
        - If there is a conduction block and the stimulation is proximal to the block, the amplitudes will be reduced.
        - Although temporal dispersion and phase cancellation resulting in smaller proximal amplitudes are primarily seen in sensory nerve conduction studies, similar changes may also occur in motor studies if the conduction slowing is severe. Severe conduction slowing can cause pathologic temporal dispersion and phase cancellation, leading to smaller or absent amplitudes, even in the absence of conduction block. However, conduction slowing alone never results in an area drop of >50%. An area drop of >50% indicates unequivocal conduction block.
- Inherited demyelinating neuropathy
  - Because inherited demyelinating neuropathy affects all myelin, symmetric (bilateral and nearby nerves) and uniform slowing in the demyelinating range are the key features. In this type of neuropathy, conduction block or temporal dispersion is not present.
  - The prototype of inherited demyelinating diseases is Charcot-Marie-Tooth type 1.

## 🔑 KEY POINT

In inherited demyelinating neuropathy especially Charcot-Marie-Tooth type 1 (CMT1), key feature in NCS is **"uniform slowing."**

- Acquired demyelinating neuropathy
  - Because demyelination is multifocal and occurs randomly, asymmetry (between left and right sides, and nearby nerves), conduction block, and pathological temporal dispersion are the key features.
  - The prototype acquired demyelinating diseases are the acute inflammatory demyelinating polyneuropathy (AIDP) type of Guillain-Barré syndrome and chronic inflammatory demyelinating polyneuropathy (CIDP).

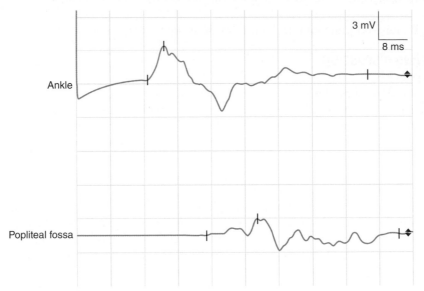

**Fig. 6.1 Demyelinating features.** Slowed nerve conduction is a main feature of demyelination. This tracing demonstrates a tibial motor study in a subject with chronic inflammatory demyelinating polyneuropathy (CIDP) when stimulating at the ankle and popliteal fossa, and recording at the abductor hallucis. **Severely prolonged distal motor latency** (17 ms, >130% of upper normal limit)* and **slowed conduction velocity** (28 m/s, <75% of lower normal limit)* are key electrophysiologic features of demyelination. **Conduction block** (drop of amplitudes and areas by 51%, >50%)* and **temporal dispersion** are features of acquired demyelination. *Numbers indicate parameters in this tracing.

- Differential diagnosis of major inherited demyelinating diseases
  - Inherited disorders with uniform conduction slowing
    - Charcot-Marie-Tooth disease type 1
    - Charcot-Marie-Tooth disease type 4
    - Charcot-Marie-Tooth disease X
    - Dejerine-Sottas syndrome
    - Refsum disease
    - Metachromatic and other leukodystrophies
    - Cockayne syndrome
  - Inherited disorders with multifocal conduction slowing or block at common entrapment and compression sites (which may be misdiagnosed as acquired neuropathy)
    - Hereditary neuropathy with liability to pressure palsy (HNPP)
- Differential diagnosis of major acquired demyelinating diseases
  - Acute inflammatory demyelinating polyneuropathy (AIDP)
  - Chronic inflammatory demyelinating polyneuropathy (CIDP)
  - Multifocal motor neuropathy (MMN) with conduction block
  - Diphtheria
  - Toxic neuropathies e.g., from arsenic, amiodarone

**QUESTION 3.** Demyelinating features on nerve conduction studies may be seen in which of the following conditions?
- A. Diabetic polyneuropathy
- B. Charcot-Marie-Tooth type 2
- C. Cisplatin-induced polyneuropathy
- D. Mononeuritis multiplex
- E. Multifocal motor neuropathy

**ANSWER:** E. Multifocal motor neuropathy

## COMMENTS AND DISCUSSION

- See also comment and discussion from Question 2 for the differential diagnosis of the major primary demyelinating neuropathies.
- Multifocal motor neuropathy (MMN) is a unique demyelinating neuropathy that involves only motor nerves. Conduction blocks are typically present in this disorder.
- Diabetic polyneuropathy, cisplatin-induced polyneuropathy, and mononeuritis multiplex are axonal neuropathies.
- Charcot-Marie-Tooth type 2 is an axonal type of hereditary neuropathy.

**QUESTION 4.** A 30-year-old woman presents with gait imbalance for 5 years. On examination, there is pes cavus bilaterally, as well as areflexia. You suspect Charcot-Marie-Tooth type 1. Which of the following features is **NOT** expected on the nerve conduction study of this patient?
  A. Prolonged distal motor latencies of all studied nerves
  B. Slowed conduction velocities at all sites within the 10–20 m/s range
  C. Absent sensory nerve action potentials (SNAPs) in the lower extremities
  D. Conduction block on the median motor study
  E. Absent H reflexes

**ANSWER:** D. Conduction block on the median motor study

## COMMENTS AND DISCUSSION

- Charcot-Marie-Tooth type 1 (CMT1) is the most common hereditary motor and sensory neuropathy.
- The key feature of CMT1 is uniform conduction slowing on nerve conduction study (NCS) due to uniform and diffuse demyelination. This can be seen as prolonged distal latencies and slowed conduction velocities at all sites.
- Conduction block, which is often a sign of acquired demyelination, is not typically seen in CMT1. It is important to note that conduction block may also occur in a few inherited demyelinating neuropathies, most commonly in hereditary neuropathy with liability to pressure palsy (HNPP).
- In CMT1, SNAPs are often absent in the lower extremities due to pathologic slowing leading to temporal dispersion and phase cancellation.
- H reflexes are also absent or prolonged in CMT.

**QUESTION 5.** A 45-year-old woman presents with progressive proximal muscle weakness. In addition, she has had numbness and paresthesia in both feet and all fingers for 3 months. On examination, she has weakness, Medical Research Council (MRC) grade 3 in the proximal lower extremities and grade 4 in the proximal upper extremities. Hyperesthesia is noted in all toes and fingers. Reflexes are all absent. Nerve conduction study demonstrates the finding in the tracing below. What is the **MOST LIKELY** diagnosis?

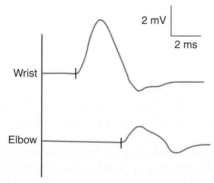

From Preston DC, Shapiro BE. *Electromyography and Neuromuscular Disorders: Clinical-electrophysiologic-ultrasound Correlations.* 4th ed. Philadelphia: Elsevier; 2020:89.

  A. Charcot-Marie-Tooth type 1
  B. Acute motor axonal neuropathy
  C. Chronic inflammatory demyelinating polyneuropathy
  D. Hypothyroidism
  E. Vasculitic neuropathy

**ANSWER:** C. Chronic inflammatory demyelinating polyneuropathy

**COMMENTS AND DISCUSSION**

- This tracing demonstrates a prominent drop in the amplitude and area (>50%) recording from the proximal stimulation site compared to the distal stimulation. This finding is called conduction block.
  - Conduction block is one of the key features of demyelination on nerve conduction study, and typically indicates acquired demyelination.
  - Among the disorders listed, only chronic inflammatory demyelinating polyneuropathy (CIDP) is an acquired demyelinating neuropathy which may demonstrate conduction block on nerve conduction study.
  - Charcot-Marie-Tooth disease type 1 is a hereditary demyelinating neuropathy that demonstrates uniform slowing without conduction block or temporal dispersion on nerve conduction study.
  - Acute motor axonal neuropathy (AMAN) is an axonal variant of Guillain-Barré syndrome. Therefore, demyelinating features are not expected in this variant.
  - Hypothyroidism can cause secondary entrapment neuropathy, polyneuropathy, or myopathy. Conduction block is not expected in any of these.
  - Vasculitic neuropathy typically leads to axonal loss in a mononeuritis multiplex pattern, and does not result in conduction block. In rare cases, pseudo-conduction block may be observed when nerve conduction studies are performed very early before Wallerian degeneration is completed.

**QUESTION 6.** Which of the following statements is **CORRECT** regarding the median motor study below?

| Nerve-recording | Stimulating site | Latency (ms) | Amplitude (mV) | Conduction velocity (m/s) |
|---|---|---|---|---|
| Median-APB | Wrist | 4.4 | 1.2 | |
| | Elbow | | 1.0 | 45 |

*APB,* abductor pollicis brevis

A. There is a significantly prolonged distal latency, which indicates demyelination.
B. Reduction in the amplitude indicates axonal degeneration.
C. The decrease in amplitudes between the distal and proximal sites represents conduction block.
D. Conduction velocity is slowed within the demyelinating range.
E. This is a normal nerve conduction study.

**ANSWER:** B. Reduction in the amplitude indicates axonal degeneration.

**COMMENTS AND DISCUSSION**

- This nerve conduction study demonstrates an axonal loss pattern.
  - Borderline distal latency
  - Slightly slowed conduction velocity
  - Reduced compound muscle action potential (CMAP) amplitudes
  - The drop in amplitude between the elbow and wrist is normal, small and does not meet the criteria for conduction block (>50% drop in amplitude and area).
- Axonal loss
  - When an axon is injured, it undergoes the process of Wallerian degeneration.
  - The major finding on nerve conduction studies is reduced amplitudes, reflecting the reduced number of axons.
  - Distal latency and conduction velocity are generally preserved. However, these measures may be affected slightly if the fastest axons are lost. These changes are not as severe as those observed in the primary demyelinating process.
  - Features of axonal loss include (Fig. 6.2):
    - Reduction of CMAP and SNAP amplitudes
    - Conduction velocity: normal or slightly slowed (not slower than 75% of the lower normal limit)
    - Distal latencies: normal or slightly prolonged (not longer than 130% of the upper normal limit)

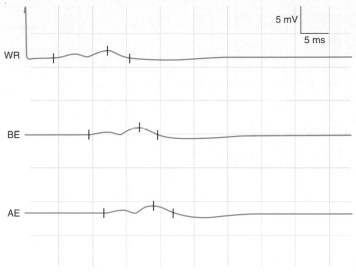

**Fig. 6.2 Reduced amplitude in axonal degeneration.** This is an ulnar motor study in a severe ulnar neuropathy. There is reduced amplitude (1.2 mV)*, which is a primary feature of axonal loss. There is a slightly prolonged distal latency (4.1 ms)* and a slightly slowed conduction velocity (45 m/s)*, although these values do not meet the demyelinating criteria. These features are compatible with axonal degeneration. *Numbers indicate parameters in this tracing.

 **KEY POINT**

One crucial aspect of NCS interpretation is to distinguish between primary demyelination and primary axonal loss.

- Axonal loss has a much wider range of differential diagnoses compared to demyelinating diseases.
  - Differential diagnosis of inherited axonal neuropathy includes:
    - Charcot-Marie-Tooth type 2
    - Hereditary motor neuropathies
    - Hereditary sensory and autonomic neuropathies
    - Some subtypes of hereditary spastic paraplegia (e.g., SPG10, SPG17)
  - Differential diagnosis of acquired axonal neuropathy is extensive, and includes:
    - Metabolic disorders (e.g., diabetes)
    - Endocrine disorders (e.g., hypothyroidism)
    - Toxin/drugs (e.g., alcohol, antiretroviral nucleoside analogues, platinum-based chemotherapeutic agents)
    - Immune-mediated (e.g., acute motor axonal neuropathy [AMAN], acute motor and sensory axonal neuropathy [AMSAN], and vasculitis)
    - Infection (e.g., syphilis)
    - Paraproteinemia (e.g., Waldenström macroglobulinemia, amyloidosis)

**QUESTION 7.** A 19-year-old man presents with right wrist drop that he noticed upon awakening. He attended a party last night. You suspect Saturday night palsy. What is the earliest time after the onset for nerve conduction studies to determine the prognosis of wrist drop?
A. Day 1
B. Day 3
C. Day 7
D. Day 14
E. Day 21

**ANSWER:** C, Day 7

**COMMENTS AND DISCUSSION**
- Wallerian degeneration in axonal loss
  - When the axon is injured, the remaining axon distal to the injury site will degenerate. This process is known as "Wallerian degeneration."
  - Motor fibers are the first to undergo degeneration, beginning on day 3 after the injury, and the process is typically completed by day 7 (Fig. 6.3). Hence, assessing wallerian degeneration of motor fibers could be assessed at day 7 if needed.

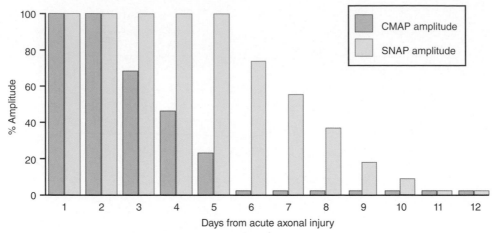

**Fig. 6.3 Changes in compound muscle action potential (CMAP) and sensory nerve action potential (SNAP) in Wallerian degeneration.** After an axonal injury, Wallerian degeneration begins at the site of the lesion, and progresses distally. This process takes several days. If nerve conduction study is performed immediately after the injury, both CMAP and SNAP are still normal, since the nerve distal to the injury site has not yet degenerated. Following the injury, the drop in CMAP amplitudes occurs first, around day 3, potentially, due to failure first of the neuromuscular junction. It is completed on days 5–7. The drop in SNAP amplitudes begins later on days 6–7, and is completed around days 10–12. From Katirji B. *Electromyography in Clinical Practice: A Case Study Approach*. 3rd ed. Oxford University Press; 2018:120.

- Sensory fibers begin to degenerate on day 5, with the process completed on approximately day 10 (Fig. 6.3).
- Therefore, if the nerve conduction study is performed prior to the completion of Wallerian degeneration, the exact pathology cannot be identified.
- If nerve conduction is performed prior to the onset of Wallerian degeneration, a *pseudo-conduction block* pattern may be seen, which can be mistaken for demyelination (Fig. 6.4).
- Nerve conduction studies before the completion of Wallerian degeneration can aid in localizing the precise location of a lesion by revealing a pseudo-conduction block.

## ◎ HIGH-YIELD FACT

Performing the nerve conduction study prior to the onset of Wallerian degeneration can result in a **pseudo-conduction block** that mimics demyelination.

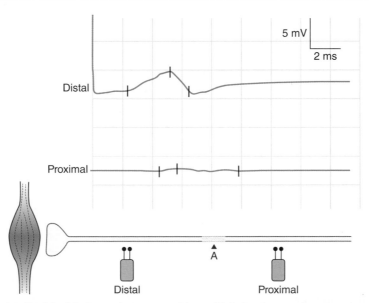

**Fig. 6.4 Pseudo-conduction block in hyperacute axonal loss.** Wallerian degeneration takes several days to complete. If nerve conduction study is performed in the hyperacute period after the injury but before Wallerian degeneration has completed, a pseudo-conduction block is seen. The distal compound muscle action potential (CMAP) remains normal, since Wallerian degeneration has not yet occurred. However, when stimulating proximal to the site of nerve injury (A), the conduction fails, resulting in small or absent potential. This pattern mimics conduction block and can be mistaken for demyelination, if the timing of the study is not considered. Therefore, the pathology of the nerve injury cannot be determined in the hyperacute period, but a nerve conduction study can still be useful for localization of the nerve injury. Adapted from Preston DC, Shapiro BE. Electromyography and Neuromuscular Disorders: Clinical-electrophysiologic-ultrasound Correlations. 4th ed. Philadelphia: Elsevier; 2020;3:25.

- One limitation of the nerve conduction study is that the electrophysiological changes may not be detectable during the early phase of nerve injury.
- To accurately determine nerve pathology and prognosis, nerve conduction studies should be performed at least 14 days following the injury to ensure completion of Wallerian degeneration, to reach a plateau in compound muscle action potential (CMAP) and sensory nerve action potential (SNAP) amplitudes. If nerve conduction studies are performed prior to completion of the degeneration, pseudo-conduction block due to preservation of the distal fibers can be mistaken for demyelination.

**QUESTION 8.** Which of the following patients carries the **BEST** prognosis?
A. Mr. A presents with right foot drop. Nerve conduction study (NCS) on day 30 shows reduced amplitudes of right peroneal compound muscle action potential (CMAP).
B. Mr. B presents with weakness of the right intrinsic hand muscles. NCS on day 21 shows focal slowing of the right ulnar motor conduction velocity across the elbow.
C. Mr. C develops weakness of the left leg. Needle electromyography (EMG) reveals fibrillation potentials in the left tensor fascia latae with markedly reduced recruitment.
D. Mr. D presents with left wrist drop for 4 weeks. Needle EMG reveals fibrillation potentials with inability to activate any motor unit action potentials (MUAPs) in the extensor digitorum communis.
E. Mr. E presents with weakness of the right arm and leg for 6 weeks. He has known atrial fibrillation but is not on anticoagulation. Needle EMG reveals decreased activation but normal recruitment of muscles in the right arm.

**ANSWER:** B. Mr. B presents with weakness of the right intrinsic hand muscles. NCS on day 21 shows focal slowing of the right ulnar motor conduction velocity across the elbow.

**COMMENTS AND DISCUSSION**
- In general, demyelination carries the better prognosis due to rapid remyelination, compared to axonal loss.
- Axonal loss is associated with Wallerian degeneration, and nerve regeneration occurs slowly, at a rate of ~1 mm/day. As a result, axonal loss has a poorer prognosis in terms of recovery time and the extent of recovery. that can be achieved.
- To determine nerve pathology, NCS must be done at least 14 days after the injury, to ensure that Wallerian degeneration has already been completed.
- Among all options, only Mr. B has demyelinating feature (focal slowing), and therefore has the best prognosis. Mr. A has reduced CMAP amplitudes on NCS, indicating axonal loss of the right peroneal nerve. Both Mr. C and Mr. D have fibrillation potentials (active denervation) on needle EMG representing ongoing axonal loss. Mr. E has only decreased activation on needle EMG but normal recruitment, which denotes poor cooperation or a central etiology including a stroke. This patient may have weakness from ischemic stroke in the clinical context of right hemiparesis and known atrial fibrillation without anticoagulation.

**QUESTION 9.** Which of the following statements is **CORRECT** regarding Wallerian degeneration?
A. It occurs in both demyelination and axonal loss.
B. It occurs in retrograde fashion from the site of the injury to the neuronal cell body.
C. It takes ~5 days to complete.
D. Sensory fibers degenerate first due to their smaller size.
E. It indicates poorer prognosis compared to an isolated loss of the myelin sheath.

**ANSWER:** E. It indicates poorer prognosis compared to an isolated loss of the myelin sheath.

**COMMENTS AND DISCUSSION**
- Wallerian degeneration occurs only in axonal loss (not in demyelination) and indicates a poorer prognosis.
- When there is an axonal injury, Wallerian degeneration occurs in anterograde fashion from the site of the injury down to the axon terminal, not in retrograde fashion.
- In pure demyelination without axonal injury, there is no Wallerian degeneration.
- The process of Wallerian degeneration takes up to 10–14 days to complete. Motor fibers typically degenerate first on day 3, before sensory fibers, due to neuromuscular junction failure (Fig. 6.3).
- Sensory fibers begin to degenerate later on day 5 (Fig. 6.3).

**QUESTION 10.** Distal compound muscle action potential (CMAP) amplitude is most likely normal in which of the following conditions?
A. Submaximal stimulation
B. Stimulator slipping off from the studied nerve
C. Distal demyelinating conduction block
D. Proximal demyelinating conduction block
E. Axonal loss

**ANSWER:** D. Proximal demyelinating conduction block

### COMMENTS AND DISCUSSION
- Axonal injury is the most common cause of reduction of CMAP amplitudes at all testing sites.
- However, there are also other less common conditions including some technical factors that can mimic axonal loss, including:
  ○ Submaximal stimulation can result in an erroneously low CMAP amplitude that can be mistaken for axonal loss.
  ○ When the stimulator slips off the nerve, the recording responses will be falsely small.
  ○ In cases of distal demyelination where there is a conduction block distal to the distal stimulation site, the CMAP amplitudes from both proximal and distal stimulation may be small, mimicking axonal loss. An example of distal demyelination is carpal tunnel syndrome, in which demyelination can occur more distal to the wrist and elbow stimulation sites typically used in nerve conduction studies.
  ○ In cases of proximal demyelination, where demyelination occurs between the proximal and distal stimulation sites, there can be either focal slowing and/or conduction block. Conduction block is indicated by a drop of 50% or greater in the area or ampltidue of CMAP from proximal stimulation compared to distal stimulation. In these cases, the distal CMAP amplitude remains normal.

**QUESTION 11.** A 68-year-old man has difficulty lifting the right arm above his head for the past 3 months. In addition, he has a tingling sensation from the right shoulder down to the thumb. Examination reveals weakness of the right deltoid and biceps, Medical Research Council (MRC) grade 4. Sensory exam reveals decreased pinprick sensation in the right C5 through C6 distribution. Reflexes are 1+ in the right biceps and brachioradialis and 2+ in the other sites. You suspect right C5-6 radiculopathy. Which of the following findings is expected on the nerve conduction study?
A. Reduced median compound muscle action potential (CMAP) amplitude
B. Reduced ulnar CMAP amplitude
C. Reduced median sensory nerve action potential (SNAP) amplitude recording index finger
D. Reduced ulnar SNAP amplitude recording little finger
E. None of the above

**ANSWER:** E. None of the above

### COMMENTS AND DISCUSSION
- In radiculopathy where the lesion is proximal to dorsal root ganglion (i.e., pre-ganglionic), all SNAPs are preserved. Sensory neurons within the dorsal root ganglion are pseudo-unipolar neurons that have both proximal and distal branches. Pre-ganglionic lesions affect only the proximal branch, while the distal branch remains intact and does not degenerate since the neuronal cell bodies within the dorsal root ganglion are unaffected. Consequently, the SNAP typically obtained from distal extremity stimulation remains normal in pre-ganglionic lesions, even though there can be sensory impairment on clinical examination.
- Median SNAP recording the index finger (in C6 dermatomal distribution) remains normal, since the lesion is pre-ganglionic in a C5-6 radiculopathy.
- In radiculopathy, CMAP recordings the affected muscles can show abnormalities, whereas the SNAPs are preserved. However, in C5-6 radiculopathy, the median motor study recording abductor pollicis brevis (C8, T1) and ulnar motor study recording abductor digiti minimi (C8, T1) remain normal, since these muscles are not supplied by the C5-6 myotomes.
- Ulnar SNAP recording the little finger (in C8 dermatomal distribution) should be normal.

> ## 🗝 KEY POINT
>
> When the lesion involves nerve roots proximal to the dorsal root ganglion (i.e., radiculopathy), the SNAP is normal, mimicking a pure motor neuropathy on electrophysiology studies. However, sensory loss presents on clinical examination.

**QUESTION 12.** A 25-year-old man presents with right wrist drop upon awakening for 1 day. He went to a party last night. He reports numbness and tingling over the dorsum of the right hand. You suspect right radial neuropathy at the spiral groove. Nerve conduction study performed on the same day demonstrates normal radial compound muscle action potential (CMAP) amplitude with stimulation at the elbow and below the spiral groove, but a reduced CMAP amplitude with stimulation above the spiral groove. Which of the following statements is **CORRECT**?

A. Reduced CMAP amplitude proximally represents axonal loss.

B. Conduction block over the spiral groove represents focal demyelination.

C. Martin-Gruber anastomosis at the forearm segment is suspected.

D. Co-stimulation at the proximal site causes pseudo-conduction block.

E. The pathology cannot be determined with certainty due to the time course.

**ANSWER:** E. The pathology cannot be determined with certainty due to the time course.

### COMMENTS AND DISCUSSION

- Normal CMAP amplitudes below the spiral groove, but a reduced CMAP amplitude above it represents "conduction block" at the spiral groove. In most cases, this finding reflects focal demyelination. However, if the nerve conduction study (NCS) is performed only 1 day after the injury (i.e., hyperacute nerve injury) as in this case, the drop in amplitude can be due to "pseudo-conduction block" (Fig. 6.4) caused by axonal pathology, as Wallerian degeneration has not yet begun. In this scenario, the drop in the CMAP amplitude from proximal stimulation occurs because the electrical activity cannot travel through the site of the nerve injury. Thus, performing nerve conduction studies in the hyperacute period before the onset of Wallerian degeneration can make it difficult to distinguish "pseudo-conduction block" caused by axonal pathology from true conduction block due to demyelinating pathology.
- If the lesion was axonal, the CMAP amplitudes from the distal stimulation would remain normal, as Wallerian degeneration has not yet occurred in the distal nerve segment. While "pseudo-conduction block" in the hyperacute period of nerve injury may be helpful for localizing the lesion, it is not possible to determine the true pathology (i.e., demyelination versus axonal process) at this stage.
- Nerve conduction study performed 10–14 days after the nerve injury can distinguish between demyelinating process (resulting in true conduction block) and axonal loss. If the amplitudes obtained from the distal stimulation sites are reduced, the pathology is axonal loss. If the amplitudes obtained from the distal stimulation remain normal, the process is likely demyelination (with conduction block due to conduction failure).
- Martin-Gruber anastomosis is an anomalous innervation where the median motor nerve fibers travels to the ulnar nerve. This anomaly does not involve the radial nerve.
- Co-stimulation at the proximal site would cause a higher (not lower) CMAP amplitude, compared to the distal stimulation.

**QUESTION 13.** A 68-year-old man is referred for an evaluation of bilateral leg weakness for 3 months. Recently, when walking for a long distance, he has to stop because of pain radiating from the back to the anterior thighs. The pain is relieved after bending or sitting. Examination reveals decreased tone in both legs. Motor exam shows intact strength of the lower extremities with normal sensation. Reflexes are 1+ in bilateral knees and 2+ elsewhere. Which of the following electrodiagnostic findings is **MOST LIKELY** seen in this patient?

A. Reduced tibial motor compound muscle action potential (CMAP) amplitudes

B. Absent superficial peroneal sensory neuron action potentials (SNAPs)

C. Active denervation in vastus medialis

D. Large motor unit action potentials (MUAPs) in the iliacus

E. Normal or equivocal study

**ANSWER:** E. Normal or equivocal study

### COMMENTS AND DISCUSSION

- Based on the clinical history and examination, this patient has neurogenic claudication.
- The diagnosis is most likely lumbar spinal stenosis at the L2-3 levels.

- In neurogenic claudication, symptoms occur with prolonged walking or standing and are relieved by bending or sitting (not resting while standing, which relieves vascular claudication).
- Because the compression is intermittent, it is not unusual that the clinical exam is normal or equivocal. Likewise, the electrodiagnostic study is often normal or equivocal.

**QUESTION 14.** A 26-year-old woman is referred for an evaluation of numbness and weakness of the right hand for 3 months. Nerve conduction study shows a markedly prolonged distal latency of a normal amplitude right median compound muscle action potential (CMAP) with an absent right median sensory nerve action potential (SNAP). Needle electromyography (EMG) of the right abductor pollicis brevis muscle shows normal spontaneous activity and normal motor unit action potential (MUAP) morphology, but markedly reduced recruitment. Which of the following statements is **CORRECT**?

A. The study needs to be repeated in the next 4 weeks when active denervation appears.
B. The reinnervation process is complete, so only reduced recruitment is seen.
C. This patient has a pure demyelinating lesion.
D. Reduced recruitment represents poor cooperation.
E. This study is inadequate for interpretation.

**ANSWER:** C. This patient has pure demyelinating lesion.

**COMMENTS AND DISCUSSION**
- Prolonged distal motor latency of the right median CMAP along with absent median SNAP on the nerve conduction study indicates median nerve pathology. If the distal latency is >130% the upper limit of normal, this denotes demyelination (i.e., demyelination between the stimulator and recording electrodes—thus at the wrist).
- Along with clinical presentation, the diagnosis is most likely carpal tunnel syndrome. In entrapment neuropathy, the primary pathology is often demyelination, although secondary axonal loss may also occur.
- On needle EMG, presence of signs of active denervation such as fibrillation potentials or positive sharp waves indicate axonal loss. Denervation refers to the separation of axons from the innervated muscles. However, it is important to note that these signs of active denervation may take 3-4 weeks to emerge after the onset of axonal loss. Needle EMG in this patient is performed 3 months after the onset, and there are still no signs of active denervation. Likewise, there is no evidence of reinnervation but only reduced recruitment.
- Markedly reduced recruitment with normal CMAP and without evidence of active denervation or reinnervation is most consistent with conduction block, which is a sign of demyelination.
- In this case, the nerve conduction study was performed 3 months after the onset. The timing is already adequate for an evaluation of signs of active denervation. No repeat study is required.
- Reinnervation in a chronic neurogenic process will result in changes in the MUAP morphology. When reinnervation is complete, MUAPs are large in amplitude and long in duration.
- Poor cooperation is a "central" process and results in reduced activation, not recruitment, on needle EMG.

**QUESTION 15.** A 24-year-old man presents with right arm weakness and numbness from a traumatic brachial plexopathy. On nerve conduction study (NCS), all the sensory nerve action potentials (SNAPs) in the arm are absent; the motor studies show reduced amplitudes with normal latencies and conduction velocities. On needle electromyography (EMG), there are fibrillations and positive sharp waves in all muscles. Motor unit action potential (MUAP) morphology is normal, but the recruitment is moderately decreased in all weak muscles. How old is the lesion?

A. Hyperacute (<1 week)
B. Acute (2–3 weeks)
C. Subacute (3–5 weeks)
D. Subacute to chronic (>6 weeks)
E. Very chronic (>2 years)

**ANSWER:** C. Subacute (3–5 weeks)

**COMMENTS AND DISCUSSION**
- This section will discuss temporal evolution of NCS and EMG findings.

- Evidence of axonal loss on NCS occurs with Wallerian degeneration, which starts on days 2–3 for motor studies and days 5–6 for sensory studies. It is complete at approximately days 10–11.
- Spontaneous activity on needle EMG
  - Fibrillation potentials and positive sharp waves indicate active denervation.
  - The onset of fibrillation potentials and positive sharp waves is dependent on the length of the nerve between the injury and the muscle. In general, it can take a few weeks to appear after an axonal injury.
  - For example, in a lumbar radiculopathy, fibrillation potentials and positive sharp waves appear:
    - 10–14 days in the paraspinal muscles
    - 2–3 weeks in the gluteal and thigh muscles
    - 3–4 weeks in the lower leg
    - 4–5 weeks in the foot
  - Eventually, when reinnervation is complete, active denervation disappears.
  - Motor unit action potential (or MUAP) changes on needle EMG
    - Acute phase: MUAP morphology is normal but recruitment is reduced.
    - After denervation occurs (typically 2–5 weeks after an axonal injury), reinnervation begins and there are subsequent changes in MUAP morphology.
      - First, there are satellites and increased polyphasia from collateral sprouting. Recruitment continues to be reduced.
      - After a period of denervation, reinnervated motor units result in MUAPs that become larger in amplitude, longer in duration, and polyphasic with ongoing reduced recruitment.
      - In the late stage, motor units are completely remodeled, and MUAPs become large and long, with less prominent polyphasia, but still with reduced recruitment.
    - In cases of severe denervation, where no nearby intact motor units remain, collateral sprouting is not possible. The only possibility for reinnervation is for the original axon to regrow the entire length of nerve. At some point during this process, the new axon may attach to a few muscle fibers but will not have had enough time to fully reinnervate all denervated muscle fibers. These newly formed motor units are called "nascent units", characterized by small, short, and polyphasic morphology with markedly reduced recruitment (Fig. 6.5).

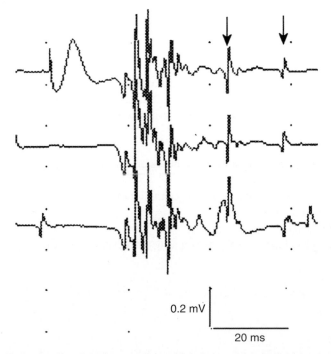

**Fig. 6.5  Nascent units.** Nascent motor unit action potentials are immature motor units that have recently reinnervated muscle fibers. Due to their immaturity, the morphology is very complex and polyphasic, resembling myopathic units. However, in contrast to myopathic units, the recruitment is reduced. Nascent units are unstable. Satellite units (*arrows*) can also be a part of nascent units as seen in this figure. From Katirji B. *Electromyography in Clinical Practice: A Case Study Approach*. 3rd ed. Oxford University Press; 2018:82.

**QUESTION 16.**  A 67-year-old man presented with weakness of his right ankle and toe dorsiflexion along with foot eversion weakness 3 weeks ago. In addition, he noted numbness on the top of his right foot. Yesterday, he developed weakness of his left-hand grip along with numbness of the ring and little fingers. How would you characterize this pattern of abnormalities?

A.  Mononeuropathy
B.  Polyneuropathy
C.  Multiple mononeuropathies
D.  Polyradiculopathy
E.  Pure motor neuropathy

**ANSWER:** C. Multiple mononeuropathies

**COMMENTS AND DISCUSSION**

- Patterns of abnormalities on nerve conduction study based on the types of nerve involvement
  - Involvement of both motor and sensory nerves
    - Mononeuropathy
      - Involvement of only one nerve
      - Most common etiology is entrapment neuropathy
    - Multiple mononeuropathies
      - Involvement of several individual (named) nerves
      - Also called "mononeuritis multiplex," since the main etiology is "vasculitis"
    - Polyneuropathy
      - The most common pattern in clinical practice
      - Demyelinating polyneuropathy has a narrow list of differential diagnoses (e.g., acute inflammatory demyelinating polyneuropathy [AIDP] and chronic inflammatory demyelinating polyneuropathy [CIDP]).
      - In contrast, axonal polyneuropathy has a broad differential diagnosis including diabetic, toxic, metabolic, nutritional, chemotherapy-related, and drug-induced neuropathies.
  - Pure motor neuropathy
    - The prototypic disorders are acute motor axonal neuropathy (AMAN) and multifocal motor neuropathy with conduction block (MMN-CB).
    - It can also be seen if the lesion involves the pure motor branch (e.g., anterior interosseous nerve [AIN] or posterior interosseous nerve [PIN])
    - Caveat:
      - A lesion involving nerve roots proximal to dorsal root ganglion (DRG) can mimic pure motor neuropathy on electrophysiologic studies. However, the clinical examination demonstrates both motor and sensory impairment, since both motor and sensory nerve roots are affected.
  - Pure sensory involvement
    - The lesion can involve the sensory nerve fibers or dorsal root ganglion
    - Differential diagnoses include:
      - Anti-Hu (ANNA1)–associated sensory ganglionopathy
      - Sjogren syndrome
      - Vitamin B6 toxicity
      - Chemotherapy-related sensory neuropathy (especially cisplatin)

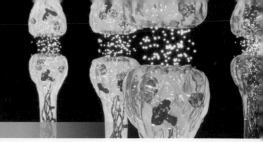

# CHAPTER 7

# Electrodiagnostic Medicine V: Electrodiagnosis of Neuromuscular Junction

## PART 1 | PRACTICE TEST

**Q1.** The ultrastructural homologue of the miniature endplate potential (MEPP) is the:
- A. quantum.
- B. safety factor.
- C. quantal release.
- D. endplate potential.
- E. synaptic vesicle.

**Q2.** A decremental response on slow repetitive nerve stimulation does **NOT** occur in which of the following:
- A. Botulism
- B. Amyotrophic lateral sclerosis
- C. Myasthenia gravis
- D. Corticosteroid myopathy
- E. Lambert-Eaton myasthenic syndrome (LEMS)

**Q3.** After short exercise, a post-exercise stimulation to look for a compound muscle action potential (CMAP) increment, is often used as an alternative to painful rapid repetitive nerve stimulation in diagnosing Lambert-Eaton myasthenic syndrome (LEMS). The optimal exercise duration for this test is:
- A. 10 seconds.
- B. 10 minutes.
- C. 1 minute.
- D. 3 minutes.
- E. 30 seconds.

**Q4.** Which condition has the highest possibility of being detected by routine electrodiagnostic studies?
- A. Acute (<1 week) Guillain-Barré syndrome
- B. Chronic (>6 months) lumbar radiculopathy
- C. Acute (<1 week) peroneal nerve palsy at the fibular neck
- D. Ocular seronegative myasthenia gravis
- E. Acute (<1 week) cervical radiculopathy

**Q5.** In patients with suspected ocular myasthenia, which test is the most sensitive in establishing the diagnosis?
- A. Serum acetylcholine receptor antibody
- B. Single-fiber jitter study of the frontalis muscle
- C. Slow repetitive stimulation of the facial nerve
- D. Slow repetitive stimulation of the spinal accessory nerve
- E. Single-fiber jitter study of the extensor digitorum communis

**Q6.** Regarding single-fiber needle electromyography:
- A. Abnormal jitter is specific for myasthenia gravis.
- B. Blocking indicates abnormalities of neuromuscular junction transmission.
- C. Normal subjects demonstrate no jitter.
- D. Blocking usually occurs when the jitter is normal.
- E. Fiber density in a normal subject is usually greater than three.

**Q7.** The **greatest** drop in compound muscle action potential (CMAP) amplitude and area in myasthenia gravis following slow repetitive nerve stimulation occurs:
- A. between the first and the second responses.
- B. between the first and sixth responses.
- C. between the second and fifth responses.
- D. between the first and ninth responses.
- E. between the first and tenth responses.

**Q8.** Following slow repetitive nerve stimulation in patients with myasthenia gravis, the decrement of the compound muscle action potential (CMAP) is usually **maximal** when comparing:
- A. the first and the fourth CMAPs.
- B. the first and second CMAPs.
- C. the first and ninth CMAPs.
- D. the second and fifth CMAPs.
- E. the first and tenth CMAPs.

**Q9.** Factors that increase the utility of slow repetitive stimulation in myasthenia gravis include all of the following **EXCEPT**:
A. Slow repetitive stimulation, recording weak muscles
B. Immobilization of the limb including the recording and stimulating electrodes
C. Slow repetitive stimulation, recording a proximal muscle
D. Slow repetitive stimulation soon after taking pyridostigmine
E. Slow repetitive stimulation on warm limbs

**Q10.** Which statement is **TRUE** of decrementing responses?
A. Not the usual finding in presynaptic disorders at high rates of stimulation
B. Best seen with high rates of stimulation
C. Not seen in amyotrophic lateral sclerosis (ALS) or myopathies
D. Not usually repaired with short bursts of exercise
E. Is not a feature of postsynaptic disorders

**Q11.** One of the following statements is **TRUE** regarding rapid repetitive nerve stimulation (RNS) in botulism and Lambert-Eaton myasthenic syndrome (LEMS).
A. Botulism is easier to diagnose by RNS than LEMS.
B. Botulism increments are always evident from any muscle.
C. Botulism shows more prominent increments than LEMS.
D. LEMS increments occur mostly from proximal muscles.
E. Botulism and LEMS are presynaptic disorders.

**Q12.** The minimal percentage decrement necessary to be diagnostic of a neuromuscular transmission abnormality is:
A. 5%.
B. 10%.
C. 30%.
D. 25%.
E. 50%.

**Q13.** Nerve conduction studies (NCSs) in Lambert–Eaton myasthenic syndrome (LEMS) are characterized by:
A. normal baseline amplitude of compound muscle action potentials on routine NCS.
B. an incrementing response following slow (2–3 Hz) repetitive nerve stimulation of the median nerve.
C. low baseline amplitude of compound muscle action potentials on routine NCS.
D. abnormalities in symptomatic muscles only.
E. a decrementing response to high-frequency rapid (20–50 Hz) repetitive nerve stimulation of the ulnar nerve.

**Q14.** One of the following is **NEVER** seen in myasthenia gravis on needle electromyography:
A. Fibrillation potentials
B. Varying motor unit action potential amplitude and morphology
C. Low-amplitude and short-duration motor unit morphology
D. Increased jitter and blocking of muscle fibers
E. High-amplitude and long-duration motor unit morphology

**Q15.** A 55-year-old man presents with generalized fatigue and weakness, along with occasional double vision. His examination shows generalized weakness and areflexia. His sensory and nerve conduction studies are normal except for low-amplitude compound muscle action potentials (CMAPs). The best next appropriate step in establishing a diagnosis is:
A. post-brief exercise CMAP evaluation of the median and ulnar nerves.
B. slow repetitive stimulations of the spinal accessory nerve.
C. single-fiber electromyography (EMG) of the extensor digitorum communis.
D. slow repetitive stimulations of the facial nerve.
E. serum acetylcholine receptor antibodies.

---

## PART 2 | QUESTIONS WITH ANSWERS AND DISCUSSION

**QUESTION 1.** The ultrastructural homologue of the miniature endplate potential (MEPP) is the:
A. quantum.
B. safety factor.
C. quantal release.
D. endplate potential.
E. synaptic vesicle.

**ANSWER:** E. synaptic vesicle.

### COMMENTS AND DISCUSSION
- Quantum. A quantum is the amount of acetylcholine (ACh) packaged in a *single synaptic vesicle*, accounting for ~5000 to 10,000 ACh molecules.

- Miniature endplate potential (or MEPP). Each quantum (vesicle) released into the synaptic cleft results in a *1-mV change* in postsynaptic membrane potential. This phenomenon occurs spontaneously and continuously at rest.
- Primary (immediately available) store. This comprises ACh-containing synaptic vesicles located beneath the presynaptic nerve terminal membrane.
- Acetylcholine release. The number of ACh quanta released as the result of a nerve action potential depends on the number of quanta in the primary store and the release probability of quanta. This can be defined by the equation $m = p \times n$, where $m$ = the number of quanta released during each stimulation, $p$ = the probability of release (effectively proportional to the concentration of calcium and typically about 0.2, or 20%), and $n$ = the number of quanta in the immediately available store. Under normal conditions, a single nerve action potential triggers the release of 50–300 quanta (average of about 60 quanta).
- Secondary (or mobilization) store. This usually starts to replenish the immediately available store after 1–2 seconds of sequential nerve action potentials.
- Tertiary (or reserve) store. This large storage is available in the axon and cell body.
- Endplate potential (EPP). The EPP is the potential generated at the postsynaptic membrane following a presynaptic nerve action potential and neuromuscular transmission. Because each released quantum results in a 1-mV change in the postsynaptic membrane potential (MEPP), the ACh release after a nerve action potential results in an average of a 60-mV change in the amplitude of the membrane potential. The resultant electrical-chemical-electrical transmission is fleeting, as the enzyme acetylcholinesterase quickly breaks down ACh at the postsynaptic basal lamina.
- Safety factor. Under normal conditions, the number of quanta (vesicles) released at the neuromuscular junction (NMJ) by the presynaptic terminal (average 60 vesicles with a range of 50–300 vesicles) far exceeds the postsynaptic membrane potential change required to reach the *threshold* needed to generate a postsynaptic muscle action potential (*7 to 20 mV*). The safety factor allows for every EPP to always reach threshold, results in an all-or-none muscle fiber action potential (MFAP), and prevents neuromuscular transmission failure despite the depletion of ACh stores with repetitive action potentials (Fig. 7.1 and Fig. 7.2). In addition to quantal release, several other factors contribute to the safety factor and EPP including ACh receptor conduction properties, ACh receptor density, acetylcholinesterase activity, synaptic architecture, and sodium channel density at the NMJ.

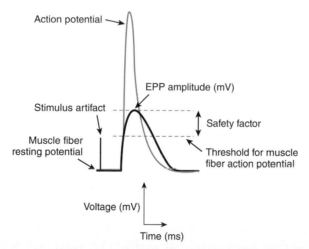

**Fig. 7.1** Safety factor, endplate potential (EPP), and muscle fiber action potential (MFAP). The EPP is a potential that arises at the postsynaptic membrane as a result of the presynaptic nerve action potential and subsequent neuromuscular transmission. In normal conditions, a sufficient number of vesicles are released at the neuromuscular junction by the presynaptic terminal to generate a MFAP. The safety factor ensures that all EPPs reach the necessary threshold for generating an all-or-none MFAP.

- Calcium influx into the terminal axon. Following depolarization of the presynaptic terminal, voltage-gated calcium channels (VGCCs) open leading to calcium influx. Through a calcium-dependent intracellular cascade, vesicles are docked at active release sites (called active zones) and release ACh molecules. Calcium then diffuses slowly away from the vesicle release site in *100–200 ms*. The rate at which motor nerves are repetitively stimulated in the electrodiagnosis (EDX) laboratory dictates whether calcium accumulation plays a role in enhancing the release of ACh or not, that is, influencing "p" in $m = p \times n$.
- Compound muscle action potential (CMAP). The CMAP is obtained during motor NCS with supramaximal stimulation of a motor nerve while recording via a surface electrode placed over the belly of a muscle. The CMAP represents the summation of all MFAPs generated in a muscle following stimulation of all motor axons in its supplying nerve.

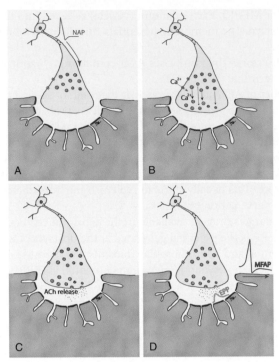

**Fig. 7.2 Neuromuscular junction and transmission.** This figure depicts the process of neuromuscular transmission at the neuromuscular junction (NMJ). (A) First, a nerve action potential (NAP) travels down the axon of the neuron. (B) When the NAP reaches the presynaptic terminal, calcium channels open, allowing calcium to flow into the terminal. The calcium influx triggers the mobilization of acetylcholine (ACh) vesicles to move to the synaptic terminal, where they fuse with the presynaptic membrane. (C) This fusion causes ACh to diffuse across the synaptic cleft and bind to acetylcholine receptors (AChR) on the postsynaptic membrane of the muscle fiber. (D) When ACh binds to AChR, ion channels open, allowing sodium ions (Na+) to flow into the muscle fiber. This influx of Na+ results in depolarization of the muscle fiber, creating an endplate potential (EPP). If the EPP reaches a certain threshold, a muscle fiber action potential (MFAP) occurs, ultimately causing the muscle to contract.

**QUESTION 2.** A decremental response on slow repetitive nerve stimulation does **NOT** occur in which of the following:

A. Botulism
B. Amyotrophic lateral sclerosis
C. Myasthenia gravis
D. Corticosteroid myopathy
E. Lambert-Eaton myasthenic syndrome (LEMS)

**ANSWER:** D. Corticosteroid myopathy

### COMMENTS AND DISCUSSION

- Decremental response on slow repetitive nerve stimulation may occur when there is any dysfunction in the neuromuscular junction, due to reduction of the safety factor. This may be due to a presynaptic defect (such as with Lambert-Eaton myasthenic syndrome [or LEMS] and botulism) or postsynaptic defect (such as with myasthenia gravis).
- Decremental response on slow repetitive nerve stimulation may occur in neurogenic disorders associated with active denervation and reinnervation such as amyotrophic lateral sclerosis.
- Decremental response on slow repetitive nerve stimulation is not seen with corticosteroid myopathy.

**QUESTION 3.** After short exercise, a post-exercise stimulation to look for a compound muscle action potential (CMAP) increment, is often used as an alternative to painful rapid repetitive nerve stimulation in diagnosing Lambert-Eaton myasthenic syndrome (LEMS). The optimal exercise duration for this test is:

A. 10 seconds.
B. 10 minutes.
C. 1 minute.
D. 3 minutes.
E. 30 seconds.

**ANSWER:** A. 10 seconds.

## COMMENTS AND DISCUSSION

- Rapid repetitive nerve stimulation (RNS) at 30 to 50 Hz is painful. In patients who have fair to good muscle power, it can be replaced by brief exercise looking for a post-exercise increment.
- Brief periods of maximal voluntary isometric exercise have the same effect as rapid RNS, are much less painful, and are a good substitute in cooperative subjects.
- A single supramaximal stimulus is applied to generate a baseline compound muscle action potential (CMAP); then the patient performs a 10-second, maximal isometric voluntary contraction, which is followed by another stimulus that produces a post-exercise CMAP.
- Calculation of a CMAP increment after brief (10-second) voluntary contraction is similar to the calculation of the increment following rapid RNS, as follows:

$$\% \ increment = \frac{Amplitude \ of \ post\text{-}exercise \ response - Amplitude \ of \ pre\text{-}exercise \ response}{Amplitude \ of \ pre\text{-}exercise \ response} \times 100$$

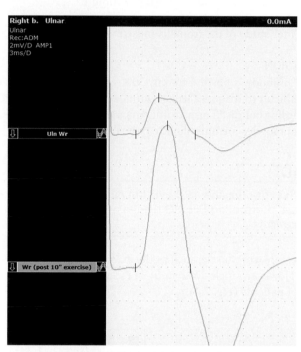

**Fig. 7.3 Post 10-second exercise response in patient with Lambert-Eaton myasthenic syndrome (LEMS).** This upper tracing displays the baseline compound muscle action potential (CMAP) before exercise, while the lower tracing displays the CMAP after 10 seconds of exercise. In LEMS, the post 10-second exercise CMAP exhibits a characteristic increase in amplitude of over 200% when compared to the baseline amplitude.

- Brief exercise is usually done following 5–30 seconds with most robust increment occurring at 10 seconds in patients with LEMS (Fig. 7.3).

**QUESTION 4.**   Which condition has the highest possibility of being detected by routine electrodiagnostic studies?
- A. Acute (<1 week) Guillain-Barré syndrome
- B. Chronic (>6 months) lumbar radiculopathy
- C. Acute (<1 week) peroneal nerve palsy at the fibular neck
- D. Ocular seronegative myasthenia gravis
- E. Acute (<1 week) cervical radiculopathy

**ANSWER:** C. Acute (<1 week) peroneal nerve palsy at the fibular neck

## COMMENTS AND DISCUSSION

- Routine electrodiagnostic studies, which include nerve conduction study (NCS), needle electromyography (EMG), and repetitive nerve stimulation (RNS), are best to diagnose focal demyelinating peripheral nerve lesions. In acute compressive peroneal neuropathy at the fibular neck, there is a likely a conduction block across the fibular neck that would be easily diagnosed on peroneal NCSs in the first week.
- Chronic lumbar radiculopathy may go unnoticed if reinnervation is mild and the compression is mostly on the sensory roots, leading only to pain and numbness.

- The diagnosis of acute cervical radiculopathy will depend on the presence of fibrillation potentials, which appears 2–3 weeks after acute axonal loss.
- Acute Guillain-Barré syndrome (GBS) in the first 1–2 weeks of illness is often non-diagnostic, since the pathology may be predominantly proximal or very distal.
- Ocular myasthenia gravis is difficult to diagnose when seronegative, since RNS results are normal in more than 50% of patients, often requiring more advanced tests such a single-fiber EMG.

**QUESTION 5.**  In patients with suspected ocular myasthenia, which test is the most sensitive in establishing the diagnosis?
- A.  Serum acetylcholine receptor antibody
- B.  Single-fiber jitter study of the frontalis muscle
- C.  Slow repetitive stimulation of the facial nerve
- D.  Slow repetitive stimulation of the spinal accessory nerve
- E.  Single-fiber jitter study of the extensor digitorum communis

**ANSWER:** B. Single-fiber jitter study of the frontalis muscle

**COMMENTS AND DISCUSSION**
- Acetylcholine receptor antibody is positive in only 50%–60% of patients with ocular myasthenia.
- Ocular myasthenia is difficult to diagnose using routine electrodiagnostic studies. Repetitive nerve stimulation (RNS) recordings of distal or proximal muscles are positive in about 50% of patients and RNS recordings of facial muscles are only slightly more useful.

## ◎ HIGH YIELD FACT

> SFEMG is highly sensitive for myasthenia gravis but can lack specificity due to abnormalities in other conditions. Thus, interpreting SFEMG results with clinical and diagnostic findings is crucial for a reliable diagnosis.

- Single-fiber study of the forearm muscle, such as the extensor digitorum communis, is positive in about 80% of patients. However, single-fiber study of facial muscles, such as the frontalis, shows abnormal jitter in ~95% of patients (Fig. 7.4).

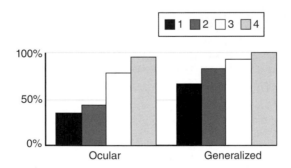

1 = Slow RNS recording distal (hand) muscle
2 = Slow RNS recording proximal (shoulder) muscle
3 = Single-fiber EMG of forearm muscle (extensor digitorum communis)
4 = Single-fiber EMG of facial muscle (frontalis)

**Fig. 7.4**  The diagnostic sensitivity of slow repetitive nerve stimulation (RNS) and single-fiber electromyography (EMG) in the diagnosis of myasthenia gravis (MG). This figure demonstrates the sensitivities of the diagnosis of MG using slow RNS recording the distal (hand) and proximal (shoulder) muscles, as well as single-fiber EMG of the forearm (extensor digitorum communis) and facial (frontalis) muscles. From Geiger C, Katirji B. *Electrodiagnosis of neuromuscular transmission disorders. In: Kaminski HJ, Kusner LL, eds. Myasthenia Gravis and Related Disorders.* 3rd ed. Springer; 2018:249–279.

- It is important to note that while single-fiber electromyography is highly sensitive for the diagnosis of neuromuscular junction disorders, it is not specific and may also be observed in various neuropathic and myopathic conditions.

**QUESTION 6.** Regarding single-fiber needle electromyography:
- A. Abnormal jitter is specific for myasthenia gravis.
- B. Blocking indicates abnormalities of neuromuscular junction transmission.
- C. Normal subjects demonstrate no jitter.
- D. Blocking usually occurs when the jitter is normal.
- E. Fiber density in a normal subject is usually greater than three.

**ANSWER:** B. Blocking indicates abnormalities of neuromuscular junction transmission.

## COMMENTS AND DISCUSSION

- Single-fiber electromyography (SFEMG) is used for the evaluation of neuromuscular transmission, such as in patients with suspected myasthenia gravis.
- SFEMG is the selective recording of a small number (usually two or three) of muscle fiber action potentials (MFAPs) innervated by a single motor unit.
- SFEMG jitter study aims to analyze the effects of the variation in the time it takes the endplate potentials (EPPs) to reach threshold and generate MFAPs. With disorders of the neuromuscular junction (NMJ), there is an increased variation in the time to attain an EPP capable of reaching threshold. Although the examination may be applied to many neuromuscular disorders, SFEMG jitter study is most useful in clinical practice in the diagnosis of NMJ disorders, particularly myasthenia gravis.
- SFEMG jitter studies may be performed with two distinct types of needle electrodes (Fig. 7.5):
  - A specialized single-fiber concentric EMG needle. These needles have a small circular recording surface (25 x 25 μm), which is located on a side port and has a recording volume of ~300 μm³. However, the cost of these electrodes is prohibitive, with a single needle costing several hundred dollars or more. In addition, reusing autoclaved single-fiber electrodes raises concerns regarding the risk of infection transmission and may render them dull, thereby affecting patient comfort.
  - A small concentric "facial" needle. This electrode has an oval recording surface of 80 x 300 μm and a larger catchment area of roughly 1 cm³. This needle is affordable, disposable, and has the same sensitivity and specificity as single-fiber electrodes when assessing neuromuscular disease. Given the standard distance between muscle fibers (200 μm), it is possible that a captured potential with a concentric facial needle is not a true representation of a single muscle fiber, but possibly a summation of two to three neighboring fibers.

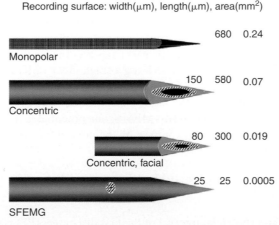

Recording surface: width(μm), length(μm), area(mm²)

| | | | | |
|---|---|---|---|---|
| Monopolar | | | 680 | 0.24 |
| Concentric | | 150 | 580 | 0.07 |
| Concentric, facial | | 80 | 300 | 0.019 |
| SFEMG | | 25 | 25 | 0.0005 |

**Fig. 7.5** Comparison of monopolar, concentric, concentric facial, and single-fiber needle electrodes. This figure demonstrates the shape and dimensions of the recording surface, including width, length and area, of various types of electrodes. From Stålberg Erik V, Sanders Donald B Jitter recordings with concentric needle electrodes. *Muscle Nerve.* 2009;40(3):331–339.

- Certain other requirements that are essential for the accurate interpretation of jitter studies using a disposable needle.
  - Although jitter analysis may be obtained from any skeletal muscle, the orbicularis oculi, frontalis, and extensor digitorum muscles are ideal because of their frequent involvement in NMJ disorders and the ability of most patients to voluntarily control and sustain activity to a minimum level as required for the test.
  - Filter settings should be set at 1000 Hz for the low-frequency (high-pass) filter when using concentric needle electrode, and at 500 Hz when using a single-fiber electrode. Filter settings should be set at 10,000 Hz for the high-frequency (low-pass) filter.

- Selected single MFAPs should have mainly one positive and one negative peak, a rise time of 300 μs with a constant slope and, preferably, a peak-to-peak amplitude of 200 μV or more.
- An amplitude threshold triggers a delay line to allow recording from a single spike by triggering on it on a screen with a delay line capability.
- Computerized equipment assists in calculating individual and mean interpotential intervals (IPIs) and jitters.
- There are two techniques commonly used in SFEMG jitter recordings.
  - *Volitional (recruitment) SFEMG.* Here, the patient activates and maintains the firing rate of the motor unit. This technique is not possible if the patient cannot cooperate (e.g., a child or a patient with cognitive impairment, encephalopathy, coma, or severe weakness). The study is also difficult if the patient is unable to maintain a constant and stable voluntary muscle contraction (e.g., in patients with parkinsonism, tremor, dystonia, or spasticity). An amplitude threshold is used to trigger the oscilloscope trace on the closest potential (the action potential with the sharpest rise time and the greatest amplitude), whereas potentials from other motor units are excluded from the oscilloscope screen. With minimal voluntary activation, the needle is positioned until two time-locked spikes (a pair) from a single motor unit are recognized. When a pair is identified, one potential triggers the oscilloscope (*triggering potential*) and the second precedes or follows the first (*slave potential*). After recording multiple consecutive firings of these two potentials (usually about 50–100 consecutive discharges), the electromyographer determines, usually with the aid of a computerized system, the consecutive IPIs and calculates the difference between consecutive IPIs. Comparison of IPIs illustrates the slight variation in transmission time at the NMJ, named the *neuromuscular jitter*.
  - *Stimulation (axonal stimulation) SFEMG.* This is performed by inserting an additional monopolar needle electrode near the intramuscular nerve twigs and stimulating at a low current and constant rate. Then the recording needle electrode is moved slightly until one or more potentials are recorded. This technique requires that the electromyographer manipulates two electrodes, a stimulating and recording electrode. Percutaneous (surface) stimulation can substitute for the needle electrode stimulations in anatomic areas where the motor branch is superficial and easily accessible, such as stimulating the zygomatic branch of the facial nerve while recording the frontalis muscle. Stimulation SFEMG has the advantage of not requiring patient participation and, thus, may be performed on patients who may not be able to fully cooperate or complete a volitional study. Another advantage of this technique is that the rate of stimulation may be adjusted from slow rate (2–3 Hz) to a rapid rate (20–50 Hz). This is helpful in differentiating presynaptic from postsynaptic disorders, since the jitter improves significantly with rapid RNS in LEMS while it does not change or worsens in myasthenia gravis. In stimulation SFEMG, the IPI is measured as the latency between the stimulus artifact and a single MFAP and, thus, only one endplate is involved in the analysis. Consequently, stimulation SFEMG jitter normal values are smaller than volitional SFEMG. To calculate the normal stimulation jitter value using a single-fiber EMG needle, it is recommended that the reference data for volitional SFEMG is multiplied by 0.80.
- Jitter is most accurately determined by calculating a *mean consecutive difference (MCD)*. The jitter is calculated as the variation in IPIs between two MFAPs; one potential is time-locked by the trigger, and all the variation of both endplates is expressed by the jitter of the slave potential.
  - It is calculated as follows:

$$MCD = \frac{(IPI1 - IPI2) + (IPI2 - IPI3) + ... + (IPI(N-1) - IPIN)}{N-1}$$

  Where IPI1 is the interpotential interval of the first discharge, IPI2 is of the second discharge, etc., and N is the number of discharges recorded.

  - Normal subjects have a small jitter, which varies among different muscles. The mean jitter of the muscle sampled is reported after analyzing 20 pairs (Table 7.1).
  - Abnormal jitter is a very sensitive measure of impaired neuromuscular transmission but is non-specific, since it may occur with neurogenic and myopathic disorders as well.
  - Blocking is measured as the percentage of discharges in which the slave single-fiber potential does not fire (Fig. 7.6). For example, in 100 discharges of the pair, if a slave potential is missing 30 times, the blocking is 30%. In general, blocking occurs when the jitter values are significantly abnormal.
  - Blocking indicates a significant impairment of NMJ transmission and is always seen when the jitter values are abnormal.
  - A number of different variables, including the muscle examined, the type of recording electrode used, the mode of muscle fiber activation, and age of the subject, may affect normal values for jitter.

**TABLE 7.1** Reference values for jitter measurements during volitional muscle activation by recording with adisposable concentric facial EMG needle.

| Volitional | Orbicularis oculi | Frontalis | Extensor digitorum |
|---|---|---|---|
| Mean MCD, μs, mean (SD) | 22.9 (3.9) | 20.6 (3.6) | 23.4 (3.0) |
| Upper limit | 31 | 28 | 30 |
| 18th MCD, μs, mean (SD)* | 29.0 (7.6) | 25.8 (5.6) | 30.0 (6.1) |
| Upper limit | 45 | 38 | 43 |

*EMG,* electromyography; *MCD,* mean consecutive difference; *SD,* standard deviation.
*18th MCDs (volitional) were determined to be the cutoff jitter values for any particular muscle fiber pair in a given muscle, with a reading above this value considered an "outlier."

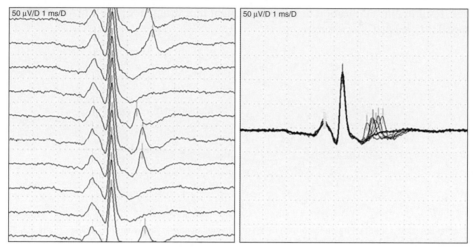

**Fig. 7.6 Abnormal jitter and blocking.** Single-fiber study showing three potentials (*left panel:* 10 rastered discharges; *right panel:* 10 superimposed discharges). Middle potential is the triggering potential. In the right panel, the potential on the left (yellow) has normal jitter, whereas the potential on the right (green) has abnormal jitter and blocking.

- The final results of SFEMG jitter study are expressed by (1) the mean jitter of all muscle pairs studied, (2) the percentage of pairs with impulse blocking, and (3) the percentage of pairs with abnormal jitter. The study is abnormal when one or more of the following criteria are met:
  - Mean consecutive difference (or MCD) exceeds an upper limit (normal mean + 2 standard deviations [SD] for a given muscle).
  - More than two (10%) pairs have jitter considered to be in an outlier range when 20 individual muscle fiber pairs are analyzed.
  - Impulse blocking is seen frequently in the majority of fiber pairs in a muscle.
- Fiber density is measured by sampling 20 different sites in a muscle and counting the number of fibers seen in each site. An average number of single muscle fiber potentials per recording site can be calculated. In reinnervation, fiber density increases due to sprouting. Fiber density values differ between muscles and tend to increase with age, particularly over the age of 50 years. Fiber density values range between 1.5 and 2.5 in normal subjects. In reinnervation, fiber density will increase.

**QUESTION 7.** The **greatest** drop in compound muscle action potential (CMAP) amplitude and area in myasthenia gravis following slow repetitive nerve stimulation occurs:
  A. between the first and the second responses.
  B. between the first and sixth responses.
  C. between the second and fifth responses.
  D. between the first and ninth responses.
  E. between the first and tenth responses.

**ANSWER:** A. between the first and the second responses.

**COMMENTS AND DISCUSSION**
- Slow repetitive nerve stimulation (RNS) is usually performed by applying five supramaximal stimuli to a mixed or motor nerve at a rate of 2–3 Hz. Calculation of the decrement with slow RNS includes

comparing the baseline CMAP amplitude to the third or fourth CMAP amplitude. Slow RNS at rest should be repeated after an interval of 1–2 minutes to confirm a normal (or abnormal) response. The CMAP decrement is expressed as a percentage and calculated as follows:

$$\% \ decrement = \frac{Amplitude\,(1st\,response) - Amplitude\,(3rd\,or\,4th\,response)}{Amplitude\,(1st\,response)} \times 100$$

- In myasthenia gravis, the CMAP decrement with slow RNS initially worsens for the first few stimuli, which then plateaus or even improves, due to the mobilization store re-supplying the immediately available store. Although the greatest drop in CMAP amplitude and area occurs between the first and the second responses, the decrement usually continues and is typically maximal when comparing the first and fourth CMAPs (Fig. 7.7). Often, after the fifth or sixth stimulus, the secondary stores are mobilized, resulting in stabilization or sometimes slight improvement of the CMAP, giving rise to the characteristic "U-shaped" decrement.

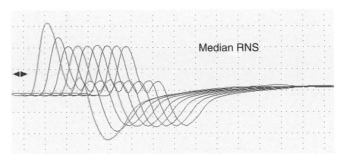
Median RNS

**Fig. 7.7** Decrement on slow repetitive nerve syndrome (RNS) of the median nerve. Note that the largest drop is usually between the first and second responses, whereas the maximal drop is usually between the first and third or fourth responses.

**QUESTION 8.** Following slow repetitive nerve stimulation in patients with myasthenia gravis, the decrement of the compound muscle action potential (CMAP) is usually **maximal** when comparing:
  A. the first and the fourth CMAPs.
  B. the first and second CMAPs.
  C. the first and ninth CMAPs.
  D. the second and fifth CMAPs.
  E. the first and tenth CMAPs.

**ANSWER:** A. The first and the fourth CMAPs

**COMMENTS AND DISCUSSION:** (see also comments and discussion from Question 7 and Fig. 7.7)

**QUESTION 9.** Factors that increase the utility of slow repetitive stimulation in myasthenia gravis include all of the following **EXCEPT**:
  A. Slow repetitive stimulation, recording weak muscles
  B. Immobilization of the limb including the recording and stimulating electrodes
  C. Slow repetitive stimulation, recording a proximal muscle
  D. Slow repetitive stimulation soon after taking pyridostigmine
  E. Slow repetitive stimulation on warm limbs

**ANSWER:** D. Slow repetitive stimulation soon after taking pyridostigmine

## COMMENTS AND DISCUSSION
- Repetitive nerve stimulation (RNS) requires the following:
  - Patients taking acetylcholinesterase inhibitors (such as pyridostigmine) should be asked, if possible, to withhold their medication, preferably for 6–12 hours before RNS. These agents improve neuromuscular transmission and may mask a compound muscle action potential (CMAP) decrement resulting in a false-negative RNS.

○ Limb temperature should be maintained at around 33°C at the recording site. A cool limb enhances neuromuscular transmission and may mask a CMAP decrement, resulting in a false-negative RNS. This may be due to decreased functional effectiveness of the enzyme acetylcholinesterase, resulting in increased amount of acetylcholine available at the neuromuscular junction (NMJ).

○ Movement at either the stimulation or recording site may result in a variable waveform baseline, giving the appearance of a CMAP amplitude decay or increment. To ensure minimal movement, especially at the stimulation or recording sites, the limb undergoing testing should be securely immobilized to a board using either tape or Velcro.

○ Supramaximal stimulation and CMAP is required to ensure that all nerve fibers are activated. Unnecessarily high intensity or long-duration stimuli should be avoided to prevent movement artifacts and excessive pain.

○ The choice of nerve to be stimulated and the muscle to be recorded depends on the patient's symptom manifestations. Useful nerves for RNS are the median and ulnar nerves, recording the abductor pollicis brevis and abductor digiti minimi, respectively. Because the upper limb is easily immobilized, these RNSs are well tolerated and accompanied by minimal movement artifact. However, since distal muscles are often spared in postsynaptic NMJ disorders (such as myasthenia gravis), recording from a proximal muscle is often necessary. Slow RNS of the spinal accessory nerve, recording the trapezius muscle, is the most common study of a proximal nerve. It is relatively well tolerated and subject to less movement artifact when compared to RNS of other proximal nerves such as the musculocutaneous or axillary nerves, recording the biceps or deltoid muscles, respectively. Finally, slow RNS of the facial nerve, recording nasalis or orbicularis oculi muscles, is indicated in patients with ocular, bulbar, or facial weakness when myasthenia gravis is suspected and other RNSs are normal or equivocal. However, the normal facial CMAP is often low in amplitude and often plagued by large stimulation artifacts. This renders measurement of facial CMAP decrement more difficult and subject to error.

**QUESTION 10.** Which statement is **TRUE** of decrementing responses?
A. Not the usual finding in presynaptic disorders at high rates of stimulation
B. Best seen with high rates of stimulation
C. Not seen in amyotrophic lateral sclerosis (ALS) or myopathies
D. Not usually repaired with short bursts of exercise
E. Is not a feature of postsynaptic disorders

**ANSWER:** A. Not the usual finding in presynaptic disorders at high rates of stimulation

**COMMENTS AND DISCUSSION**
- During repetitive nerve stimulation (RNS), compound muscle action potentials (CMAPs) are evaluated for evidence of amplitude/area decrement or increment.
- Rate of motor nerve stimulation influences calcium physiology and accumulation in enhancing acetylcholine (ACh) release.
  ○ Calcium diffuses from the presynaptic terminal in about 100–200 ms after a single stimulus.
  ○ Slow RNS (a stimulation rate of <5 Hz) causes depletion of the primary or immediately available store of ACh but does not effectively increase the concentration of calcium. This, in turn, results in fewer endplate potentials (EPPs) reaching the threshold needed to generate an action potential in muscle fiber, which then leads to the typical CMAP decrement seen in postsynaptic disorders. Slow RNS is usually done at a rate 2–3 Hz. A total of five stimuli is sufficient, since the maximal decrease in ACh release occur after the first four stimuli. Increasing stimulation to 9–10 stimuli can be done but is not necessary. Decrements with slow RNS are seen in all types of neuromuscular junction (NMJ) disorders, including both presynaptic and postsynaptic disorders.
  ○ In addition, rapid RNS (stimulation rate >10 Hz) causes depletion of the primary or immediately available store of ACh but also increases the concentration of calcium and the probability of ACh release. The increase in probability in ACh release usually wins out, allowing more EEPs to reach threshold, and is ultimately responsible for the CMAP increment seen in presynaptic disorders. A frequency of 20–50 Hz in rapid RNS ensures the accumulation of calcium in the presynaptic terminal. However, this is usually quite painful. A train of 1–3 s is needed. A brief period of maximal isometric voluntary exercise, best at 10 s, has the same effect as rapid RNS at 20–50 Hz. The patient is effectively firing their motor unit action potentials (MUAPs) at 20–50 Hz, which is the normal maximal rate of activation. This is much less painful than rapid RNS and, given its tolerability,

allows for examination of multiple motor nerves. Brief exercise could substitute for rapid RNS in most cooperative subjects. However, rapid RNS is necessary in patients who cannot produce a strong isometric exercise such as in young children, unresponsive patients, or patients with severe weakness.

o Increments, not decrements, are seen in presynaptic disorders with rapid rates of stimulation (typically 30–50 Hz). Slow rates of stimulation are optimal to bring out a decrement, as they deplete the primary store of ACh but do not result in calcium accumulation within the presynaptic terminal.

o If slow RNS shows a decrement (≥10%) at rest, the same test should be repeated after the patient exercises for 10 seconds to demonstrate *repair* of the decrement ("*post-exercise facilitation*"). This is due to increased release of ACh quanta and a greater number of EPPs reaching the threshold needed to generate action potential.

o Any disorder associated with denervation (e.g., ALS or inflammatory myopathies) will have resultant reinnervation. When that occurs, new NMJs are formed, which, when immature, may demonstrate impaired transmission and abnormal decrements with slow RNS.

**QUESTION 11.** One of the following statements is **TRUE** regarding rapid repetitive nerve stimulation (RNS) in botulism and Lambert-Eaton myasthenic syndrome (LEMS).
A. Botulism is easier to diagnose by RNS than LEMS.
B. Botulism increments are always evident from any muscle.
C. Botulism shows more prominent increments than LEMS.
D. LEMS increments occur mostly from proximal muscles.
E. Botulism and LEMS are presynaptic disorders.

**ANSWER:** E. Botulism and LEMS are presynaptic disorders.

**COMMENTS AND DISCUSSION**
- Botulism and LEMS are presynaptic disorders, whereas myasthenia gravis is a postsynaptic disorder (see Table 7.2).
- In patients with LEMS, post-tetanic facilitation exceeds 60% in all muscles and 100% in at least one muscle in 80% of cases. In addition, it is common to have robust increments exceeding 200% in many LEMS patients, particularly those with elevated voltage-gated calcium channel antibody.
- The electrodiagnostic (EDX) findings in botulism are compatible with a presynaptic defect of neuromuscular transmission and are somewhat similar to the findings in LEMS. However, the results of EDX testing are more variable and dependent on the amount and type of toxic exposure, degree and distribution of muscle weakness, and the timing of the study. During the early course of the disease, the EDX abnormalities may be limited and often change significantly from day to day, particularly as the muscle weakness worsens.
- Low compound muscle action potential (CMAP) amplitudes, obtained during routine motor nerve conduction studies (NCSs), are the most consistent finding, present in 85% of patients with botulism, particularly when recording from weak muscles (usually proximal). Diminished CMAP amplitudes are the result of the inadequate release of synaptic vesicles, which in turn render many endplate potentials (EPPs) unable to reach threshold after a single stimulus. Rarely, the CMAPs are diffusely absent in severe cases of botulism, consistent with total blockade of acetylcholine (ACh) release.
- Rapid RNS in patients with botulism results in CMAP increment. The CMAP increment occurs also following a brief (10 s) period of isometric exercise. With tetanic stimulation, calcium accumulation is greatly enhanced resulting in larger releases of quanta. This leads to an increasing number of muscle fibers reaching the threshold required for the generation of muscle fiber action potentials. The increment in botulism is modest, and sometimes evident only with recording proximal or weak muscles. The increment ranges between 50% to 100%, when compared to the increment in LEMS, which often surpasses 200%. The increment may occasionally be absent, especially in severe cases, presumably due to the degree of presynaptic blockade.
- Slow RNS in patients with botulism may cause a decrement of CMAP amplitude. However, this is infrequent and mild, often not exceeding 8% to 10% of baseline. It is caused by the progressive depletion of the immediately available ACh stores without accumulation of calcium in the presynaptic terminals.

**TABLE 7.2** Baseline CMAP and repetitive stimulation findings in common neuromuscular junction disorders

| NMJ disorder | NMJ defect | CMAP amplitude | Slow RNS | Rapid RNS or 10-second exercise |
|---|---|---|---|---|
| Myasthenia gravis | Postsynaptic | Normal | Decrement | Normal or decrement |
| Lambert-Eaton myasthenic syndrome | Presynaptic | Low in all muscles | Decrement | Marked increment: >100% in at least one muscle and >60% in all muscles |
| Botulism | Presynaptic | Low in proximal and weak muscles | Decrement | Modest increment: in weak muscles (50%–100%) |

*CMAP*, compound muscle action potential; *NMJ*, neuromuscular junction; *RNS*, repetitive nerve stimulation.

**QUESTION 12.** The minimal percentage decrement necessary to be diagnostic of a neuromuscular transmission abnormality is:
   A. 5%.
   B. 10%.
   C. 30%.
   D. 25%.
   E. 50%.

**ANSWER:** B. 10%.

**COMMENTS AND DISCUSSION**
- A reproducible decrement of more than 10% is considered abnormal and reduces false positives. Decrements of 5% to 10% are considered equivocal and not diagnostic. If there is a reproducible decrement at rest ($\geq$10%), slow repetitive nerve stimulation (RNS) should be repeated after the patient exercises for 10 seconds to demonstrate repair of the decrement (*"post-exercise facilitation"*).
- If there is no or equivocal decrement (<10%) with slow RNS at rest, the patient should perform maximal voluntary exercise for 1 minute. Immediately following the period of exercise, slow RNS is repeated during the subsequent 1, 2, 3, 4, and 5 minutes. Because the amount of acetylcholine (ACh) released with each stimulus is at its minimum 2 to 5 minutes after exercise, slow RNS after exercise provides a high chance of detecting a defect in the neuromuscular junction (NMJ) by demonstrating a worsening compound muscle action potential (CMAP) decrement (*"post-exercise exhaustion"*). Post-exercise slow RNS studies increase the yield of RNS by about 5% to 7%.
- Slow RNS results in a decrease in quantal release due to the depletion of the immediate (primary) ACh stores. In myasthenia gravis, this stresses the NMJ to a point where many endplate potentials (EPPs) fail to reach the threshold needed to generate an action potential. The loss of many muscle fiber action potentials (MFAPs) is reflected as a decremental CMAP on slow RNS. The diagnostic sensitivity of slow RNS in myasthenia gravis is increased when recording from symptomatic muscles such as the proximal muscles (e.g., the trapezius in generalized myasthenia gravis), and facial muscles (e.g., the orbicularis oculi or nasalis in ocular or bulbar myasthenia gravis). Slow RNS of the facial and spinal accessory nerves increases the diagnostic sensitivity of the study by about 5% to 20%, compared to recording distal muscles (e.g., the abductor digiti minimi).

**QUESTION 13.** Nerve conduction studies (NCSs) in Lambert-Eaton myasthenic syndrome (LEMS) are characterized by:
   A. normal baseline amplitude of compound muscle action potentials on routine NCS.
   B. an incrementing response following slow (2–3 Hz) repetitive nerve stimulation of the median nerve.
   C. low baseline amplitude of compound muscle action potentials on routine NCS.
   D. abnormalities in symptomatic muscles only.
   E. a decrementing response to high-frequency rapid (20–50 Hz) repetitive nerve stimulation of the ulnar nerve.

**ANSWER:** C. low baseline amplitude compound muscle action potentials on routine NCS.

**COMMENTS AND DISCUSSION**

- The following triad characterizes LEMS: (1) Low baseline amplitude of compound muscle action potential (CMAP) on routine NCS, (2) a decrementing response following slow (2–3 Hz) repetitive nerve stimulation, and (3) an incrementing response to high rapid (20–50 Hz) repetitive nerve stimulation or following 10 seconds of brief exercise.
- The CMAPs, obtained during routine motor NCSs, are usually low in amplitude in patients with LEMS, since many endplate potentials (EPPs) do not reach threshold after a single stimulus due to inadequate release of synaptic vesicles. Thus a low number of muscle fiber action potentials (MFAPs) are generated, leading to low-amplitude CMAPs. Low CMAP amplitudes are usually present universally in all muscles.
- The optimal frequency is 20–50 Hz for 2–5 seconds. Typical rapid repetitive nerve stimulation (RNS) applies 200 stimuli at a rate of 50 Hz (i.e., 50 Hz for 4 seconds). Calculation of CMAP increment after rapid RNS is as follows:

$$\% \ increment = \frac{Amplitude\,(Highest\,response) - Amplitude\,(1st\,response)}{Amplitude\,(1st\,response)} \times 100$$

- A CMAP increment of more than 50%–100% (i.e., 150%-200% of the baseline amplitude) is considered abnormal. A modest increment of 25%–40% may occur in normal individuals. This is likely caused by increased synchrony of MFAPs following tetanic stimulation ("*physiologic post-tetanic facilitation or pseudofacilitation*").
- Rapid RNS (usually 20–50 Hz) or brief (10 seconds) isometric exercise results in a CMAP amplitude increment. This rate of stimulation or type of exercise enhances calcium influx into the presynaptic terminal, which results in larger releases of quanta and larger EPPs. Although many EPPs do not reach threshold after the first stimulus, many muscle fibers achieve threshold required for the generation of MFAPs with the subsequent stimuli. In patients with LEMS, post-tetanic facilitation can exceed 60% in all muscles and 100% in at least one muscle in 80% of cases. It is also common to observe robust CMAP increments can exceed 200% in many patients with LEMS, particularly those with elevated voltage-gated calcium channel antibody.
- Slow RNS results in >10 % CMAP decrement in all patients with LEMS. With slow RNS, ACh release is reduced further because of the depletion of the immediately available stores, and, at this slow rate of stimulation, calcium does not accumulate in the presynaptic terminal. The end result is further loss of many MFAPs and a decrement of CMAP amplitude. Slow RNS cannot distinguish LEMS from the decrement seen in postsynaptic disorders, such as myasthenia gravis, rendering it not useful in LEMS diagnosis.

**QUESTION 14.**  One of the following is **NEVER** seen in myasthenia gravis on needle electromyography:
- A.  Fibrillation potentials
- B.  Varying motor unit action potential amplitude and morphology
- C.  Low-amplitude and short-duration motor unit morphology
- D.  Increased jitter and blocking of muscle fibers
- E.  High-amplitude and long-duration motor unit morphology

**ANSWER:** E. High-amplitude and long-duration motor unit morphology

**COMMENTS AND DISCUSSION**

- Abnormal jitter on single-fiber studies is common in myasthenia gravis.
- Routine needle electromyography (EMG) is usually normal in neuromuscular junction (NMJ) disorders. However, in moderate to severe cases, the needle EMG may occasionally show:
  - Moment-to-moment variation and instability of motor unit action potentials (MUAPs). In healthy subjects, individual MUAP amplitude, duration, and phases are stable with little, if any, morphology variation. However, individual MUAP amplitude and morphology in NMJ disorders may vary significantly during activation due to intermittent NMJ blockade, slowing, or both.
  - Short-duration, low-amplitude, and polyphasic MUAP are usually seen primarily in proximal muscles and are similar in morphology to those seen in myopathies. In NMJ disorders, "myopathic" MUAPs are caused by physiological blocking and slowing of neuromuscular transmission at endplates during voluntary activation. This is due to exclusion of muscle fiber action potentials (MFAPs) from the MUAP leading to short-duration and low-amplitude MUAPs, and asynchrony of neuromuscular transmission of muscle fibers leading to polyphasic MUAPs. In contrast, high-amplitude and long-duration motor unit morphology does not accompany myasthenia gravis.

○ Fibrillation potentials are rarely encountered in NMJ disorders, and when present, they are usually inconspicuous and observed mostly in proximal muscles. They are likely a result of chronic neuromuscular transmission blockade, loss of endplates, or loss of presynaptic terminals, leading to "effective" denervation of individual muscle fibers. In contrast to myasthenia gravis and Lambert–Eaton myasthenic syndrome (LEMS), fibrillation potentials are commonly seen in botulism on weak muscles if needle EMG is performed several weeks after exposure.

**QUESTION 15.** A 55-year-old man presents with generalized fatigue and weakness, along with occasional double vision. His examination shows generalized weakness and areflexia. His sensory and nerve conduction studies are normal except for low-amplitude compound muscle action potentials (CMAPs). The best next appropriate step in establishing a diagnosis is:

A. post-brief exercise CMAP evaluation of the median and ulnar nerves.
B. slow repetitive stimulations of the spinal accessory nerve.
C. single-fiber electromyography (EMG) of the extensor digitorum communis.
D. slow repetitive stimulations of the facial nerve.
E. serum acetylcholine receptor antibodies.

**ANSWER:** A. post-brief exercise CMAP evaluation of the median and ulnar nerves.

## COMMENTS AND DISCUSSION

- This patient has findings consistent with Lambert-Eaton myasthenic syndrome (LEMS).
- The electrodiagnostic (EDX) strategy in a patient with a suspected neuromuscular junction (NMJ) disorder should start with a detailed history and comprehensive neurological examination.
- Sensory and motor nerve conduction studies (NCSs) in two limbs (preferably an upper and a lower extremity) should be the initial studies.
  ○ Sensory NCSs are normal in NMJ disorders, unless there is an additional entrapment mononeuropathy or peripheral polyneuropathy.
  ○ Motor NCSs are helpful in the evaluation of all disorders affecting the motor unit, including NMJ disorders. *CMAP amplitude* is the most useful parameter in NMJ disorders, since the motor distal latencies, conduction velocities, F-wave minimal latencies, and H reflexes are normal.
    - CMAP amplitudes are usually normal in postsynaptic disorders (such as myasthenia gravis), following a single supramaximal stimulus of all motor nerves, due to the effect of the safety factor. Despite partial acetylcholine (ACh) receptor blockade, endplate potentials (EPPs) achieve threshold and generate muscle fiber action potentials (MFAPs) in all muscle fibers, resulting in normal CMAP.
    - CMAP amplitudes are often low in presynaptic disorders (such as LEMS), since many EPPs do not reach threshold and many muscle fibers do not depolarize.
- The clinical situation and baseline CMAP amplitudes dictate the next steps:
  ○ If the CMAP amplitudes are low or the diagnosis of LEMS is clinically suspected, as in this patient with weakness, fatigue, diplopia, and areflexia, a sufficient screening test is to measure the baseline and post-exercise CMAPs of at least two distal motor nerves (such as the median and ulnar nerves). In LEMS, CMAP increment is usually robust and may surpass 200%. A rapid repetitive nerve stimulation (RNS) of one distal nerve for 3–5 seconds can be performed for confirmation if there are definite CMAP increments after brief exercise, although this test is extremely painful.
  ○ If the diagnosis of botulism is considered, the choice of muscle should include clinically weak muscles. In botulism, the CMAP increment is usually 50%–100%. In addition, the study may be repeated in 1–2 days, particularly if the initial evaluation was done during the early phase of the illness.
  ○ If the diagnosis of myasthenia gravis is clinically suspected, slow RNS should be performed on at least two motor nerves. The selection of nerves and muscles is dependent on the clinical manifestations, with the goal to record from clinically weak muscles. One should start by performing slow RNS on a distal hand muscle (such as the abductor digiti minimi or abductor pollicis brevis) and move on to a proximal muscle such as the upper trapezius. If a decrement is found, RNS should be repeated following 10 seconds of exercise to confirm that the decrement "improves" (or is less marked) as would be expected in true NMJ disorders. If no decrement is discovered on routine RNS studies, the study should be repeated after 1-minute of exercise at 1-minute intervals for the next 4–5 minutes to assess for the development of a significant decrement (post-exercise exhaustion).

- Facial RNS should be reserved for patients with oculobulbar manifestations and normal slow RNS recording from distal and proximal muscles.
- Single-fiber EMG (SFEMG) of one or two muscles (such as the frontalis, orbicularis oculi, or extensor digitorum communis) should be considered if the diagnosis of myasthenia gravis is still considered despite normal RNS studies in seronegative patients.
- If the CMAPs obtained on motor NCSs in a patient with suspected myasthenia gravis are low or borderline, post-exercise CMAP screening should be done to exclude LEMS and botulism. A misdiagnosis of myasthenia gravis is often made if post-exercise CMAP evaluation is not done and a slow RNS shows a CMAP decrement.
- Post-exercise CMAP screening is recommended for patients with weakness associated with a malignancy (particularly small-cell lung cancer), or if the clinical situation does not clearly differentiate between LEMS and myasthenia gravis.
- Slow RNS and SFEMG cannot routinely discriminate between pre- and post-synaptic diseases.
- In addition, ACh receptor antibodies are usually elevated in myasthenia gravis, whereas voltage-gated calcium channel receptor antibodies are elevated in LEMS.

## SUGGESTED READINGS

Geiger CD, Katirji B. Electrodiagnosis of Neuromuscular Junction Disorders. In: Kaminski H, Kusner L, eds. *Myasthenia Gravis and Related Disorders. Current Clinical Neurology. New Jersey:* 3rd ed. Humana Press, Cham.; 2018:249-279.

Hatanaka Y, Oh SJ. Ten-second exercise is superior to 30-second exercise for post-exercise facilitation in diagnosing Lambert-Eaton myasthenic syndrome. *Muscle Nerve.* 2008;37:572-575.

Howard JF, Sanders DB, Massey JM. The electrodiagnosis of myasthenia gravis and the Lambert-Eaton syndrome. *Neurol Clin.* 1994;12:305-330.

Katirji B, Kaminski HJ, Ruff RL, eds. *Neuromuscular Disorders in Clinical Practice.* 2nd ed. New York: Springer; 2014:153-163.

Oh SJ, Kim DE, Kuruoglu R, et al. Diagnostic sensitivity of the laboratory tests in myasthenia gravis. *Muscle Nerve.* 1992;15:720-724.

Plomp JJ. Neuromuscular junction: physiology and pathophysiology. In: Kaminski HJ, Kusner LL, eds. *Myasthenia Gravis and Related Disorders. Current Clinical Neurology.* New Jersey: 3rd ed. Humana Press, Cham.; 2018:1-12.

Stålberg EV, Sanders DB. Jitter recordings with concentric needle electrodes. *Muscle Nerve.* 2009;40(3):331–339.

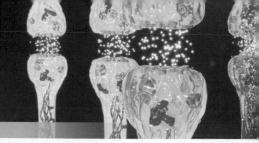

# CHAPTER 8

# Electrodiagnostic Medicine VI: Electrodiagnostic Technical Factors

**Q1.** An 85-year-old woman has numbness in both feet for 2 years. The nerve conduction study (NCS) shows normal peroneal, tibial, and median compound muscle action potentials (CMAPs) and normal median and radial sensory nerve action potentials (SNAPs), but sural SNAP amplitudes of 2 μV. Needle electromyography (EMG) shows no active denervation, with normal motor unit action potentials (MUAPs) in the extensor hallucis longus, tibialis anterior, and tibialis posterior. Which of the following is most **CORRECT**?
A. This patient has a demyelinating polyneuropathy.
B. Abnormal sural SNAPs always indicate an axonal polyneuropathy.
C. Lumbosacral radiculopathy can be ruled out.
D. This patient has a lumbosacral plexopathy.
E. Reduced/absent sural SNAPs can be a normal finding in the very elderly.

**Q2.** Which of the following features on nerve conduction studies is seen in newborns when compared to adults?
A. Similar amplitudes as adults
B. Similar conduction velocities as adults
C. Reduced conduction velocities compared to adults
D. Increased conduction velocities compared to adults
E. Nerve conduction studies cannot be performed in newborns.

**Q3.** Nerve conduction study on a 15-day-old neonate showed that all motor conduction velocities are between 25 and 30 m/s. Sensory nerve action potential (SNAP) and compound muscle action potential (CMAP) amplitudes are normal. Needle EMG is normal. Given the nerve conduction and needle EMG study results, what is the next best step of management in this patient?
A. *SMN1* gene detection test
B. Nerve biopsy to search for onion bulb formation
C. Oral corticosteroids
D. Intravenous immunoglobulin
E. No evidence of peripheral polyneuropathy

**Q4.** A nerve conduction study is performed on a 48-year-old woman who presents with right hand numbness. Sensory conduction study of the right upper extremity is shown in the table below.

| Nerve-recording | Latency (ms) | Amplitude (μV) | Conduction velocity (m/s) |
|---|---|---|---|
| Median-index finger | 3.6 | 120 | 39 |
| Ulnar-little finger | 3.1 | 100 | 40 |
| Radial-dorsum of thumb | 2.9 | 98 | 42 |

Which of the following statements is **CORRECT**?

A. Conduction velocities are normal for this age.
B. This study results are due to cool temperature.
C. There is co-stimulation of adjacent nerves.
D. She likely has carpal tunnel syndrome.
E. The diagnosis is hereditary motor and sensory neuropathy.

**Q5.** Which of the following statements is **CORRECT** regarding the effect of cold temperature on the peripheral nerve?
A. Detachment of the myelin sheath from the nerve
B. Delayed opening of potassium channels
C. More sodium influx into the cell
D. Decreased motor and sensory nerve conduction amplitudes
E. More prominent changes in motor than sensory responses

**Q6.** A median sensory study is performed with a hand temperature of 28°C. The conduction velocity is 46 m/s. What is the corrected conduction velocity for 34°C?
A. 38 m/s
B. 42 m/s
C. 46 m/s
D. 58 m/s
E. 72 m/s

**Q7.** A 28-year-old woman presents with ptosis and proximal muscle weakness. Myasthenia gravis is suspected, and repetitive nerve stimulation is performed. Before starting the study, you find that the temperature of her hand is 27°C. If warming is not done, which of the following findings is expected on slow repetitive nerve stimulation of the extremity?
A. No difference from a normothermic hand
B. More prominent decremental response
C. Less decremental response
D. Incremental response
E. Decremental response in the first train and incremental response after exercise

**Q8.** Which of the following can explain slowed conduction velocities in extremely tall subjects?
A. Smaller diameter of the nerve distally
B. Wider nodes of Ranvier distally
C. Demyelination distally
D. Less blood supply distally
E. Less sodium influx into the cell distally

**Q9.** You perform a nerve conduction study on a 20-year-old woman who presents with numbness of the right hand. The right ulnar motor study is shown in the table below. What is the next best step?

| Nerve-recording | Stimulating site | Distal latency (ms) | Amplitude (mV) | Conduction velocity (m/s) |
|---|---|---|---|---|
| Ulnar-abductor digiti minimi | Wrist | 3.1 | 6.5 | |
| | Below elbow | | 3.2 | 58 |
| | Above elbow | | 3.2 | 65 |

A. Reposition the G1 recording electrode on the abductor digiti minimi (ADM) muscle.
B. Warm the tested limb.
C. Stimulate ulnar proximal sites (axilla and Erb's point).
D. Keep the recording electrodes at the same position, and stimulate the median nerve at the wrist and antecubital fossa.
E. No further action is needed.

**Q10.** Which of the following muscles is the most commonly innervated by the median fibers that cross-over through a Martin-Gruber anastomosis?
A. First dorsal interosseous
B. Fourth lumbrical
C. Abductor digiti minimi
D. Flexor pollicis brevis
E. Flexor carpi ulnaris

**Q11.** A 61-year-old man is referred to your electromyography (EMG) lab for an evaluation of numbness in the right hand. Carpal tunnel syndrome is suspected clinically. The median motor study recording the abductor pollicis brevis is shown in the following figure. Which of the following statements is **CORRECT**?

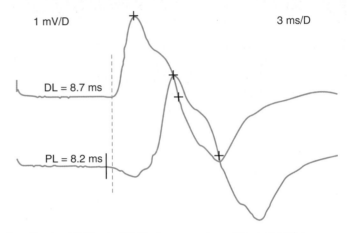

From Preston DC, Shapiro BE. *Electromyography and Neuromuscular Disorders: Clinical-electrophysiologic-ultrasound Correlations.* 4th ed. Philadelphia, PA: Elsevier; 2021:67.

A. There is co-stimulation at the wrist.
B. The stimulation at the antecubital fossa is submaximal.
C. This extremity is colder than 32°C.
D. There is a combination of carpal tunnel syndrome and Martin-Gruber anastomosis.
E. This study represents distal acquired demyelinating symmetric (DADS) neuropathy.

**Q12.** The peroneal motor conduction study is performed (see the following figure). Which of the following can explain this tracing?

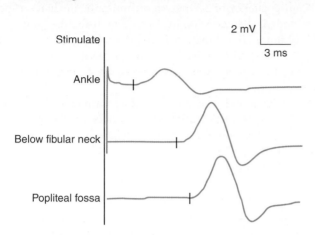

From Preston DC, Shapiro BE. *Electromyography and Neuromuscular Disorders: Clinical-electrophysiologic-ultrasound Correlations.* 4th ed. Philadelphia, PA: Elsevier; 2021.

   A. Co-stimulation at the ankle
   B. Submaximal stimulation at the popliteal fossa
   C. Cold temperature of the tested limb
   D. Accessory branch of the superficial peroneal nerve
   E. Conduction block between the ankle and below the fibular neck

**Q13.** You accidentally decrease the high-frequency (low-pass) filter on the electromyography (EMG) machine. Which of the following changes in sensory responses would be the most apparent?
   A. Increased area
   B. Decreased duration
   C. Decreased amplitude
   D. Decreased onset latency
   E. No change

**Q14.** You accidentally increase the low-frequency (high-pass) filter on the electromyography (EMG) machine. Which of the following changes in motor unit action potentials (MUAPs) would be the most apparent?
   A. Increased duration
   B. Increased amplitude
   C. Decreased amplitude
   D. Increased onset latency
   E. No change

**Q15.** While performing an ulnar sensory study, you notice a large artifact at the beginning of the recording (as shown in the following figure), which interferes with the measurement of the take-off of the response. Which of the following can improve the recording quality of the waveform?

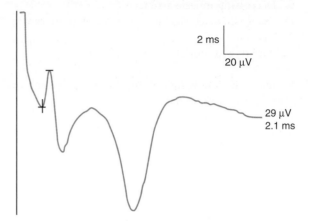

From Preston DC, Shapiro BE. *Electromyography and Neuromuscular Disorders: Clinical-electrophysiologic-ultrasound Correlations.* 4th ed. Philadelphia, PA: Elsevier; 2021:85.

   A. Moving the ground electrode to the opposite limb
   B. Decreasing the distance between the stimulator and the recording electrodes
   C. Rotating the anode around while maintaining the cathode at the same location
   D. Using a higher stimulus intensity
   E. Increasing the distance between the recording (G1) and the reference (G2) electrodes

**Q16.** While performing a median motor study (recording the abductor pollicis brevis [APB] and stimulating the wrist), you encounter the waveform as shown in the following figure. Which of the following statements is **CORRECT**?

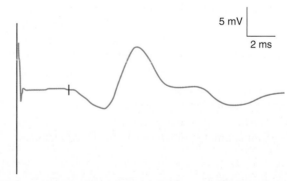

From Preston DC, Shapiro BE. *Electromyography and Neuromuscular Disorders: Clinical-electrophysiologic-ultrasound Correlations.* 4th ed. Philadelphia, PA: Elsevier; 2021:91.

   A. This median motor response has a prolonged distal latency.
   B. The recording (G1) electrode is off the muscle belly.
   C. The reference (G2) electrode is off the tendon.
   D. The distance between the G1 and G2 electrodes is too short.
   E. There is an anodal block.

**Q17.** Which of the following is the reason for the preferred inter-electrode distance of 3–4 cm in sensory and mixed nerve studies?
  A. Avoiding phase cancellation from both electrodes
  B. Decreasing stimulus artifact
  C. Decreasing muscle artifact
  D. Decreasing electrical noises that can interfere with the baseline
  E. Avoiding an initial positive deflection

**Q18.** Which of the following can improve the recording quality of this sensory potential?

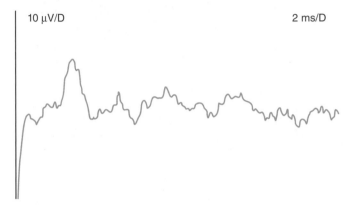

10 µV/D                                        2 ms/D

From Preston DC, Shapiro BE. *Electromyography and Neuromuscular Disorders: Clinical-electrophysiologic-ultrasound Correlations.* 4th ed. Philadelphia, PA: Elsevier; 2021.

  A. Increasing the high-frequency filter
  B. Decreasing the low-frequency filter
  C. Averaging 10 stimuli
  D. Rotating the anode
  E. Increasing the distance between the stimulating and recording electrodes

**Q19.** A routine median motor study is performed. The compound muscle action potential (CMAP) amplitude stimulating the wrist is 14 mV, but when the antecubital fossa is stimulated, the CMAP amplitude is 6 mV. This finding **CANNOT** be explained by which of the following:
  A. Conduction block
  B. Co-stimulation at the wrist
  C. Martin-Gruber anastomosis
  D. Submaximal stimulation at the antecubital fossa

**Q20.** A routine median sensory study is performed using the antidromic method to the index finger. The sensory nerve action potential (SNAP) amplitude is 20 µV, with an onset latency of 2.2 ms. An orthodromic median sensory study is then done on the same digit using the same distance. The amplitude is 10 µV and the onset latency is 2.2 ms. Which of the following is **CORRECT**?
  A. There is an axonal loss pattern on the orthodromic study.
  B. The limb is cool and should be warmed up.
  C. Co-stimulation affected the antidromic study.
  D. Lack of supramaximal stimulation was present for the orthodromic study.
  E. This is a normal study.

**Q21.** A routine ulnar motor study is performed recording the abductor digiti minimi (ADM). With the elbow in the straight position, the conduction velocity (CV) in the forearm is 55 m/s and across the elbow it is 45 m/s. Performing the study with the elbow in the bent (flexed) position, the CV in the forearm is 55 m/s and 60 m/s across the elbow. Which of the following is **CORRECT**?
  A. There is evidence of demyelination in the straight position.
  B. The limb is warmer in the bent position.
  C. A Martin-Gruber anastomosis is present.
  D. Submaximal stimulation occured at the above-elbow site in the straight position.
  E. This is a normal study.

**Q22.** Nerve conduction study (NCS) and needle electromyography (EMG) are uniformly safe procedures and not associated with any complications, similar to electrocardiography (ECG).
  A. True
  B. False

**QUESTION 1.** An 85-year-old woman has numbness in both feet for 2 years. The nerve conduction study (NCS) shows normal peroneal, tibial, and median compound muscle action potentials (CMAPs) and normal median and radial sensory nerve action potentials (SNAPs), but sural SNAP amplitudes of 2 $\mu$V. Needle electromyography (EMG) shows no active denervation, with normal motor unit action potentials (MUAPs) in the extensor hallucis longus, tibialis anterior, and tibialis posterior. Which of the following is most **CORRECT**?
A. This patient has a demyelinating polyneuropathy.
B. Abnormal sural SNAPs always indicate an axonal polyneuropathy.
C. Lumbosacral radiculopathy can be ruled out.
D. This patient has a lumbosacral plexopathy.
E. Reduced/absent sural SNAPs can be a normal finding in the very elderly.

**ANSWER:** E. Reduced/absent sural SNAPs can be a normal finding in the very elderly.

**COMMENTS AND DISCUSSION**
- Age is an important physiologic factor that affects both NCS and needle EMG.
  - Conduction velocity (CV) depends on the presence and amount of myelin.
  - Myelination begins in utero and is not complete until age 3–5.
  - At birth, CV is only 50% of the adult values, and by the age 1 reaches 75% of adult values.
  - In patients 60 years or older, CV as well as CMAP and SNAP amplitudes drop due to loss of neurons from aging.
  - In patients 60 years or older, CV drops approximately 0.5–4.0 m/s per decade.
  - Sensory fibers are more affected than motor fibers by aging.
  - In the normal elderly, sural SNAPs can be low or sometimes even absent. Thus caution is advised when interpreting a reduced or absent sural SNAP in the elderly, especially without other NCS or needle EMG evidence of polyneuropathy.
  - On needle EMG, MUAP duration increases during childhood due to the physical increase of muscle fibers and motor units.
  - In the elderly, the number of motor units decreases due to aging. There is subsequent compensatory reinnervation with a slight increase in MUAP amplitude and duration.
- The isolated finding of low amplitude sural SNAPs in this elderly patient is not consistent with a demyelinating or axonal polyneuropathy, or lumbosacral radiculopathy, since this finding is common in the elderly and not associated with other NCS or needle EMG abnormalities.
- A lumbosacral radiculopathy cannot be ruled out with certainty despite normal needle EMG because the symptoms may consist of only pain and sensory manifestations.

**QUESTION 2.** Which of the following features on nerve conduction studies is seen in newborns when compared to adults?
A. Similar amplitudes as adults
B. Similar conduction velocities as adults
C. Reduced conduction velocities compared to adults
D. Increased conduction velocities compared to adults
E. Nerve conduction studies cannot be performed in newborns

**ANSWER:** C. Reduced conduction velocities compared to adults

**COMMENTS AND DISCUSSION**
- Normal ranges of conduction velocity (CV) depend on age.
- At birth, conduction velocity is only half of the normal adult value: 25–30 m/s.
- Myelination starts in utero.
- CV increases dramatically and reaches 75% of the normal adult value by age 1 year, and eventually reaches the normal adult range by age 3–5 years.
- Sensory nerve action potential (SNAP) and compound muscle action potential (CMAP) amplitudes in newborns are also smaller than in adults.

**QUESTION 3.** Nerve conduction studies on a 15-day-old neonate showed that all motor conduction velocities are between 25 and 30 m/s. Sensory nerve action potential (SNAP) and compound muscle action potential (CMAP) amplitudes are normal. Needle EMG is normal. Given the nerve conduction and needle EMG study results, what is the next best step of management in this patient?

A. *SMN1* gene detection test
B. Nerve biopsy to search for onion bulb formation
C. Oral corticosteroids
D. Intravenous immunoglobulin
E. No evidence of peripheral polyneuropathy

**ANSWER:** E. No evidence of peripheral polyneuropathy

**COMMENTS AND DISCUSSION**

- The normal ranges of conduction velocity (CV) depend on age. For newborns, the conduction velocity is only half of the normal adult values: approximately 25–30 m/s.
- Given the normal nerve conduction study in this patient, there is no evidence of either an inherited or acquired demyelinating peripheral polyneuropathy.
- *SMN1* gene (survival motor neuron 1 gene) detection is a test for spinal muscular atrophy. This is an inherited motor neuron disease. Needle EMG will demonstrate marked neurogenic changes with active denervation and especially large, long-duration motor unit action potentials (MUAPs) with reduced recruitment.
- Onion bulb formation on nerve biopsy indicates repeated bouts of demyelination and remyelination. This finding can be seen in chronic demyelinating neuropathies such as Charcot-Marie-Tooth disease. Hence, corticosteroids and intravenous immunoglobulin are not indicated.

**QUESTION 4.** A nerve conduction study is performed on a 48-year-old woman who presents with right hand numbness. Sensory conduction study of the right upper extremity is shown in the table below.

| Nerve-recording | Latency (ms) | Amplitude (μV) | Conduction velocity (m/s) |
| --- | --- | --- | --- |
| Median-index finger | 3.6 | 120 | 39 |
| Ulnar-little finger | 3.1 | 100 | 40 |
| Radial-dorsum of thumb | 2.9 | 98 | 42 |

Which of the following statements is **CORRECT**?

A. Conduction velocities are normal for this age.
B. This study results are due to cool temperature.
C. There is co-stimulation of adjacent nerves.
D. She likely has carpal tunnel syndrome.
E. The diagnosis is hereditary motor and sensory neuropathy.

**ANSWER:** B. This study is due to cool temperature.

**COMMENTS AND DISCUSSION**

- This sensory studies show that the right median, ulnar, and radial sensory potentials have borderline latencies and slowed conduction velocities, but very large amplitudes.
- Technical factors affecting all nerves should be suspected. This pattern can be due to the effects of cool temperature.
- Temperature is the **MOST** important physiologic factor that affects nerve conduction study (NCS).
- Temperature also affects motor unit action potential (MUAP) morphology on needle electromyography (EMG).
- Cool temperatures affect the sodium channels along the nerve and neuromuscular junction.
  - Cool temperature delays inactivation of sodium channels → prolonged depolarization time → slowed conduction of the nerve

○ Prolonged depolarization time → more sodium influx into the cell → larger and longer muscle/sensory fiber action potentials → larger amplitudes and longer durations of compound muscle action potentials (CMAPs) and sensory nerve action potentials (SNAPs)

- The effect is more pronounced in SNAPs compared to CMAPs, given the dramatically smaller responses (μV in SNAPs and mV in CMAPs).
- On needle EMG, MUAPs can have longer duration and larger amplitude (due to summation of longer and larger muscle fiber action potentials), and also more phases (due to slower conduction of terminal nerve twigs and more temporal dispersion of the muscle fiber action potentials)

 **HIGH-YIELD FACT**

For every 1°C decrease in temperature, conduction velocity in normal nerve slows by 1.5–2.5 m/s and distal latency is prolonged by 0.2 ms for both motor and sensory studies.

 **KEY POINT**

An electromyographer can misinterpret normal nerve conductions as peripheral neuropathy in a cool limb due to prolonged distal latencies and slowed conduction velocities.

**QUESTION 5.** Which of the following statements is **CORRECT** regarding the effect of cold temperature on the peripheral nerve?
A. Detachment of the myelin sheath from the nerve
B. Delayed opening of potassium channels
C. More sodium influx into the cell
D. Decreased motor and sensory nerve conduction amplitudes
E. More prominent changes in motor than sensory responses

**ANSWER:** C. More sodium influx into the cell

**COMMENTS AND DISCUSSION (see also comments and discussion from Question 4)**
- Cold temperature delays inactivation of the sodium channels at the nodes of Ranvier, resulting in more prolonged depolarization time and slower conduction velocity.
- More prolonged depolarization time also results in more sodium influx into cells and potentials with larger amplitude and longer duration.
- Temperature does not cause structural changes or detachment of the myelin sheath.

**QUESTION 6.** A median sensory study is performed with a hand temperature of 28°C. The conduction velocity is 46 m/s. What is the corrected conduction velocity for 34°C?
A. 38 m/s
B. 42 m/s
C. 46 m/s
D. 58 m/s
E. 72 m/s

**ANSWER:** D. 58 m/s

**COMMENTS AND DISCUSSION**
- When performing a nerve conduction study (NCS), it is preferred to keep the temperaure of the tested limb within the range between 32–34°C.
- A cool limb should be warmed up.
- If the limb cannot be warmed, the correction factor of 1.5–2.5 m/s/°C for the conduction velocity may be used.
- Because 2 m/s/°C is the average correction factor, the corrected conduction velocity in this case is 46°C + (2 m/s/°C x 6°C) = 58 m/s.

**QUESTION 7.** A 28-year-old woman presents with ptosis and proximal muscle weakness. Myasthenia gravis is suspected, and repetitive nerve stimulation is performed. Before starting the study, you find that the temperature of her hand is 27°C. If warming is not done, which of the following findings is expected on slow repetitive nerve stimulation of the extremity?

A. No difference from a normothermic hand
B. More prominent decremental response
C. Less decremental response
D. Incremental response
E. Decremental response in the first train and incremental response after exercise

**ANSWER:** C. Less decremental response

**COMMENTS AND DISCUSSION**

- Cold temperature affects the neuromuscular junction by decreasing the enzymatic activity of acetylcholinesterase at the synaptic cleft.
- This results in more acetylcholine available to bind to the postsynaptic receptors.
- In slow repetitive nerve stimulation, the compound muscle action potential (CMAP) decrement may be diminished, and sometimes masked, if the muscle is cold.
- It is crucial for an electromyographer to warm the limb before repetitive nerve stimulation to avoid a false-negative result (falsely absent decremental response).

**QUESTION 8.** Which of the following can explain slowed conduction velocities in extremely tall subjects?

A. Smaller diameter of the nerve distally
B. Wider nodes of Ranvier distally
C. Demyelination distally
D. Less blood supply distally
E. Less sodium influx into the cell distally

**ANSWER:** A. Smaller diameter of the nerve distally

**COMMENTS AND DISCUSSION**

- Height affects conduction velocity (CV) and is especially important in very tall individuals.
  - Taller subjects have longer limbs.
  - Nerve roots start out with similar diameters among individuals.
  - A nerve tapers as it runs down a limb.
  - Thus individuals with longer limbs will have more tapered and small diameter nerves distally.
  - CV is proportional to nerve diameter.
  - Nerves with smaller diameters → slower CVs
  - Longer limbs → slower CVs
  - This also explains why CVs in the lower extremities are slower than CVs in the upper extremities.
- Height also affects late responses (F responses and H-reflexes).
  - The length of nerve traveled is simply farther for tall individuals.
  - Thus normal values for late responses must be based on height or limb length.
- In contrast to height, wider nodes of Ranvier, less blood supply, less sodium influx into the cell, or demyelination distally are not the explanation for reduced conduction velocities in tall individuals.

**QUESTION 9.** You perform a nerve conduction study on a 20-year-old woman who presents with numbness of the right hand. The right ulnar motor study is shown in the table below. What is the next best step?

| Nerve-recording | Stimulating site | Distal latency (ms) | Amplitude (mV) | Conduction velocity (m/s) |
|---|---|---|---|---|
| Ulnar-abductor digiti minimi | Wrist | 3.1 | 6.5 | |
| | Below elbow | | 3.2 | 58 |
| | Above elbow | | 3.2 | 65 |

A. Reposition the G1 recording electrode on the abductor digiti minimi (ADM) muscle.
B. Warm the tested limb.
C. Stimulate ulnar proximal sites (axilla and Erb's point).
D. Keep the recording electrodes at the same position, and stimulate the median nerve at the wrist and antecubital fossa.
E. No further action is needed.

**ANSWER:** D. Keep the recording electrodes at the same position, and stimulate the median nerve at the wrist and antecubital fossa.

### COMMENTS AND DISCUSSION

- Anomalous innervations can result in several important patterns that can impact the nerve conduction study (NCS) and electromyography (EMG) study interpretation.
  - The Martin-Gruber anastomosis (MGA) is the most common anomaly in the upper extremity.
    - Cross-over of median **motor** fibers to the ulnar nerve in the forearm (Fig. 8.1)
    - Is recognized as an apparent conduction block in the forearm during a routine ulnar motor conduction study
    - In an MGA, ulnar-innervated intrinsic hand muscles are partially median innervated, including the first dorsal interosseous (FDI), abductor digiti minimi (ADM), adductor pollicis, deep head of the flexor pollicis brevis, or a combination.
    - Confirmed by stimulating the median nerve (at the wrist and antecubital fossa), **while recording the ulnar-innervated muscles (ADM or FDI)**

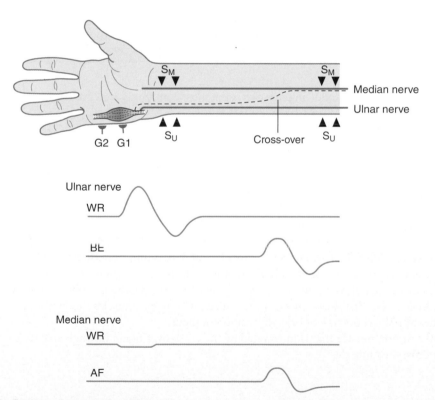

**Fig. 8.1 Martin-Gruber anastomosis (MGA).** MGA is a cross-over of median motor fibers to the ulnar nerve in the forearm segment. When performing the ulnar motor study $(S_u)$ recording the abductor digiti minimi *(ADM)*, the compound muscle action potential (CMAP) from stimulation at the wrist *(WR)* shows a normal amplitude; however, there is a drop in the CMAP amplitudes when stimulating below the elbow *(BE)*. In order to confirm MGA, an electromyographer continues recording the ADM, but changes the stimulation to the median nerve $(S_m)$. When stimulating at WR, there is no response, since the median fibers at this point all supply median innervated muscles, which depolarize at a distance to the ADM. However, when stimulating at the antecubital fossa (AF), the median fibers that cross-over to the ulnar nerve are also stimulated, and a CMAP appears. The CMAP amplitude from the ulnar stimulation BE plus the CMAP amplitude from the median stimulation at the AF is often almost equal to the CMAP amplitude from ulnar stimulation at WR. From Preston DC, Shapiro BE. Electromyography and Neuromuscular Disorders: Clinical-electrophysiologic-ultrasound Correlations. 4th ed. Philadelphia, PA: Elsevier; 2021:71.

- If MGA is present to the ADM (Fig. 8.1):
  - When stimulating the median nerve at the wrist, there is usually no response.
  - But when stimulating at the median nerve at the antecubital fossa, there will be a compound muscle action potential (CMAP) response
- If MGA is present to the FDI
  - When stimulating the median nerve at the wrist, there will be a small CMAP (from co-recording the ulnar thenar muscles).
  - But when stimulating the median nerve at the antecubital fossa, there will be a much larger CMAP response.
  - The CMAP amplitude difference between the elbow and wrist stimulations of the median nerve represents the cross-over.
- There is a possible conduction block of the ulnar nerve in the forearm segment between the wrist and below-elbow stimulation sites.
- However, whenever this pattern is seen on an ulnar motor conduction study, one must assess for an MGA.
  - If an MGA is present, stimulating the median nerve proximally at the antecubital fossa will result in a CMAP being present.
  - Changing the recording electrode (G1) to the belly should be done when there is a positive deflection at the beginning of the recorded waveform. This finding can be seen when the recording electrode (G1) is off the belly of the recorded muscle.
  - This ulnar motor study has a normal distal amplitude and latency, arguing against effects from cool temperature.
  - When an acquired demyelinating neuropathy is suspected, stimulating at very proximal sites (e.g., axilla and Erb's point) can be helpful to demonstrate a proximal conduction block.

##  KEY POINT

Martin-Gruber anastomosis may result in pseudo-conduction block of the ulnar motor nerve conduction study, usually in the forearm segment, which may be mistaken for ulnar neuropathy.

**QUESTION 10.** Which of the following muscles is the most commonly innervated by the median fibers that cross-over through a Martin-Gruber anastomosis?
A. First dorsal interosseous
B. Fourth lumbrical
C. Abductor digiti minimi
D. Flexor pollicis brevis
E. Flexor carpi ulnaris

**ANSWER:** A. First dorsal interosseous

### COMMENTS AND DISCUSSION (see also comments and discussion from Question 9)
- Median fibers that cross-over to the ulnar nerve in a Martin-Gruber anastomosis (MGA) can innervate any of the following ulnar innervated muscles: (1) hypothenar muscles (abductor digiti minimi [ADM]), (2) first dorsal interosseous muscle, (3) thenar muscles (adductor pollicis, deep head of flexor pollicis brevis), or (4) combination of these.
- The most common muscle that is innervated by the cross-over fibers through an MGA is the first dorsal interosseous muscle.

**QUESTION 11.** A 61-year-old man is referred to your electromyography (EMG) lab for an evaluation of numbness in the right hand. Carpal tunnel syndrome is suspected clinically. The median motor study recording the abductor pollicis brevis is shown in the following figure. Which of the following statements is **CORRECT**?

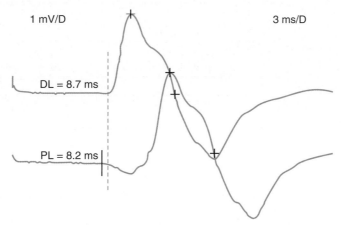

From Preston DC, Shapiro BE. *Electromyography and Neuromuscular Disorders: Clinical-electrophysiologic-ultrasound Correlations.* 4th ed. Philadelphia, PA: Elsevier; 2021:67.

    A. There is co-stimulation at the wrist.
    B. The stimulation at the antecubital fossa is submaximal.
    C. This extremity is colder than 32°C.
    D. There is a combination of carpal tunnel syndrome and Martin-Gruber anastomosis.
    E. This study represents distal acquired demyelinating symmetric (DADS) neuropathy.

**ANSWER:** D. There is a combination of carpal tunnel syndrome and Martin-Gruber anastomosis.

**COMMENTS AND DISCUSSION**
- Carpal tunnel syndrome in individuals with Martin-Gruber anastomosis (MGA) (Fig. 8.2)
  - Very important pattern to recognize on routine median motor study
  - When stimulating at the wrist, the latency is prolonged due to carpal tunnel syndrome.
  - However, when stimulating at the antecubital fossa, the median fibers that cross-over through the MGA bypass the carpal tunnel by traveling instead with the ulnar nerve.
  - Thus the proximal stimulation arrives at the muscle faster than normal by bypassing the slowing at the carpal tunnel. This results in the following pattern:
    - Initial positive deflection (dip) of median compound muscle action potential (CMAP) from the proximal stimulating site
    - Factiously fast conduction velocity of the median nerve in the forearm segment
- In this question, the median motor study demonstrates a very prolonged distal latency (normal distal median motor latency <4.4 ms). On proximal stimulation, an initial positive deflection of the CMAP is seen. In addition, the proximal latency is actually shorter than the distal latency!
  - Technical errors, especially co-stimulation at the antecubital fossa, need to be excluded—not submaximal stimulation.
  - Co-stimulation can cause an unusually large amplitude due to stimulation of an adjacent nerve. In contrast, submaximal stimulation results in a waveform that is smaller than the actual one.
  - After exclusion of technical factors, this pattern is also seen in a marked median neuropathy at the wrist with a coexistent MGA.
    - The severely prolonged distal motor latency is due to the carpal tunnel syndrome.
    - When the proximal site is stimulated, a latency is demonstrated with initial positive dip at proximal stimulation that is faster than the latency from the distal stimulation. This is because the electrical activity that travels along cross-over median fibers bypasses the slowing at the carpal tunnel.
  - Cool temperature can cause slow conduction velocities and prolonged latencies due to delayed inactivation of sodium channels, and larger waveforms due to prolonged depolarization time and more sodium influx. The proximal latency that is shorter than the distal one cannot be due to a cool temperature.

- Distal acquired demyelinating symmetric (DADS) neuropathy is one of the chronic inflammatory demyelinating polyneuropathy (CIDP) variants. The key electrodiagnostic feature of DADS is markedly prolonged distal motor latencies due to distal demyelination. However, the proximal latency is not shorter than the distal one.

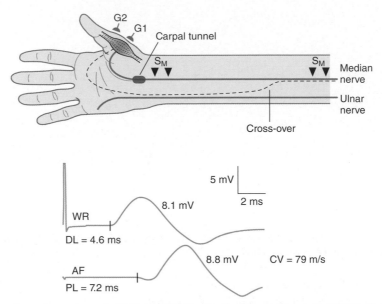

**Fig. 8.2 Carpal tunnel syndrome in an individual with Martin-Gruber anastomosis (MGA).** On the median motor study, when stimulating at the wrist, the latency is prolonged due to carpal tunnel syndrome. However, when stimulating at the ante-cubital fossa, the median fibers that cross-over through MGA have a normal velocity, since they bypass the carpal tunnel and travel with the ulnar nerve instead. When conduction velocity is calculated, the latency in the forearm segment is abnormally fast, as it bypasses the slowing through the carpal tunnel. Adapted from Preston DC, Shapiro BE. *Electromyography and Neuromuscular Disorders: Clinical-electrophysiologic-ultrasound Correlations*. 4th ed. Philadelphia, PA: Elsevier; 2021.

**QUESTION 12.** The peroneal motor conduction study is performed (see the following figure). Which of the following can explain this tracing?

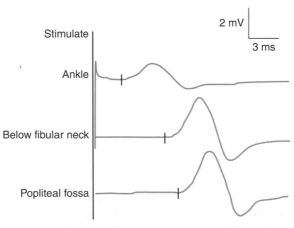

From Preston DC, Shapiro BE. *Electromyography and Neuromuscular Disorders: Clinical-electrophysiologic-ultrasound Correlations*. 4th ed. Philadelphia, PA: Elsevier; 2021.

    A. Co-stimulation at the ankle
    B. Submaximal stimulation at the popliteal fossa
    C. Cold temperature of the tested limb
    D. Accessory branch of the superficial peroneal nerve
    E. Conduction block between the ankle and below the fibular neck

**ANSWER:** D. Accessory branch of the superficial peroneal nerve

## COMMENTS AND DISCUSSION

- Waveforms from distal stimulation normally have the largest amplitude, with waveforms from proximal stimulation being slightly smaller due to physiological temporal dispersion and phase cancellation. In this tracing, the waveform recording from distal stimulation (ankle) is smaller than the ones stimulating at the proximal sites (below the fibular neck and popliteal fossa). This can result from:
  - Submaximal stimulation at the distal site (ankle)
  - Co-stimulation of adjacent nerves at the proximal stimulation sites
  - Presence of an accessory peroneal nerve (APN) as a normal variation
- Cool temperature can cause slow conduction velocities and prolonged latencies due to delayed inactivation of sodium channels, and larger waveforms due to prolonged depolarization time and more sodium influx. Cool temperature usually affects the distal parts of the limb. In this figure, the smaller distal response argues against the effect from cool temperature.
- Conduction block is recognized as a significant drop of compound muscle action potential (CMAP) amplitude and area between distal and proximal stimulation sites. In this tracing, the amplitudes increased from the distal to the proximal stimulations, in reverse from what is present in a conduction block.
- Accessory peroneal nerve (APN) (Fig. 8.3)
  - Most common anomaly in the lower extremity
  - Extensor digitorum brevis muscle (EDB) is normally innervated by the deep peroneal nerve.
  - The APN arises from the superficial peroneal nerve, traveling behind the lateral malleolus to supply the lateral EDB.
  - This results in a larger CMAP when stimulating the peroneal nerve at the proximal sites (fibular neck and knee), compared to when stimulating at the ankle. This can be mistaken for a technical error.
  - To confirm an APN, one needs to stimulate behind the lateral malleolus while recording the EDB. If an APN is present, the stimulation will result in a CMAP.
  - The CMAP amplitude from the stimulation at the ankle plus the CMAP amplitude from the stimulation behind the lateral malleolus will be approximately equal to the CMAP amplitude from the proximal stimulating sites.

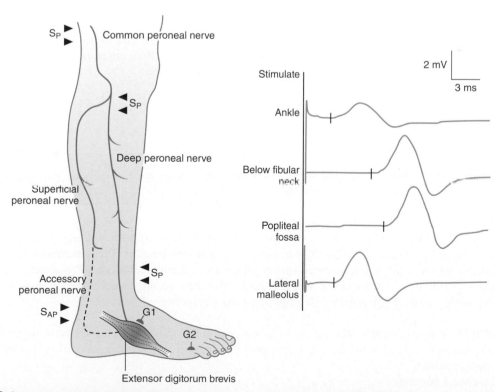

**Fig. 8.3 Accessory peroneal nerve.** The peroneal compound muscle action potential (CMAP) amplitude recording at the extensor digitorum brevis (EDB) muscle is smaller when stimulating at the ankle as compared to proximal stimulation sites. This may be mistaken for a technical error but is most often due to an accessory peroneal nerve. To confirm, one stimulates below the lateral malleolus where the accessory peroneal nerve runs. The CMAP amplitude from the stimulation at the ankle plus the CMAP amplitude from the stimulation behind the lateral malleolus is approximately equal to the CMAP amplitude from proximal stimulating sites. From Preston DC, Shapiro BE. *Electromyography and Neuromuscular Disorders: Clinical-electrophysiologic-ultrasound Correlations.* 4th ed. Philadelphia, PA: Elsevier; 2021.

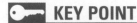 **KEY POINT**

Larger amplitudes with peroneal nerve stimulation at the proximal sites compared to the distal site (ankle) can be due to accessory peroneal nerve.

**QUESTION 13.** You accidentally decrease the high-frequency (low-pass) filter on the electromyography (EMG) machine. Which of the following changes in sensory responses would be the most apparent?
A. Increased area
B. Decreased duration
C. Decreased amplitude
D. Decreased onset latency
E. No change

**ANSWER:** C. Decreased amplitude

**COMMENTS AND DISCUSSION**
- There are a variety of non-physiologic factors that affect electrodiagnostic data acquisition and interpretation. One of the most important are the filters that are used both for the nerve conduction study (NCS) and needle EMG.
  - Three main filters: high-frequency (low-pass), low-frequency (high-pass), and band-pass (notch) filters
    - **Low**-frequency filter:
      - Attenuates low-frequency signals below the setting
      - Allows high-frequency signals to pass through
      - Normally set at 10 Hz
      - However, it can affect **duration (primarily)**, area, and peak latency (**not onset latency**) of the signal of interest (especially sensory potentials, which are smaller than motor).
    - **High**-frequency filter:
      - Excludes high-frequency signals above the setting
      - Allows low-frequency signals to pass through
      - Normally set at 10 kHz for motor studies and needle EMG; 2 kHz for sensory studies
      - However, it can affect **amplitude (primarily)** and latency (**both onset and peak**) of the signal of interest (especially sensory potentials).
    - Notch filter:
      - Attenuates certain frequencies (e.g., 60 Hz)

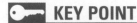 **KEY POINTS**

| ↓ **low**-frequency filter → ↑**duration** | ↑amplitude | ↑area | ↑peak latency |
| ↓ **high**-frequency filter → ↑**amplitude** | ↑duration | ↓area | ↑onset/peak latency |

- In the question, the high-frequency (low-pass) filter blocks high-frequency noise. If a high-frequency filter is lowered, more high-frequency noise will be blocked. This can affect the waveforms, especially the sensory potentials, which are in the **microvolt** range as compared to motor potentials which are in the **millivolt** range. The largest change would be a decrease in amplitude, as amplitude is primarily a high-frequency response.

**QUESTION 14.** You accidentally increase the low-frequency (high-pass) filter on the electromyography (EMG) machine. Which of the following changes in motor unit action potentials (MUAPs) would be the most apparent?
A. Increased duration
B. Increased amplitude
C. Decreased amplitude
D. Increased onset latency
E. No change

**ANSWER:** A. Increased duration

**COMMENTS AND DISCUSSION (see also comments and discussion from Question 13)**
- Low-frequency (high-pass) filter blocks low-frequency noise.
- Low-frequency noise can result in wandering of the baseline.
- If the low-frequency filter is increased, more low frequencies will pass through. This can affect waveforms by increasing their durations, as duration is predominantly a low-frequency response.
- MUAPs are easily made shorter and longer by changing the low-frequency filter up and down, respectively.

**QUESTION 15.** While performing an ulnar sensory study, you notice a large artifact at the beginning of the recording (as shown in the following figure), which interferes with the measurement of the take-off of the response. Which of the following can improve the recording quality of the waveform?

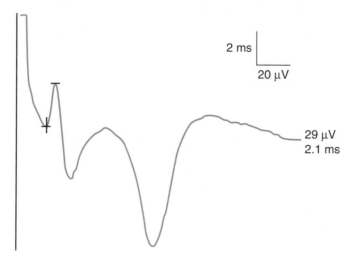

From Preston DC, Shapiro BE. *Electromyography and Neuromuscular Disorders: Clinical-electrophysiologic-ultrasound Correlations.* 4th ed. Philadelphia, PA: Elsevier; 2021:85.

A. Moving the ground electrode to the opposite limb
B. Decreasing the distance between the stimulator and the recording electrodes
C. Rotating the anode around while maintaining the cathode at the same location
D. Using a higher stimulus intensity
E. Increasing the distance between the recording (G1) and the reference (G2) electrodes

**ANSWER:** C. Rotating the anode around while maintaining the cathode at the same location

**COMMENTS AND DISCUSSION**
- This waveform is contaminated by a stimulus artifact.
- Stimulus artifact:
  - Far-field potentials from distant stimulation and are always present
  - Sometimes the artifact will be positive (coming from below) and other times it will be negative (coming from above).
    - These can affect the take-off point of the potential, resulting in either an early or delayed onset latency.
    - These can also affect amplitude, especially when the stimulus artifact is negative and cuts off the signal, especially when the signal of interest is small (e.g., sensory nerve action potential [SNAP]).
- Artifacts are much more of an issue in sensory as compared to motor studies, given the dramatically smaller responses (μV in sensory studies and mV in motor studies).
  - Can be improved by:
    - Placing a ground electrode between the stimulator and the recording electrodes
    - Cleaning the skin and using enough conducting paste to reduce electrode—impedance mismatch
    - Using coaxial recording cables
    - Avoiding excessively high-stimulation currents

- Rotating the anode while keeping the cathode fixed
- Increasing the distance between the stimulator and recording electrodes
- Ensuring that the stimulator cable does not overlap with the recording cable

**QUESTION 16.** While performing a median motor study (recording the abductor pollicis brevis [APB] and stimulating the wrist), you encounter the waveform as shown in the following figure. Which of the following statements is **CORRECT**?

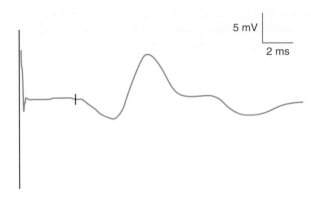

Figure from Preston DC, Shapiro BE. *Electromyography and Neuromuscular Disorders: Clinical-electrophysiologic-ultrasound Correlations.* 4th ed. Philadelphia, PA: Elsevier; 2021:91.

A. This median motor response has a prolonged distal latency.
B. The recording (G1) electrode is off the muscle belly.
C. The reference (G2) electrode is off the tendon.
D. The distance between the G1 and G2 electrodes is too short.
E. There is an anodal block.

**ANSWER:** B. The recording (G1) electrode is off the muscle belly.

**COMMENTS AND DISCUSSION**
- This median motor response has a prominent initial positive deflection.
- This finding indicates that the recording (G1) electrode is off the muscle belly (Answer B).
  - This occurs when the initial depolarization does not start immediately under the G1 electrode.
    - A depolarization at a distance is recorded as a positive deflection.
    - When the depolarization later travels under G1, the trailing negative deflection occurs.
    - When G1 is properly placed at the muscle belly, depolarization occurs right underneath the electrode, resulting in an initial negative deflection.
    - For motor studies, the belly-tendon montage is used.
      - Active electrode (G1) is placed at the belly of the recording muscle.
      - Reference electrode (G2) is placed at a distal tendon, which is usually (but not always) a neutral point.
      - When G1 is off from the muscle belly, **an initial positive dip** can be seen on the waveform as the depolarization first occurs off from G1.

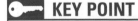 **KEY POINT**

When G1 is off the belly of the stimulating muscle, there is an initial positive dip on CMAP.

  - A true onset latency cannot be measured in motor responses with initial negative deflections.
  - If the reference (G2) electrode is not over the tendon, it does not result in an initial positive deflection.
  - When the inter-electrode distance (between G1 and G2) is less than 3–4 cm, it does not result in an initial positive deflection. However, when performing sensory studies, if G1 and G2 are too close, both electrodes may record the depolarization at the same time, which then cancels out some of the response resulting in a reduced amplitude.

○ Anodal block can theoretically occur when the cathode and the anode are reversed: the anode (instead of the cathode) is located closer to the recording electrode. The depolarization occurs underneath the cathode, and hyperpolarization that occurs underneath the anode can create a block. Thus depolarization cannot propagate further. However, this occurs rarely in practice. Reversal of the cathode and the anode affects the latency of the waveform, since the distance between the cathode and the recording electrode is actually longer than what is measured.

 **KEY POINT**

In motor studies, the active (G1) and reference (G2) electrodes are placed in the belly-tendon montage.
In sensory studies, the active (G1) and reference (G2) electrodes are placed 3–4 cm from each other.

**QUESTION 17.** Which of the following is the reason for the preferred inter-electrode distance of 3–4 cm in sensory and mixed nerve studies?
A. Avoiding phase cancellation from both electrodes
B. Decreasing stimulus artifact
C. Decreasing muscle artifact
D. Decreasing electrical noises that can interfere with the baseline
E. Avoiding an initial positive deflection

**ANSWER:** A. Avoiding phase cancellation from both electrodes

**COMMENTS AND DISCUSSION**
• For sensory studies, both active (G1) and reference (G2) electrodes are placed over the nerve.
   ○ If G1 and G2 are too close to each other, they will capture the same response at the same time, resulting in a cancellation effect → smaller potentials (Fig. 3.9).
   ○ The preferable separation inter-electrode distance is **3-4 cm** to avoid this.

**QUESTION 18.** Which of the following can improve the recording quality of this sensory potential?

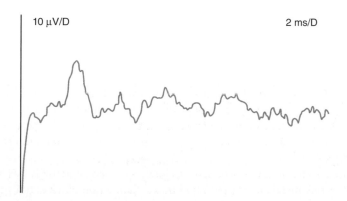

10 μV/D                                    2 ms/D

From Preston DC, Shapiro BE. *Electromyography and Neuromuscular Disorders: Clinical-electrophysiologic-ultrasound Correlations.* 4th ed. Philadelphia, PA: Elsevier; 2021.

A. Increasing the high-frequency filter
B. Decreasing the low-frequency filter
C. Averaging 10 stimuli
D. Rotating the anode
E. Increasing the distance between the stimulating and recording electrodes

**ANSWER:** C. Averaging 10 stimuli

**COMMENTS AND DISCUSSION**
- There is high-frequency background noise in this sensory potential recording.
- To improve the quality of this recording, averaging from multiple stimulations (e.g., 10 stimulations) is a useful technique.
  - Averaging will cancel out electric noise, which occurs at random leaving the signal of interest (Answer C).
  - An averaged waveform is obtained from multiple stimuli.
  - It is most useful for small signals (e.g., sensory potentials).
- Increasing the high-frequency filter will actually increase high-frequency noise.
- Decreasing the low-frequency filter does not affect the high-frequency noise.
- Rotating the anode can reduce or eliminate the stimulus artifact and improve the take-off of the response. However, in this case, there is no stimulus artifact interfering with the take-off of the response.
- Increasing the distance between the stimulating and the recording electrodes likewise can improve the take-off from the stimulus artifact, but this would not reduce the background noise.

**QUESTION 19.** A routine median motor study is performed. The compound muscle action potential (CMAP) amplitude stimulating the wrist is 14 mV, but when the antecubital fossa is stimulated, the CMAP amplitude is 6 mV. This finding **CANNOT** be explained by which of the following:
A. Conduction block
B. Co-stimulation at the wrist
C. Martin-Gruber anastomosis
D. Submaximal stimulation at the antecubital fossa

**ANSWER:** C. Martin-Gruber anastomosis

**COMMENTS AND DISCUSSION**
- A marked drop in amplitude/area between a distal and proximal stimulation site during motor studies is the pattern seen in a conduction block from demyelination, provided the study was performed correctly.
- Martin-Gruber anastomosis results in apparent conduction block in the forearm during *routine ulnar*, not median, motor conduction studies.
- Supramaximal stimulation
  - Supramaximal stimulation is required to ensure that the stimulation is high enough that all fibers are depolarized and a maximal response is obtained.
  - When stimulation is submaximal, the waveform will be lower in amplitude than what is true.
    - When this occurs at a proximal stimulation site, it results in the mistaken interpretation of a conduction block.
    - When this occurs at a distal stimulation site, it results in the mistaken interpretation an axonal loss pattern.
- Co-stimulation
  - Co-stimulation occurs when the stimulation is excessive and spreads to nearby nerves.
  - If co-stimulation occurs, the waveform will be larger in amplitude than what is true.
  - Co-stimulation of an adjacent nerve may result in a response that is larger than what is true.
    - When this occurs at a distal stimulation site, it results in the mistaken interpretation of a conduction block.
    - When this occurs at a proximal stimulation site in a nerve that actually has a conduction block, it may result in the mistaken interpretation that a conduction block is not present.

**QUESTION 20.** A routine median sensory study is performed using the antidromic method to the index finger. The sensory nerve action potential (SNAP) amplitude is 20 μV, with an onset latency of 2.2 ms. An orthodromic median sensory study is then done on the same digit using the same distance. The amplitude is 10 μV and the onset latency is 2.2 ms. Which of the following is **CORRECT**?
A. There is an axonal loss pattern on the orthodromic study.
B. The limb is cool and should be warmed up.
C. Co-stimulation affected the antidromic study.
D. Lack of supramaximal stimulation was present for the orthodromic study.
E. This is a normal study.

**ANSWER:** E. This is a normal study.

## COMMENTS AND DISCUSSION

- This is a normal study.
  - The main advantage of antidromic recording is that the responses are larger as the nerve is closer to the recording electrodes.
  - Otherwise, antidromic and orthodromic sensory studies have the same latency and conduction velocity.
- Antidromic versus orthodromic sensory recording
  - In sensory studies, recording electrodes are placed over the nerve.
  - Two techniques can be used: antidromic and orthodromic recording.
  - Orthodromic recording follows the physiologic sensory conduction: stimulating distally and recording proximally.
  - Antidromic recording is reversed: stimulating proximally and recording distally.
  - Each technique has advantages and disadvantages (Table 8.1).

**TABLE 8.1** Comparison between the orthodromic and antidromic sensory nerve conduction studies

| Orthodromic | Antidromic |
| --- | --- |
| Same direction as physiologic conduction | Opposite to physiologic conduction |
| Stimulate only sensory nerve | Stimulate both sensory and motor nerves |
| Unlikely to result in volume conduction | Higher tendency for volume conduction |
| More tissue between the nerve and the recording site (e.g., at the wrist) | The recording site is closed to the nerve (e.g., at the digit) |
| Smaller amplitude | Larger amplitude |
| More difficult to stimulate | Easier to stimulate |
| More prone to noise and artifacts due to smaller size | Subject to volume conduction muscle artifacts |
| Onset latency may be more difficult to mark due to smaller size | Clear onset and peak latency |

**QUESTION 21.** A routine ulnar motor study is performed recording the abductor digiti minimi (ADM). With the elbow is in the straight position, the conduction velocity (CV) in the forearm is 55 m/s and across the elbow is 45 m/s. Performing the study with the elbow in the bent (flexed) position, the CV in the forearm is 55 m/s and 60 m/s across the elbow. Which of the following is **CORRECT?**

A. There is evidence of demyelination in the straight position.
B. The limb is warmer in the bent position.
C. A Martin-Gruber anastomosis is present.
D. Submaximal stimulation is present at the above-elbow site for the study in the straight position.
E. This is a normal study.

**ANSWER:** E. This is a normal study.

## COMMENTS AND DISCUSSION

- This is a normal study.
- Limb position can affect nerve conduction study (NCS), especially for the ulnar nerve when measuring distance across the elbow.
  - Usually the distance of the underlying nerve is assumed from the distance measured from the surface between the stimulating and recording sites.
  - At the elbow, the ulnar nerve lies over the epicondylar groove.
  - When the arm is extended, the nerve becomes slack.
  - When the elbow is flexed, the nerve is no longer slack.
    - The surface distance measured in the straight position underestimates the true nerve length.
      - CV = measured distance/time
      - When the measured distance is erroneously short (e.g., in the straight-elbow position), the conduction velocity is erroneously slow.

- Calculated conduction velocity obtained with the elbow straight will result in a calculated CV across the elbow approximately 10 m/s slower than when performed with the elbow flexed.
- Thus when an NCS is performed of the ulnar nerve at the elbow, the elbow flexed results in a more anatomically correct CV.

**QUESTION 22.** Nerve conduction study (NCS) and needle electromyography (EMG) are uniformly safe procedures and not associated with any complications, similar to electrocardiography (ECG).
  A. True
  B. False

**ANSWER:** B. False

**COMMENTS AND DISCUSSION**
- Electrodiagnostic studies (NCS and needle EMG) are generally safe and minimally invasive procedures. However, there are some instances where they are contraindicated and complications can occur.
- Electrical safety procedures to follow
  - Using a grounding receptacle or a three-prong outlet
  - Always checking ground system and all electrical wires
  - Maintenance of the EMG machine regularly
  - Using non–electrical-conducted bed (preferred) (e.g., wood bed)
  - No unnecessary electrical equipment in the same EMG room
  - Keeping the equipment, devices, and wires dry and clean
  - Avoiding contact between the patient and parts of the machine
- Patients at risk during the nerve conduction study
  - Patients with central lines
    - Study of the limb contralateral to the side of the central line is preferred.
    - If examination of the ipsilateral limb is needed, do not stimulate at proximal sites near the central line (e.g., axilla and Erb's point).
  - Patients with external wires
    - Do not perform a study in patients with external pacing or instruments with a guidewire.
    - These form a direct conduit to conduct electricity to the heart.
  - Patients with implanted cardiac pacemaker or defibrillators
    - Do not perform a study close to the device (e.g., Erb's point, axilla).
    - Avoid using high-intensity stimulation (stimulus pulse $\leq$0.2 ms and rate $\leq$1 Hz).
- Patients at risk during the needle EMG
  - Risk of pneumothorax
    - Depends on the areas tested (e.g., supraspinatus, rhomboid, serratus anterior, and lower cervical/thoracic paraspinal muscles have a higher risk)
    - Needle EMG can still be performed but with caution.
    - Ensure the appropriate landmark and stay superficial.
  - Risk for bleeding
    - Rare if no bleeding risks; more concerned in patients taking anticoagulants; patient with severe thrombocytopenia or some particular medical history with bleeding tendency
    - Needle EMG can still be performed on patients with coagulopathy but these muscles should be avoided.
      - Muscles close to major blood vessels (e.g., pronator teres, iliacus, and flexor digitorum longus)
      - Muscles in which a hematoma could result in compartment syndrome (e.g., tibialis posterior, gluteus maximus, and pronator teres)
      - Deep muscles on which tamponade cannot be obtained from surface pressure.
- Risk for infection
  - Applies to both patients and electromyographers
  - Uses disposable needles
  - Universal precautions: handwashing, gloving while performing needle EMG study, using alcohol to clean the skin before application of the surface electrode or needle EMG
  - Do not recap the needle with the contralateral hand.

## SUGGESTED READINGS

Al-Shekhlee A, Shapiro BE, Preston DC. Iatrogenic complications and risks of nerve conduction studies and needle electromyography. *Muscle Nerve.* 2003;27(5):517-526.

Boon AJ, Gertken JT, Watson JC, et al. Hematoma risk after needle electromyography. *Muscle Nerve.* 2012;45:9-12.

Katirji B. *Electromyography in Clinical Practice.* 3th ed. New York, NY: Oxford University Press; 2018.

Mallik A, Weir AI. Nerve conduction studies: essentials and pitfalls in practice. *J Neurol Neurosurg Psychiatry.* 2005;76(suppl II):ii23-ii31.

Preston DC, Shapiro BE. *Electromyography and Neuromuscular Disorders: Clinical-electrophysiologic-ultrasound Correlations.* 4th ed. Philadelphia, PA: Elsevier; 2021.

Zachary NI. Safety and pain in electrodiagnostic studies. *Muscle Nerve.* 2017;55:149-159.

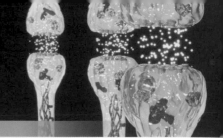

# CHAPTER 9

# Electrodiagnostic Medicine VII: Autonomic Testing

## PART 1 | PRACTICE TEST

**Q1.** In the sympathetic nervous system, which organ is mediated by acetylcholine as a neurotransmitter from the postganglionic neuron?
A. Pupil
B. Lacrimal gland
C. Sweat gland
D. Smooth muscle in blood vessels
E. Heart

**Q2.** Which statement is **CORRECT** regarding acetylcholine (ACh) and norepinephrine (NE) in the parasympathetic nervous system?
A. Neurotransmitter for preganglionic neuron is ACh, and postganglionic neuron is ACh.
B. Neurotransmitter for preganglionic neuron is ACh, and postganglionic neuron is NE.
C. Neurotransmitter for preganglionic neuron is NE, and postganglionic neuron is ACh.
D. Neurotransmitter for preganglionic neuron is NE, and postganglionic neuron is NE.
E. None of the above.

**Q3.** Quantitative sudomotor axon reflex test (QSART) is performed to assess patients with suspected small fiber neuropathy. Which neurotransmitter or chemical substance is essential to activate the response?
A. Acetylcholine
B. Dopamine
C. Glutamate
D. Iodine
E. Norepinephrine

**Q4.** A 55-year-old woman with a history of type 2 diabetes presents with burning feet for 5 months. Neurological examination shows normal motor power and sensation in all modalities except for hyperesthesia in both soles. Electromyography (EMG) is unremarkable. Quantitative sudomotor axon reflex test (QSART) shows reduced sweat output in the foot and distal leg but normal output in the hand. Which of the following statements is **CORRECT** regarding this condition?
A. Myelin is abnormal.
B. Sensory ataxia is a common presentation.
C. Nerve biopsy is a gold standard test.
D. Thermoregulatory sweat test (TST) should be normal.
E. Pathology is confined to the C fibers.

**Q5.** Which medication should be withheld prior to performing a quantitative sudomotor axon reflex test (QSART)?
A. Propranolol
B. Ondansetron
C. Nortriptyline
D. Valproic acid
E. Verapamil

**Q6.** Which of the following conditions can cause an abnormal thermoregulatory sweat test (TST) but a normal quantitative sudomotor axon reflex test (QSART)?
A. Multiple system atrophy
B. Diabetic polyneuropathy
C. Amyloid light chain (AL) amyloidosis
D. Postural tachycardia syndrome
E. None of the above

**Q7.** Which autonomic testing best assesses cardiovagal function?
A. Heart rate response to deep breathing
B. Blood pressure response to the Valsalva maneuver
C. Tilt table testing
D. Quantitative sudomotor axon reflex test
E. Thermoregulatory sweat test

**Q8.** Which of the following statements can influence the result of heart rate response to deep breathing?
A. Age
B. Rate of breathing
C. Depth of breathing
D. Medications
E. All of the above

**Q9.** Which of the following statements is **CORRECT** regarding the beat-to-beat blood pressure (BP) response to Valsalva maneuver?
A. Phases I and IV represent intrathoracic pressure changes from mechanical variation.
B. Early phase II drop-off in BP is due to vagal overactivity.
C. Late phase II recovery of BP is a result of sympathetic surge.
D. Vasodilation occurs in phase III.
E. Phase IV overshoot of BP is associated with tachycardia

**Q10.** A 58-year-old man presents with recurrent syncopal episodes upon standing several times for 3 months. His daughter notices the patient walks slower than his baseline in the past 6 months. On examination, he has parkinsonism signs with a wide-based gait. Dysmetria is noted on the finger-to-nose test. You suspect multiple system atrophy. Which of the following statements is **CORRECT** regarding the autonomic testing result in this patient?
A. This disorder predominantly affects the parasympathetic nervous system.
B. Spared phase $II_L$ in Valsalva maneuver is a key feature for central dysautonomia.
C. Decreased systolic blood pressure (SBP) >20 mmHg upon 70-degree tilt is diagnostic of orthostatic hypotension.
D. Abnormal quantitative sudomotor axon reflex test (QSART) in all sites is a mandatory feature in multiple system atrophy (MSA).
E. Thermoregulatory sweat test (TST) shows normal sweat pattern.

**Q11.** A 22-year-old woman presents with dizziness and palpitation upon standing for 4 months. She has episodes of dizziness, light-headedness, palpitation, and near syncope once she stands. Her neurological examination is normal. You suspect postural tachycardia syndrome (POTS). Which of the following statements is **CORRECT** regarding autonomic testing for this patient?
A. Thermoregulatory sweat test is a sensitive test for POTS.
B. Blood pressure drops along with increases in heart rate are changes in POTS.
C. Peripheral sympathetic sudomotor dysfunction does not accompany POTS.
D. In POTS, heart rate increases within the first 10 minutes after head tilt.
E. Ictal discharges captured on electroencephalography (EEG) can be seen during the attack of POTS.

**Q12.** The diagnosis of postural tachycardia syndrome is confirmed on tilt table testing by an increase in heart rate of more than 30 bpm **AND**:
A. an increase in systolic blood pressure of more than 20 mmHg.
B. a gradual drop of systolic blood pressure of more than 20 mmHg.
C. a gradual drop in diastolic blood pressure of more than 10 mmHg.
D. a sudden drop in blood pressure.
E. clinical symptoms such as dizziness, nausea, and palpitation.

**Q13.** Postural tachycardia syndrome is **NOT** associated with:
A. vasodepressor syncope.
B. reduced quantitative sudomotor axon reflex test (QSART).
C. orthostatic hypotension.
D. elevated standing plasma norepinephrine.
E. migraine.

**Q14.** A characteristic of delayed orthostatic hypotension is which of the following:
A. It affects older patients.
B. It occurs beyond 3 minutes of head-up tilt.
C. It is more severe than early (<3 minutes) orthostatic hypotension.
D. It is due to neurally mediated reflex (vasovagal) syncope.
E. It is a manifestation of severe sympathetic adrenergic failure.

**Q15.** Orthostatic hypotension does **NOT** usually accompany which of the following disorders?
A. Lambert-Eaton myasthenic syndrome
B. Diabetic polyneuropathy
C. Parkinson disease
D. Amyotrophic lateral sclerosis
E. Multiple system atrophy

**Q16.** Which of the following factors may interfere with the sympathetic skin response (SSR)?
A. Low-frequency filter (high-pass) setting
B. Anxiety
C. Distraction
D. Amitriptyline
E. All of the above

## PART 2 | QUESTIONS WITH ANSWERS AND DISCUSSION

**QUESTION 1.** In the sympathetic nervous system, which organ is mediated by acetylcholine as a neurotransmitter from the postganglionic neuron?
A. Pupil
B. Lacrimal gland
C. Sweat gland
D. Smooth muscle in blood vessels
E. Heart

**ANSWER:** C. Sweat gland

### COMMENTS AND DISCUSSION
- Sympathetic nervous system (Fig. 9.1)
  - System for *"fight or flight"*
  - Maintenance of blood pressure, local regulation of blood flow, thermoregulation, and response to exercise and internal or external stressors
  - Preganglionic neurons: Intermediolateral cell column (lamina VII) at the T1–L2 spinal segments
  - Neurotransmitter in sympathetic preganglionic neurons is acetylcholine (ACh) (see Fig. 2.12)
  - Sympathetic ganglia are located close to the spinal cord, except the adrenal gland
    - Paravertebral ganglia supply all organs except abdomen, pelvis, and perineum
    - Prevertebral ganglia supply viscera and blood vessels of abdomen and pelvis
    - Adrenal medulla releases epinephrine to bloodstream
  - Primary neurotransmitter in sympathetic ganglionic neurons is norepinephrine **EXCEPT** for acetylcholine in sweat glands (see Fig. 2.12)
- Receptors for norepinephrine and epinephrine (adrenoreceptors)
  - $\alpha 1$: mediates excitation of smooth muscle in blood vessels, iris, vas deferens, bladder neck, and internal sphincter of rectum
  - $\alpha 2$: autofeedback loop in presynaptic terminals
  - $\beta 1$: heart, stimulate automatism of the sinus node, excitability of the His-Purkinje system, contractility of the myocardium
  - $\beta 2$: elicits smooth muscle relaxation; vasodilation, bronchodilation, and relaxation of smooth muscle in the bladder and uterus

**QUESTION 2.** Which statement is **CORRECT** regarding acetylcholine (ACh) and norepinephrine (NE) in the parasympathetic nervous system?
A. Neurotransmitter for preganglionic neuron is ACh, and postganglionic neuron is ACh.
B. Neurotransmitter for preganglionic neuron is ACh, and postganglionic neuron is NE.
C. Neurotransmitter for preganglionic neuron is NE, and postganglionic neuron is ACh.
D. Neurotransmitter for preganglionic neuron is NE, and postganglionic neuron is NE.
E. None of the above.

**ANSWER:** A. Neurotransmitter for preganglionic neuron is ACh, and postganglionic neuron is ACh.

### COMMENTS AND DISCUSSION
- **Parasympathetic nervous system (Table 9.1 and Fig. 9.1)**
  - System for *"rest and digest"*
  - Preganglionic neurons: brain stem (cranial nerves [CN] III, VII, and X) and intermediolateral cell column at the S2–S4 spinal segments
  - Neurotransmitter in parasympathetic preganglionic neurons is acetylcholine (ACh), similar to the preganglionic neurons in the sympathetic nervous system (see Fig. 2.12)
  - Parasympathetic ganglia are located near the target organs (just outside or within the wall of the organ) → provide organ-specific reflexes
  - Primary neurotransmitters in parasympathetic ganglionic neurons are acetylcholine (ACh) and nitric oxide (NO) (see Fig. 2.12)
  - Seventy-five percent of parasympathetic nervous system are innervated by the vagus nerve (CN X) (Table 9.1).

**Sympathetic nervous systems**

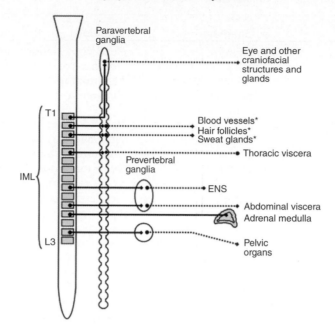

**Parasympathetic nervous system**

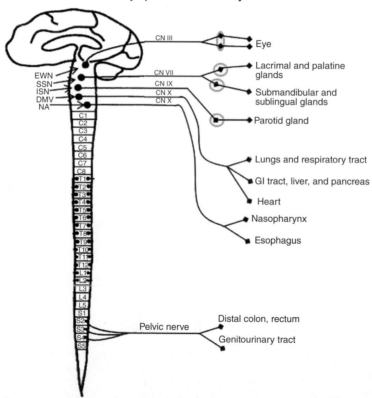

**Fig. 9.1** Sympathetic and parasympathetic nervous system: **Upper panel** is the **sympathetic** nervous system. Sympathetic preganglionic neurons are located in the intermediolateral cell column in the T1–L2-3 spinal segments, which project to pre- and paravertebral ganglia located close to the spinal cord. The postganglionic fibers travel to the targeted organs. **Lower panel** is the **parasympathetic** nervous system. Parasympathetic preganglionic neurons are located at the craniosacral level, which project the fibers to ganglia located close to the organs. The postganglionic fibers run in a very short distance to the targeted organs. Adapted from Illigens BMW, Gibbons CH. Autonomic testing, methods and techniques. In: Levin KH, Chauvel P, eds. *Handbook of Clinical Neurology*. Philadelphia, PA: Elsevier; 2019:419–433. CN, Cranial nerve; DMV, Dorsal motor nucleus of the vagus; ENS, Enteric nervous system; EWN, Edinger-Westphal nucleus; IML, Intermediolateral nucleus; ISN, Inferior salivatory nucleus; NA, Nucleus ambiguous; SSN, Superior salivatory nucleus.

**TABLE 9.1** Parasympathetic nervous system

|  | Ganglion | Function |
|---|---|---|
| CN III | Ciliary | Pupil constriction and accommodation reflexes |
| CN VII | Pterygopalatine | Lacrimation, cranial vasodilation |
|  | Submaxillary and submandibular | Salivation |
| CN IX | Otic | Parotid gland secretion |
| Dorsal motor nucleus of the vagus | Cardiac | Negative chronotropic and negative ionotropic action |
|  | Tracheal | Pulmonary gland secretion, broncho-constriction, bronchodilation |
|  | Enteric | Acid secretion, gastric relaxation/contraction, pancreatic exocrine function |
|  | Intramural ganglion of gallbladder | Gallbladder contraction |
| Nucleus ambiguous | Intrinsic cardiac ganglion | Controlling sinus node |
| Sacral parasympathetic system | Pelvic (hypogastric) | Vasodilation, genital organs and uterus |
|  | Pelvic | Glands of genital organs |
|  | Pelvic and intramural ganglion of bladder | Micturition |

- Receptors for parasympathetic postganglionic organs are muscarinic receptors.
  - M2: Receives inhibitory effects from the vagus nerve; this receptor controls automatism of the sinus and atrioventricular nodes
  - M3: Most excitatory effects of ACh on the visceral targets; this receptor has a role in smooth muscle contraction, exocrine gland secretion, endothelial synthesis of nitric oxide, and secretion of sweat. Of note, M3 receptors in the sweat glands are innervated by the sympathetic nervous system, not the parasympathetic.

 **HIGH-YIELD FACT**

The neurotransmitter in both sympathetic and parasympathetic preganglionic neurons is acetylcholine (ACh) but neurotransmitters in postganglionic neurons are different.

**QUESTION 3.** Quantitative sudomotor axon reflex test (QSART) is performed to assess patients with suspected small fiber neuropathy. Which neurotransmitter or chemical substance is essential to activate the response?
A. Acetylcholine
B. Dopamine
C. Glutamate
D. Iodine
E. Norepinephrine

**ANSWER:** A. Acetylcholine

**COMMENTS AND DISCUSSION**
- Sweat is controlled by the sympathetic autonomic nervous system.
  - However, the neurotransmitter at postganglionic neuron is acetylcholine, rather than norepinephrine or epinephrine (see Fig. 2.12).
- Sudomotor testing: Quantitative sudomotor axon reflex test (QSART) and thermoregulatory sweat test (TST) are two main tests for assessing sudomotor or sweat dysfunction.
- Quantitative sudomotor axon reflex test (QSART) (Fig. 9.2)
  - Testing postganglionic sympathetic sudomotor axon
  - Measuring sweat production (sudomotor function)
  - Iontophoresis of *acetylcholine* over skin surface → activate axon reflex (retrograde stimulation via an axon twig to nearby axons) → stimulate adjacent sweat glands

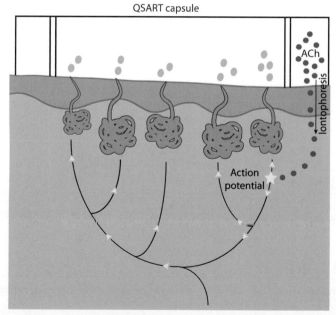

**Fig. 9.2 QSART loop.** QSART capsule has a multicompartment ring. The most outer ring is filled with acetylcholine, and where iontophoretic stimulation takes place. The most inner ring is the area where sweat is measured. The middle layer is kept empty to prevent direct stimulation from leakage of the iontophoresis. Acetylcholine is pushed through the skin layer by iontophoresis, which induces action potentials at postsynaptic fibers. Action potentials travel both orthodromically and antidromically. Sweat glands are stimulated by both direct stimulation and axon reflex from antidromic action potentials and produce sweat. *ACh*, acetylcholine.

**QUESTION 4.** A 55-year-old woman with a history of type 2 diabetes presents with burning feet for 5 months. Neurological examination shows normal motor power and sensation in all modalities except for hyperesthesia in both soles. Electromyography (EMG) is unremarkable. Quantitative sudomotor axon reflex test (QSART) shows reduced sweat output in the foot and distal leg but normal output in the hand. Which of the following statements is **CORRECT** regarding this condition?

A. Myelin is abnormal.
B. Sensory ataxia is a common presentation.
C. Nerve biopsy is a gold standard test.
D. Thermoregulatory sweat test (TST) should be normal.
E. Pathology is confined to the C fibers.

**ANSWER:** E. Pathology is confined to the C fibers.

**COMMENTS AND DISCUSSION**
- Quantitative sudomotor axon reflex test (QSART):
  - Assesses postganglionic sympathetic sudomotor axons, which are small unmyelinated C fibers
  - Is abnormal with disruption of these sympathetic axons to sweat glands, as in small fiber neuropathies
- Thermoregulatory sweat test (TST) (Fig. 9.3)
  - Evaluates the anatomic pattern of sweat response over the entire body
  - Performed under controlled temperature (45°–50°C) and humidity (35%–40%)
  - Alizarin powder is applied over the subject's body.
  - Dye changes color from sandy yellow to purple when exposed to sweat.
  - Pattern of sweat is determined.
  - This test assesses both central and peripheral sympathetic sudomotor pathway
- Diagnosing small fiber neuropathy
  - There is no one gold standard test for small fiber neuropathy.
  - In clinical practice, at least *two tests* should be abnormal to confirm diagnosis, including quantitative sensory test (QST), QSART, or intraepidermal nerve fiber density (IENFD).
  - Nerve biopsy is not useful to diagnose small fiber neuropathy.

 **KEY POINT**

QSART is sensitive in detecting small fiber neuropathy.

 **KEY POINT**

If QSART is abnormal, TST is often also abnormal.

 **HIGH-YIELD FACT**

QSART may be normal when TST is abnormal in disorders affecting **central sympathetic sudomotor pathways.**

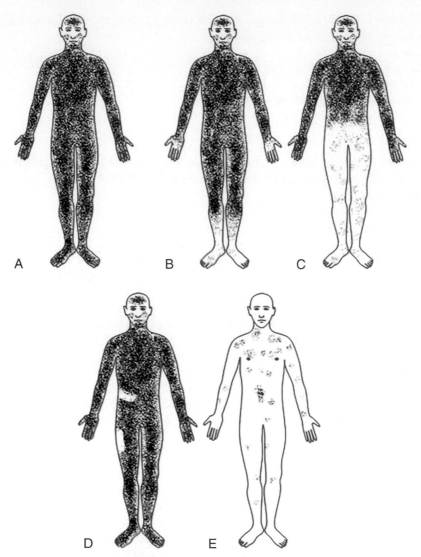

**Fig. 9.3 Thermoregulatory sweat testing (TST).** *The black area* represents the area of color change of the powder in response to sweat. (A) Normal sweat pattern in high temperature. (B) Pattern with decreased sweat production in length dependent polyneuropathy. (C) Pattern of decreased sweat in the case of spinal cord injury with sensory level deficit. (D) Patchy area of decreased sweat pattern in a patient with meralgia paresthetica and right T10 radiculopathy. (E) Pattern of no/almost no sweat production in global anhidrosis. Courtesy of Ben, M.W. Illigens, Gibbons CH. Autonomic testing, methods and techniques. In: Levin KH, Chauvel P, eds. *Handbook of Clinical Neurology.* Philadelphia, PA: Elsevier; 2019:419–433.

**QUESTION 5.** Which medication should be withheld prior to performing a quantitative sudomotor axon reflex test (QSART)?
   A. Propranolol
   B. Ondansetron
   C. Nortriptyline
   D. Valproic acid
   E. Verapamil

**ANSWER:** C. Nortriptyline

**COMMENTS AND DISCUSSION**
- Quantitative sudomotor axon reflex test (QSART) results are frequently influenced by medications.
- It is crucial to perform QSART without the effects of medications that can cause hypohidrosis to avoid misinterpretation.
- The main medications that can cause hypohidrosis are *anticholinergic agents* (e.g., amitriptyline, nortriptyline, glycopyrrolate, and hyoscyamine).

- Other medications with central adrenergic, antimuscarinic, or carbonic anhydrase inhibition effects may also influence sudomotor functions including:
  - ○ topiramate and zonisamide
  - ○ clonidine
  - ○ carbamazepine
  - ○ cyproheptadine, diphenhydramine
  - ○ clozapine, olanzapine, quetiapine
  - ○ scopolamine

**QUESTION 6.** Which of the following conditions may cause an abnormal thermoregulatory sweat test (TST) but a normal quantitative sudomotor axon reflex test (QSART)?
  A. Multiple system atrophy
  B. Diabetic polyneuropathy
  C. Amyloid light chain (AL) amyloidosis
  D. Postural tachycardia syndrome
  E. None of the above

**ANSWER:** A. Multiple system atrophy

**COMMENTS AND DISCUSSION (see also comments and discussion from Question 4)**
- Thermoregulatory sweat test (TST)
  - ○ Evaluates the anatomic pattern of the sweat over the entire body
  - ○ Determines central and peripheral sympathetic sudomotor pathways
- Multiple system atrophy may result in normal QSART and abnormal TST.
- Diabetic polyneuropathy, amyloid light chain (AL) amyloidosis, and postural tachycardia syndrome are associated with peripheral neuropathy, often including the small fibers resulting in abnormal TST and QSART.

 **KEY POINT**

- Abnormal QSART localizes the lesion to the periphery involving postganglionic sudomotor neurons or axons.
- In contrast, lesions anywhere in the thermoregulatory pathway (from central to peripheral pathway) may cause abnormal TST.

 **KEY POINT**

In peripheral sudomotor lesions, both TST and QSART are abnormal.
In central sudomotor lesions, only TST is abnormal.

**QUESTION 7.** Which autonomic testing assesses cardiovagal function?
  A. Heart rate response to deep breathing
  B. Blood pressure response to the Valsalva maneuver
  C. Tilt table testing
  D. Quantitative sudomotor axon reflex test
  E. Thermoregulatory sweat test

**ANSWER:** A. Heart rate response to deep breathing

**COMMENTS AND DISCUSSION**
- Autonomic tests for cardiovagal or cardiovascular parasympathetic system include heart rate response to deep breathing (HR-DB) and Valsalva ratio (VR).

- Heart rate response to deep breathing (HR-DB) (Fig. 9.4)
  - Determines cardiovagal system by assessing heart rate response
  - Measurement:
    - Mean heart rate range (maximum-minimum) of the five consecutive largest responses from eight breathing cycles
    - Normal value is based on age
  - Method:
    - Heart rate recording while patient is in the supine position for 20 minutes
    - Patient is asked to breathe slowly at a rate of 6 breaths per minutes (5 s in and 5 s out).
    - From electrocardiography (ECG) recording, R-R interval is converted to heart rate and monitored continuously.

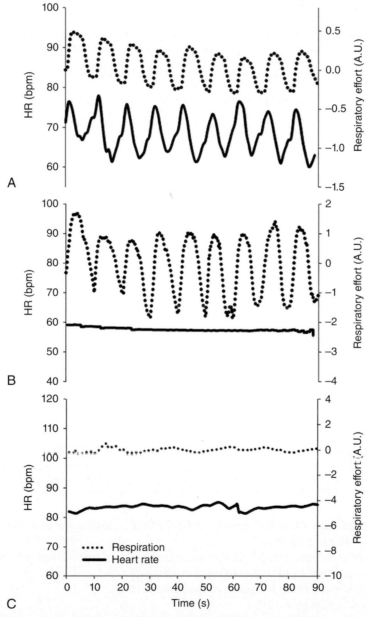

**Fig. 9.4 Tracing from heart rate response to deep breathing (HR-DB).** *Dotted lines* are respiratory capacity (higher number indicates a greater chest wall excursion and lung volume or inspiration and lower number occurs in expiration [right Y-axis]). *Solid lines* are heart rate, which is variable with the breathing (left Y-axis). (A) This is an HR-DB, where the heart rate variability has time locked to the breathing pace. (B) This is an abnormal HR DB in a patient with Parkinson's disease with dysautonomia. The breathing pattern is adequate; however, the heart rate line is flat without variability due to a loss of cardiovagal function. (C) This is an inadequate tracing. The breathing line is flat and represents poor effort. Courtesy of Ben, M.W. Illigens, Gibbons CH. Autonomic testing, methods and techniques. In: Levin KH, Chauvel P, eds. *Handbook of Clinical Neurology.* Philadelphia, PA: Elsevier; 2019:419–433.

- Valsalva ratio (VR)
  - Measuring heart rate response, similar to HR-DB, but in VR testing, Heart rate is measured while patient performs Valsalva maneuver
  - Measurement:
    - Valsalva ratio = maximum heart rate/minimum heart rate following the peak heart rate within 30 seconds
  - Method:
    - Patient is in the recumbent position.
    - Patient is asked to blow, maintaining a column of mercury at 30–40 mmHg for 12–15 seconds via a bugle with an air leak (ensuring the opening of the glottis).
    - Repeat 2–4 times with interval baseline rest of at least 3 minutes.

## 🔑 KEY POINT

Valsalva ratio (**heart rate** response to Valsalva) represents only the cardiovagal **parasympathetic** system; however, **BP response** to Valsalva can represent **noradrenergic (sympathetic)** cardiovascular function.

**QUESTION 8.** Which of the following statements can influence the result of heart rate response to deep breathing?
- A. Age
- B. Rate of breathing
- C. Depth of breathing
- D. Medications
- E. All of the above

**ANSWER:** E. All of above

### COMMENTS AND DISCUSSION

- Both heart rate response to deep breathing (HR-DB) and to Valsalva maneuver are affected by multiple factors.
  - Age
  - Posture
  - Body mass index (BMI)
  - Rate of breathing
  - Depth of breathing
  - Pulmonary disease (emphysema, chronic obstructive pulmonary disease [COPD])
  - Medications (tricyclic antidepressants and anticholinergic, sympathomimetic, and antispasmodic agents)
- Normal values of HR-DB and Valsalva ratio are dependent on a subject's age.

## 🔑 KEY POINT

It is crucial to stop medications that can interfere with autonomic testing to avoid misinterpretation.

**QUESTION 9.** Which of the following statements is **CORRECT** regarding the beat-to-beat blood pressure (BP) response to Valsalva maneuver?
- A. Phase I and IV represent intrathoracic pressure changes from mechanical variation.
- B. Early phase II drop-off in BP is due to vagal overactivity.
- C. Late phase II recovery of BP is a result of sympathetic surge.
- D. Vasodilation occurs in phase III.
- E. Phase IV overshoot of BP is associated with tachycardia

**ANSWER:** C. Late phase II recovery of BP is a result of sympathetic surge.

### COMMENTS AND DISCUSSION

- Autonomic test for vasomotor adrenergic system is the change in beat-to-beat blood pressure during the Valsalva maneuver.
- During Valsalva maneuver, the dynamic changes in blood pressure are divided into four phases (Table 9.2 and Fig. 9.5).

**TABLE 9.2** Blood pressure (BP) phases in Valsalva maneuver

| Phases | BP changes | Mechanisms |
|---|---|---|
| **Phase I** | Mechanically increased BP | Increased intrathoracic pressure during inhalation |
| **Phase II - Early (Phase II$_E$)** | Decreased BP | Decreasing in venous return, stroke volume, and cardiac output |
| **Phase II - Late (Phase II$_L$)** | BP stops declining and recovering | Decreased BP from early phase II triggers withdrawal of vagal tone, result in **sympathetic response** → vasoconstriction, increased heart rate, and inotropic force |
| **Phase III** | Mechanically decreased BP | Normalization of intrathoracic pressure during exhalation |
| **Phase IV** | BP rapidly returning back to baseline, followed by overshoots | Normalization of venous return and cardiac output in a setting of vasoconstriction (overshoots) from **sympathetic response in phase II$_L$** <br> Increase in aortic pressure → reflex decrease in heart rate (**parasympathetic response**) |

## 🔑 KEY POINT

In Valsalva maneuver
→ BP changes during **late phase II (phase II$_L$) and phase IV** represent **sympathetic** function
→ HR changes during **phase IV** represent **parasympathetic** function

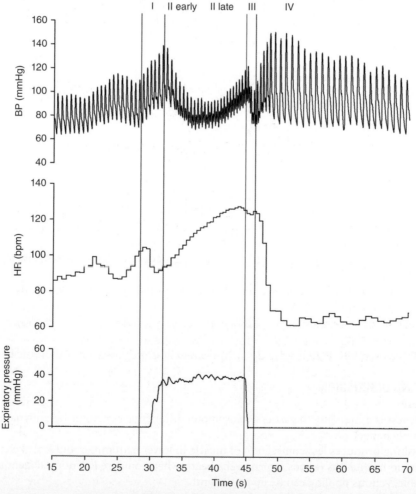

**Fig. 9.5 Blood pressure (BP) and heart rate responses to the Valsalva maneuver.** Tracing and phases of the Valsalva maneuver. The *upper trace* is blood pressure responses; the *middle trace* is heart rate responses to a Valsalva maneuver. The *lower trace* is an expiratory pressure to visualize the effort. The BP responses are divided into phase I, II$_E$, late II$_L$, III, and IV. Phase II$_L$ and IV represent adrenergic or sympathetic function. the tachycardia from the heart rate tracing is an appropriate response during Valsalva maneuver and is calculated to Valsalva ratio to determine cardiovagal or parasympathetic function. Courtesy of Ben, M.W. Illigens, Gibbons CH. Autonomic testing, methods and techniques. In: Levin KH, Chauvel P, eds. *Handbook of Clinical Neurology.* Philadelphia, PA: Elsevier; 2019:419–433.

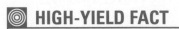

## HIGH-YIELD FACT

| ↑ Degree of adrenergic failure | ↓ responses during phase II$_L$ and phase IV (Fig. 9.6) |

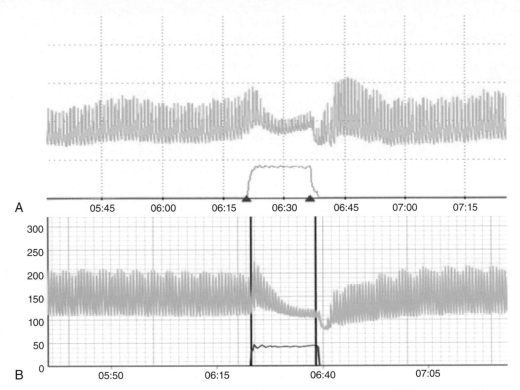

**Fig. 9.6** Blood pressure (BP) responses to Valsalva maneuver. (A) Normal Valsalva maneuver. (B) BP responses to Valsalva maneuver in a 65-year-old man with pure autonomic failure. Note the absence of phase II late (II$_L$), no phase IV, and long BP recovery time. Lower curve = respiratory pressure. Courtesy of Ali Arvantaj.

**QUESTION 10.** A 58-year-old man presents with recurrent syncopal episodes upon standing several times for 3 months. His daughter notices the patient walks slower than his baseline in the past 6 months. On examination, he has signs of parkinsonism with a wide-based gait. Dysmetria is noted on the finger-to-nose test. You suspect multiple system atrophy. Which of the following statements is **CORRECT** regarding the autonomic result in this patient?
A. This disorder predominantly affects the parasympathetic nervous system.
B. Spared phase II$_L$ in Valsalva maneuver is a key feature for central dysautonomia.
C. Decreased systolic blood pressure (SBP) >20 mmHg upon 70-degree tilt is diagnostic of orthostatic hypotension.
D. Abnormal quantitative sudomotor axon reflex test (QSART) in all sites is a mandatory feature in multiple system atrophy (MSA).
E. Thermoregulatory sweat test (TST) shows normal sweat pattern.

**ANSWER:** C. Decreased SBP >20 mmHg upon 70-degree tilt is diagnostic of orthostatic hypotension.

### COMMENTS AND DISCUSSION
- Tilt table test
  - Tilt table test is a modality that assesses vasomotor adrenergic system or hemodynamic response to postural change.
  - Passive tilting produces less contraction of muscle in lower extremities and less skeletal muscle activation in facilitating venous return to the heart, when compared to normal standing.
  - In tilt table, venous pooling can be up to 1000 mL.
  - Venous pooling → drop in BP → trigger withdrawal signal from baroreceptors → increase in heart rate (HR) (parasympathetic withdrawal) and increase in BP (increased sympathetic tone)
  - Measurement
    - Blood pressure trend and symptoms at baseline and upon 70-degree tilt.

- Method
  - Baseline continuous beat-to-beat blood pressure and heart rate are monitored in the supine position.
  - Passive head-up tilting to 70 degrees is performed.
- In multiple system atrophy, orthostatic hypotension is usually severe, and treatment is frequently complicated by supine hypertension. There is usually pan-dysautonomia affecting both sympathetic and parasympathetic nervous systems. QSART is usually normal while TST is often abnormal.

**QUESTION 11.** A 22-year-old woman presents with dizziness and palpitation upon standing for 4 months. She has episodes of dizziness, light-headedness, palpitation, and near syncope once she stands. Her neurological examination is normal. You suspect postural tachycardia syndrome (POTS). Which of the following statements is **CORRECT** regarding autonomic testing for this patient?
  A. Thermoregulatory sweat test is a sensitive test for POTS.
  B. Blood pressure drops along with increases in heart rate are changes in POTS.
  C. Peripheral sympathetic sudomotor dysfunction does not accompany POTS.
  D. In POTS, heart rate increases within the first 10 minutes after head tilt.
  E. Ictal discharges captured on electroencephalography (EEG) can be seen during the attack of POTS.

**ANSWER:** D. In POTS, heart rate increases within the first 10 minutes after head tilt.

**COMMENTS AND DISCUSSION**
- Tilt table testing (Fig. 9.7) is sensitive in assessing the hemodynamic responses to postural changes.
  - Tilt table testing is sensitive to evaluate the following conditions:
    - Syncope
    - Orthostatic hypotension
    - Postural tachycardia syndrome (POTS)
    - Orthostatic intolerance
- In neurogenic orthostatic hypotension
  - Blood pressure (BP) drops more than 20 mmHg systolic and/or 10 mmHg diastolic within 3 minutes of standing or tilting.
  - Often occurs in the first 5–10 minutes of tilt.
  - Heart rate (HR) fails to rise despite the drop in BP.
- In POTS
  - HR increases from baseline more than 30 bpm within 10 minutes of standing or tilting.
  - BP is stable (no evidence of orthostatic hypotension).
  - In half of patients, peripheral sympathetic sudomotor dysfunction accompanies POTS and manifests by abnormal QSART.
  - POTS is a syndrome that may result from several underlying mechanisms.
  - Main mechanisms in POTS include:
    - Impaired sympathetically mediated vasoconstriction in the lower extremities
    - Excessive cardiac sympathoexcitatory responses
    - Volume dysregulation
    - Joint hypermobility
    - Physical deconditioning
- POTS is not associated with ictal electroencephalography (EEG).

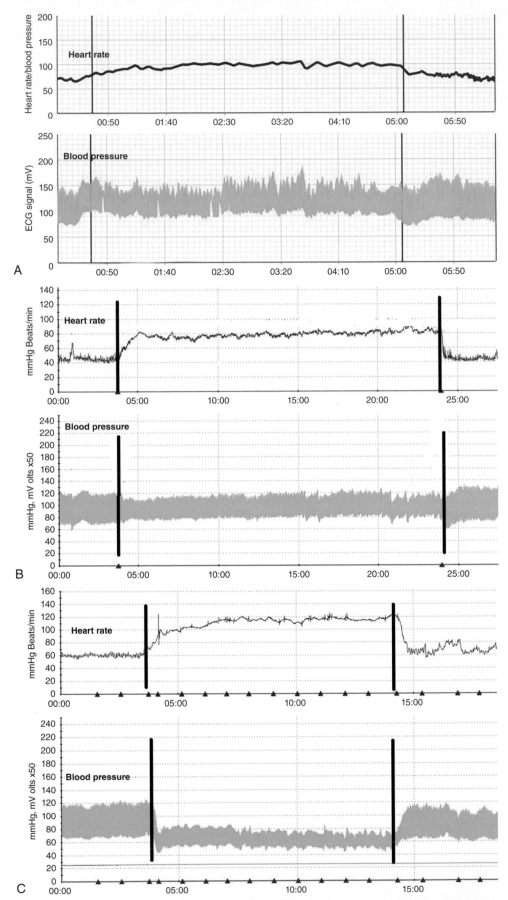

**Fig. 9.7 Tilt table testing**. Tilt table recording in (A) normal subject; (B) in a 21-year-old woman with postural tachycardia syndrome (note the rapid rise in heart rate from a baseline of about 35 bpm with a 70-degree tilt followed by a rapid return of heart rate to baseline while the blood pressure remains stable without any significant change in blood pressure). (C) In a 55-year-old woman with orthostatic hypotension (note the abrupt drop in blood pressure from a baseline of about systolic 120 mmHg to systolic 80 mmHg and ultimately reaching 70 mmHg). *Vertical lines* represent the beginning and end of 70-degree tilt. Courtesy of Ali Arvantaj.

**QUESTION 12.** The diagnosis of postural tachycardia syndrome is confirmed on tilt table testing by an increase in heart rate of more than 30 bpm AND:

A. an increase in systolic blood pressure of more than 20 mmHg.
B. a gradual drop of systolic blood pressure of more than 20 mmHg.
C. a gradual drop in diastolic blood pressure of more than 10 mmHg.
D. a sudden drop in blood pressure.
E. clinical symptoms such as dizziness, nausea, and palpitation.

**ANSWER:** E. clinical symptoms such as dizziness, nausea, and palpitation.

**COMMENTS AND DISCUSSION (see also comments and discussion from Question 11)**

- Postural tachycardia syndrome (POTS) is defined by a symptomatic increase of heart rate of more than 30 bpm during the first 10 minutes of tilt in the absence of any drop in blood pressure (Fig. 9.7B and 9.8).
- Gradual drops in systolic blood pressure of more than 20 mmHg or in diastolic blood pressure of more than 10 mmHg are signs of orthostatic hypotension (Fig. 9.7C).
- A sudden drop in blood pressure is a feature of reflex syncope (vasodepressor syncope).

**QUESTION 13.** Postural tachycardia syndrome is **NOT** associated with:

A. vasodepressor syncope.
B. reduced quantitative sudomotor axon reflex test (QSART).
C. orthostatic hypotension.
D. elevated standing plasma norepinephrine.
E. migraine.

**ANSWER:** C. orthostatic hypotension

**COMMENTS AND DISCUSSION**

- POTS often manifests with lightheadedness, palpitations, headache, and vasodepressor syncope (in about 1/3 of patients).
- Patients have an elevated plasma norepinephrine concentration of 600 pg/mL or more on standing.
- POTS may be associated with small fiber neuropathy and/or abnormal QSART, termed neuropathic POTS.
- POTS is associated with several comorbidities including migraine, chronic fatigue syndrome, sleep disturbance, Raynaud's syndrome, and chronic pain.

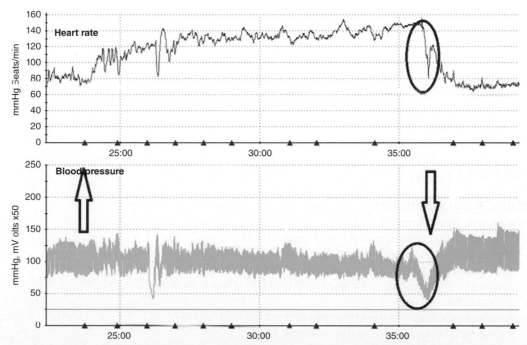

**Fig. 9.8** Tilt table testing in postural tachycardia syndrome. Tilt table study in a 25-year-old man with postural tachycardia syndrome (POTS) and vasodepressor syncope. Note the increase in heart rate with 70-degree tilt followed by a sudden drop in blood pressure and heart rate *(circles)*. *Arrows* denote the beginning and end of tilt. Courtesy of Ali Arvantaj.

**QUESTION 14.** A characteristic of delayed orthostatic hypotension is which of the following:
  A. It affects older patients.
  B. It occurs beyond 3 minutes of head-up tilt.
  C. It is more severe than early (<3 minutes) orthostatic hypotension.
  D. It is due to neurally mediated reflex (vasovagal) syncope.
  E. It is a manifestation of severe sympathetic adrenergic failure.

**ANSWER:** B. It occurs between beyond 3 minutes of head up tilt.

**COMMENTS AND DISCUSSION (see also comments and discussion from Questions 12 and 13)**
- Delayed orthostatic hypotension affects relatively younger patients, and is a sign of mild sympathetic adrenergic failure.
- It occurs beyond 3 minutes of tilt table testing. The magnitude of the blood pressure (BP) fall does not differ between those with early hypotension. Therefore, the tilt table testing should be monitored at least 10 minutes of standing.
- Neurally mediated reflex (vasovagal) syncope is not a manifestation of autonomic failure and is often associated with bradycardia and abrupt drop in BP.

**QUESTION 15.** Orthostatic hypotension does **NOT** usually accompany which of the following disorders?
  A. Lambert-Eaton myasthenic syndrome
  B. Diabetic polyneuropathy
  C. Parkinson disease
  D. Amyotrophic lateral sclerosis
  E. Multiple system atrophy

**ANSWER:** D. Amyotrophic lateral sclerosis

**COMMENTS AND DISCUSSION**
- Lambert-Eaton myasthenic syndrome is an autoimmune, often paraneoplastic, disorder that associated with autoantibodies against voltage-gated calcium channels at the presynaptic terminals of muscarinic *and* nicotinic synapses. This manifests as fatigable weakness and areflexia but also dysautonomia including dry mouth, impotence, and orthostatic hypotension.
- Diabetic autonomic neuropathy is a frequent complication of long-standing diabetes mellitus. Denervation of autonomic nerves results in autonomic neuropathy, often manifesting as tachycardia, postural hypotension, reduced heart rate variability or fixed heart rate.
- Parkinson disease and multiple system atrophy are often associated with orthostatic hypotension.
- Amyotrophic lateral sclerosis is not associated with orthostatic hypotension.

**QUESTION 16.** Which of the following factors can interfere with the sympathetic skin response (SSR)?
  A. Low-frequency filter (high-pass) setting
  B. Anxiety
  C. Distraction
  D. Amitriptyline
  E. All of the above

**ANSWER:** E. All of above

**COMMENTS AND DISCUSSION**
- Sympathetic skin response (SSR)
  - A response that is generated by sweat from stimuli.
  - Assessment of peripheral sympathetic function.
  - Less commonly performed due to its variability of response
  - Quantitative sudomotor axon reflex test (QSART) is much more reproducible.
  - Measurement
    - Amplitude (peak-to-peak) measuring from the evoked potentials is the most sensitive indicator but variable and habitable from multiple trials.
    - Latency which is more reproducible compared to amplitude; however, it can be variable due to central conduction delay.

- Method
  - Apply electrical shock as a stimulus.
  - Other stimuli, for example, tactile, startle, cough, and magnetic stimulation also can be used, depending on individual laboratory protocols.
  - Record responses over the palms and soles.
  - Because responses are of very low frequency compared to other responses, low-frequency (high-pass) filter is set much lower than the usual setting.
  - If the low-frequency filter is increased, amplitude is affected and is much smaller.
  - Normal values depends on the lab, since the amplitude of the responses can vary witih different filter settings and numbers of trials.
- Factors that can interfere responses from SSR:
  - Multiple trials may habituate the response.
  - Low-frequency filter setting
  - Anxiety
  - Distraction
  - Anticholinergic medications

## SUGGESTED READINGS

Illigens BMW, Gibbons CH. Autonomic testing, methods and techniques. In: Levin KH, Chauvel P, eds. *Handbook of Clinical Neurology*. Elsevier; 2019:419-433.

Cheshire WP, Fealey RD. Drug-induced hyperhidrosis and hypohidrosis: incidence, prevention and management. *Drug Saf*. 2008;31:109-126.

Devigili G, Rinaldo S, Lombardi R, et al. Diagnostic criteria for small fiber neuropathy in clinical practice and research. *Brain*. 2019;142(12):3728-3736.

Gibbons CH. Small fiber neuropathies. *Continuum (Minneap Minn)*. 2014;20(5):1398-1412.

Gibbons CH, Freeman R. Delayed orthostatic hypotension: a frequent cause of orthostatic intolerance. *Neurology*. 2006;67:28-32.

Low PA, Benarroch EE. *Clinical Autonomic Disorders*. 3rd ed. LWW; 2008.

Thaisetthawatkul P, Fernandes Filho JA, Herrmann DN. Contribution of QSART to the diagnosis of small fiber neuropathy. *Muscle Nerve*. 2013;48(6):883-888.

Zhou L. Small fiber neuropathy. *Semin Neurol*. 2019;39(5):570-577.

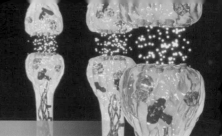

# CHAPTER 10

# Muscle and Nerve Biopsies

## PART 1 | PRACTICE TEST

**Q1.** A muscle biopsy is **NOT** indicated in which of the following scenarios?
A. A woman with proximal weakness and dysphagia
B. A teenager with two attacks of exercise-induced rhabdomyolysis
C. A man with progressive leg weakness and spasticity
D. A man with quadriceps and hand flexor weakness
E. A woman with myalgia and high creatine kinase

**Q2.** A 13-year-old boy has proximal symmetrical muscle weakness starting at age 6 years. Motor power examination reveals Medical Research Council (MRC) grade 4 weakness of biceps muscles, minimal weakness of triceps muscles, grade 1 weakness of quadriceps muscles, and grade 2 weakness of hip adductors. In addition, there is pseudohypertrophy of the bilateral calves. Biopsy of which of the following muscles would give the highest diagnostic yield?
A. Biceps
B. Triceps
C. Quadriceps
D. Hip adductors
E. Gastrocnemius

**Q3.** Which of the following statements is **CORRECT** regarding internalized nuclei within muscle fibers?
A. In normal muscle biopsy, there should be no internalized nuclei in muscle fibers.
B. In myotonic dystrophy type 1, there is an increase in internalized nuclei, mainly in type 1 muscle fibers.
C. In myotonic dystrophy type 2, there is an increase in internalized nuclei in both types 1 and 2 muscle fibers.
D. In centronuclear myopathy, there is an increase in central nuclei, mainly in type 2 muscle fibers.
E. In muscle biopsy of neurogenic disorders there should be no internalized nuclei.

**Q4.** Which of the following disorders shows pathological findings on deltoid muscle biopsy that are different from the others?
A. Amyotrophic lateral sclerosis
B. C5 radiculopathy
C. Chronic inflammatory demyelinating polyneuropathy
D. Parsonage-Turner syndrome
E. Thyrotoxic proximal weakness

**Q5.** An 11-month-old infant presents with muscle weakness and hypotonia. Muscle biopsy reveals the finding as in the following figures (top with hematoxylin and eosin (H&E) staining and bottom with adenosine triphosphatase pH 4.3). Which of the following findings is expected on the electrodiagnostic study in this patient?

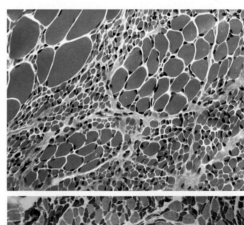

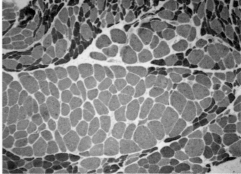

Adapted from Miles JD, Cohen ML. In: Prayson RA, Goldblum JR, eds. *Neuropathology*. 2nd ed. Elsevier; 2012;11:563.

A. Myotonic discharges
B. Neuromyotonic discharges
C. Reduced recruitment
D. Small polyphasic motor unit action potentials
E. Double compound muscle action potentials following a single stimulus

**Q6.** A 23-year-old woman presents with muscle weakness. Muscle biopsy reveals the finding as shown in the following figure (modified Gomori trichrome stain). What is the most likely diagnosis?

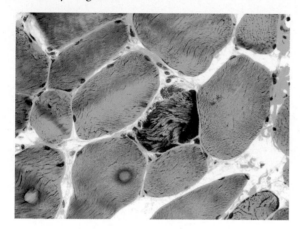

Courtesy Mark Cohen, MD.

A. Emery-Dreifuss muscular dystrophy
B. Mitochondrial encephalomyopathy, lactic acidosis, and stroke-like episodes
C. Myofibrillar myopathy
D. Nemaline myopathy
E. Pompe disease

**Q7.** A 25-year-old woman presents with muscle weakness. Muscle biopsy is performed and sent for electron microscopy which shows the findings in the following figure. What is the most likely diagnosis in this patient?

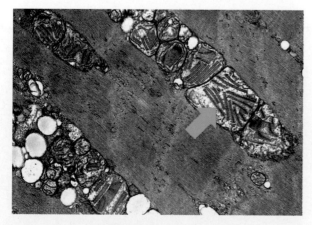

From frontalcortex.com

A. Dermatomyositis
B. Inclusion body myositis
C. Myoclonic epilepsy with ragged-red fibers
D. Nemaline myopathy
E. Oculopharyngeal muscular dystrophy

**Q8.** Which of the following pathological findings is expected in zidovudine (AZT)–induced myopathy?
A. Intranuclear tubulofilamentous inclusions
B. Nemaline rods
C. Perifascicular atrophy
D. Ragged-red fibers
E. Rimmed vacuoles

**Q9.** A 15-year-old girl presents with proximal muscle weakness. Muscle biopsy is performed and reveals the findings in the following figure (modified Gomori trichrome stain). The mutation in which of the following genes is **MOST LIKELY** to be found?

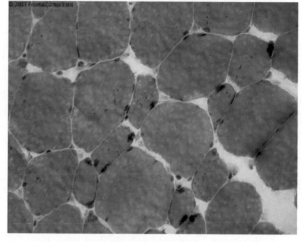

From frontalcortex.com

A. *ACTA1*
B. *FHL1*
C. *MTM1*
D. *POLG*
E. *RYR1*

**Q10.** A 13-year-old boy presents with proximal muscle weakness. Electron microscopic examination of a muscle biopsy demonstrates the finding in the following figure. The muscle disease in this patient is classified as a:

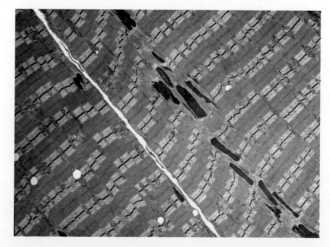

From Dowling JJ, North KN, Goebel HH, et al. In: Darras BT, Jones HR, Ryan MM, et al., eds. *Neuromuscular Disorders of Infancy, Childhood, and Adolescence.* 2nd ed. Elsevier; 2015;28:509.

A. congenital myopathy.
B. metabolic myopathy.
C. mitochondrial myopathy.
D. muscular dystrophy.
E. toxic myopathy.

**Q11.** Which of the following statements is **CORRECT** regarding rimmed vacuoles?
A. Rimmed vacuoles are a specific finding for inclusion body myositis (IBM), distal myopathy with rimmed vacuoles (DMRVs), and oculopharyngeal muscular dystrophy (OPMD).
B. Rimmed vacuoles cannot be seen on hematoxylin and eosin staining but can be seen on modified Gomori trichrome staining.
C. Rimmed vacuoles stain positive for periodic acid–Schiff (PAS).
D. Rimmed vacuoles in OPMD contain amyloid.
E. Rimmed vacuoles in IBM contain autophagic materials.

**Q12.** A 65-year-old man presents with muscle weakness. Muscle biopsy with Congo red staining under polarized light shows the following finding. What is the most likely diagnosis?

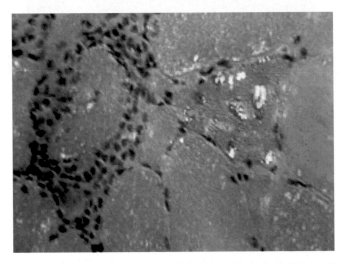

From Doughty CT, Amato AA. In: Jankovic J, Maziotta JC, Pomeroy SL, Newman NJ, eds. *Bradley and Daroff's Neurology in Clinical Practice*. 8th ed. Elsevier; 2022; 109:2018.

A. Polymyositis
B. Dermatomyositis
C. Inclusion body myositis
D. Necrotizing myopathy
E. Overlap myositis syndrome

**Q13.** A 67-year-old man presents with weakness of bilateral finger flexors and quadriceps. The muscle biopsy demonstrates the finding in the following figure (modified Gomori trichrome stain). Which of the following pathological findings is **NOT** expected to be seen on the muscle biopsy of this patient?

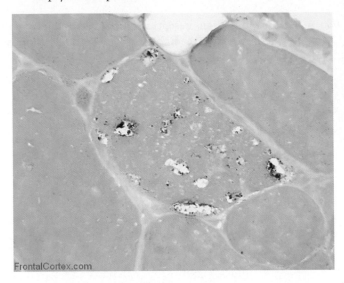

From frontalcortex.com

A. Amyloid deposition
B. TAR DNA-binding protein (TDP-43) accumulation
C. Positive SMI-31 staining
D. Cytochrome oxidase (COX)–deficient fibers
E. Strong succinic dehydrogenase (SDH)–positive vessels

**Q14.** An 11-month-old male infant presents with generalized hypotonia and develops respiratory failure requiring intubation. Muscle biopsy reveals findings as in the figure below. The left panel is hematoxylin and eosin staining and the right panel is periodic acid–Schiff staining. Which of the following stains would be most useful for the diagnosis?

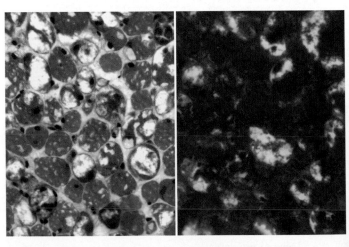

From Dubowitz V, Sewry CA, Oldfors A. *Muscle Biopsy*. 5th ed. Elsevier; 2021;17:391.

A. Acid phosphatase
B. Alkaline phosphatase
C. ATPase
D. Modified Gomori trichrome
E. NADH-TR

**Q15.** Which of the following disorders have muscle histopathological findings most similar to Pompe disease?
A. Danon disease
B. Debrancher enzyme deficiency
C. McArdle disease
D. Niemann-Pick type C
E. Tarui disease

**Q16.** A 23-year-old man presents with proximal muscle weakness. Muscle biopsy shows the finding below. The upper and lower panels are hematoxylin and eosin, and Oil Red O stains, respectively. What is the most likely diagnosis?

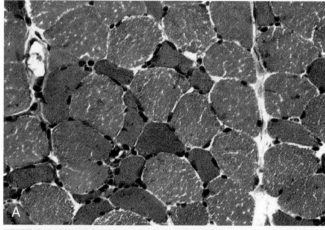

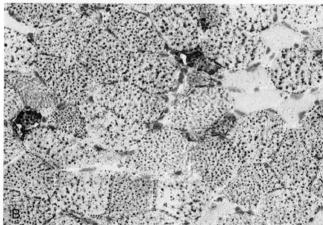

From Angelini C, Nascimbeni AC, Semplicini C. *Ther Adv Neurol Disord.* 2013;6(5):311-321.

A. Acid maltase deficiency
B. Debrancher enzyme deficiency
C. Multiple acyl-CoA dehydrogenase deficiency
D. Myophosphorylase deficiency
E. Phosphofructokinase deficiency

**Q17.** A 9-month-old infant presents with hypotonia. Muscle biopsy is performed, and on reduced nicotinamide adenine dinucleotide-tetrazolium reductase (NADH-TR) staining reveals the finding in the figure below (scale bar: 100 μm). Which of the following conditions is associated with this disorder?

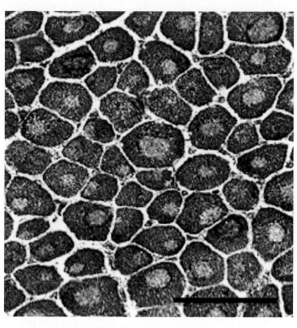

From Marks S, van Ruitenbeek E, Fallon P, et al. *Neuromuscul Disord.* 2018;28(5): 422-426.

A. Adrenal insufficiency
B. Cardiac conduction block
C. Malignant hyperthermia
D. Pulmonary fibrosis
E. Thyroid storm

**Q18.** The finding in the muscle biopsy below (nicotinamide adenine dinucleotide-tetrazolium reductase (NADH-TR) staining) is most likely seen in which of the following disorders?

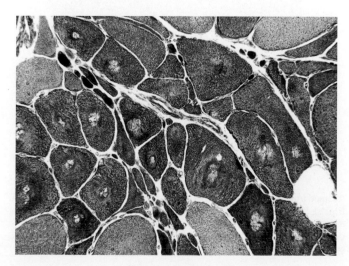

From frontalcortex.com

A. Amyotrophic lateral sclerosis
B. Central core disease
C. Myofibrillar myopathy
D. X-linked myotubular myopathy
E. None of the above, since this is an artifact

**Q19.** A 23-year-old man presents with muscle weakness. Muscle biopsy reveals the findings in the following figure (A: modified Gomori trichrome stain; B: cytochrome oxidase stain; C: succinic dehydrogenase stain. What is the most likely diagnosis?

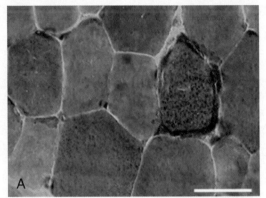

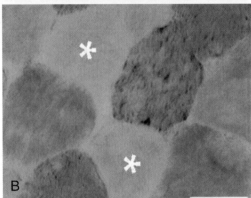

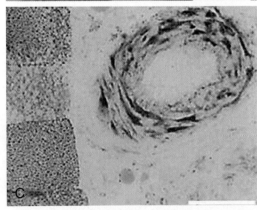

Adapted from (A and B) Lorenzoni PJ, Scola RH, Kay CS, Arndt RC, Freund AA, Bruck I, Santos ML, Werneck LC. *Arq Neuropsiquiatr.* 2009 Sep;67(3A):668-76. doi: 10.1590/s0004-282x2009000400018. PMID: 19722047. (C) Lorenzoni PJ, Werneck LC, Kay CS, Silvado CE, Scola RH. *Arq Neuropsiquiatr* 2015;73(11): 959-67. doi: 10.1590/0004-282X20150154. PMID: 26517220.

A. Adult-onset nemaline myopathy
B. Amyloid myopathy
C. Inclusion body myositis
D. McArdle disease
E. Mitochondrial encephalomyopathy, lactic acidosis, and stroke-like episodes (MELAS)

**Q20.** A 34-year-old woman presents with muscle weakness. Electron microscopic examination of muscle biopsy demonstrates the finding as shown in the following figure. Which of the following histopathologic findings is also expected to be seen?

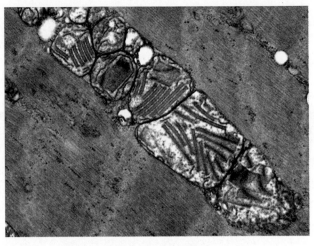

From fronalcortex.com

A. Amyloid within muscle fibers
B. Nemaline rods
C. Perifascicular atrophy
D. Ragged-red fibers
E. Rimmed vacuoles

**Q21.** A 44-year-old woman presents with proximal muscle weakness. Muscle biopsy demonstrates the finding in the following figure (Hematoxylin and eosin stain). Which of the following antibodies is **MOST LIKELY** to be positive in this patient?

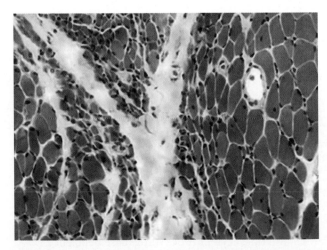

From Uruha A, Suzuki S, Nishino I. *Clin Exp Neuroimmunol.* 2017;8:302-312.

A. Anti-3-hydroxy-3-methylglutaryl-CoA reductase (HMGCR)
B. Anti-LDL receptor-related protein 4 (LRP4)
C. Anti-Mi2
D. Anti-cytosolic 5′-nucleotidase 1A (NT5c1A)
E. Anti-signal recognition particle (SRP)

**Q22.** Which of the following is the histopathologic feature that is most likely found in immune-mediated necrotizing myopathy?
A. Perifascicular atrophy
B. Rimmed vacuoles
C. Prominent endomysial lymphocytic infiltration
D. Macrophage infiltration of necrotic fibers
E. Increased major histocompatibility complex (MHC) class II expression

**The following vignette is for QUESTIONS 23 and 24.**

> A 65-year-old man with coronary artery disease, hypertension, diabetes, and dyslipidemia has had severe left hemiparesis since an ischemic stroke of the right middle cerebral artery territory 3 months ago. He shows no improvement after the stroke and does not participate in rehabilitation.

**Q23.** If the biopsy is performed in the left biceps muscle, which of the following findings is most likely to be found?
A. Large group atrophy
B. Type 1 muscle fiber atrophy
C. Type 2 muscle fiber atrophy
D. Fiber type grouping
E. Wedge-shaped infarct within muscle fascicles

**Q24.** If the electrodiagnostic study is performed in the left arm, including the needle electromyography (EMG) of the left biceps muscle, which of the following findings is expected to be seen?
A. Poor activation of motor unit action potentials (MUAPs)
B. Early recruitment of MUAPs
C. Slow nerve conduction velocity
D. Conduction block
E. Small polyphasic MUAPs

**The following options are for QUESTIONS 25 through 29.**
Match one disorder with each electron microscopic finding.
A. Dermatomyositis
B. Inclusion body myositis
C. Oculopharyngeal muscular dystrophy
D. Myoclonic epilepsy with ragged-red fibers
E. Nemaline myopathy

**Q25.**

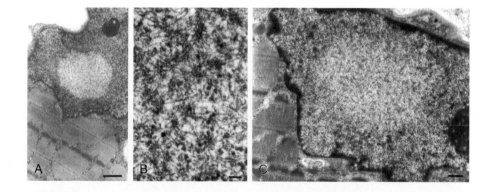

Scale bars in the left, middle, and right panels represent 1, 0.1, and 0.5 μm, respectively. From Uyama E, Nohira O, Chateau D, et al. *Neurology.* 1996;46(3): 773-778.

**Q26.**

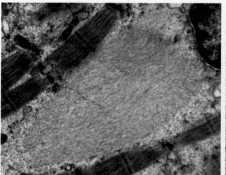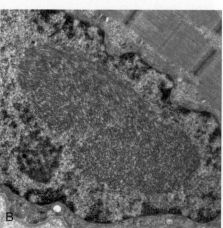

Scale bars in the left, and right panels represent 0.1 μm. From Amato AA, Russell J. *Neuromuscular Disease.* New York: McGraw-Hill; 2016;17:847.

**Q27.**

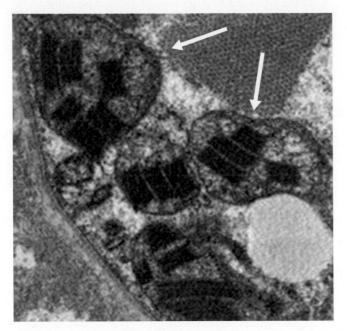

From Amati-Bonneau P, Valentino ML, Reynier P, Gallardo ME, Bornstein B, Boissière A, et al. *Brain*. 2007;131(2):345.

**Q28.**

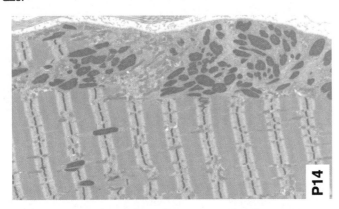

Adapted from Malfatti, E., Lehtokari, VL., Böhm, J. et al. *Acta Neuropathol Commun*. 2, 44 (2014). https://doi.org/10.1186/2051-5960-2-44.

**Q29.**

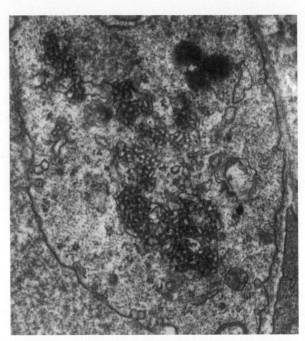

From Goebel HH, Trautmann F, Dippold W. *Pathol Res Pract*. 1985;180(1):1-9.

**The following options are for QUESTIONS 30 through 33.**
Match one histopathologic finding with each agent.
    A.  Type 2 fiber atrophy
    B.  Ragged-red fibers
    C.  Necrotizing myopathy
    D.  Vacuolar myopathy

**Q30.** Chloroquine
**Q31.** Simvastatin
**Q32.** Prednisone
**Q33.** Zidovudine

**Q34.** Which of the following histopathologic findings is a feature of critical illness myopathy?
    A.  Loss of thin filaments
    B.  Loss of thick filaments
    C.  Streaming of Z-discs
    D.  Tubulofilamentous inclusions
    E.  Paracrystalline inclusions

**Q.35.** A sural nerve biopsy is **MOST** suitable in which of the following situations:
A. An alcoholic patient with distal sensorimotor polyneuropathy
B. A diabetic patient with painful small fiber sensory neuropathy
C. A patient with pure motor multifocal mononeuropathies
D. A patient with severe subacute asymmetrical sensorimotor neuropathy
E. A patient with pes cavus and possible hereditary polyneuropathy

**Q.36.** A nerve biopsy performed in a 27-year-old woman demonstrates the finding in the following figure (hematoxylin and eosin staining). Which of the following is the most pathognomonic clinical presentation of this disorder?

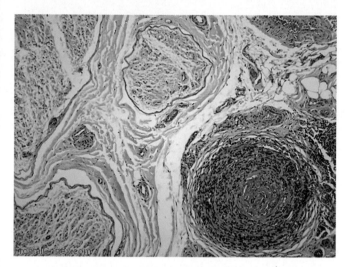

From frontalcortex.com

A. Bilateral facial diplegia
B. Mononeuropathy
C. Mononeuropathy multiplex
D. Distal symmetric polyneuropathy, length-dependent pattern
E. Distal symmetric polyneuropathy, non–length-dependent pattern

**Q.37.** The teased fiber preparation of the nerve biopsy in a 22-year-old woman with a demyelinating polyneuropathy reveals the finding in the following figure. Which of the following genetic abnormalities is expected to be seen in this patient?

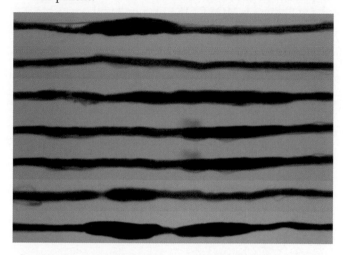

From Kim SM, Chung KW, Choi BO, et al. *Exp Mol Med.* 2004;36(1):28-35.

A. *GJB1* mutation
B. *MFN2* mutation
C. *MPZ* mutation
D. *PMP22* deletion
E. *PMP22* duplication

**Q.38.** A 6-year-old girl presents with weakness and numbness in all extremities, more prominent in both legs. A sural nerve biopsy is performed and the finding is shown in the following figure. Which of the following genetic abnormalities is **MOST LIKELY** to be seen in this patient?

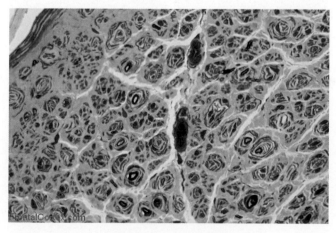

From www.frontalcortex.com

A. *MFN2* mutation
B. *PMP22* deletion
C. *PMP22* duplication
D. *SCN9A* mutation
E. Exon 7 deletion in the *SMN1* gene

**Q39.** A 70-year-old man presents for an evaluation of numbness in both hands and feet. A nerve biopsy is performed and demonstrates the findings shown in the following figure (Congo red staining in upper and left lower panels and polarized light in right lower panel). Which of the following findings is **MOST LIKELY** found in this patient?

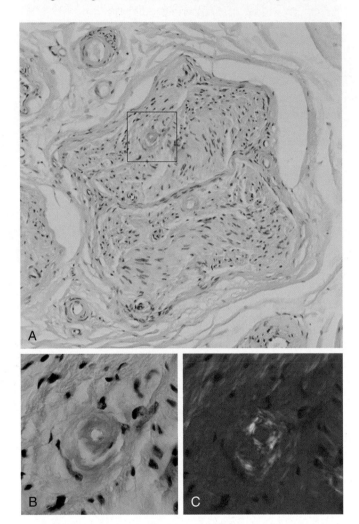

From Asiri MMH, Engelsman S, Eijkelkamp N, Höppener JWM. *Cells.* 2020;9(6):1553.

A. Angiokeratoma
B. Orange-colored tonsils
C. Hypertrophic cardiomyopathy
D. Leukodystrophy
E. Pes cavus

**Q40.** A nerve biopsy is performed in a patient as part of an evaluation of neuropathy and demonstrates the electron microscopic finding as in the following figure. Which of the following laboratory findings is most likely found in this patient?

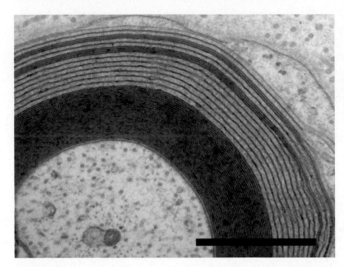

From Kawagashira Y, Koike H, Ohyama K, et al. *J Neurol Sci.* 2015;348(1-2):67-73.

A. Anti-GM1 antibody
B. IgM monoclonal gammopathy
C. Lambda (λ) free light chain
D. Positive antineutrophil cytoplasmic antibody
E. *PMP22* duplication

**Q41.** A 35-year-old woman presents with numbness and burning, which started in her feet and ascended into her hands. She has been in good health except for mild migratory arthralgias. Neurological examination is normal. Which of the following studies is **LEAST** likely to be useful in making a final diagnosis?
A. Needle electromyography
B. Sensory nerve conduction studies in legs
C. Skin biopsy to assess intraepidermal nerve fiber density
D. Lip biopsy to evaluate salivary glands
E. Quantitative sudomotor axon reflex test

- An excessively increased number of muscle fibers with internalized nuclei can be seen in centronuclear myopathy and myotonic dystrophies.
  - In myotonic dystrophy type 1, there are increased internalized nuclei in type 1 fibers.
  - In myotonic dystrophy type 2, there are increased internalized nuclei in type 2 fibers.

## MNEMONICS

In myotonic dystrophy **type 1**, there are increased internalized nuclei in **type 1** muscle fibers.
In myotonic dystrophy **type 2**, there are increased internalized nuclei in **type 2** muscle fibers.

- Each muscle fiber of a motor unit intermingles with fibers of other motor units.
  - This is best demonstrated on ATPase staining as a normal mosaic or "checkerboard" pattern.
- In normal muscle, only very little endomysial connective tissue can be seen around muscle fibers.

##  HIGH-YIELD FACT

Increased internalized nuclei (greater than 3% of all muscle fibers) is mainly seen in:
1. centronuclear myopathy
2. myotonic dystrophies

**QUESTION 4.** Which of the following disorders shows pathological findings on deltoid muscle biopsy that are different from the others?
A. Amyotrophic lateral sclerosis
B. C5 radiculopathy
C. Chronic inflammatory demyelinating polyneuropathy
D. Parsonage-Turner syndrome
E. Thyrotoxic proximal weakness

**ANSWER:** E. Thyrotoxic proximal weakness

## COMMENTS AND DISCUSSION

- Neurogenic findings on muscle biopsy are seen when the lesion is at the anterior horn cell (e.g., spinal muscular atrophy or amyotrophic lateral sclerosis), nerve root (e.g., C5 radiculopathy), plexus (e.g., Parsonage-Turner syndrome), or peripheral nerve (e.g., chronic inflammatory demyelinating polyneuropathy). In contrast, thyrotoxic proximal weakness shows myopathic findings, which is different from the other disorders.
- Neurogenic findings include (Fig. 10.1 and Table 10.1):
  - Group atrophy: large group atrophy or small group atrophy
  - Atrophic fibers
    - Both group atrophy and atrophic fibers are evidence of denervation.
  - Hypertrophic fibers
  - Muscle fiber splitting
  - Target or targetoid fibers
    - Evidence of denervation and reinnervation
    - Demonstrated well on NADH and SDH staining
    - Three concentric zones: the innermost zone, located in the central region of the muscle fibers, is devoid of NADH, SDH, and ATPase activity.
    - Target fibers can be distinguished from cores in central core myopathy.
    - In target fibers, there is a peripheral dark rim around the central clear region.
    - Target fibers occur in both type 1 and type 2 fibers, whereas cores mainly affect type 1 fibers.
    - The central clear region in the target fibers does not extend along the length of muscle fibers, whereas cores do.

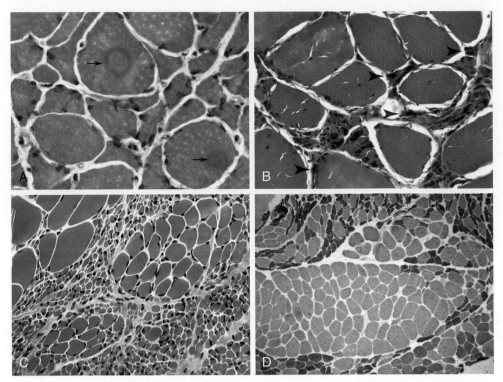

**Fig. 10.1** **Muscle biopsy findings in neurogenic diseases.** (A) Hematoxylin and eosin (H&E) staining demonstrates atrophic and angular fibers, as well as target fibers (*arrows*). (B) H&E staining demonstrates groups of atrophic muscle fibers. The remaining nuclei are clumped together, giving an appearance of "nuclear bags (*arrowheads*)." (C) H&E staining demonstrates large groups of muscle atrophy. (D) ATPase staining demonstrates fiber type grouping, and also atrophic fibers. Adapted from Miles JD, Cohen ML. Skeletal muscle and peripheral nerve disorders. In: Prayson RA, Goldblum JR, eds. *Neuropathology.* 2nd ed. Elsevier; 2012;11:562-563.

**TABLE 10.1**  Summary of neurogenic versus myopathic findings on muscle biopsy.

| Neurogenic findings | Myopathic findings |
| --- | --- |
| Small or large group atrophy | Variation of muscle fiber size |
| Fiber type grouping (seen on ATPase staining) | In case of muscular dystrophy and inflammatory myopathy |
| Angular fibers | • Necrotic fibers |
| Target or targetoid fibers | • Regenerating fibers |
| Hypertrophic fibers | • Increased endomysial collagen |
| Muscle fiber splitting | and fibrous tissue |

- ○ Fiber type grouping (Fig. 10.2)
  - • One of the most important neurogenic findings
  - • Best demonstrated on ATPase staining
  - • This is evidence of both denervation and reinnervation.
    - • Muscle fibers that are denervated receive reinnervation by axon sprouting from a nearby motor neuron.
    - • Thus these denervated muscles will change their fiber type to the one of the new motor unit.
    - • The new motor unit that is controlled by the survived motor neuron will become a larger motor unit in which muscle fibers of the same fiber type are adjacent to each other.
    - • This gives a feature of fiber type grouping.
  - • This finding correlates with large motor unit action potentials (MUAPs) on needle electromyographic studies.

## ◎ HIGH-YIELD FACT

Fiber type grouping indicates reinnervation (which occurs after denervation) of the neurogenic process. This correlates with large MUAPs on needle EMG.

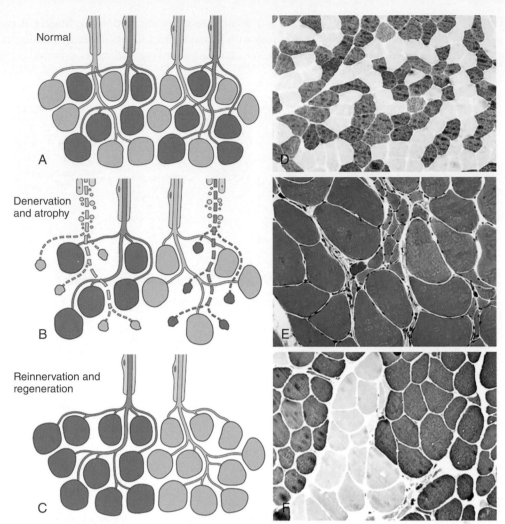

**Fig. 10.2 Denervation and reinnervation in the neurogenic process results in fiber type grouping.** (A, D) In normal muscle, type 1 and type 2 muscle fibers are interspersed with each other, giving a checkerboard appearance on ATPase staining (D). Of note, muscle fibers from the same motor units have the same fiber type. (B, E) In this example, two of four motor units are affected, resulting in denervation of the muscle fibers. Denervation leads to atrophy of muscle fibers with an angular shape (E). (C, F) Following denervation, reinnervation occurs from nearby motor neurons. Reinnervated muscle fibers adopt the fiber type of the rescuing motor units (i.e., reinnervated muscle fibers will become the same type as the new motor units), resulting in fiber type grouping, which is demonstrated on ATPase staining (F). From Pytel P, Anthony DC. Peripheral nerves and skeletal muscles. In: Kumar V, Abbas AK, Aster JC, eds. *Robbins & Cotran Pathologic Basis of Disease*. 10th ed. Elsevier; 2021:27;1227.

**QUESTION 5.** An 11-month-old infant presents with muscle weakness and hypotonia. Muscle biopsy reveals the finding as in the following figures (top with hematoxylin and eosin (H&E) staining and bottom with adenosine triphosphatase pH 4.3). Which of the following findings is expected on the electrodiagnostic study in this patient?

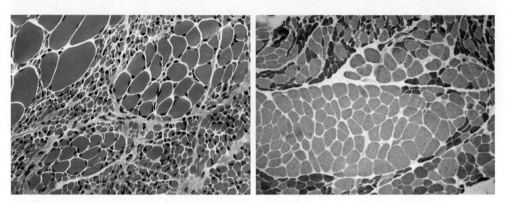

Adapted from Miles JD, Cohen ML. Skeletal muscle and peripheral nerve disorders. In: Prayson RA, Goldblum JR, eds. *Neuropathology.* 2nd ed. Elsevier; 2012;11:563.

A. Myotonic discharges
B. Neuromyotonic discharges
C. Reduced recruitment
D. Small polyphasic motor unit action potentials
E. Double compound muscle action potentials following a single stimulus

**ANSWER:** C. Reduced recruitment

**COMMENTS AND DISCUSSION**
- The left panel is a hematoxylin and eosin (H&E) stain demonstrating large group atrophy. The right panel is an ATPase stain showing fiber type grouping. Loss of the normal mosaic or checkerboard pattern is evident, and muscle fibers of the same type, which are normally interspersed, become adjacent to each other. These findings are indicative of neurogenic diseases in which the lesion can be at the anterior horn cell, the nerve root, the plexus, or the peripheral nerve, but not at the muscle itself.
- Small and large group atrophy indicates denervation, and fiber type grouping reflects reinnervation from the remaining nearby motor neurons.
- Of all choices, reduced recruitment is the electrodiagnostic finding seen in neurogenic diseases. In addition, large, long-duration motor unit action potentials (MUAPs) can be seen, indicating larger motor units after reinnervation, and correlating with fiber type grouping.
- Small polyphasic MUAPs are myopathic findings, not neurogenic. Double or repetitive compound muscle action potentials (CMAPs) following a single stimulus can be seen in some congenital myasthenic syndromes such as slow channel syndrome and acetylcholine esterase deficiency (due to *COLQ* mutations). Myotonic discharges and neuromyotonia are not expected in neurogenic diseases.

**QUESTION 6.** A 23-year-old woman presents with muscle weakness. Muscle biopsy reveals the finding as shown in the following figure (modified Gomori trichrome stain). What is the most likely diagnosis?

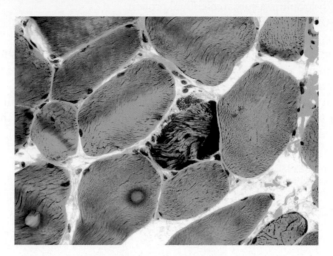

Courtesy Mark Cohen, MD.

A. Emery-Dreifuss muscular dystrophy
B. Mitochondrial encephalomyopathy, lactic acidosis, and stroke-like episodes
C. Myofibrillar myopathy
D. Nemaline myopathy
E. Pompe disease

**ANSWER:** B. Mitochondrial encephalomyopathy, lactic acidosis, and stroke-like episodes

**COMMENTS AND DISCUSSION**

- This muscle biopsy shows a ragged-red fiber on modified Gomori trichrome (mGT) stain. with subsarcolemmal accumulation of red material indicating abnormal mitochondria. Ragged-red fibers are a hallmark of mitochondrial myopathies caused by mutations in the mitochondrial or nuclear genome, including mitochondrial encephalomyopathy, lactic acidosis, and stroke-like episodes (MELAS), myoclonic epilepsy with ragged-red fibers (MERRF), Kearns-Sayre syndrome, mitochondrial neurogastrointestinal encephalomyopathy (MNGIE), and many others.
- A general feature that is common to all myopathies is *variation of muscle fiber size.*
- Muscle findings specific to *muscular dystrophies*
  ○ Dystrophic pattern: necrosis and regeneration (Fig. 10.3)
  ○ Necrotic muscle fibers
    • Breakdown of normal muscle fibers
    • Macrophages can be seen around necrotic fibers; these help in clearance of necrotic fibers.
    • After necrosis, pyknotic nuclear clumps, which are an aggregation of remaining nuclei, can be seen.
  ○ Regenerating fibers
    • Small bluish fibers on H&E stain
    • These fibers can be highlighted on alkaline phosphatase stain.

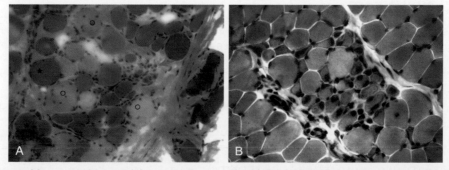

**Fig. 10.3 Dystrophic muscle biopsy.** (A) Hematoxylin and eosin (H&E) stain demonstrates pale necrotic muscle fibers *(open circles)*, hypercontracted fibers *(*)* that have a rounded shape (instead of polygonal shape) and appear darker than normal, and basophilic fibers *(green arrow)*. (B) Regenerating fibers are seen as small bluish fibers on H&E stain. From Dubowitz V, Sewry CA, Oldfors A. *Muscle Biopsy.* 5th ed. Elsevier; 2021:10;216, 219.

- ○ Special immunohistochemical staining can be useful for demonstrating deficient proteins.
  - • Dystrophin staining (Fig. 10.4)
    - • Reacts to dystrophin, a subsarcolemmal protein.
    - • Staining is absent or reduced in dystrophinopathies.
      - • Staining is typically absent in Duchenne muscular dystrophy.
      - • Staining is typically reduced or uneven in Becker muscular dystrophy.
    - • Three stainings: antibodies to N (amino)-terminal domain, rod domain, and C (carboxy)-terminal domain
    - • C-terminal antibody staining has highest sensitivity, since the C-terminal domain is translated after N-terminal and rod domains during mRNA translation. If the dystrophin protein is truncated, C-terminal is most likely to be absent.

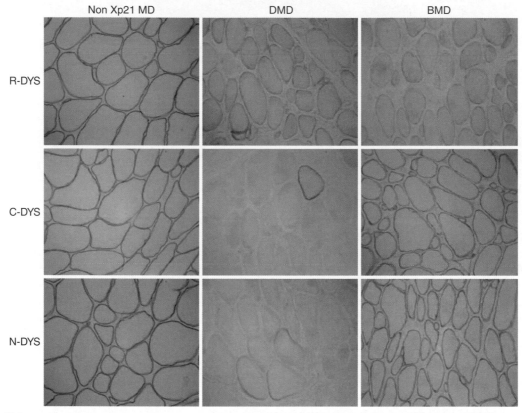

**Fig. 10.4 Dystrophin immunostaining.** The *left column* displays muscle biopsy from a case with non-dystrophinopathy muscular dystrophy used as a control, with normal immunostaining of the C-terminal *(C-DYS)*, rod domain *(R-DYS)*, and N-terminal *(N-DYS)*. The middle column displays the muscle biopsy in Duchenne muscular dystrophy *(DMD)* with absent C-DYS and N-DYS immunostaining, and markedly reduced. R-DYS staining compared to control. One revertant fiber, with paradoxically intense staining, is also demonstrated on the C-DYS staining. The *right column* displays the muscle biopsy in Becker muscular dystrophy *(BMD)*, with reduced R-DYS staining, but preserved C-DYS and N-DYS staining. From Vogel H, Zamecnik J. Diagnostic immunohistology of muscle diseases. *J Neuropathol Exp Neurol.* 2005;64(3):181-193.

### ◎ HIGH-YIELD FACT

Immunostaining of the C-terminal of the dystrophin protein has the highest sensitivity to detect reduced or absent staining. This is because the C-terminal domain is translated after the N-terminal and rod domains, and is most likely affected by the premature stop codon.

- • In some limb-girdle muscular dystrophies (LGMDs), special immunohistochemical stains of the deficient protein are available.
  - • Examples include γ-sarcoglycan (absent in LGMD2C), α-sarcoglycan (absent in LGMD2D), β-sarcoglycan (absent in LGMD2E), and δ-sarcoglycan (absent in LGMD2F).
- • Emery-Dreifuss muscular dystrophy (EDMD)
  - • X-linked recessive form due to *EMD* mutations encoding emerin protein
    - • Emerin is a nuclear protein.

- There is absent nuclear immunostaining of emerin in X-linked EDMD.
- There are also mutations in other proteins, including lamin A/C (located at the inner nuclear membrane and associated with autosomal dominant ADMD) and Nesprin-1 (located at the nuclear envelope, mainly associated with the autosomal dominant form of the disease).
- Muscle findings specific to *congenital myopathies*
  - Nemaline myopathy
    - Presence of nemaline rods, which are best demonstrated on modified Gomori trichrome (mGT) stain
    - On electron microscopy (EM), streaming of Z-discs is seen.
  - Central core myopathy (Fig. 10.5)
    - Core is seen as devoid of staining, best demonstrated on nicotinamide adenine dinucleotide-tetrazolium reductase (NADH-TR) stain
  - Centronuclear myopathy (aka myotubular myopathy) (Fig. 10.5)
    - Marked increase in internalized (central) nuclei
    - Centronuclear myopathy due to mutations of the *DNM2* gene encoding for dynamin can show radial stranding of the intermyofibrillary network, resulting in a spoke-like appearance.
  - Congenital fiber type disproportion (CFTD) (Fig. 10.5)
    - Type 1 muscle fibers are disproportionately smaller than type 2 fibers.

## ◎ HIGH-YIELD FACT

Nemaline rods are best visualized on modified Gomori trichrome (mGT) stain.
Central cores are best visualized on NADH-TR stain.

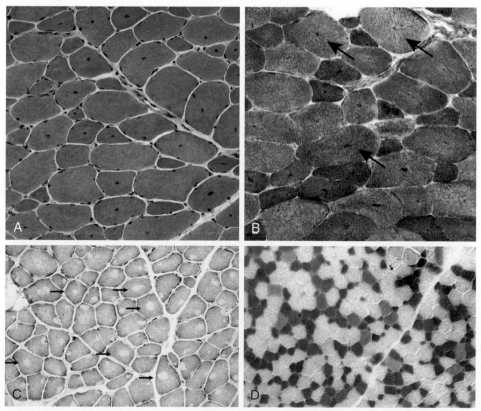

**Fig. 10.5 Muscle biopsy from various congenital myopathies.** (A, B) Centronuclear myopathy. Parts A and B are muscle biopsy from the same patient. Hematoxylin and eosin (H&E) stain (A) demonstrates variation of muscle fiber size and an increased number of muscle fibers with internalized nuclei. NADH-TR stain (B) demonstrates a radial spoke around the internalized nuclei (*large arrow*). This feature is seen in centronuclear myopathy due to *DNM2* mutations. (C) Central core disease. NADH-TR stain demonstrates an area devoid of staining at the center of most muscle fibers (*small arrows*). (D) Congenital fiber type disproportion. ATPase staining at pH 4.3 demonstrates small type 1 muscle fibers, which are darkly stained. Note that the image for nemaline myopathy is in Fig. 10.14, and not included in this figure. (A) and (B) From Dubowitz V, Sewry CA, Oldfors A. *Muscle Biopsy*. 5th ed. Elsevier; 2021:337. (C) From frontalcortex.com (D) From Angelini C. Congenital fiber-type disproportion. In: *Genetic Neuromuscular Disorders*. Springer; 2014:146.

**HIGH-YIELD FACT**

Type 1 fibers are smaller than type 2 fibers in congenital fiber type disproportion.
Type 2 fiber atrophy is seen in steroid myopathy and disuse atrophy.

 **HIGH-YIELD FACT**

Type 2 fiber atrophy (such as in steroid myopathy, disuse atrophy) is not detected on needle EMG. Type 1 fibers, but not type 2, are recruited mainly during voluntary activity assessment of needle EMG.

- Muscle findings specific to *mitochondrial myopathies*
  - Ragged-red fibers on mGT stain
  - Cytochrome oxidase (COX)–negative fibers on COX stain
  - Succinic dehydrogenase (SDH)–reactive COX-negative (deficient) fibers indicate mitochondrial myopathy due to mutations in the mitochondrial genome.
  - Strong SDH-reactive blood vessels (SSVs) can be seen in some mitochondrial myopathy such as mitochondrial encephalopathy, lactic acidosis, and stroke-like episodes (MELAS).
  - Electron microscopy (EM) reveals paracrystalline inclusions (often described as "parking lot" pattern) in ragged-red fibers

 **HIGH-YIELD FACT**

Key muscle biopsy findings in mitochondrial myopathies include ragged-red fibers (on mGT stain) and COX-negative fibers.
Ragged-red fibers are seen as paracrystalline inclusions on electron microscopy.

- Muscle findings specific to *metabolic myopathies*
  - Glycogen storage myopathy
    - General features
      - Vacuoles are seen in muscle fibers on H&E stain.
      - These vacuoles stain positive for periodic acid–Schiff (PAS), since they contain glycogen.
    - Pompe disease (acid maltase or alpha-1,4 glucosidase deficiency or glycogen storage disease [GSD] type II)
      - Acid phosphatase staining, which indicates lysosomal accumulation, can also be positive
    - McArdle disease (myophosphorylase deficiency or GSD V)
      - Absent myophosphorylase immunostaining
    - Tarui disease (phosphofructokinase deficiency or GSD VII)
      - Absent phosphofructokinase immunostaining
- Muscle findings specific to *inflammatory myopathies* (Fig. 10.6 and Table 10.2)
  - Polymyositis (PM)
    - Lymphocytic infiltration in endomysium. These lymphocytes surround but do not invade muscle fibers.
    - These lymphocytes are mainly CD8+ T cells.
    - Increased major histocompatibility complex (MHC) class I expression on muscle fiber membrane (sarcolemmal membrane)

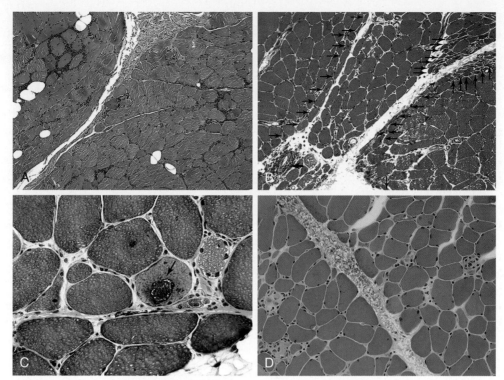

**Fig. 10.6 Muscle biopsy in inflammatory myopathies.** (A) Polymyositis. Hematoxylin and eosin (H&E) stain demonstrates marked variation of muscle fiber size, endomysial lymphocytic infiltration, and lymphocytic invasion of non-necrotic muscle fibers. There is also endomysial fibrosis. (B) **Dermatomyositis.** H&E stain demonstrates the characteristic feature of perifascicular atrophy (*arrows*) in which muscle fibers at the periphery of the fascicles are small. There is also evidence of vasculitis of the blood vessel in perimysium, seen as intramural lymphocytic infiltration of the blood vessel wall. This perimysial vasculitis results in muscle fiber necrosis at the periphery of the muscle fascicles. (C) *Inclusion body myositis.* Modified Gomori trichrome (mGT) stain demonstrates rimmed vacuoles *(arrow)* containing inclusions within muscle fibers. Note that these vacuoles contain amyloid, phosphorylated tau, and TDP-43, which can be demonstrated on additional immunostaining *(not shown)*. (D) Immune-mediated necrotizing myopathy. There is variation of muscle fiber size and necrotic muscle fibers without evidence of lymphocytic infiltration. However, there are macrophages present at the necrotic fibers, which have a role in scavenging these fibers. (A and C) courtesy Mark Cohen, MD. (B) from Miles JD, Cohen ML. Skeletal muscle and peripheral nerve disorders. In: Prayson RA, Goldblum JR, eds. *Neuropathology.* 2nd ed. Elsevier; 2012;11:593. (D) from Dubowitz V, Sewry CA, Oldfors A. *Muscle Biopsy.* 5th ed. Elsevier; 2021:496.

**TABLE 10.2** Summary of key muscle biopsy findings in inflammatory myopathies.

| Subtype of inflammatory myopathies | Key muscle biopsy findings |
| --- | --- |
| Polymyositis | Endomysial lymphocytic infiltration |
| | Mainly CD8+ lymphocytes |
| | Increased MHC class I expression |
| Dermatomyositis | Perifascicular atrophy |
| | Lymphocytic infiltration (mainly CD4+) in perimysium or perimysial vessel wall |
| | EM: tubuloreticular inclusions in capillary endothelium |
| Inclusion body myositis | Rimmed vacuoles |
| | Amyloid deposition (Congo red stain) |
| | Increased accumulation of p62, SMI-31 (tau), and TDP-43 |
| | EM: 15-18 nm filamentous inclusion in muscle |
| Necrotizing autoimmune myopathy | Muscle fiber necrosis without lymphocytic infiltration |

*EM,* electron microscopy.

- Dermatomyositis (DM)
  - Key feature is perifascicular atrophy, which refers to atrophy of muscle fibers at the rim of muscle fascicles.
  - Lymphocytic infiltration at perimysium and perimysial vessels
  - These lymphocytes are mainly CD4+ T cells.
  - Increased MHC class I expression on muscle fiber membrane
  - Expression of myxovirus-resistance protein A (MxA) in sarcoplasm
  - EM shows tubuloreticular inclusions within capillary endothelial cells.
- Inclusion body myositis (IBM)
  - Presence of rimmed vacuoles on H&E stain
  - These vacuoles contain amyloid, which can be demonstrated on Congo red, crystal violet, or thioflavin T/S staining
    - On Congo red stain, amyloid shows apple green birefringence under polarized light.
  - Accumulation of abnormal proteins including p62 (sequestosome-1, an autophagosome cargo protein involved in autophagy), SMI-31 (paired helical filament [PHF]-tau), or TDP-43
  - EM shows accumulation of 15-18 nm filamentous inclusions in muscle fibers
- Necrotizing autoimmune myopathy (NAM) (aka immune-mediated necrotizing myopathy [IMNM])
  - Presence of necrotic muscle fibers with no or minimal evidence of lymphocytic infiltration
  - Macrophage infiltration can be seen, which has a role in clearing necrotic muscle tissue.

## ◎ HIGH-YIELD FACT

> In immune-mediated necrotizing myopathy, there is no or minimal evidence of (lymphocytic) inflammation, but macrophages that scavenge the necrotic fibers can be seen.

- Muscle findings specific to *toxic myopathies*
  - Zidovudine (AZT) myopathy
    - Ragged-red fibers can be seen, since zidovudine is toxic to mitochondria
  - Drug-induced myopathy with presence of autophagic vacuoles within muscle fibers (Fig. 10.7)
    - Chloroquine
    - Colchicine
      - Of note, colchicine can also affect both nerves and muscles, called "neuromyopathy"

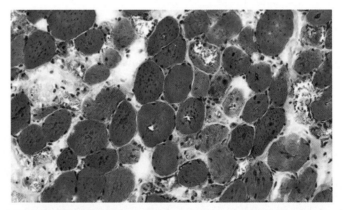

**Fig. 10.7 Hydroxychloroquine-induced myopathy.** This muscle biopsy demonstrates marked variation of muscle fiber size and the presence of vacuoles within muscle fibers. These vacuoles contain autophagic material and can be positively stained for acid phosphatase *(not shown)*. From Shukla S, Gultekin SH, Saporta M. Pearls & Oysters: Hydroxychloroquine-induced toxic myopathy mimics Pompe disease: Critical role of genetic test. *Neurology.* 2019;92(7):e742-e745.

**QUESTION 7.** A 25-year-old woman presents with muscle weakness. Muscle biopsy is performed and sent for electron microscopy which shows the findings in the following figure. What is the most likely diagnosis in this patient?

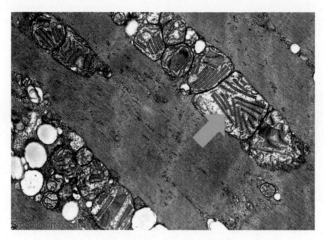

From frontalcortex.com

A. Dermatomyositis
B. Inclusion body myositis
C. Myoclonic epilepsy with ragged-red fibers
D. Nemaline myopathy
E. Oculopharyngeal muscular dystrophy

**ANSWER:** C. Myoclonic epilepsy with ragged-red fibers

**COMMENTS AND DISCUSSION (see also comments and discussion from Question 6)**

- On electron microscopy, this muscle demonstrates paracrystalline inclusions arranged in a "parking lot" pattern. These inclusions represent abnormal accumulation of mitochondria in the subsarcolemmal region. This finding is found in mitochondrial myopathy and correlates with ragged-red fibers on modified Gomori trichrome stain. Among the choices, myoclonic epilepsy with ragged-red fibers (MERRF) is the only mitochondrial myopathy.
- Below are important electron microscopic findings in various myopathies:
  - Nemaline rods in nemaline myopathy
    - Streaming of Z-discs
  - Mitochondrial myopathy
    - Paracrystalline inclusions arranged in a "parking lot" pattern can be demonstrated in ragged-red fibers.
  - Critical illness myopathy (Fig. 10.8)
    - Loss of thick filaments (myosin)

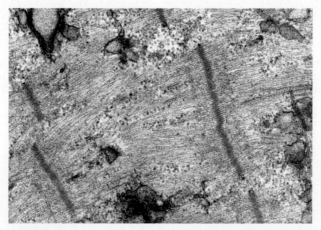

**Fig. 10.8 Critical illness myopathy.** Electron microscopic examination of the longitudinal section of this muscle biopsy demonstrates marked loss of thick filaments (myosin) with preserved thin filaments. Courtesy Mark Cohen, MD.

- Oculopharyngeal muscular dystrophy (OPMD) (Fig. 10.9)
  - Intranuclear tubulofilamentous inclusions, 8.5 nm in external diameter
- Inclusion body myositis (Fig. 10.10)
  - Intranuclear and intracytoplasmic tubulofilamentous inclusions, 15–18 nm in diameter
- Dermatomyositis (Fig. 10.11)
  - Tubuloreticular inclusions within endothelial cells

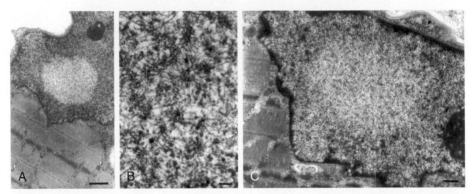

**Fig. 10.9 Electron microscopic findings in oculopharyngeal muscular dystrophy (OPMD).** Left, middle, and right panels represent low, middle, and high magnification, respectively. This figure demonstrates intranuclear tubulofilamentous inclusions, measuring 8.5 nm in external diameter. Scale bars in the left, middle, and right panels represent 1, 0.5, and 0.1 μm, respectively. From Uyama E, Nohira O, Chateau D, et al. Oculopharyngeal muscular dystrophy in two unrelated Japanese families. *Neurology.* 1996;46(3):773-778.

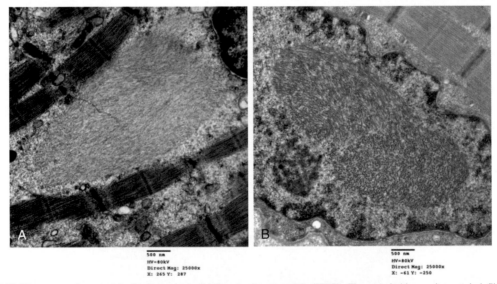

**Fig. 10.10 Electron microscopic findings in inclusion body myositis (IBM).** The muscle biopsy shows tubulofilamentous inclusions in both intranuclear and intracytoplasmic locations. The diameters of these inclusions are 15–18 nm, larger than those seen in oculopharyngeal muscular dystrophy (OPMD). From Amato AA, Russell J. *Neuromuscular Disease.* New York: McGraw-Hill; 2016:847.

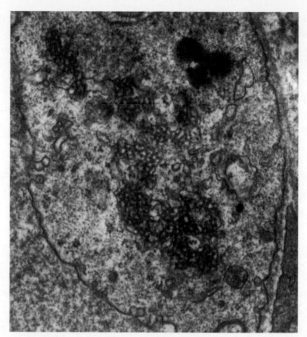

**Fig. 10.11 Electron microscopic findings in dermatomyositis (DM).** The muscle biopsy shows tubuloreticular inclusions in the endothelial cell. From frontalcortex.com

 **HIGH-YIELD FACT**

Tubulofilmentous inclusions in:
- Oculopharyngeal muscular dystrophy: intranuclear, 8.5 nm in diameter
- Inclusion body myositis: intranuclear and intracytoplasmic, 15–18 nm in diameter

**QUESTION 8.** Which of the following pathological findings is expected in zidovudine (AZT)–induced myopathy?
  A. Intranuclear tubulofilamentous inclusions
  B. Nemaline rods
  C. Perifascicular atrophy
  D. Ragged-red fibers
  E. Rimmed vacuoles

**ANSWER:** D. Ragged-red fibers

**COMMENTS AND DISCUSSION (see comments and discussion from Question 6)**
- In zidovudine (AZT)–induced myopathy, there is an abnormal accumulation of mitochondria. Thus ragged-red fibers can be seen, as in other mitochondrial myopathies. Multiple mechanisms including impairment of respiratory chain and mitochondrial DNA depletion due to inhibition of mitochondrial polymerase-γ have been proposed.

 **HIGH-YIELD FACT**

Zidovudine is toxic to MITOCHONDRIA. Thus ragged-red fibers are seen, as in mitochondrial myopathy.

- Intranuclear tubulofilamentous inclusions can be seen in inclusion body myositis (IBM) and oculopharyngeal muscular dystrophy (OPMD) (Fig. 10.9 and 10.10).
  - However, the sizes are different: diameters of 15–18 nm in IBM and 8.5 nm in OPMD.
  - In OPMD, the inclusions can be intranuclear or intracytoplasmic, whereas in IBM, the inclusions are intranuclear.
- Nemaline rods are typically found in nemaline myopathy (Fig. 10.14).
- Perifascicular atrophy is a classic finding in dermatomyositis (Fig. 10.6).
- Rimmed vacuoles can be seen in distal myopathy with rimmed vacuoles (aka Nonaka myopathy), OPMD, and IBM.

**QUESTION 9.** A 15-year-old girl presents with proximal muscle weakness. Muscle biopsy is performed and reveals the finding in the following figure (modified Gomori trichrome stain). The mutation in which of the following genes is most likely to be found?

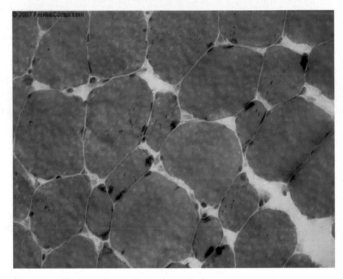

From frontalcortex.com

A. *ACTA1*
B. *FHL1*
C. *MTM1*
D. *POLG*
E. *RYR1*

**ANSWER:** A. *ACTA1*

**COMMENTS AND DISCUSSION**
- The figure demonstrates nemaline bodies, seen as dark purplish inclusions at the periphery of muscle fibers on modified Gomori trichrome stain. Nemaline bodies are typically seen in nemaline myopathy. The genes responsible for Nemaline myopathy include *ACTA1, TPM2, TPM3, TNNT1, CFL2, KBTBD13, KLHL40, KLHL41*, among others.
- Mutations in the *FHL1* gene are found in reducing body myopathy and Emery-Dreifuss muscular dystrophy.
- Mutations in the *MTM1* gene are found in an X-linked form of centronuclear (aka myotubular) myopathy.
- Mutations in the nuclear *POLG* gene are responsible for mitochondrial disorders with the phenotypes of chronic progressive ophthalmoplegia (CPEO) or Kearns-Sayre syndrome (KSS).
- Mutations in the *RYR1* gene are mainly responsible for central core myopathy.

**QUESTION 10.** A 13-year-old boy presents with proximal muscle weakness. Electron microscopic examination of a muscle biopsy demonstrates the finding in the following figure. The muscle disease in this patient is classified as a:

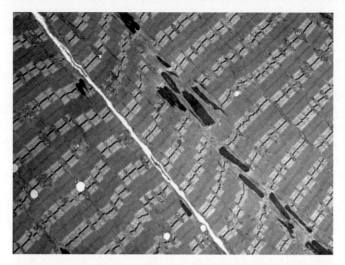

From Dowling JJ, North KN, Goebel HH, et al. Congenital and other structural myopathies. In: Darras BT, Jones HR, Ryan MM, et al., eds. *Neuromuscular Disorders of Infancy, Childhood, and Adolescence.* 2nd ed. Elsevier; 2015;28:509.

    A. congenital myopathy.
    B. metabolic myopathy.
    C. mitochondrial myopathy.
    D. muscular dystrophy.
    E. toxic myopathy.

**ANSWER:** A. congenital myopathy.

**COMMENTS AND DISCUSSION**

- The electron microscopic examination in this figure demonstrates streaming of nemaline rods as thread-like structures ("nema" is derived from Greek—meaning rods). These nemaline rods have the same density as the Z-discs, from which they are derived.
- Nemaline rods are typically seen in nemaline myopathy, which is a form of congenital myopathy. On modified Gomori trichrome stain, nemaline rods are demonstrated as dark purplish structures at the periphery of muscle fibers (Fig. 10.14).

 **HIGH-YIELD FACT**

Nemaline rods are seen as streaming of Z-discs on electron microscopic examination.

**QUESTION 11.** Which of the following statements is **CORRECT** regarding rimmed vacuoles?
    A. Rimmed vacuoles are a specific finding for inclusion body myositis (IBM), distal myopathy with rimmed vacuoles (DMRVs), and oculopharyngeal muscular dystrophy (OPMD).
    B. Rimmed vacuoles cannot be seen on hematoxylin and eosin staining but can be seen on modified Gomori trichrome staining.
    C. Rimmed vacuoles stain positive for periodic acid–Schiff (PAS).
    D. Rimmed vacuoles in OPMD contain amyloid.
    E. Rimmed vacuoles in IBM contain autophagic materials.

**ANSWER:** E. Rimmed vacuoles in IBM contain autophagic materials.

**COMMENTS AND DISCUSSION**

- Rimmed vacuoles are seen as areas devoid of staining material on H&E and modified Gomori trichrome (mGT) stains. These vacuoles are surrounded by a rim that is basophilic on H&E stain and dark purple on mGT stain (Fig. 10.15).

- Rimmed vacuoles can be seen in inclusion body myositis (IBM), distal myopathy with rimmed vacuoles (aka Nonaka myopathy, quadriceps sparing myopathy or GNE myopathy), and oculopharyngeal muscular dystrophy (OPMD).
- However, rimmed vacuoles are not specific to these three disorders, and have also been described in several other muscle diseases such as four-and-a-half-LIM domain 1 (FHL1)-related Emery-Dreifuss muscular dystrophy, titin distal myopathy, facioscapulohumeral dystrophy, and telethoninopathy, among others.
- Rimmed vacuoles typically contain autophagic materials such as p62/SQSTM1 (sequestosome 1).
- In IBM, rimmed vacuoles also contain abnormal protein such as amyloid, TAR DNA-binding protein (TDP-43), or phosphorylated neurofilament/tau (stained with SMI-31). This amyloid deposition can be seen on Congo red stain and has apple green birefringence under polarized light. Thus IBM is also recognized as "Alzheimer's disease of the muscle."
- PAS stains glycogen or polysaccharides within vacuoles, as seen in glycogen storage myopathies such as Pompe disease. It is important to note that these vacuoles are different from rimmed vacuoles, as there is no rim seen on H&E or mGT staining.

**QUESTION 12.** A 65-year-old man presents with muscle weakness. Muscle biopsy with Congo red staining under polarized light shows the following finding. What is the most likely diagnosis?

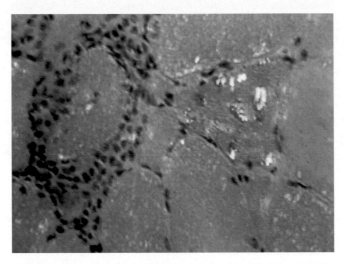

From Doughty CT, Amato AA. Disorders of skeletal muscle. In: Jankovic J, Maziotta JC, Pomeroy SL, Newman NJ, eds. *Bradley and Daroff's Neurology in Clinical Practice.* 8th ed. Elsevier; 2022:109;2018.

    A. Polymyositis
    B. Dermatomyositis
    C. Inclusion body myositis
    D. Necrotizing myopathy
    E. Overlap myositis syndrome

**ANSWER:** C. Inclusion body myositis

**COMMENTS AND DISCUSSION**
- This muscle biopsy shows apple green birefringence under polarized light on Congo red staining. This is due to amyloid deposition within the muscle fiber, typically within the rimmed vacuoles. This finding is seen in inclusion body myositis. In addition, there is evidence of endomysial lymphocytic infiltration in this biopsy specimen.
- In polymyositis, dermatomyositis, and immune-mediated necrotizing myopathy, there is no amyloid deposition.
- In overlap syndromes, the clinical manifestations are mixed between connective tissue disorders (such as systemic lupus erythematosus, rheumatoid arthritis, and mixed connective tissue disease) and inflammatory myopathy. Muscle pathology in overlap syndromes usually shows findings similar to dermatomyositis or polymyositis. However, there is no amyloid deposition in overlap syndrome.

**QUESTION 13.**   A 67-year-old man presents with weakness of bilateral finger flexors and quadriceps. The muscle biopsy demonstrates the finding in the following figure (modified Gomori trichrome stain). Which of the following pathological findings is **NOT** expected to be seen on the muscle biopsy of this patient?

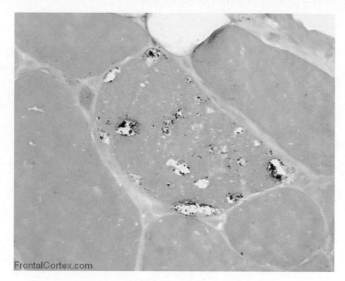

From frontalcortex.com

A. Amyloid deposition
B. TAR DNA-binding protein (TDP-43) accumulation
C. Positive SMI-31 staining
D. Cytochrome oxidase (COX)–deficient fibers
E. Strong succinic dehydrogenase (SDH)–positive vessels

**ANSWER:** E. Strong succinic dehydrogenase (SDH)–positive vessels

**COMMENTS AND DISCUSSION**

- This muscle biopsy demonstrates multiple rimmed vacuoles within the muscle fiber at the center of the figure on modified Gomori trichrome (mGT) staining. These vacuoles have dark purple rims on mGT staining. Along with the clinical features, this muscle biopsy supports the diagnosis of inclusion body myositis (IBM).

- In IBM, there is an accumulation of several proteins including amyloid (which can be demonstrated on Congo red staining with apple green birefringence under polarized light), tau (which can be demonstrated on immunostaining with antibodies to SMI-31), and TDP-43 (which can be demonstrated on immunostaining with antibodies to TDP-43). There may also be positive staining of antibodies to p62/sequestosome-1 (SQSTM), an autophagosome cargo protein involved in the autophagic process. In addition, cytochrome oxidase (COX)–negative fibers can be seen in IBM, demonstrating the evidence of mitochondrial dysfunction in IBM.

- Strong succinic dehydrogenase (SDH)–positive vessels (SSVs) can be seen in some mitochondrial myopathies such as mitochondrial encephalomyopathy, lactic acidosis, and stroke-like episodes (MELAS), but this finding is not seen in IBM.

**QUESTION 14.** An 11-month-old male infant presents with generalized hypotonia and develops respiratory failure requiring intubation. Muscle biopsy reveals findings as in the figure below. The left panel is hematoxylin and eosin staining and the right panel is periodic acid–Schiff staining. Which of the following stains would be most useful for the diagnosis?

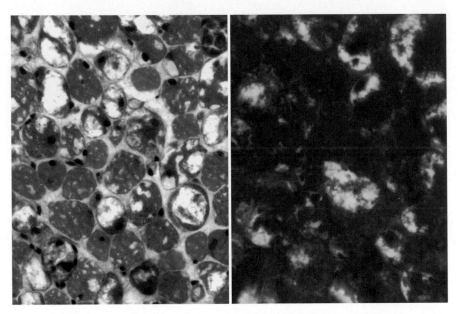

From Dubowitz V, Sewry CA, Oldfors A. *Muscle Biopsy.* 5th ed. Elsevier; 2021:17;391.

A. Acid phosphatase
B. Alkaline phosphatase
C. ATPase
D. Modified Gomori trichrome
E. NADH-TR

**ANSWER:** A. Acid phosphatase

**COMMENTS AND DISCUSSION**

- This muscle biopsy reveals numerous large vacuoles in the muscle fibers on hematoxylin and eosin (H&E) staining. Periodic acid–Schiff (PAS) staining reveals a lot of intense pink material within these muscle fibers, which is glycogen. From the clinical presentation of infantile-onset hypotonia and respiratory failure, Pompe disease is suspected. Pompe disease is caused by a deficiency of the acid maltase or α-1,4-glucosidase enzyme, which helps in the breakdown of glycogen within the lysosomes. Pompe disease is not only a glycogen storage disease (glycogen storage disease type II) but also a lysosomal storage disease. Due to lysosomal accumulation within muscle fibers, there is strong positivity of acid phosphatase (a lysosomal enzyme) staining within muscle fibers. Thus acid phosphatase staining is very helpful in the diagnosis of Pompe disease.
- Modified Gomori trichrome and nicotinamide adenine dinucleotide-tetrazolium reductase (NADH-TR) staining do not provide further information for the diagnosis of Pompe disease.

## ◎ HIGH-YIELD FACT

Pompe disease is both a glycogen storage and a lysosomal storage disease.
Abnormal glycogen accumulation is demonstrated on periodic acid–Schiff (PAS) staining.
Abnormal lysosomal accumulation is demonstrated on acid (not alkaline) phosphatase staining.

- Staining battery of frozen muscle tissue includes the following (Fig. 10.12):
  ○ Hematoxylin and eosin (H&E)
    - For general inspection of muscle architecture
    - It is important to examine H&E before examining other stains.
    - H&E staining is used to examine muscle fiber size including variation of muscle fiber size, endomysial and perimysial connective tissue, and vacuoles. Sometimes abnormal accumulation can be seen faintly on H&E, and this prompts further examination with other stains.

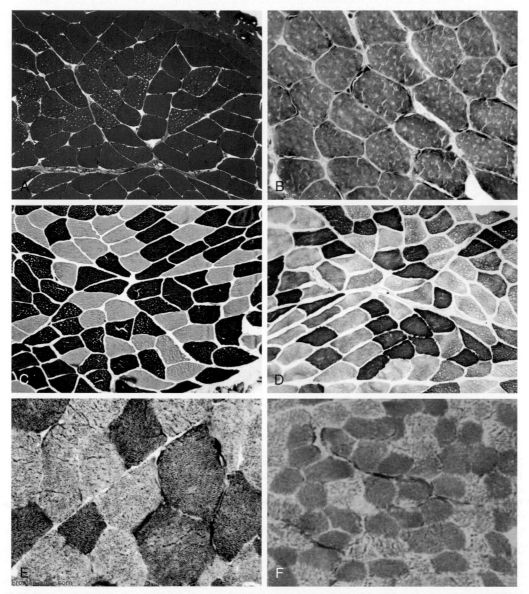

**Fig. 10.12 Selected stains of normal frozen muscle tissue from the staining battery.** (A) Hematoxylin and eosin (H&E) stain. Note ice crystal artifacts in several muscle fibers. (B) Modified Gomori trichrome (mGT) stain. (C) ATPase stain. (D) Cytochrome oxidase (COX) stain. (E) Nicotinamide adenine dinucleotide-tetrazolium reductase (NADH-TR) stain. (F) Succinic dehydrogenase (SDH) stain (x100 magnification in A, C, and D). A–E from frontalcortex.com. F from Gaspar BL, Vasishta RK, Radotra BD. Histochemistry and immunochemistry of normal muscle. In: *Myopathology.* Singapore: Springer. 2019.

○ Modified Gomori trichrome (mGT)
- Useful for demonstrating abnormal accumulation within muscle fibers especially
  - Ragged-red fibers (Fig. 10.13)
    - Accumulation of abnormal mitochondria, typically at the periphery of the muscle fibers
    - Seen in mitochondrial myopathies such as
      - Mitochondrial encephalomyopathy, lactic acidosis, and stroke-like episodes (MELAS)
      - Myoclonic epilepsy with ragged-red fibers (MERRF)
      - Kearns-Sayre syndrome (KSS)
      - Mitochondria neurogastrointestinal encephalomyopathy (MNGIE), and others
    - On electron microscopy, these abnormal mitochondria are seen as paracrystalline inclusion arranged in a "parking lot" pattern.

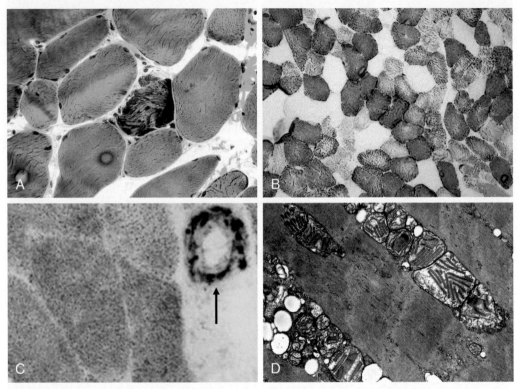

**Fig. 10.13 Histopathologic features of mitochondrial myopathies.** (A) Ragged-red fibers on modified Gomori trichrome (mGT) stain. (B) Cytochrome oxidase (COX)–deficient fibers. (C) Strong succinic dehydrogenase (SDH)–reactive vessels which can be seen in some mitochondrial myopathies such as mitochondrial encephalomyopathy, lactic acidosis, and stroke-like episodes (MELAS). (D) Electron microscopy showing paracrystalline inclusions arranged in a "parking lot" pattern. These inclusions correlate with ragged-red fibers on mGT stain. (A, B) Courtesy Mark Cohen, MD. (C) Adapted from Lorenzoni PJ, Scola RH, Kay CS, et al. MELAS: clinical features, muscle biopsy and molecular genetics. *Arq Neuropsiquiatr.* 2009;67(3A):668-676. (D) adapted from frontalcortex.com

- Nemaline bodies or rods ("nema" from Greek, meaning *thread*) (Fig. 10.14)
  - Stain dark purplish or red on mGT, usually at periphery of the muscle fiber, which represents an accumulation of rod- or thread-like bodies
  - Seen in nemaline myopathy, but can also rarely be seen in other conditions such as central core myopathy
  - On EM, nemaline bodies are demonstrated as streaming of Z-discs.

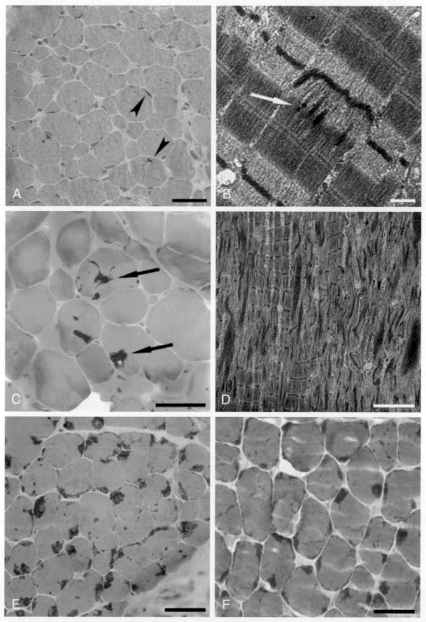

**Fig. 10.14 Nemaline rods in nemaline myopathy.** Nemaline rods in three patients (Patient 1-A, B; Patient 2-C, D; Patient 3-E at age 15-years-old, F at age 29-years-old). Panels A, C, E, F demonstrate nemaline rods on modified Gomori trichrome (mGT) stain (*arrowheads and black arrows*). Panels B and D demonstrate electron microscopic findings of nemaline (thread-like) rods (*white arrow*) of Patients 1 (B) and 2 (D). These rods have the same density as Z-discs. Scale bar = 50 μm in A, C, E, F; 1 μm in B, D. From Moreno CAM, Abath Neto O, Donkervoort S, et al. Clinical and histologic findings in ACTA1-related nemaline myopathy: case series and review of the literature. *Pediatr Neurol.* 2017;75:11-16.

- Rimmed vacuoles (Fig. 10.15)
  - These vacuoles are characterized by an area devoid of the mGT staining with purple rims.
  - Can also be seen on H&E as vacuoles with basophilic rims
  - Contain autophagic vacuoles and lysosomes
  - Rimmed vacuoles can be seen in
    - Inclusion body myositis (IBM)
    - Distal myopathy with rimmed vacuoles (DMRV; aka GNE myopathy, Nonaka myopathy, quadriceps sparing myopathy, hereditary inclusion body myopathy)
    - Oculopharyngeal muscular dystrophy (OPMD)
    - Can also be seen in other several muscle diseases

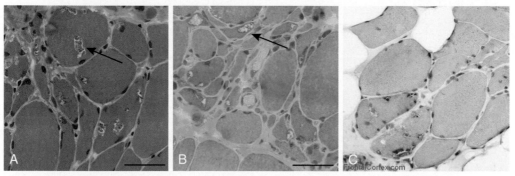

**Fig. 10.15 Rimmed vacuoles.** (A) H&E stain and (B) modified Gomori trichrome [mGT] stain are from the same patient with *GNE* myopathy (aka distal myopathy with rimmed vacuoles or Nonaka myopathy). Note the presence of autophagic materials within the vacuoles (*arrows*) in Panel A and B. (C) mGT stain from a patient with inclusion body myositis. (A, B) From Estephan EP, Moreno CAM, et al. Muscle biopsy with dystrophic pattern and rimmed vacuoles: *GNE* myopathy in a Brazilian patient. *Arq Neuropsiquiatr.* 2017;75(1):72–73. (C) From frontalcortex.com

- Others
  - Tubular aggregates: present in tubular aggregate myopathy
  - Reducing bodies: present in reducing body myopathy
  - Lesions in myofibrillar myopathy
    - Hyaline lesion: amorphous material, dark blue green in color
    - Non-hyaline lesion: dark green color, denser than hyaline lesions
- Periodic acid–Schiff (PAS) (Fig. 10.16)
  - Glycogen vacuoles are dark pink on PAS staining
  - Glycogen accumulation is seen in glycogen storage diseases (GSD) or glycogenoses such as
    - Pompe disease (acid maltase or alpha-1,4 glucosidase deficiency or GSD type II)
    - Debrancher enzyme deficiency (Cori-Forbes disease or GSD III)
    - Brancher enzyme deficiency (Andersen disease or GSD IV)
    - McArdle disease (myophosphorylase deficiency or GSD V)
    - Tarui disease (phosphofructokinase deficiency or GSD VII)

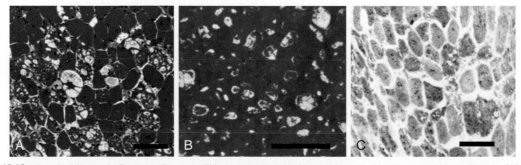

**Fig. 10.16 Muscle biopsy in Pompe disease.** This muscle biopsy is from an 11-year-old patient with Pompe disease. (A) H&E stain demonstrates marked variation of muscle fiber size and numerous vacuoles within muscle fibers. (B) Periodic acid–Schiff (PAS) staining demonstrates intense PAS positivity, indicating glycogen accumulation within muscle fibers. (C) Acid phosphatase staining is positive, indicating the accumulation of abnormal lysosomes within muscle fibers. Scale bar = 100 μm. From Werneck LC, Lorenzoni PJ, Kay CS, Scola RH. Muscle biopsy in Pompe disease. *Arq Neuropsiquiatr.* 2013;71(5):284-289.

- Oil red O (Fig. 10.17)
  - Stains neutral lipids
  - Lipid droplets are stained red on Oil red O and black on Sudan black staining.
  - Lipid droplets are seen in lipid storage myopathy. Examples include:
    - Carnitine palmitoyltransferase II (CPT II) deficiency
    - Multi-acyl-CoA dehydrogenase deficiency (MADD)
    - Neutral lipid storage disease
      - Neutral lipid storage disease with myopathy (NLSDM)
      - Neutral lipid storage disease with ichthyosis (NLSDI; aka Chanarin-Dorfman syndrome)

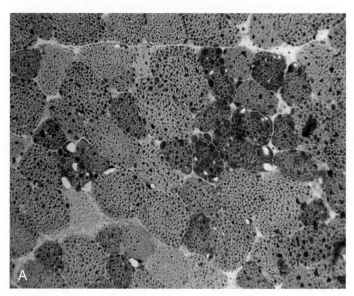

**Fig. 10.17  Muscle pathology in lipid storage myopathy.**  This muscle biopsy shows positive Oil Red O staining indicating the presence of lipid accumulation within muscle fibers as red droplets. This patient is diagnosed with neutral lipid storage disease. From Laforêt P, Vianey-Saban C. Disorders of muscle lipid metabolism: diagnostic and therapeutic challenges. *Neuromuscular Disorders.* 2010;20(11):693-700.

- Reduced nicotinamide adenine dinucleotide-tetrazolium reductase (NADH-TR) (Fig. 10.18)
  - Useful for assessing myofibrillary network and its disruption
  - Can demonstrate core in central core myopathy
    - Core is an area devoid of NADH-TR staining at the center of muscle fibers.

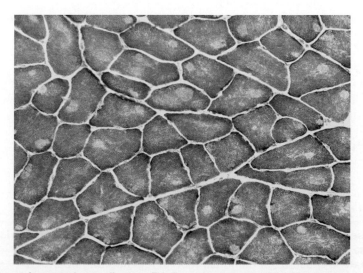

**Fig. 10.18  Muscle biopsy in central core disease.**  This figure demonstrates NADH-TR staining of the muscle biopsy. There are areas devoid of enzymatic activity mainly located at the center of the muscle fibers. From Dubowitz V, Sewry CA, Oldfors A. *Muscle Biopsy.* 5th ed. Elsevier; 2021:63.

- o Adenosine triphosphatase (ATPase) (Fig. 10.19)
  - Useful for assessing muscle fiber types
  - In acidic pH (e.g., pH 4.3 or 4.6), type 1 fibers are dark brown; type 2A fibers are light brown, and type 2B fibers have an intermediate brown color.
  - In basic pH (e.g., pH 9.4), colors are reversed from the acidic pH: type 1 fibers are light brown and type 2 fibers are dark brown.
  - ATPase staining can demonstrate pathological findings, including:
    - Fiber type grouping (Fig. 10.27): seen in neurogenic diseases
    - Disproportionate size between type 1 and 2 muscle fibers: seen in congenital fiber type disproportion and other congenital myopathies (small type 1 fibers), as well steroid myopathy and disuse atrophy (small type 2 fibers)

## MNEMONICS

In **acidic** pH, **type 1** fibers are dark brown. In **basic** pH, **type 2** fibers are dark brown. Mnemonic – "**a**" comes before "**b**", or pH is lower in acidic and higher in basic.

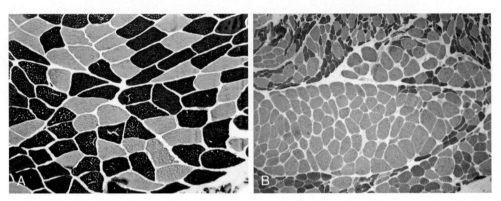

**Fig. 10.19 ATPase staining.** (A) ATPase staining of the normal muscle at pH 4.3. Note that type 1 muscle fibers are dark brown, whereas type 2 muscle fibers are light brown. (B) ATPase staining of muscles in neurogenic diseases demonstrates fiber type grouping. Groups of atrophic fibers are also present. A from frontalcortex.com. B from Miles JD, Cohen ML. Skeletal muscle and peripheral nerve disorders. In: Prayson RA, Goldblum JR, eds. *Neuropathology*. 2nd ed. Elsevier; 2012:563.

- o Cytochrome oxidase (COX)
  - Is complex IV of mitochondrial electron transport chain
  - COX-negative fibers
    - Are fibers devoid of COX staining
    - Seen in mitochondrial myopathies; can also be seen in inclusion body myositis
- o Succinic dehydrogenase (SDH)
  - Is complex II of mitochondrial electron transport chain
  - All SDH subunits are encoded from the nuclear gene, whereas subunits of COX are encoded from both the nuclear and mitochondrial genomes. Thus the presence of muscle fibers that have SDH-positive but COX-negative staining is suggestive of mitochondrial myopathy from mutations in the mitochondrial genome.
  - Strong SDH-reactive blood vessels (SSVs) can be seen in MELAS.
- o Alkaline phosphatase
  - Useful for identification of regenerating fibers

## ◎ HIGH-YIELD FACT

**Acid phosphatase** staining is useful for demonstration of **abnormal accumulation of lysosomes**, such as in Pompe disease.
**Alkaline phosphatase** is useful for demonstration of **regenerating fibers**.

**QUESTION 15.** Which of the following disorders have muscle histopathological findings most similar to Pompe disease?

A. Danon disease
B. Debrancher enzyme deficiency
C. McArdle disease
D. Niemann-Pick type C
E. Tarui disease

**ANSWER:** A. Danon disease

**COMMENTS AND DISCUSSION**

- Danon disease is an X-linked dominant lysosomal storage disease. Given an X-linked dominant inheritance, clinical presentation is usually more severe in males, compared to females. Males typically have earlier age at onset, in childhood or adolescence, whereas affected females can present at later ages.
- Clinical manifestations of Danon disease include myopathy, hypertrophic cardiomyopathy, and intellectual disability. It is due to mutations in the *LAMP2* gene encoding for lysosomal-associated membrane protein 2.
- Muscle histopathology in Danon disease is almost identical to Pompe disease, with glycogen vacuoles seen on H&E and PAS staining, and strongly positive staining for acid phosphatase indicating excessive accumulation of lysosomes.
- Danon disease should be suspected if muscle histopathology is compatible with Pompe disease, but further biochemical or genetic testing does not confirm the diagnosis of Pompe disease.
- Debrancher enzyme deficiency, McArdle disease, and Tarui disease are also glycogen storage diseases in which skeletal muscles are affected. Thus glycogen accumulation can also be seen in muscle histopathology in these disorders. However, unlike Pompe disease, these disorders are not lysosomal storage diseases, and do not demonstrate excessive lysosomal accumulation on acid phosphatase staining.
- Niemann-Pick type C does not typically affect skeletal muscles.

## ◎ HIGH-YIELD FACT

> When muscle biopsy findings are compatible with Pompe disease, but genetic or biochemical testing does not confirm this diagnosis, one has to think about Danon disease.

**QUESTION 16.** A 23-year-old man presents with proximal muscle weakness. Muscle biopsy shows the finding below. The left and right panels are hematoxylin and eosin, and Oil Red O stains, respectively. What is the **MOST LIKELY** diagnosis?

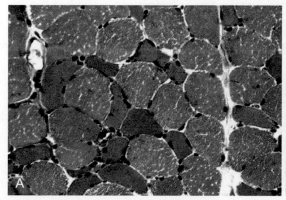 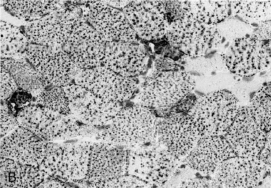

From Angelini C, Nascimbeni AC, Semplicini C. Therapeutic advances in the management of Pompe disease and other metabolic myopathies. *Ther Adv Neurol Disord.* 2013;6(5):311-321.

A. Acid maltase deficiency
B. Debrancher enzyme deficiency
C. Multiple acyl-CoA dehydrogenase deficiency
D. Myophosphorylase deficiency
E. Phosphofructokinase deficiency

**ANSWER:** C. Multiple acyl-CoA dehydrogenase deficiency

**COMMENTS AND DISCUSSION**

- This muscle biopsy demonstrates multiple small vacuoles within muscle fibers on hematoxylin and eosin (H&E) staining. Oil Red O staining demonstrates multiple lipid droplets in red color within these muscle fibers. The diagnosis is, therefore, lipid storage myopathy. Among all choices, only multiple acyl-CoA dehydrogenase deficiency (MADD) is a lipid storage myopathy. Other examples of lipid storage myopathy include primary carnitine deficiency, carnitine palmitoyltransferase II (CPT II) deficiency, and neutral lipid storage disease, among others. Of note, muscle biopsy in CPT II deficiency may demonstrate only minimal or no increased lipid droplets within muscle fibers on Oil Red O staining.
- Acid maltase deficiency (aka Pompe disease), debrancher enzyme deficiency, myophosphorylase deficiency, and phosphofructokinase deficiency are glycogen storage myopathies. Muscle biopsies in these disorders would reveal glycogen vacuoles, which are PAS positive, but are not stained red on Oil Red O.

**MNEMONICS**

OIL RED O indicates accumulation of LIPID droplets which are seen in RED.
OIL = lipid

**QUESTION 17.** A 9-month-old infant presents with hypotonia. Muscle biopsy is performed, and on reduced nicotinamide adenine dinucleotide-tetrazolium reductase (NADH-TR) staining reveals the finding in the figure below (scale bar: 100 μm). Which of the following conditions is associated with this disorder?

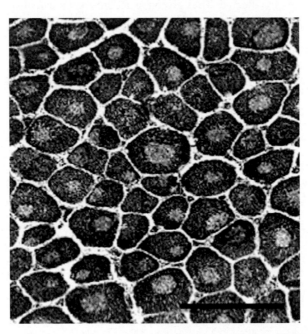

From Marks S, van Ruitenbeek E, Fallon P, et al. Parental mosaicism in RYR1-related central core disease. *Neuromuscul Disord.* 2018;28(5):422-426.

A. Adrenal insufficiency
B. Cardiac conduction block
C. Malignant hyperthermia
D. Pulmonary fibrosis
E. Thyroid storm

**ANSWER:** C. Malignant hyperthermia

**COMMENTS AND DISCUSSION**

- This muscle biopsy demonstrates central cores, which appear as areas devoid of staining at the center of muscle fibers on reduced nicotinamide adenine dinucleotide-tetrazolium reductase (NADH-TR) staining.

- The diagnosis in this patient is central core myopathy, a type of congenital myopathy. Central core myopathies are mainly associated with mutations in the *RYR1* gene.
- In central core myopathy due to RYR1 mutations, there is a risk of malignant hyperthermia after receiving depolarizing neuromuscular blocking agents for anesthesia.
- Central core myopathy is not associated with adrenal insufficiency, cardiac conduction block, pulmonary fibrosis, or thyroid storm.

**QUESTION 18.** The finding in the muscle biopsy below (nicotinamide adenine dinucleotide-tetrazolium reductase (NADH-TR) staining) is most likely seen in which of the following disorders?

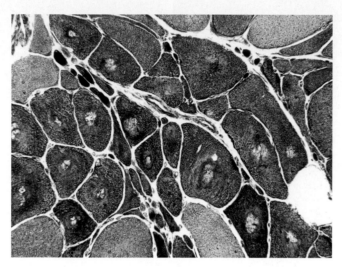

From frontalcortex.com

A. Amyotrophic lateral sclerosis
B. Central core disease
C. Myofibrillar myopathy
D. X-linked myotubular myopathy
E. None of the above, since this is an artifact

**ANSWER:** A. Amyotrophic lateral sclerosis

**COMMENTS AND DISCUSSION**
- This muscle biopsy shows target fibers, on nicotinamide adenine dinucleotide-tetrazolium reductase (NADH-TR) staining. These fibers show central areas devoid of staining, surrounded by peripheral rims with dark intense staining.
- Target and targetoid fibers indicate denervation and reinnervation, thus are seen in neurogenic diseases.
- Target and targetoid fibers can be confused with cores in central core myopathy. However, cores usually lack the peripheral dark rim, involve mainly type 1 muscle fibers (in contrast to target fibers which involve both types 1 and 2 fibers), and in the longitudinal section, extend along muscle fibers (whereas central clear regions in target fibers do not). Of all choices, only amyotrophic lateral sclerosis is a neurogenic disorder. In addition to target fibers, small, angulated fibers, small and large group atrophy, and fiber type grouping can be seen in neurogenic disorders.
- X-linked myotubular myopathy or centronuclear myopathy should have increased internalized nuclei, not clear central regions.
- Freezing or ice crystal artifact can be seen as vacuolar changes of variable sizes and shapes on H&E staining.

 **HIGH-YIELD FACT**

Target or targetoid fibers indicate denervation and reinnervation.

**QUESTION 19.** A 23-year-old man presents with muscle weakness. Muscle biopsy reveals the findings in the following figure (A: modified Gomori trichrome stain; B: cytochrome oxidase stain; C: succinic dehydrogenase stain). What is the most likely diagnosis?

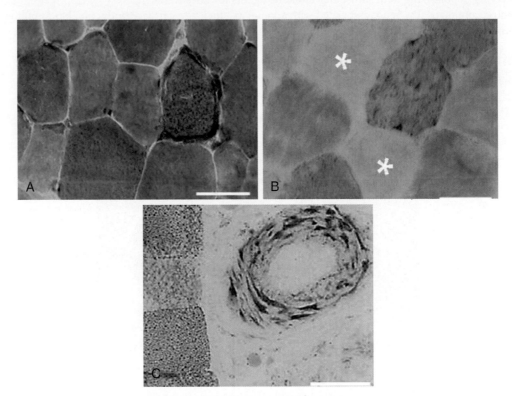

Adapted from (A and B) Lorenzoni PJ, Scola RH, Kay CS, Arndt RC, Freund AA, Bruck I, Santos ML, Werneck LC. MELAS: clinical features, muscle biopsy and molecular genetics. *Arq Neuropsiquiatr.* 2009 Sep;67(3A):668-76. doi: 10.1590/s0004-282x2009000400018. PMID: 19722047. (C) Lorenzoni PJ, Werneck LC, Kay CS, Silvado CE, Scola RH. When should MELAS (Mitochondrial myopathy, Encephalopathy, Lactic Acidosis, and Stroke-like episodes) be the diagnosis? *Arq Neuropsiquiatr* 2015;73(11):959-67. doi: 10.1590/0004-282X20150154. PMID: 26517220.

    A. Adult-onset nemaline myopathy
    B. Amyloid myopathy
    C. Inclusion body myositis
    D. McArdle disease
    E. Mitochondrial encephalomyopathy, lactic acidosis, and stroke-like episodes (MELAS)

**ANSWER:** E. Mitochondrial encephalomyopathy, lactic acidosis, and stroke-like episodes (MELAS)

**COMMENTS AND DISCUSSION**

- This muscle biopsy demonstrates ragged-red fibers on modified Gomori trichrome staining (left upper panel), and cytochrome oxidase (COX)–negative fibers (right upper panel). In addition, strong succinic dehydrogenase (SDH)–strong reactive vessel (SSV) is also seen (lower panel). These findings are suggestive of mitochondrial myopathy. SSV can be seen in some mitochondrial myopathies such as mitochondrial encephalomyopathy, lactic acidosis, and stroke-like episodes (MELAS).
- COX-negative fibers can be found in inclusion body myositis (IBM), but ragged-red fibers and SSV are not expected to be seen. In addition, this patient is too young for IBM.
- There are no nemaline rods, amyloid, or glycogen vacuoles demonstrated in the figure.

**QUESTION 20.** A 34-year-old woman presents with muscle weakness. Electron microscopic examination of muscle biopsy demonstrates the finding as shown in the following figure. Which of the following histopathologic findings is also expected to be seen?

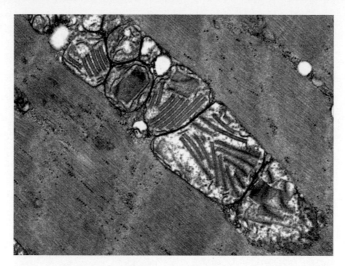

From frontalcortex.com

A. Amyloid within muscle fibers
B. Nemaline rods
C. Perifascicular atrophy
D. Ragged-red fibers
E. Rimmed vacuoles

**ANSWER:** D. Ragged-red fibers

**COMMENTS AND DISCUSSION**

- This electron microscopic examination demonstrates paracrystalline inclusions arranged in a "parking lot" pattern. This finding correlates with ragged-red fibers on modified Gomori trichrome staining, suggesting a mitochondrial myopathy. Other findings that can be seen in mitochondrial myopathies include cytochrome oxidase (COX)–negative fibers and strong succinic dehydrogenase (SDH) strong reactive vessel (SSV).
- There are no amyloid fibrils seen in this muscle biopsy.
- Nemaline rods would be demonstrated as streaming of thread-like structures with the same density as Z-discs.
- Perifascicular atrophy is a classic histopathologic feature in dermatomyositis. In this disorder, there are tubuloreticular inclusions within endothelial cells on electron microscopy.
- Rimmed vacuoles can be seen in several disorders such as inclusion body myositis (IBM), distal myopathy with rimmed vacuoles (DMRV or Nonaka disease), and oculopharyngeal muscular dystrophy (OPMD). In IBM, intranuclear and intracytoplasmic tubulofilamentous inclusions, 15–18 nm in diameter, can be seen on electron microscopy.

 **HIGH-YIELD FACT**

The classic electron microscopic finding in mitochondrial myopathy is paracrystalline inclusions. These are arranged in a "parking lot" pattern.

**QUESTION 21.** A 44-year-old woman presents with proximal muscle weakness. Muscle biopsy demonstrates the finding in the following figure (Hematoxylin and eosin stain). Which of the following antibodies is **MOST LIKELY** to be positive in this patient?

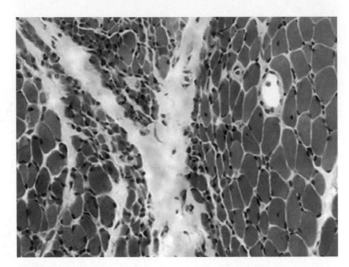

From Uruha A, Suzuki S, Nishino I. *Clin Exp Neuroimmunol.* 2017;8:302-312.

A. Anti-3-hydroxy-3-methylglutaryl-CoA reductase (HMGCR)
B. Anti-LDL receptor-related protein 4 (LRP4)
C. Anti-Mi2
D. Anti-cytosolic 5′-nucleotidase 1A (NT5c1A)
E. Anti-signal recognition particle (SRP)

**ANSWER:** C. Anti-Mi2

**COMMENTS AND DISCUSSION**

- This muscle biopsy demonstrates perifascicular atrophy, which is a classic finding in dermatomyositis. Microvasculitis of perimysial vessels, characterized by lymphocytic infiltration of the vessel wall, can also be observed. Perifascicular atrophy is thought to be associated with the disruption of blood flow resulting from microvasculitis. The diagnosis in this case is dermatomyositis.
- Of all choices, anti-Mi2 is associated with classic dermatomyositis. Other antibodies associated with dermatomyositis include anti-NXP2 and anti-TIF1-γ. Anti-SAE and anti-MDA5 are typically associated with amyopathic dermatomyositis.
- Anti-HMGCR and anti-signal recognition particle (SRP) are associated with immune-mediated necrotizing myopathy.
- Anti-LRP4 is associated with myasthenia gravis, not myopathy.
- Anti-NT5c1A is associated with inclusion body myositis.

**QUESTION 22.** Which of the following is the histopathologic feature that is most likely found in immune-mediated necrotizing myopathy?
A. Perifascicular atrophy
B. Rimmed vacuoles
C. Prominent endomysial lymphocytic infiltration
D. Macrophage infiltration of necrotic fibers
E. Increased major histocompatibility complex (MHC) class II expression

**ANSWER:** D. Macrophage infiltration of necrotic fibers

**COMMENTS AND DISCUSSION**

- In immune-mediated necrotizing myopathy (IMNM), also named necrotizing autoimmune myopathy (NAM), muscle biopsy typically shows scattered necrotic fibers with regenerating fibers but without or with only minimal lymphocytic infiltration. However, macrophage infiltration into necrotic muscle fibers for phagocytosis can be seen.

- Useful immunomarkers in inflammatory myopathies are the following:
  - CD3: T cells
  - CD4: helper T cells
  - CD8: cytotoxic T cells
  - CD20: B cells
  - CD56: regenerating fibers
  - CD68: macrophages
- In addition, there can be increased major histocompatibility complex (MHC) class I expression in IMNM, but not class II and membrane attack complex (MAC) expression.
- Prominent endomysial lymphocytic infiltration is not a feature of IMNM, but can be seen in other inflammatory myopathies mostly polymyositis, and inclusion body myositis (IBM).
- Perifascicular atrophy is a classic feature of dermatomyositis.
- Rimmed vacuoles are seen in several disorders such as IBM, distal myopathy with rimmed vacuoles (DMRV or Nonaka myopathy), and oculopharyngeal muscular dystrophy, among others.

### The following vignette is for QUESTIONS 23 and 24.

A 65-year-old man with coronary artery disease, hypertension, diabetes, and dyslipidemia has had severe left hemiparesis since an ischemic stroke of the right middle cerebral artery territory 3 months ago. He does shows no improvement after the stroke and does not participate in rehabilitation.

**QUESTION 23.** If the biopsy is performed in the left biceps muscle, which of the following findings is **MOST LIKELY** to be found?
  A. Large group atrophy
  B. Type 1 muscle fiber atrophy
  C. Type 2 muscle fiber atrophy
  D. Fiber type grouping
  E. Wedge-shaped infarct within muscle fascicles

**ANSWER:** C. Type 2 muscle fiber atrophy

### COMMENTS AND DISCUSSION
- After prolonged disuse of muscles, type 2 muscle fiber atrophy is seen. In addition to disuse atrophy, type 2 muscle fiber atrophy can also occur in steroid myopathy.
- Type 1 muscle fiber atrophy is seen in several conditions such as congenital myopathies including congenital fiber type disproportion, nemaline myopathy and myotonic dystrophy, among others, but is not a feature of disuse atrophy.
- Large and small group atrophy and fiber type grouping are features of neurogenic diseases, where the lesion is at the anterior horn cell (lower motor neuron), nerve root, plexus or peripheral nerve, not the upper motor neuron lesion as in this case.
- Wedge-shaped muscle infarcts are not expected to be seen in disuse atrophy. Typically biopsy of infarcted muscle shows widespread necrosis of entire muscle fascicles rather than wedge-shaped infarct within each muscle fascicle.

###  HIGH-YIELD FACT

Type 2 muscle fiber atrophy is seen in:
1. steroid myopathy
2. disuse atrophy

**QUESTION 24.** If the electrodiagnostic study is performed in the left arm, including the needle electromyography (EMG) of the left biceps muscle, which of the following findings is expected to be seen?
  A. Poor activation of motor unit action potentials (MUAPs)
  B. Early recruitment of MUAPs
  C. Slow nerve conduction velocity
  D. Conduction block
  E. Small polyphasic MUAPs

**ANSWER:** A. Poor activation of motor unit action potentials (MUAPs)

## COMMENTS AND DISCUSSION

- In type 2 muscle fiber atrophy (such as disuse atrophy or steroid myopathy), electrodiagnostic study is typically normal. In rare situations, low compound muscle action potential (CMAP) amplitudes can occur on nerve conduction study (NCS) when there is severe muscle atrophy.
- On needle EMG, poor activation can be seen in central process, such as in upper motor neuron weakness or functional (psychogenic) weakness, and would be expected in this patient with weakness from his stroke.
- Needle EMG typically first recruits only type 1 or slow muscle fibers, and type 2 muscle fibers are not recruited. Thus type 2 muscle abnormalities are not detected on needle EMG during low levels of activation. Hence, motor unit action potentials should not be small or polyphasic in type 2 muscle atrophy.
- Early recruitment is a feature of myopathy associated with dysfunction of type 1 muscle fibers.
- On NCS, slow nerve conduction velocity and conduction block are features of demyelinating neuropathy, which is not the case in this patient.

**The following options are for QUESTIONS 25 through 29.** Match one disorder with each electron microscopic finding.

- A. Dermatomyositis
- B. Inclusion body myositis
- C. Oculopharyngeal muscular dystrophy
- D. Myoclonic epilepsy with ragged-red fibers
- E. Nemaline myopathy

### QUESTION 25.

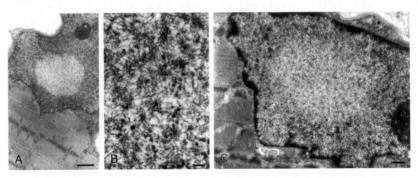

Scale bars in the left, middle, and right panels represent 1, 0.1, and 0.5 μm, respectively. From Uyama E, Nohira O, Chateau D, et al. *Neurology.* 1996;46(3):773-778.

**ANSWER:** C. Oculopharyngeal muscular dystrophy

### QUESTION 26.

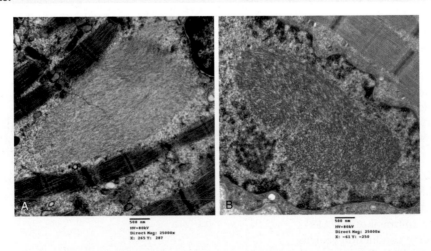

Scale bars in the left, and right panels represent 0.1 μm. From Amato AA, Russell J. *Neuromuscular Disease.* New York: McGraw-Hill; 2016;17:847.

**ANSWER:** B. Inclusion body myositis

**QUESTION 27.**

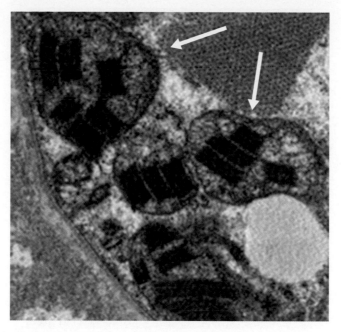

From Amati-Bonneau P, Valentino ML, Reynier P, Gallardo ME, Bornstein B, Boissière A, et al. OPA1 mutations induce mitochondrial DNA instability and optic atrophy 'plus' phenotypes. *Brain.* 2007;131(2):345.

**ANSWER:** D. Myoclonic epilepsy with ragged-red fibers

**QUESTION 28.**

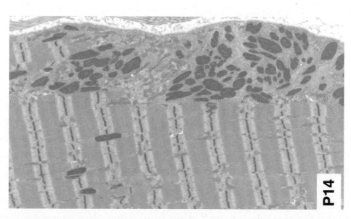

Adapted from Malfatti E, Lehtokari VL, Böhm J, et al. Muscle histopathology in *nebulin*-related nemaline myopathy: ultrastrastructural findings correlated to disease severity and genotype. *Acta Neuropathol Commun.* 2014;2:44.

**ANSWER:** E. Nemaline myopathy

**QUESTION 29.**

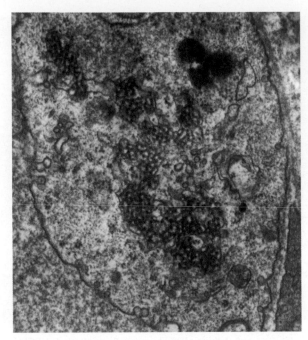

From Goebel HH, Trautmann F, Dippold W. Recent advances in the morphology of myositis. *Pathol Res Pract.* 1985;180(1):1-9.

**ANSWER:** A. Dermatomyositis

**COMMENTS AND DISCUSSION**

- On electron microscopic examination, oculopharyngeal muscular dystrophy (OPMD) demonstrates intranuclear tubulofilamentous inclusions, 8.5 nm in external diameter (Question 25). Tubulofilamentous inclusions can also be seen in inclusion body myositis (IBM, Question 26). In IBM, the inclusions can be present in both intranuclear and intracytoplasmic locations, and the diameters are larger (15–18 nm) than those seen in OPMD.
- In dermatomyositis, tubuloreticular inclusions are usually seen in the endothelial cells (Question 29).
- Paracrystalline inclusions are abnormal mitochondria that typically localize in the subsarcolemmal region and arrange in a "parking lot" pattern. They are seen as the ragged-red portion in ragged-red fibers, which are classic features of mitochondrial myopathies such as mitochondrial encephalomyopathy, lactic acidosis, and stroke-like episodes (MELAS), myoclonic epilepsy with ragged-red fibers (MERRF, Question 27), Kearns-Sayre syndrome (KSS), and mitochondrial neurogastrointestinal encephalomyopathy (MNGIE).
- Nemaline rods are thread-like materials ("nema" is derived from Greek, meaning *thread*) within muscle fibers that have the same density as Z-discs from which they originate. Nemaline rods are seen in nemaline myopathy (Question 28).

---

**The following options are for QUESTIONS 30 through 33.** Match one histopathologic findings with each agent.

   A.  Type 2 fiber atrophy
   B.  Ragged-red fibers
   C.  Necrotizing myopathy
   D.  Vacuolar myopathy

**QUESTION 30.** Chloroquine
**ANSWER:** D. Vacuolar myopathy

**QUESTION 31.** Simvastatin
**ANSWER:** C. Necrotizing myopathy

**QUESTION 32.**  Prednisone
**ANSWER:** A. Type 2 fiber atrophy

**QUESTION 33.**  Zidovudine
**ANSWER:** B. Ragged-red fibers

## COMMENTS AND DISCUSSION

- Chloroquine myopathy shows autophagic vacuoles within muscle fibers on biopsy (Question 30). Vacuoles within muscle fibers can also be seen in colchicine myopathy. Colchicine can affect both nerves and muscles, resulting in neuromyopathy.
- Simvastatin can cause immune-mediated necrotizing myopathy (Question 31) and is associated with anti-3-hydroxy-3-methylglutaryl-coenzyme A reductase (anti-HMGCR) antibodies.
- Prednisone and other corticosteroids can result in steroid myopathy, which demonstrates type 2 muscle fiber atrophy on biopsy (Question 32).
- Zidovudine (aka AZT) can result in mitochondrial dysfunction in muscle fibers due to respiratory chain dysfunction and mitochondrial DNA depletion. Thus zidovudine myopathy can demonstrate ragged-red fibers, a feature of mitochondrial myopathy, on muscle biopsy (Question 33).

**QUESTION 34.**  Which of the following histopathologic findings is a feature of critical illness myopathy?
A. Loss of thin filaments
B. Loss of thick filaments
C. Streaming of Z-discs
D. Tubulofilamentous inclusions
E. Paracrystalline inclusions

**ANSWER:** B. Loss of thick filaments

## COMMENTS AND DISCUSSION

- One characteristic pathological feature of critical illness myopathy is loss of myosin or thick filaments on electron microscopic examination.
- Streaming of Z-discs is seen in nemaline myopathy.
- Tubulofilamentous inclusions can be seen in inclusion body myositis (intranuclear and intracytoplasmic locations, 15–18 nm in diameter) and oculopharyngeal muscular dystrophy (intranuclear, 8.5 nm in diameter) (Fig. 10.9 and 10.10).
- Paracrystalline inclusions are accumulation of abnormal mitochondria seen in mitochondrial myopathies.

**QUESTION 35.**  A sural nerve biopsy is **MOST** suitable in which of the following situations:
A. An alcoholic patient with distal sensorimotor polyneuropathy
B. A diabetic patient with painful small fiber sensory neuropathy
C. A patient with pure motor multifocal mononeuropathies
D. A patient with severe subacute asymmetrical sensorimotor neuropathy
E. A patient with pes cavus and possible hereditary polyneuropathy

**ANSWER:** D. A patient with severe subacute asymmetrical sensorimotor neuropathy

## COMMENTS AND DISCUSSION

- Nerve biopsy of a superficial sensory nerve is often done when a vasculitic neuropathy or an amyloid neuropathy is suspected.
- A superficial sensory nerve with an absent or reduced sensory action potential should be biopsied.
- The most common nerve for biopsy is the sural nerve, as it is:
  - Easily identified, unlikely to be affected by compression injury
  - Pure sensory nerve: biopsy does not result in motor deficits
- Other nerves such as superficial peroneal and superficial radial nerves are much less commonly biopsied.

- Typically, nerve biopsy is not performed in other peripheral nerve disorders such as hereditary or demyelinating neuropathies, since the diagnosis can be confirmed by other methods such as electrophysiologic or genetic testing.
- Motor nerves are rarely biopsied, and typically patients with suspected hereditary or acquired demyelinating neuropathies (such as chronic inflammatory demyelinating polyneuropathy [CIDP]) or multifocal motor neuropathy do not require biopsy.
- Nerve biopsy in alcoholic or diabetic polyneuropathies is not useful because the information often does not add to the clinical and electrophysiologic findings.
- Nerve biopsy requires special expertise in techniques, staining, and interpretation.
- The biopsied nerve is divided into three parts
  - Fixed in formaldehyde (formalin)
    - For paraffin section and teasing
      - Paraffin section is used for H&E staining, as well as for modified trichrome and Congo red staining
      - Teased nerve fiber is useful for demonstration of
        - Segmental demyelination in acquired demyelinating neuropathies:
        - Myelin ovoids in axonal neuropathy
  - Fixed in 4% glutaraldehyde
    - For semithin section and electron microscopy
    - Toluidine blue staining
  - Fixed in isopentane in liquid nitrogen
    - For frozen section
- Normal findings on nerve biopsy are (Fig. 10.20):
  - Connective tissue
    - Epineurium: outermost; covering all nerve fascicles
    - Perineurium: covering each nerve fascicle
    - Endoneurium: covering axons within each nerve fascicle
  - Nerve fibers of various sizes are mixed within nerve fascicles.
    - Large size: axon with thick myelin sheath
    - Intermediate size: axon with intermediate thickness of myelin sheath
    - Small size: unmyelinated nerve fibers
    - On semi-thin section, myelin sheath has a dark blue color, giving a "donut" appearance.

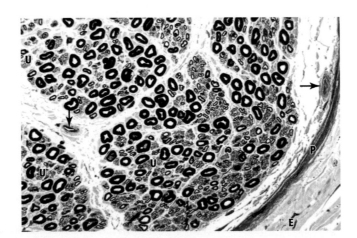

**Fig. 10.20 Normal nerve biopsy.** Toluidine blue staining of this semi-thin section of the nerve demonstrates a nerve fascicle surrounded by perineurium (*P*) and epineurium (*E*). Myelin sheath is stained dark blue, so are nuclei of endothelial cells (*arrow*). The nerve fascicle contains large, myelinated fibers, small, myelinated fibers, and unmyelinated fibers (*U*). From Miles JD, Cohen ML. Skeletal muscle and peripheral nerve disorders. In: Prayson RA, Goldblum JR, eds. *Neuropathology.* 2nd ed. Elsevier; 2012;11:599.

- The findings on nerve biopsy in vasculitic neuropathy include (Fig. 10.21):
  ○ Transmural infiltration of mononuclear inflammatory cells (lymphocytes and monocytes) into the vessel wall
  ○ There can be fibrinoid necrosis of the blood vessel wall.
  ○ Myelin ovoids can be seen, which represent axonal degeneration.
  ○ Selective nerve fiber degeneration (SNFD) can be seen as wedge-shaped loss of myelinated nerve fibers within nerve fascicles.

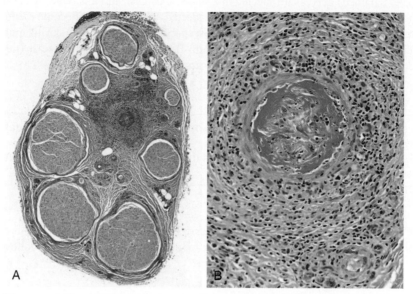

**Fig. 10.21 Vasculitic neuropathy.** (A) H&E stain at low magnification demonstrates intramural inflammation of the epineurial vessel wall with fibrinoid necrosis and thrombosis. (B) At higher magnification, the wall of the epineurial vessel is infiltrated by inflammatory cells composed of polymorphonuclear and mononuclear cells. Fibrinoid necrosis and thrombus in the lumen are also demonstrated. From Bilbao JM, Schmidt RE. Vasculitic neuropathy. In: *Biopsy Diagnosis of Peripheral Neuropathy.* Springer; 2015;13:250.

**QUESTION 36.**    A nerve biopsy performed in a 27-year-old woman demonstrates the finding in the following figure (hematoxylin and eosin staining). Which of the following is the most pathognomonic clinical presentation of this disorder?

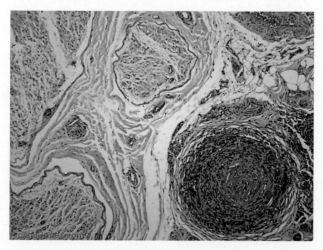

From frontalcortex.com

A. Bilateral facial diplegia
B. Mononeuropathy
C. Mononeuropathy multiplex
D. Distal symmetric polyneuropathy, length-dependent pattern
E. Distal symmetric polyneuropathy, non–length-dependent pattern

**ANSWER:** C. Mononeuropathy multiplex

**COMMENTS AND DISCUSSION** (see also comments and discussion from question 35)

- This nerve biopsy with hematoxylin and eosin (H&E) staining demonstrates intramural infiltration of inflammatory cells in the wall of epineurial vessels. This feature is characteristic of vasculitic neuropathy which can be associated with systemic vasculitis such as polyarteritis nodosa (PAN), granulomatosis with polyangiitis (GPA, aka Wegener granulomatosis), or eosinophilic granulomatosis with polyangiitis (EGPA, aka Churg-Strauss syndrome).
- The classic clinical presentation of vasculitic neuropathy is mononeuritis multiplex, where individual peripheral nerves ("named" nerves) are affected in a stepwise pattern, and it is typically painful. In chronic vasculitic neuropathy in which multiple nerves are affected, the pattern can become confluent and mimic distal symmetric polyneuropathy. However, the most specific pattern is mononeuritis multiplex.
- Bilateral facial diplegia can be associated with Guillain-Barré syndrome, Lyme disease (neuroborreliosis), and sarcoidosis, among others, but is not a classic feature of vasculitic neuropathy.

## ◎ HIGH-YIELD FACT

The key muscle biopsy finding in vasculitic neuropathy is INTRAMURAL inflammation of epineurial vessels.
INTRAMURAL inflammation means that there is infiltration of inflammatory cells WITHIN blood vessel walls.

**QUESTION 37.** The teased fiber preparation of the nerve biopsy in a 22-year-old woman with a demyelinating polyneuropathy reveals the finding in the following figure. Which of the following genetic abnormalities is expected to be seen in this patient?

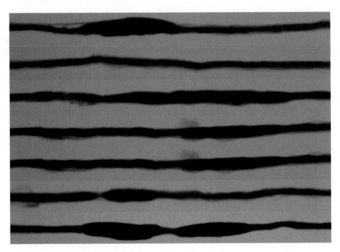

From Kim SM, Chung KW, Choi BO, et al. Hereditary neuropathy with liability to pressure palsies (HNPP) patients of Korean ancestry with chromosome 17p11.2-p12 deletion. *Exp Mol Med.* 2004;36(1):28-35.

- A. *GJB1* mutation
- B. *MFN2* mutation
- C. *MPZ* mutation
- D. *PMP22* deletion
- E. *PMP22* duplication

**ANSWER:** D. *PMP22* deletion

## COMMENTS AND DISCUSSION

- This nerve biopsy obtained via the teased-fiber technique demonstrates tomacula or focal swelling of myelin, giving a sausage-like appearance. This finding is a characteristic feature of hereditary neuropathy with liability to pressure palsy (HNPP, aka tomaculous neuropathy). HNPP is due to *deletion in the PMP22 gene* encoding for peripheral myelin protein.

- All other choices are genetic abnormalities seen in Charcot-Marie-Tooth disease (CMT).
  - The most common mutation is *PMP22 duplication* in CMT1A (autosomal dominant, demyelinating type).
  - Mutations in the *MPZ* gene encoding for P0 protein are related to CMT1B (autosomal dominant, demyelinating type).
  - Mutations in the *GJB1* gene encoding connexin 32, the gap junction protein, are responsible for CMTX (X-linked inheritance).
  - Mutations in the *MFN2* gene encoding for mitofusin 2, a protein that has a role in mitochondrial fusion, cause CMT2A (autosomal dominant, axonal type).
- Demyelinating features on nerve biopsy are seen in:
  - Hereditary neuropathies such as CMT1A
    - Loss of large, myelinated nerve fibers
    - Onion bulb formation (Fig. 10.22)
      - Represents evidence of repetitive demyelination and remyelination; not specific to CMT
      - There are proliferation of Schwann cell processes.

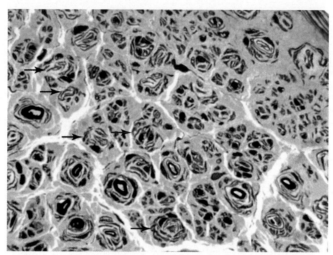

**Fig. 10.22 Nerve biopsy findings in the demyelinating type of Charcot-Marie-Tooth (CMT).** This toluidine blue staining of the semi-thin section demonstrates onion bulb formation due to proliferation of Schwann cell process. This feature represents repetitive demyelination and remyelination, and is indicative of chronic demyelinating neuropathy. From Miles JD, Cohen ML. Skeletal muscle and peripheral nerve disorders. In: Prayson RA, Goldblum JR, eds. *Neuropathology*. 2nd ed. Elsevier; 2012;11:600.

  - Hereditary neuropathy with liability to pressure palsy (HNPP)
    - Tomacula (Latin; means *sausage*): focal sausage shaped swelling of myelin sheath (Fig. 10.23)
  - Acquired demyelination (e.g., chronic inflammatory demyelinating polyneuropathy [CIDP] or acute inflammatory demyelinating polyneuropathy [AIDP])
    - Segmental demyelination can be demonstrated on teased-fiber preparation (Fig. 10.24)

## MNEMONICS

**SMALL** gene (*PMP22* DELETION) – **LARGE** nerve (**TOMACULA**) in **HNPP**
**LARGE** gene (*PMP22* DUPLICATION) – **SMALL** nerve (**DEMYELINATION**) in **CMT1A**

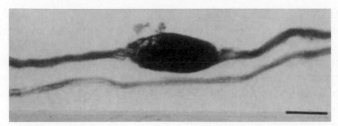

**Fig. 10.23 Nerve biopsy finding in hereditary neuropathy with liability to pressure palsy (HNPP).** This figure demonstrates a teased nerve fiber stained with osmium tetroxide. There is a focal sausage-shaped swelling of the nerve, called "tomacula." Scale bar = 20 μm. From Oda K, Miura H, Shibasaki H, et al. Hereditary pressure-sensitive neuropathy: demonstration of "tomacula" in motor nerve fibers. *J Neurol Sci.* 1990;98(2-3):139-148.

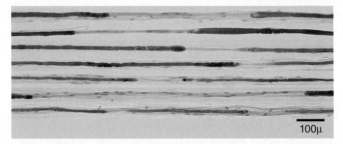

**Fig. 10.24 Segmental demyelination.** This teased nerve fiber preparation from a patient with chronic inflammatory demyelinating polyneuropathy (CIDP) demonstrates segmental loss of myelin sheath. From Piccione EA, Engelstad J, Dyck PJ, Mauermann ML, Dispenzieri A, Dyck PJ. Nerve pathologic features differentiate POEMS syndrome from CIDP. *Acta Neuropathol Commun.* 2016;4(1):116.

**QUESTION 38.** A 6-year-old girl presents with weakness and numbness in all extremities, more prominent in both legs. A sural nerve biopsy is performed and the finding is shown in the following figure. Which of the following genetic abnormalities is **MOST LIKELY** to be seen in this patient?

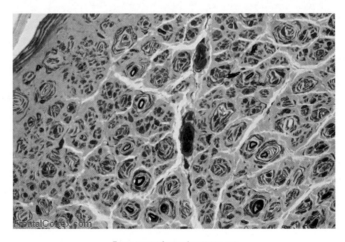

From www.frontalcortex.com

    A. *MFN2* mutation
    B. *PMP22* deletion
    C. *PMP22* duplication
    D. *SCN9A* mutation
    E. Exon 7 deletion in the *SMN1* gene

**ANSWER:** C. *PMP22* duplication

**COMMENTS AND DISCUSSION (see also comments and discussion from Question 37)**

- This nerve biopsy with toluidine blue staining demonstrates onion bulb formation. There is proliferation of Schwann cell processes. Onion bulb formation indicates repetitive demyelination and remyelination, and is hence seen in chronic demyelinating neuropathies such as Charcot-Marie-Tooth type 1A (CMT1A). Of all choices, *PMP22* duplication is found in CMT1A.

- *MFN2* mutations are associated with CMT2A, which is an axonal type of CMT.
- *PMP22* deletion is associated with hereditary neuropathy with liability to pressure palsy (HNPP) in which tomacula (i.e., focal swelling of myelin) is seen.
- *SCN9A* mutations are associated with erythromelalgia in which there are abnormalities of small fibers. Skin biopsy can demonstrate decreased intraepidermal nerve fiber density.
- Exon 7 deletion in the *SMN1* gene is responsible for spinal muscular atrophy in which the primary pathology is at the motor neurons, not the peripheral nerves.

## ◎ HIGH-YIELD FACT

Onion bulb formation represents chronic repetitive demyelination and remyelination. On the board exam, it is often associated with CMT1A, but in fact it can also be seen in other disorders associated with chronic demyelination.

**QUESTION 39.** A 70-year-old man presents for an evaluation of numbness in both hands and feet. A nerve biopsy is performed and demonstrates the findings shown the following figure (Congo red staining in upper and left lower panels and polarized light in right lower panel). Which of the following findings is **MOST LIKELY** found in this patient?

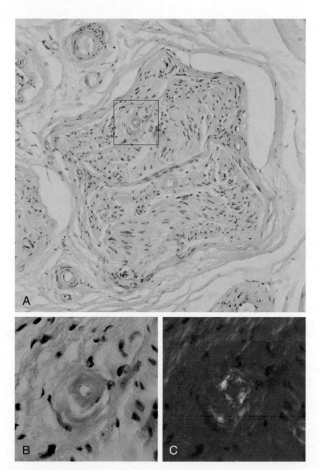

From Asiri MMH, Engelsman S, Eijkelkamp N, Höppener JWM. Amyloid Proteins and Peripheral Neuropathy. *Cells.* 2020;9(6):1553.

A. Angiokeratoma
B. Orange-colored tonsils
C. Hypertrophic cardiomyopathy
D. Leukodystrophy
E. Pes cavus

**ANSWER:** C. Hypertrophic cardiomyopathy

## COMMENTS AND DISCUSSION

- This nerve biopsy demonstrates amyloid deposition in the wall of the endoneurial vessel, which appears red on Congo red staining (upper and left lower panels). Under polarized light, the amyloid deposits exhibit an apple green birefringence (right lower panel).
- Amyloid deposition within the nerve has the following characteristics (Fig. 10.25):
  - Common site of deposition is within the wall of epineurial vessels.
  - Amyloid can also deposit within the endoneurial or perineurial space.
  - Amyloid stains red on Congo red, and it typically exhibits an apple green birefringence under the polarized light.
- The diagnosis is amyloid neuropathy.
  - Amyloid deposition can be seen in both familial and acquired amyloid neuropathies.
    - In this 70-year-old man, primary (AL) amyloidosis is more likely than the familial forms. Associated findings in primary (AL) amyloidosis include carpal tunnel syndrome, renal involvement (e.g., nephrotic syndrome), hypertrophic cardiomyopathy, hepatosplenomegaly, and small fiber involvement resulting in autonomic dysfunction, among others.

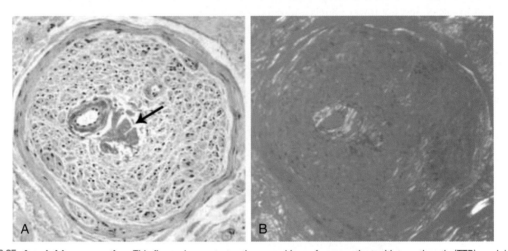

**Fig. 10.25 Amyloid neuropathy.** This figure demonstrates the nerve biopsy from a patient with transthyretin (TTR) amyloidosis. (A) Congo red staining demonstrates diffuse amyloid deposition within the nerve fascicle with high density at the wall of endoneurial vessels (*arrow*). In addition, there is loss of myelinated nerve fibers. (B) Under polarized light, amyloid deposition shows apple green birefringence. From Liepnieks JJ, Zhang LQ, Benson MD. Progression of transthyretin amyloid neuropathy after liver transplantation. *Neurology.* 2010;75(4):324-327.

## ◎ HIGH-YIELD FACT

Histopathologic findings of amyloid:
1. On Congo red staining, it appears red.
2. Under polarized light, there is apple green birefringence.

- Other neuropathies with abnormal deposits
  - Adult polyglucosan body disease (APBD)
    - Polyglucosan bodies are composed of glucose polymer with no or poor branching, in contrast to glycogen.
    - Polyglucosan bodies have the same structure as Lafora bodies and corpora amylacea.
    - In APBD, polyglucosan bodies are seen as PAS-positive material, approximately 50 μm in size, within the nerve (Fig. 10.26).

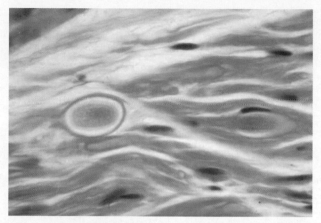

**Fig. 10.26 Polyglucosan body in adult polyglucosan body disease.** This longitudinal section of the sural nerve on H&E demonstrates two polyglucosan bodies which have an ovoid shape and basophilic staining. Reprinted from Milde P, Guccion JG, Kelly J, Locatelli E, and Jones RV "Adult Polyglucosan Body Disease: Diagnosis by Sural Nerve and Skin Biopsy" (*Arch Pathol Lab Med.* 2001;125(8):519-522) with permission from Archives of Pathology & Laboratory Medicine. Copyright 2001. College of American Pathologists.

- Fabry disease
  - Lipid inclusions in the perineurium or endothelial cells
  - Under polarized light, these lipid inclusions are seen as "Maltese cross" birefringence (Fig. 10.27).

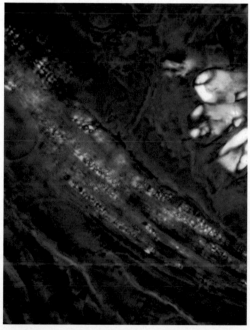

**Fig. 10.27 Nerve biopsy in Fabry disease.** Under polarized light, this unstained fresh frozen nerve demonstrates "Maltese cross" birefringence in the perineurium. From Bilbao JM, Schmidt RE. Storage diseases. In: *Biopsy Diagnosis of Peripheral Neuropathy.* Springer; 2015;20:439.

- Metachromatic leukodystrophy
  - Presence of metachromatic granules, which are sulfatide deposits within Schwann cells or macrophages (Fig. 10.28)
    - 0.5–1 μm in size
    - Brown color, not purple or blue, on toluidine blue or cresyl violet staining
    - PAS-positive
  - On electron microscopy, "tuffstone bodies" are seen (Fig. 10.28).

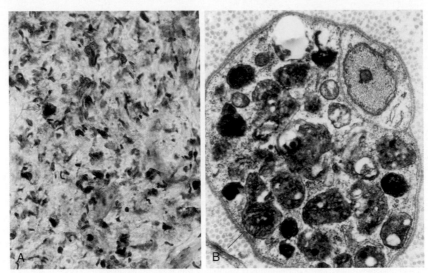

**Fig. 10.28 Nerve biopsy in metachromatic leukodystrophy.** (A) Cresyl violet staining of the nerve demonstrates metachromatic inclusions, which appear brown in color (400x). (B) On electron microscopy, "tuffstone bodies" are seen (23,660x). From Bilbao JM, Schmidt RE. Storage diseases. In: *Biopsy Diagnosis of Peripheral Neuropathy.* Springer; 2015;20:433, 435.

- Among the other options in this question, angiokeratoma, a violaceous skin lesion, usually found at the periumbilical region, is seen in Fabry disease. Orange-colored tonsils are found in Tangier disease. Leuko-dystrophy are associated with several peripheral nerve disorders such as metachromatic leukodystrophy and Krabbe disease. Pes cavus is characterized by high arch feet with shortening of the forefoot, indicating long-standing polyneuropathy present during the developmental period. This is seen in Charcot-Marie-Tooth and other hereditary neuropathies but is unlikely to be seen in acquired AL amyloidosis.

**QUESTION 40.** A nerve biopsy is performed in a patient as part of an evaluation of neuropathy and demonstrates the electron microscopic finding as in the following figure. Which of the following laboratory findings is most likely found in this patient?

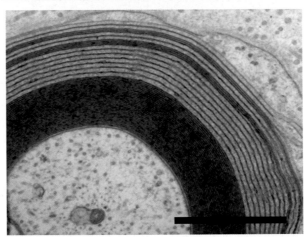

From Kawagashira Y, Koike H, Ohyama K, et al. Axonal loss influences the response to rituximab treatment in neuropathy associated with IgM monoclonal gammopathy with anti-myelin-associated glycoprotein antibody. *J Neurol Sci.* 2015;348(1-2):67-73.

    A. Anti-GM1 antibody
    B. IgM monoclonal gammopathy
    C. Lambda (λ) free light chain
    D. Positive antineutrophil cytoplasmic antibody
    E. *PMP22* duplication

**ANSWER:** B. IgM monoclonal gammopathy

**COMMENTS AND DISCUSSION**

- This electron microscopic examination of the nerve demonstrates splitting of the outer layers of myelin. This finding is a characteristic feature of anti-myelin associated glycoprotein (anti-MAG) neuropathy. Patients with anti-MAG neuropathy typically present with distal acquired demyelinating symmetric (DADS) neuropathy, since distal demyelination is prominent. It is often associated with a detectable IgM monoclonal gammopathy (IgM-DADS) (Fig. 10.29).

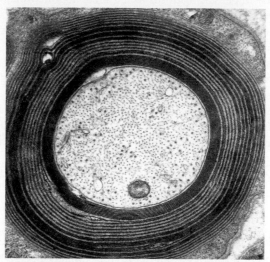

**Fig. 10.29 Electron microscopic finding in anti-myelin-associated glycoprotein (MAG) neuropathy.** This figure demonstrates splitting of outer myelin lamellae. From Miles JD, Cohen ML. Skeletal muscle and peripheral nerve disorders. In: Prayson RA, Goldblum JR, eds. *Neuropathology.* 2nd ed. Elsevier; 2012;11:605.

- Other electron microscopic findings of nerve biopsy include focally folded myelin sheath (Fig. 10.30). This is characterized as multiple redundant layers of myelin, and can be seen in CMT1B (due to mutations in the *MPZ* gene), CMT4A (due to mutations in the *GDAP1* gene), and CMT4B (due to mutations in the *MTMR2* gene).

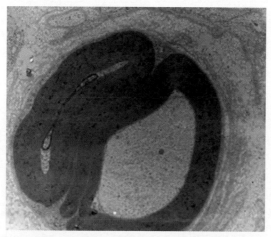

**Fig. 10.30 Focally folded myelin sheath.** This electron microscopic examination of the sural nerve is from a patient with Charcot-Marie-Tooth type 4B (CMT4B) due to the *MTMR2* mutation. There is focal folding of the myelin sheath. (20,000x) From Schenon A, Nobbio L. Inherited peripheral neuropathies. In: Gilman S, ed. *Neurobiology of Disease.* Elsevier; 2007;81.

- Among the other options in this question, anti-GM1 antibodies can be found in multifocal motor neuropathy with conduction block. Lambda (λ) free light chains are seen in amyloid neuropathy. Positive antineutrophil cytoplasmic antibody (ANCA) can be found in vasculitic neuropathy. This electron microscopic finding is not that of Charcot-Marie-Tooth (CMT) disease.

**QUESTION 41.** A 35-year-old woman presents with numbness and burning, which starts in her feet and ascended into her hands. She has been in good health except for mild migratory arthralgias. Neurological examination is normal. Which of the following studies is **LEAST** likely to be useful in making a final diagnosis?
A. Needle electromyography
B. Sensory nerve conduction studies in legs
C. Skin biopsy to assess intraepidermal nerve fiber density
D. Lip biopsy to evaluate salivary glands
E. Quantitative sudomotor axon reflex test

**ANSWER:** A. Needle electromyography

**COMMENTS AND DISCUSSION**

- This woman may have a small fiber neuropathy due to Sjogren syndrome.
- The purpose of skin biopsy in patients with suspected small fiber neuropathies is to demonstrate a reduction of intraepidermal nerve fiber density (IENFD) (Fig. 10.31).
  - Three-mm circular punch biopsy is performed from 2–3 sites including the lower calf and distal and proximal thigh.
  - Biopsy from both distal and proximal sites are useful to evaluate if there is a length-dependent pattern.
  - Samples are stained with protein gene product (PGP) 9.5, which highlights intraepidermal small nerve fibers including C-fibers and possibly Aδ-fibers.
- Sensory nerve conduction studies in legs are useful to assess large sensory fibers, whereas quantitative sudomotor axon reflex studies are useful to assess small autonomic fibers innervated sweat glands.
- Lip biopsy is useful in this patient to look for inflammation of salivary glands, which is diagnostic of Sjogren syndrome.
- Needle electromyography is the least useful, as, it only assesses large, myelinated, motor fibers of the nerve.

 **HIGH-YIELD FACT**

Skin biopsy for evaluation of intraepidermal nerve fiber density (IENFD) is used when small fiber neuropathy is suspected.

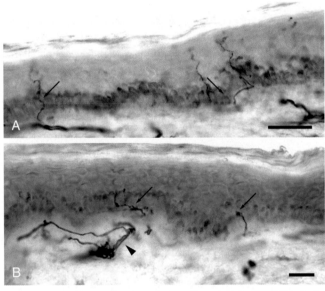

**Fig. 10.31 Skin biopsy for evaluation of intraepidermal nerve fiber density (IENFD).** Both (A) and (B) are skin biopsies from the distal leg. Proximal leg biopsy is not shown. (A) Normal IENFD, scale bar = 60 μm. (B) Reduced IENFD in small-fiber neuropathy from diabetes. *Arrows* represent intraepidermal nerve fibers. The *arrowhead* represents dermal nerve bundles. From Lauria G, Devigili G. Skin biopsy as a diagnostic tool in peripheral neuropathy. *Nat Clin Pract Neurol.* 2007;3:546-557.

## SUGGESTED READING

Amato AA, Russell JA. *Neuromuscular disorders.* 2nd ed. New York: McGraw–Hill Education Medical; 2016.

Cotta A, Carvalho E, da-Cunha-Júnior AL, et al. Muscle biopsy essential diagnostic advice for pathologists. *Surg Exp Pathol.* 2021;4:3.

Dubowitz V, Sewry CA. *A Muscle Biopsy: A Practical Approach.* 5th ed. Elsevier; 2021.

Gardner K, Hall PA, Chinnery PF, Payne BA. HIV treatment and associated mitochondrial pathology: review of 25 years of in vitro, animal, and human studies. *Toxicol Pathol.* 2014;42(5):811-822.

Gaspar BL, Vasishta RK, Radotra BD. *Histochemistry and Immunochemistry of Normal Muscle. Myopathology.* Singapore: Springer; 2019.

Laforêt P, Vianey-Saban C. Disorders of muscle lipid metabolism: diagnostic and therapeutic challenges. *Neuromuscul Disord.* 2010;20(11):693-700.

Miles JD, Cohen ML. Skeletal muscle and peripheral nerve disorders. In: Prayson RA, Goldblum JR, eds. Neuropathology. 2nd ed. Elsevier; 2012.

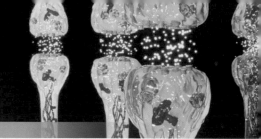

# CHAPTER 11

# Neuromuscular Ultrasound

## PART 1 | PRACTICE TEST

**Q1.** Which of the following is **TRUE** regarding the benefits and disadvantages of neuromuscular ultrasound?
A. Poorly tolerated
B. Muscle damage can occur with prolonged use.
C. Adds similar information to electrodiagnostic studies
D. Resolution is excellent, especially for deep structures
E. Can dynamically assess nerves, muscles, and tendons

**Q2.** Which of the following is **MOST LIKELY** to occur when an ultrasound wave encounters a smooth boundary between two tissues with very different acoustic impedances?
A. A bright echo is generated.
B. Back scatter
C. The ultrasound wave is absorbed as heat.
D. Posterior acoustic shadowing
E. Posterior acoustic enhancement

**Q3.** Which of the following is the **MOST CORRECT** speed of sound in soft tissue?
A. 12 m/s
B. 330 m/s
C. 550 m/s
D. 1540 m/s
E. 2500 m/s

**Q4.** What is **MOST COMMON** ultrasound image that displays anatomic information?
A. A-mode
B. B-mode
C. M-mode

**Q5.** Using color flow Doppler, the goal is to have the probe perpendicular to the blood vessel.
A. TRUE
B. FALSE

**Q6.** Power Doppler is most sensitive in looking at what structure?
A. Nerve
B. Tendon
C. Muscle
D. Blood vessels
E. Bone

**Q7.** The advantage of power Doppler is that it can pick up the direction of flow.
A. TRUE
B. FALSE

**Q8.** What is the probe frequency used for most musculoskeletal (MSK) and neuromuscular ultrasound?
A. 70 MHz
B. 15 MHz
C. 5 MHz
D. 1 MHz
E. 100 KHz

**Q9.** What step(s) could be taken to better visualize a deep structure?
A. Utilize less transmission gel.
B. Increase the gain.
C. Change to a lower frequency transducer.
D. Raise the focal zone.
E. B and C
F. C and D

**Q10.** What structure has a "honeycomb" ultrasound appearance on short axis?
A. Nerve
B. Tendon
C. Muscle
D. Blood vessels
E. Bone

**Q11.** What normal structure has a "starry night" ultrasound appearance on short axis?
A. Nerve
B. Tendon
C. Muscle
D. Blood vessels
E. Bone

**Q12.** What it is the **BEST** way to identify veins?
A. Compressibility
B. Power Doppler
C. Color Doppler
D. Posterior acoustic shadowing
E. Depth

**Q13.** How can you distinguish muscle from adipose tissue using B-mode ultrasound?
A. Utilize power Doppler to determine the more metabolically active tissue.
B. Induce anisotropy with the "heel-toe" technique.
C. Use a higher frequency transducer.
D. Image in axial and longitudinal view.

**Q14.** The cartilage type of the elbow joint and its ultrasound appearance are:
A. hyaline and hypoechoic on ultrasound.
B. hyaline and hyperechoic on ultrasound.
C. fibrous and hypoechoic on ultrasound.
D. fibrous and hyperechoic on ultrasound.

**Q15.** What structure has the **GREATEST** amount of anisotropy?
A. Nerve
B. Tendon
C. Muscle
D. Blood vessels
E. Bone

**Q16.** Posterior acoustic shadowing is **MOST LIKELY** to be seen associated with what type of tissue?
A. Cartilage
B. Bone
C. Muscle
D. Fat
E. Blood vessels

**Q17.** Posterior acoustic enhancement is **MOST LIKELY** to be seen associated with what type of tissue?
A. Cartilage
B. Bone
C. Muscle
D. Fat
E. Blood vessels

**Q18.** Reverberation artifact is **MOST LIKELY** to be seen associated with what type of tissue?
A. Needle
B. Bone
C. Muscle
D. Fat
E. Blood vessels

**Q19.** Adjusting the angle of insonation of the transducer has the greatest value in assessing which of the following tissue properties?
A. Anisotropy
B. Thickness
C. Depth
D. Stiffness
E. Acoustic impedance

**Q20.** Entrapment neuropathies are the most common indication for neuromuscular ultrasound.
A. TRUE
B. FALSE

**Q21.** The following figure is a short-axis view over the median nerve at the wrist in a patient with symptoms of carpal tunnel syndrome (CTS). What is the large structure to the left of the median nerve?

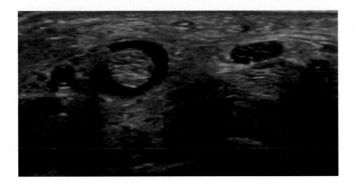

A. An enlarged flexor digitorum superficialis (FDS) muscle
B. A normal median nerve
C. An occluded radial artery
D. A bifid median nerve
E. Tenosynovitis of the flexor carpi radialis (FCR) tendon

**Q22.** In patients with common peroneal neuropathy and no obvious injury or risk factor, which of the following lesions is most likely to be detected using ultrasound?
A. Baker's cyst
B. Popliteal artery aneurysm
C. Intraneural ganglion
D. Fracture of the fibular neck
E. Tendinosis of the biceps femoris

**Q23.** Which of the following is a common ultrasound finding in carpal tunnel syndrome?
A. Increased nerve mobility
B. Decreased cross-sectional area (CSA)
C. Wrist/forearm median nerve CSA ratio >1.4
D. Decreased outlet ratio
E. Ulnar/median nerve CSA ratio >1.4

**Q24.** In carpal tunnel syndrome, the median nerve fascicular echogenicity is best described as:
A. increased when imaged deep to the transverse carpal ligament.
B. decreased when imaged just proximal to the transverse carpal ligament.
C. increased in the presence of tenosynovitis.
D. highly correlated to conduction block.
E. decreased in the forearm.

**Q25.** The image below is a long-axis view of the median nerve at the wrist of a patient with carpal tunnel syndrome who underwent carpal tunnel release 2 months ago yet has persistent disabling symptoms. Which of the following is **TRUE**?

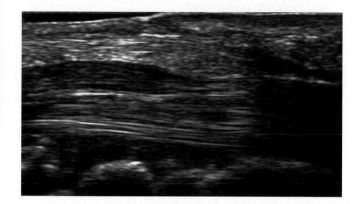

A. This is a normal finding after surgical carpal tunnel release.
B. The median nerve is scarred, so no further surgery is indicated.
C. There is persistent nerve compression, so repeat surgery is indicated to release the nerve.
D. A stump neuroma is present because the nerve was lacerated.
E. A neurofibroma was the initial cause of carpal tunnel syndrome symptoms.

**Q26.** According to evidence-based guidelines regarding the use of neuromuscular ultrasound in carpal tunnel syndrome (CTS), which statement is **CORRECT**?
A. Median nerve cross-sectional area is established as accurate for the diagnosis of CTS.
B. Median nerve echogenicity is established as accurate for the diagnosis of CTS.
C. Median nerve vascularity is established as accurate for the diagnosis of CTS.
D. When CTS is diagnosed by electrodiagnostic studies, additional ultrasound is not indicated.
E. All of the above

**Q27.** Which of the following ultrasound parameters is **NOT** commonly used to assess for median mononeuropathy at the wrist?
A. Median nerve cross-sectional area
B. Median nerve wrist-to-forearm ratio
C. Median nerve mobility
D. Median nerve echogenicity
E. Median nerve anisotropy

**Q28.** The following figure is of a short-axis view over the median nerve at the wrist with the patient extending their fingers. What is the hypoechoic structure marked by the star?

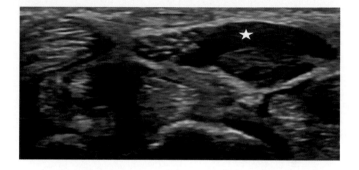

A. Ganglion cyst
B. Lumbrical muscle
C. Flexor digitorum superficialis muscle
D. "Reversed" palmaris longus muscle
E. Thrombosed persistent median artery

**Q29.** Which ultrasound finding suggests a schwannoma instead of a neurofibroma?
A. Positive on color Doppler
B. Cross-sectional area (CSA) >10 mm²
C. Eccentric location of the tumor in relationship to the nerve
D. Internal septations

**Q30.** In trauma, which is **CORRECT** about neuromuscular ultrasound?
A. Should be delayed a least a week to allow Wallerian degeneration to occur
B. Can be used to determine if the nerve is in continuity
C. Is useful in assessing the amount of axonal loss
D. Ideally used at the same time as electrodiagnostic studies

**Q31.** Which of the following are associated with hypertrophic nerves on ultrasound?
A. Chronic inflammatory demyelinating polyneuropathy (CIDP)
B. Multifocal motor neuropathy with conduction block (MMNCB)
C. Charcot-Marie-Tooth (CMT) type 1A
D. Leprosy
E. All of the above

**Q32.** Which of the following is **MOST SENSITIVE** in assessing for tongue fasciculations?
A. Clinical exam
B. Needle EMG: concentric needle
C. Needle EMG: monopolar needle
D. Ultrasound
E. Muscle impedance

**Q33.** The following are short-axis views of the tibialis anterior and extensor digitorum longus muscles adjacent to the tibia. (left, symptomatic side; right, asymptomatic side.)

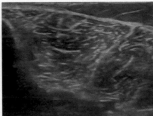

The above is most consistent with:

A. distal myopathy.
B. acute peroneal neuropathy.
C. chronic peroneal neuropathy.
D. S1 radiculopathy.
E. piriformis syndrome.

**Q34.** What is the classic ultrasound appearance of muscle in an autoimmune myositis?
A. "Moth-eaten" pattern
B. Increased muscle echogenicity with loss of bone shadows distally
C. Increased muscle echogenicity with retained bone shadows distally
D. Increased subcutaneous edema
E. Loss of fascial planes

**Q35.** The figure below is a view between the seventh and eight ribs. The arrow is pointing to:

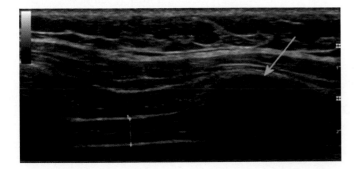

A. skin.
B. intercostal muscles.
C. rib.
D. diaphragm.
E. serratus anterior.

**Q36.** Which hemidiaphragm is easier to visualize in normal individuals?
A. Right
B. Left
C. No difference between left and right sides

**Q37.** Which is the optimal probe used to measure diaphragm thickness and the thickening ratio?
A. 15-MHz linear probe
B. 18-MHz hockey-stick probe
C. 6-MHz curvilinear probe

**Q38.** What is the best location to view the diaphragm between two ribs using ultrasound?
A. Anterior axillary line
B. Midaxillary line
C. Posterior axillary line
D. Midclavicular line
E. Subxiphoid

**Q39.** What is a normal diaphragm thickness at the end of expiration?
A. >1 mm
B. >2 mm
C. >5 mm
D. >10 mm
E. >1 cm

**Q40.** What is a normal thickening ratio of the diaphragm comparing end inspiration to end expiration?
A. >10%
B. >20%
C. >50%
D. >100%

**Q41.** Which is the optimal probe used to measure diaphragm excursion?
A. 15-MHz linear probe
B. 18-MHz hockey stick probe
C. 6-MHz curvilinear probe

**Q42.** Normal diaphragm excursion is normally greater on the left compared to the right.
A. TRUE
B. FALSE

**Q43.** How would you interpret this M-mode of the right hemidiaphragm?

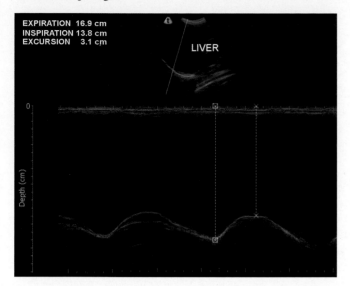

A. Normal
B. Reduced motion
C. Complete phrenic neuropathy
D. Poor patient cooperation
E. Paradoxical movement

**Q44.** How would you interpret this M-mode of the right hemidiaphragm?

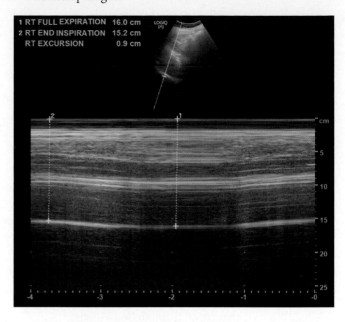

A. Normal
B. Reduced motion
C. Complete phrenic neuropathy
D. Poor patient cooperation
E. Paradoxical movement

## PART 2 | QUESTIONS WITH ANSWERS AND DISCUSSION

**QUESTION 1.** Which of the following is **TRUE** regarding the benefits and disadvantages of neuromuscular ultrasound?
A. Poorly tolerated
B. Muscle damage can occur with prolonged use.
C. Adds similar information to electrodiagnostic studies
D. Resolution is excellent, especially for deep structures.
E. Can dynamically assess nerves, muscles, and tendons

**ANSWER:** E. Can dynamically assess nerves, muscles, and tendons

**COMMENTS AND DISCUSSION**
- **Clinical benefits of neuromuscular ultrasound**
  ◦ Similar to electrodiagnostic studies, ultrasound can often localize lesions
  ◦ Adds anatomic, structural, and pathologic information that EDX studies cannot
  ◦ Painless and well tolerated
  ◦ Safe with no side effects
  ◦ Dynamic: one can visualize nerves, muscles, and tendons as a limb is moved either actively or passively to help understand the relationship between the nerves and muscles and their surrounding structures.
  ◦ Inexpensive
- **Clinical disadvantages of neuromuscular ultrasound**
  ◦ Cannot visualize behind bone.
  ◦ Resolution is poor for deep structures.
  ◦ Obese patients are difficult to image.
  ◦ Highly operator dependent

**QUESTION 2.** Which of the following is **MOST LIKELY** to occur when an ultrasound wave encounters a smooth boundary between two tissues with very different acoustic impedances?
A.  A bright echo is generated.
B.  Back scatter
C.  The ultrasound wave is absorbed as heat.
D.  Posterior acoustic shadowing
E.  Posterior acoustic enhancement

**ANSWER:** A. A bright echo is generated.

### COMMENTS AND DISCUSSION
- **Basic physics of ultrasound (U/S)**
  - Ultrasound literally means "beyond sound."
  - Sound is mechanical energy that is transmitted by longitudinal pressure waves within a medium.
  - Humans can hear sound with frequencies between 10 Hz and 20,000 Hz.
  - Most U/S probes have frequencies in the megahertz (million hertz) range between 2 MHz and 20 MHz.
  - U/S is based on piezoelectricity. Piezoelectric elements create sound waves when a voltage is applied to them. Thus they transform electrical energy into mechanical (sound) energy. However, they also do the opposite: when sound energy is absorbed into piezoelectric material, that energy is transformed into electrical energy.
  - When electricity is applied to piezoelectric elements in the U/S probe, sound waves are created that travel through body tissues.
  - In human tissue, sound travels at approximately 1540 m/s.
  - When a U/S wave travels through tissue, it can:
    - Continue and is eventually absorbed as heat (Fig. 11.1A), or
    - If the sound wave encounters an area where two tissues with different acoustic impedances lie adjacent to each other, echoes are created. These echoes are then transmitted back to the piezoelectric elements in the probe to be converted back to electrical energy.
  - The strength of the echo increases as the difference between the two acoustic impedances increases.
  - If the echoes are directed back toward the probe, they will reach the probe and can be recorded (Fig. 11.1B). By knowing the speed of the sound wave and measuring the time it takes for an echo to return after an U/S pulse is given, the distance (depth) of the tissue that created the echo can then be calculated. This information along intensity (brightness) of the returning echoes then is used to create the U/S image.
  - If the tissue is at an angle to the sound wave, it can reflect the echo back in a different direction and may never reach the probe (Fig. 11.1C).
  - If the boundary where the echo is created is irregular, echoes can scatter in many different directions. This back scattering results in "speckle" of the image, which can interfere with echoes of interest (Fig. 11.1D).

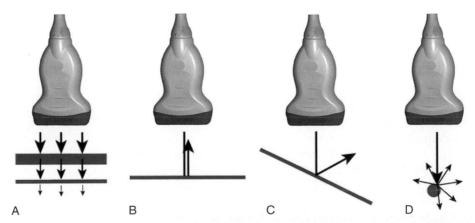

**Fig. 11.1  Echoes and attenuation.** When an ultrasound (U/S) wave travels through tissue, the energy may (A) continue and dissipate into heat; (B) create echoes, which reflect back if it encounters a boundary between two tissues that is perpendicular to the wave; (C) create echoes that reflect at an angle if the tissue is not perpendicular to the wave; and/or (D) scatter in many different directions if it reaches an irregular tissue interface. Adapted from Preston DC, Shapiro BE. *Electromyography and Neuromuscular Disorders.* 4th ed. Philadelphia, PA: Elsevier; 2020.

**HIGH-YIELD FACT**

The ultrasound probe is both the transmitter and receiver of ultrasound waves, with a much higher amount of time in the "listening" mode than in the sending mode.

**QUESTION 3.** Which of the following is the **MOST CORRECT** speed of sound in soft tissue?
   A. 12 m/s
   B. 330 m/s
   C. 550 m/s
   D. 1540 m/s
   E. 2500 m/s

**ANSWER:** D. 1540 m/s.

**COMMENTS AND DISCUSSION**
- Ultrasound waves pass through human tissue at ~1540 m/s.
- 330 m/s is the speed of sound.
- By knowing the speed of conduction through tissue, one can calculate the depth by measuring the time when the echo arrives back at the probe.

**QUESTION 4.** What is the **MOST COMMON** ultrasound image that displays anatomic information?
   A. A-mode
   B. B-mode
   C. M-mode

**ANSWER:** B. B-mode

**COMMENTS AND DISCUSSION**
- A-mode ultrasound (U/S) (Fig. 11.2)
   ○ One piezoelectric element that results in a single line of U/S is known as amplitude mode (A-mode).
   ○ In A-mode, each spike corresponds to an echo with the height of the spike corresponding to the strength of the echo, and the time of the spike correlating to the depth of the tissue that created the echo.

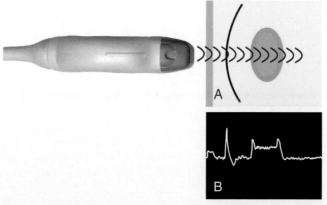

**Fig. 11.2 Amplitude mode (A-mode) ultrasound.** (A) Ultrasound transmitting a single pulse through a hypothetical structure that contains several different tissues. (B) The signal recorded from the returning echoes formed when the ultrasound pulse encountered a boundary between two different tissues. The fundamental building block of ultrasound is one piezoelectric element transmitting and recording information. This results in a single line of ultrasound information displayed on an oscilloscope, known as amplitude mode (A-mode) ultrasound. Each spike on the bottom figure corresponds to an echo. The height of the spike corresponds to the strength of the echo, and the time of the spike correlates to the depth of the tissue that created the echo. From Preston DC, Shapiro BE. *Electromyography and Neuromuscular Disorders.* 4th ed. Philadelphia, PA: Elsevier; 2020.

- **B-mode U/S (Fig. 11.3)**
   ○ U/S probes contain hundreds of piezoelectric elements that are arranged in a row.
   ○ Thus hundreds of individual lines of U/S information are recorded simultaneously, which can be stitched together digitally to create a grayscale image.

- This image is termed brightness mode (B-mode) U/S.
- The most common ultrasound image that displays anatomic information
- Areas that are bright are known as *hyperechoic*.
- Areas that are dark are *hypoechoic*.
- Complete absence of echoes resulting in complete blackness is termed *anechoic*.

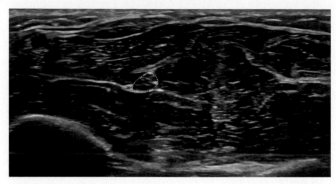

**Fig. 11.3 Brightness-mode (B-mode) ultrasound (U/S).** Standard B-mode image of the volar forearm. Hundreds of vertical lines of U/S information are digitally stitched together to create an image. From Preston DC, Shapiro BE. *Electromyography and Neuromuscular Disorders.* 4th ed. Philadelphia, PA: Elsevier; 2020.

- **M-mode U/S (Fig. 11.4)**
  - M-mode is the abbreviation for motion mode which utilizes A-mode and B-mode.
  - A standard B-mode image is displayed with a line (the index line) placed on the structure of interest.
  - At the same time, an A-mode signal is recorded from the index line.
  - The A-mode line is then recorded continuously over time to create the M-mode image.
  - M-mode is useful when assessing muscle movement over time. For example, a useful assessment of diaphragmatic function is to use M-mode to measure diaphragmatic excursion during inspiration and expiration.

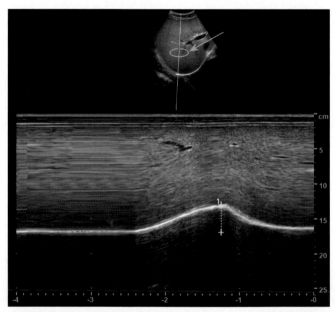

**Fig. 11.4 M-mode ultrasound (U/S).** M-mode combines A-mode and B-mode. The image on the top is a standard B-mode image of the liver. One specific index line of U/S is selected (line designated by the *green arrow*). That line of U/S (A-mode) is then recorded continuously over time. The bright line behind the liver is the echo created from the diaphragm (*red arrow*). In the M-mode trace below, note that the same line moves its position over time. This represents the excursion of the diaphragm with breathing. From Preston DC, Shapiro BE. *Electromyography and Neuromuscular Disorders.* 4th ed. Philadelphia, PA: Elsevier; 2020.

**QUESTION 5.** Using color flow Doppler, the goal is to have the probe perpendicular to the blood vessel.
  A. TRUE
  B. FALSE

**ANSWER:** B. FALSE.

## COMMENTS AND DISCUSSION

- **Doppler ultrasound (U/S) (Fig. 11.5)**
  - ○ The Doppler effect occurs when a source that is producing sound moves toward a receiver, resulting in the sound waves being compressed and an increase in frequency.
  - ○ Conversely, as the source that produces sound moves away from the receiver, the frequency decreases.
  - ○ U/S takes advantage of the Doppler effect in the assessment of moving tissues, especially flowing blood.
  - ○ When a Doppler signal is present (or positive), red indicates that the source of the sound is moving toward the probe, and blue that it is moving away (these scans are known as color Doppler).
  - ○ Blood flow in arteries is usually well seen on color Doppler, whereas blood flow in veins is typically not seen unless the amount of flow is substantial.
  - ○ For a Doppler signal to be present, the probe must be at least partially directed at an angle to the flow of the blood. If the probe is positioned at 90° to the direction of flow, there will be no Doppler effect. The probe must be tilted either toward or away from the vessel to see blood flow.
  - ○ In addition to normal blood vessels, Doppler signals are often associated with increased blood flow that occurs with:
    - Neoplastic tissue
    - Infection
    - Inflammation

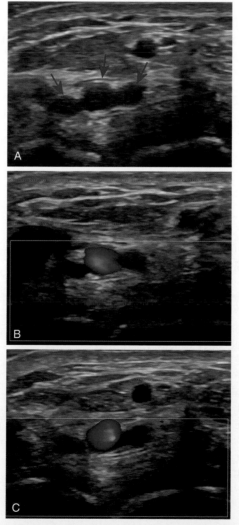

**Fig. 11.5 Color Doppler. Short-axis images of the lateral wrist, radial artery, and veins.** (A) Standard B-mode image shows three adjacent round hypoechoic structures. The radial artery is in the middle (*red arrow*) with two accompanying veins (*blue arrows*). (B) Color Doppler with the probe tilted slightly proximal. Blood flowing toward the probe results in a red signal in the artery. (C) Color Doppler with the probe tilted slightly distal. The same blood flow in the artery is now blue, indicating that the blood is now flowing away from the probe. Most veins are not positive on Doppler, as the amount and speed of the blood is too low. From Preston DC, Shapiro BE. *Electromyography and Neuromuscular Disorders.* 4th ed. Philadelphia, PA: Elsevier; 2020.

**QUESTION 6.** Power Doppler is **MOST SENSITIVE** in looking at what structure?
   A. Nerve
   B. Tendon
   C. Muscle
   D. Blood vessels
   E. Bone

**ANSWER:** D. Blood vessels

**COMMENTS AND DISCUSSION**
- A variation of color Doppler is power Doppler:
   o Power Doppler is very sensitive to the presence of movement of red blood cells.
   o It is not direction or angle specific.
   o It is particularly useful for small arteries and those vessels with low-velocity flow.
   o Power Doppler displays a characteristic deep orange color on imaging.

**QUESTION 7.** The advantage of power Doppler is that it can pick up the direction of flow.
   A. TRUE
   B. FALSE

**ANSWER:** B. FALSE

**COMMENTS AND DISCUSSION**
- The advantage of power Doppler is that it is very sensitive to the presence of blood flow and is not dependent on the angle or speed of the flow.

**QUESTION 8.** What is the probe frequency used for most musculoskeletal (MSK) and neuromuscular ultrasound?
   A. 70 MHz
   B. 15 MHz
   C. 5 MHz
   D. 1 MHz
   E. 100 KHz

**ANSWER:** B. 15 MHz

**COMMENTS AND DISCUSSION**
- Ultrasound probes and frequencies (Fig. 11.6)
   o Several types of probes are used in neuromuscular ultrasound.
      - Linear probe
         - Most common
         - Creates a rectangular image
         - Upper range of frequency usually 15–18 MHz
      - "Hockey-stick" probe
         - Small footprint
         - Creates a rectangular image
         - Useful for small structures (e.g., digits) or around bony surfaces
         - Upper range of frequency usually higher than standard linear probes
      - Curvilinear probe
         - Generates a sector image (like a piece of pie)
         - Much lower frequencies (typically in the 2–5 MHz range)
         - Useful when studying very deep structures, such as the sciatic nerve at the gluteal fold, and especially the diaphragm behind the liver

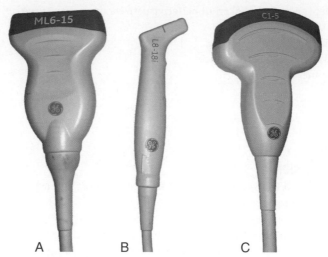

**Fig. 11.6 Ultrasound probes.** (A) Linear probe. (B) High-frequency "hockey-stick" probe. (C) Curvilinear probe. From Preston DC, Shapiro BE. *Electromyography and Neuromuscular Disorders.* 4th ed. Philadelphia, PA: Elsevier; 2020.

- Probe frequencies: pros and cons (Fig. 11.7)
  - High frequency
    - Improved resolution
    - Decreased penetration
    - Optimal for structures within a few centimeters from the surface
  - Low frequency
    - Decreased resolution
    - Increased penetration
    - Optimal for structures which are very deep (e.g., this is the standard probe for obstetric and abdominal ultrasound)

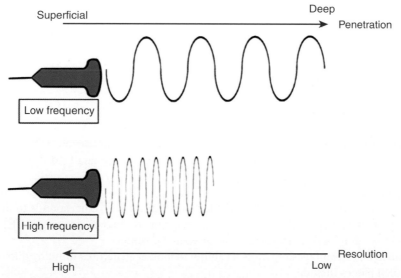

**Fig. 11.7** Low-frequency probe projects the low-frequency wavelength, which results in a deeper penetration but also decreased resolution. This is in contrast to the high-frequency probe that has better resolution but has more superficial penetration.

## ◎ HIGH-YIELD FACT

The higher the frequency the better the resolution, but the trade-off is less penetration.

**QUESTION 9.** What step(s) could be taken to better visualize a deep structure?
A. Utilize less transmission gel.
B. Increase the gain.
C. Change to a lower frequency transducer.
D. Raise the focal zone.
E. B and C
F. C and D

**ANSWER:** E. B and C

**COMMENTS AND DISCUSSION**
- Optimizing the ultrasound (U/S) image. There are several choices and adjustments that need to be done to optimize the U/S image, including:
    - Choose the correct probe.
    - Gel must be used in a sufficient amount between the probe and the skin. Any air needs to be eliminated between the probe and the skin. The probe should be held lightly against the skin, as too much pressure will displace the underlying gel.
    - The correct depth is set. If the depth is set too deep, much of the image will be taken up by black areas below the area of interest where the U/S beam has been completely attenuated. If the depth is set too shallow, one may unintentionally cut off part of the object of interest and its surrounding structures below.
    - Adjust the focus. Similar to a camera, the U/S machine can focus the sound waves at a particular depth, called the focal depth, to best see images at that depth.
    - Adjust the brightness. The brightness setting does not change the power of the U/S waves sent out but amplifies the returning echoes. The brightness setting should be adjusted so that the image is neither washed out nor too dark such that important details cannot be seen.
    - Adjust the frequency. The highest frequency will result in the best resolution. However, the higher the frequency, the more attenuation of the U/S beam as it moves deeper. If deeper structures are not well seen, one should either change the probe to a lower frequency probe or lower the frequency of the probe being used until the deeper structures of interest are well seen.
    - Normally the ultrasound beam becomes attenuated as it travels deeper. Increasing the gain may allow better utilization of deep structures. Likewise, higher frequencies are associated with less penetration. Thus decreasing the frequency will aid in better visualizing deeper structures. It is also important to adjust the focal zone to the area of interest (however, for deeper structures, the focal zone would be adjusted down).
- Image orientation (Fig. 11.8)
    - Short axis (also known as transverse)
    - Long axis (also known as longitudinal)
    - Oblique is any orientation between transverse and longitudinal
    - Orientation convention
        - For all long-axis views, the left side of the screen is always cephalad (toward the head).
        - For short-axis views, the left side of the screen is either:
            - Lateral, or
            - Most common convention is that the left side of the screen corresponds to the right side of the patient, similar to the convention for magnetic resonance imaging (MRI) and computerized tomography (CT) scans (i.e., the anatomic position)
    - One of the major advantages of U/S is its ability to look at structures in many different planes. The conventional planes include:
        - Axial
        - Sagittal
        - Coronal
    - When assessing a finding on U/S, it is good practice to image that structure in two different planes.

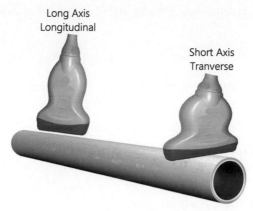

**Fig. 11.8 Short axis versus long axis orientation.** Images can also be designated by whether one is looking at the short or long axis of a structure. The short axis is also known as transverse, while the long axis is referred to as the longitudinal axis. From Preston DC, Shapiro BE. *Electromyography and Neuromuscular Disorders.* 4th ed. Philadelphia, PA: Elsevier; 2020.

**QUESTION 10.** What structure has a "honeycomb" ultrasound appearance on short axis?
  A. Nerve
  B. Tendon
  C. Muscle
  D. Blood vessels
  E. Bone

**ANSWER:** A. Nerve

**COMMENTS AND DISCUSSION**
- There are several normal tissues to recognize on neuromuscular ultrasound. Each has a specific shape, echogenicity, and pattern, in addition to other characteristics.
  - Peripheral nerve (Fig. 11.9)
    - Short axis:
      - Round or oval
      - "Honeycomb" appearance
      - Fascicles are hypoechoic
      - Epineurium is hyperechoic
      - Perineurium is hyperechoic
    - Long axis:
      - Bright epineurium is seen on the periphery of the nerve (above and below the nerve).
      - Bright parallel lines inside, which represent the perineurium

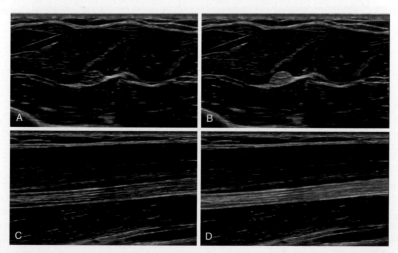

**Fig. 11.9 Ultrasound (U/S) of nerve. Median nerve in the forearm.** (A, B) Short axis. (C, D) Long axis. Same images on the right with the nerve highlighted in yellow. On short axis, nerve has a characteristic "honeycomb pattern" with the fascicles being dark and the perineurium and epineurium being bright. When the probe is oriented in long axis, the bright epineurium forms the border of the nerve above and below, while bright parallel lines run inside the nerve, which represent the layers of perineurium. From Preston DC, Shapiro BE. *Electromyography and Neuromuscular Disorders.* 4th ed. Philadelphia, PA: Elsevier; 2020.

**QUESTION 11.** What normal structure has a "starry night" ultrasound appearance on short axis?
  A. Nerve
  B. Tendon
  C. Muscle
  D. Blood vessels
  E. Bone

**ANSWER:** C. Muscle

**COMMENTS AND DISCUSSION**
- Muscle (Fig. 11.10)
  - Short axis:
    - Pattern of connective tissue is similar to nerve.
    - Individual muscle fibers packaged into fascicles are hypoechoic.
    - Perimysium and epimysium are hyperechoic.
    - Epimysium blends with the fascia over the muscle.
    - "Starry night" appearance
  - Long axis:
    - Series of linear echoes, each representing the parallel lines of connective tissue
    - If the muscle fascicles attach to an aponeurosis or central tendon, a "pennate" or feather-like pattern will be seen.
    - Muscles may have one or more internal tendons.

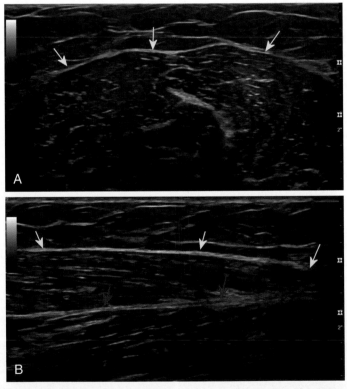

**Fig. 11.10 Ultrasound of muscle. Flexor carpi radialis.** (A) Short axis. (B) Long axis. Muscle has a classic "starry night" appearance on short axis. The actual muscle fibers are dark, with the connective tissue of the perimysium and epimysium being bright. On longitudinal images, a series of linear echoes are seen, each representing the parallel lines of connective tissue. If the muscle fascicles attach to an aponeurosis or central tendon at an angle (*red arrows*), a pennate or feather like pattern is created. The epimysium often blends with the fascia (*yellow arrows*). From Preston DC, Shapiro BE. *Electromyography and Neuromuscular Disorders.* 4th ed. Philadelphia, PA: Elsevier; 2020.

- Tendon (Fig. 11.11)
  - Tendons connect muscle to bone.
  - Each tendon has an origin and insertion.
    - The origin tends to be proximal and attaches to bone, which is more stable in position when the muscle contracts.
    - The insertion tends to be distal, and on a bone that moves with muscle contraction.
  - Made of collagen fibers that are highly packed together
  - Short axis
    - Hyperechoic, highly compact and fibrillar
    - Sometimes mistaken for nerve
    - Distinguished from nerve, as tendons do not have a honeycomb pattern and are more densely packed.
    - Tendons have prominent anisotropy (Fig. 11.11).

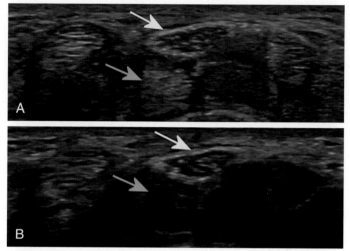

**Fig. 11.11 Tendon.** Axial scan of the median nerve at the wrist (*yellow arrows*). Tendons appear as highly compact fibrillar bundles (A, *green arrow*). On axial scans, they can sometimes be mistaken for nerve. However, unlike nerve, they do not have a honeycomb pattern, and are more densely packed. In addition, they demonstrate more prominent anisotropy than nerve. When the ultrasound probe is slightly rocked, the tendons become hypoechoic, due to anisotropy (B, *green arrow*). From Preston DC, Shapiro BE. *Electromyography and Neuromuscular Disorders.* 4th ed. Philadelphia, PA: Elsevier; 2020.

## ◎ HIGH-YIELD FACT

Assessing the amount of anisotropy is one of the key ways to differentiate tendons from nerves with tendons having very high anisotropy.

**QUESTION 12.** What it is the **BEST** way to identify veins?
- A. Compressibility
- B. Power Doppler
- C. Color Doppler
- D. Posterior acoustic shadowing
- E. Depth

**ANSWER:** A. Compressibility

## COMMENTS AND DISCUSSION

- Arteries and veins
  - Arteries and veins superficially look similar. Both are round and hypoechoic.
  - On ultrasound, arteries are:
    - Not easily compressible with probe pressure

- Are much more likely to be positive on color Doppler imaging as blood is under pressure and traveling at a higher speed than venous blood. When the probe is pointed toward an artery, the flowing blood will be red on color Doppler; when it is pointing away, it will be blue.
  - On ultrasound, veins are:
    - Associated with thinner walls then arteries
    - Less commonly positive on color Doppler unless the vein is large and/or proximal
    - May have one-way valves. These may be visible within veins when using high-frequency probes. Valves can be seen as very delicate structures, often present within slightly bulbous enlargements of a vein.
    - Commonly larger than arteries if there is a paired artery and vein. However, another common pattern is one artery surrounded by two and sometimes three smaller veins.
    - Easily compressible. If the probe is pushed down on the vein and then released, it will create a characteristic picture of the vein "blinking at you." (Fig. 11.12)

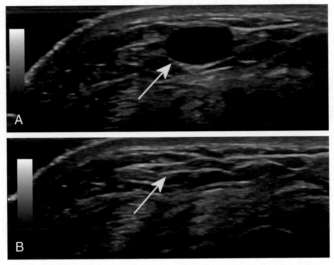

**Fig. 11.12  Vein.** Cephalic vein at the wrist, short-axis image (A, *yellow arrow*). On ultrasound, veins are recognized as circular or oval structures that are anechoic. One of the best ways to determine if the structure is a vein is to see if it is compressible with probe pressure. Most veins are easily compressible (B, *yellow arrow*). From Preston DC, Shapiro BE. *Electromyography and Neuromuscular Disorders.* 4th ed. Philadelphia, PA: Elsevier; 2020.

 **HIGH-YIELD FACT**

> Easy compressibility with minimal probe pressure is characteristic of veins. Lack of compressibility in a known vein usually indicates intraluminal clot.

**QUESTION 13.** How can you distinguish muscle from adipose tissue using B-mode ultrasound?
 A. Utilize power Doppler to determine the more metabolically active tissue.
 B. Induce anisotropy with the "heel-toe" technique.
 C. Use a higher frequency transducer.
 D. Image in axial and longitudinal view.

**ANSWER:** D. Image in axial and longitudinal view.

**COMMENTS AND DISCUSSION**
- Skin and subcutaneous tissue (Fig. 11.13)
  - Skin is seen as:
    - A thin line just under the surface
    - Slightly hyperechoic
  - Subcutaneous tissue has the following ultrasound characteristics:
    - Immediately below the skin
    - Above the muscle

- Predominantly adipose tissue, which is hypoechoic (dark)
- Has prominent connective tissue septa that run in it
- The amount of subcutaneous tissue can be quite excessive in obese patients, rendering the tissue of interest so deep that it makes ultrasound much more challenging and sometimes not possible.
- Sometimes, subcutaneous tissue can be mistaken for muscle tissue. Both can be hypoechoic with hyperechoic septi running inside them. The easiest way to separate them is to turn the probe 90°. When one is on subcutaneous tissue, the appearance will be rather similar in short and long axis. However, muscle is distinctly different. In short axis, muscle has a "starry night" appearance, whereas it has a fibular or pennate appearance on long axis.

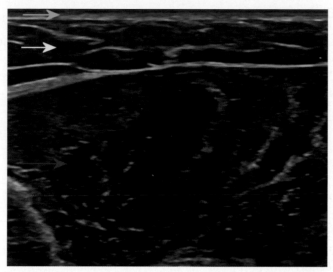

**Fig. 11.13 Axial image of the upper arm.** The skin is seen as a thin line, somewhat hyperechoic, near the surface of the image (*green arrow*). Immediately below the skin is subcutaneous tissue (*yellow arrow*). Most of the subcutaneous tissue is adipose, which is hypoechoic. Note that there are prominent connective tissue septa that run in the adipose tissue. Below the adipose tissue is muscle (*red arrow*), which has a classic "starry night" appearance. From Preston DC, Shapiro BE. *Electromyography and Neuromuscular Disorders.* 4th ed. Philadelphia, PA: Elsevier; 2020.

**QUESTION 14.** The cartilage type of the elbow joint and its ultrasound appearance are:
   A. Hyaline and hypoechoic on ultrasound.
   B. Hyaline and hyperechoic on ultrasound.
   C. Fibrous and hypoechoic on ultrasound.
   D. Fibrous and hyperechoic on ultrasound.

**ANSWER:** A. hyaline and hypoechoic on ultrasound

##  HIGH-YIELD FACT

Subcutaneous tissue can be mistaken for muscle. One easy way to identify subcutaneous tissue is to turn the probe 90 degrees—the pattern will be unchanged. If it is muscle, turning the probe 90 degrees results in a marked change—from a "starry night" appearance on the short axis to a "feather" or pennate appearance on the long axis.

## COMMENTS AND DISCUSSION
- Cartilage
  - Two types of cartilage:
    - Fibrocartilage
      - Composed of fibrous tissue (collagen)

- Densely packed and hyperechoic
- Extremely strong
- Found in joints (e.g., the triangular fibrocartilage complex in the radial-ulnar-carpal joint), and in other locations where the strength of the fibrocartilage is needed (e.g., the annulus fibrosis of the intervertebral discs, the pubis symphysis).
  - Hyaline cartilage
    - Commonly seen during neuromuscular ultrasound
    - Smooth and translucent
    - Present between most joints
    - Hypoechoic and has a characteristic wavy appearance
- Bone
  - Extremely rigid and strong
  - Easy to recognize on ultrasound
    - Very bright (hyperechoic) line and reflects the ultrasound wave back completely
    - Creates a black void below, called posterior acoustic shadowing (see also comemnts and discussion from Question 16)

**QUESTION 15.** What structure has the greatest amount of anisotropy?
A. Nerve
B. Tendon
C. Muscle
D. Blood vessels
E. Bone

**ANSWER:** B. Tendon

**COMMENTS AND DISCUSSION**
- There are many artifacts that can be encountered during ultrasound. However, they can be used to advantage to help identify both normal tissues and various pathology. The most important artifacts are the following:
  - Anisotropy (Fig. 11.14)
    - Most common artifact
    - When a sound wave encounters an acoustic barrier at 90°, the sound wave will bounce back as an echo.
    - If the sound wave is not perpendicular to the barrier, the echoes will be directed back at an angle, and only some of the echoes will reach the probe.
    - If the angle is great enough, no echoes may ever return to the probe.
    - Thus by slightly rocking the probe, the echoes will be very bright when the probe is at 90% and very dark when the probe is not.
    - This property of tissue, whereby the echoes that bounce back to the probe are dependent on the angle at which they hit the tissue, is known as anisotropy.
    - The amount of anisotropy varies among tissues. In tissues with high anisotropy, normally bright echoes will become increasing dark (hypoechoic) as the probe is tilted away from 90°. Conversely, tissues with low anisotropy will not change much in terms of brightness as the probe is tilted.
    - Anisotropy is most helpful in identifying tendons, which display high anisotropy. Indeed, one of the best ways to help confirm that a structure is tendon versus nerve is to assess the amount of anisotropy (tendon: high anisotropy; nerve: low anisotropy).

## ◎ HIGH-YIELD FACT

To assess for anisotropy, tilt the probe repetitively along the probe's long axis (rocking the probe) or along its short axis (heel-toe maneuver).

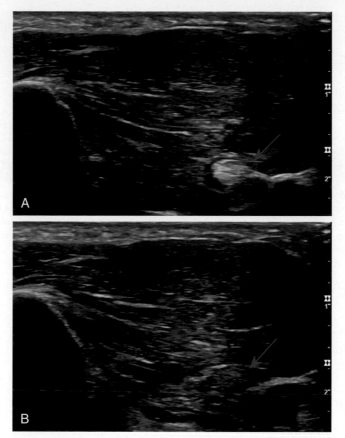

**Fig. 11.14 Anisotropy. Axial image, thenar eminence. The *red arrow* points to the tendon of the flexor pollicis longus.** (A) The ultrasound probe is perpendicular to the tendon. With the probe in this position, the tendon is bright and highly compact. (B) As the ultrasound probe is tilted slightly, the tendon becomes very dark, due to anisotropy. Although anisotropy is an "artifact," it is very useful to identify certain tissues, including tendon, which has high anisotropy. From Preston DC, Shapiro BE. *Electromyography and Neuromuscular Disorders.* 4th ed. Philadelphia, PA: Elsevier; 2020.

**QUESTION 16.** Posterior acoustic shadowing is **MOST LIKELY** to be seen associated with what type of tissue?
   A. Cartilage
   B. Bone
   C. Muscle
   D. Fat
   E. Blood vessels

**ANSWER:** B. Bone

**COMMENTS AND DISCUSSION**
- Posterior acoustic shadowing (Fig. 11.15)
   ○ Some structures are so dense that ultrasound cannot penetrate them.
   ○ A black void then occurs below that structure.
   ○ Most commonly seen with bone, other calcified lesions, surgical hardware, and foreign objects.

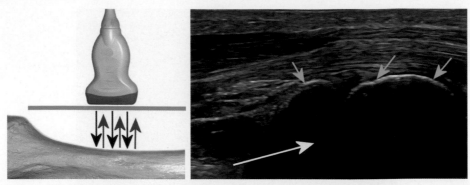

**Fig. 11.15 Posterior acoustic shadowing. Longitudinal image of the radiocarpal joint.** When ultrasound encounters a very dense tissue, it creates very bright echoes (*green arrows*). However, ultrasound energy cannot go beyond that point. When this occurs, there will be a black void below that structure (*yellow arrow*). This is most commonly seen with bone, but occurs with other calcified lesions (e.g., dystrophic calcium in tendons), surgical hardware, and foreign objects. From Preston DC, Shapiro BE. *Electromyography and Neuromuscular Disorders.* 4th ed. Philadelphia, PA: Elsevier; 2020.

**QUESTION 17.** Posterior acoustic enhancement is most likely to be seen associated with what type of tissue?
  A. Cartilage
  B. Bone
  C. Muscle
  D. Fat
  E. Blood vessels

**ANSWER:** E. Blood vessels

**COMMENTS AND DISCUSSION**
- Posterior acoustic enhancement (Fig. 11.16)
  ○ Bright echoes are seen below another structure, which is typically hypoechoic or anechoic.
  ○ Occurs because the ultrasound machine adjusts the amplified intensity of the echo depending on the depth of the echo.
  ○ In normal tissue, the strength of the ultrasound wave normally attenuates as it travels through tissue. The software counteracts this by incrementally increasing the brightness of echoes from superficial to deeper areas to create a uniform image. If this adjustment was not done, a normal ultrasound image would get progressively darker as the depth increased.
  ○ If the ultrasound wave travels through a tissue that does not attenuate the signal as much as would be expected (such as fluid), the returning echoes are brighter than expected.
  ○ Most commonly seen with cystic lesions but also seen under some arteries and veins, and can also be seen with nerve sheath and other tumors

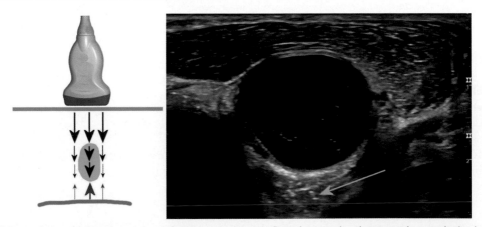

**Fig. 11.16 Posterior acoustic enhancement.** Ganglion cyst, short axis. Posterior acoustic enhancement is recognized as bright echoes below another structure (that structure is typically hypoechoic or anechoic). This occurs when the ultrasound wave travels through a tissue with very low attenuation (most commonly fluid). Because the ultrasound machine adjusts the amplified intensity of the echo depending on the depth of the echo, the signal below that area is stronger than expected. This occurs most commonly with cystic lesions. It also occurs with normal fluid-filled structures, like arteries and veins, and can also occur with nerve sheath and some other tumors. From Preston DC, Shapiro BE. *Electromyography and Neuromuscular Disorders.* 4th ed. Philadelphia, PA: Elsevier; 2020.

**QUESTION 18.** Reverberation artifact is most likely to be seen associated with what type of tissue?
A. Needle
B. Bone
C. Muscle
D. Fat
E. Blood vessels

**ANSWER:** A. Needle

**COMMENTS AND DISCUSSION**
- Reverberation artifact (Fig. 11.17)
  - When an ultrasound wave encounters two strong reflectors, echoes can bounce back and forth between the two reflectors.
  - Creates a pattern of repeating parallel lines that are separated by the same interval as the echo immediately above. As one goes deeper, there is decreasing intensity of the echoes.
  - Often seen with needles that are extremely smooth, uniform, and dense. Although it can also be seen with some normal tissues, especially bone, it is highly characteristic of metallic substances, among them surgical plates and screws.
  - If the reflector is small, a similar artifact results, which takes on a "comet tail" appearance. This can occur with
    - Gas bubbles
    - Crystalline deposits
    - Staples
    - Sutures
    - Surgical clips
  - Obscures the visualization of the tissues below the reflector. However, the tissues between the probe and the reflector are not affected.

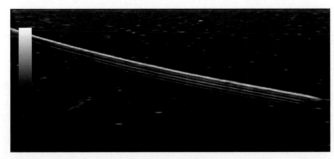

**Fig. 11.17  Reverberation artifact.** Long-axis view of a needle. When an ultrasound wave encounters two strong reflectors along the same path, echoes can bounce back and forth between the two reflectors. This creates a pattern of repeating parallel lines that are separated by the same interval as the echo immediately above. As one goes deeper, there is a decreasing intensity of the echoes. This most classically happens with needles. However, it can occur with some normal tissues, especially bone. It is also highly characteristic of metallic substances such as surgical plates and screws. From Preston DC, Shapiro BE. *Electromyography and Neuromuscular Disorders.* 4th ed. Philadelphia, PA: Elsevier; 2020.

**QUESTION 19.** Adjusting the angle of insonation of the transducer has the greatest value in assessing which of the following tissue properties?
A. Anisotropy
B. Thickness
C. Depth
D. Stiffness
E. Acoustic impedance

**ANSWER:** A. Anisotropy

## COMMENTS AND DISCUSSION

- Anisotropy is the property of tissue, where the ultrasound beam markedly attenuates when the probe is not at 90 degrees to the tissue being studied.
- Assessment of anisotropy is dependent on the angle of insonation.

**QUESTION 20.** Entrapment neuropathies are the most common indication for neuromuscular ultrasound.
- A. TRUE
- B. FALSE

**ANSWER:** A. TRUE

## COMMENTS AND DISCUSSION

- Entrapment neuropathies are the most common indication for neuromuscular ultrasound.
  - Useful in common entrapments, especially:
    - Carpal tunnel syndrome (Fig. 11.18)
    - Ulnar neuropathy at the elbow
    - Peroneal neuropathy at the fibular neck
  - Also useful in uncommon and controversial syndromes, especially:
    - Posterior interosseous neuropathy
    - Radial tunnel syndrome
    - Tarsal tunnel syndrome
    - Pronator syndrome and other high median neuropathies

## ◎ HIGH-YIELD FACT

Based on consistent Class I and Class II evidence, neuromuscular ultrasound measurement of median nerve cross-sectional area (CSA) at the wrist is established as accurate for the diagnosis of carpal tunnel syndrome (CTS). If available, neuromuscular ultrasound measurement of median nerve CSA at the wrist may be offered as an accurate diagnostic test for CTS (Level A).

- Ultrasound may be able to localize some mononeuropathies that electrodiagnostic studies cannot.
- Most frequent findings on ultrasound in an entrapment neuropathy include:
  - Increased cross-sectional area (CSA)
  - Increased ratio of CSA at the entrapment site compared to nerve segments proximally and/or distally
  - Decreased echogenicity
  - Loss of normal fascicular architecture
  - Decreased mobility

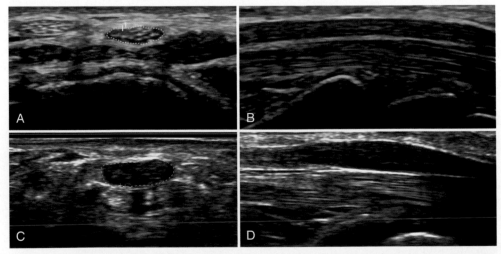

**Fig. 11.18 Entrapment neuropathy. When nerves are entrapped, they tend to swell proximal to the site of entrapment.** (A, C) Median nerve in short axis at the wrist. (B, D) Median nerve in long axis at the wrist. (A, B) from a normal patient. (C, D) from a patient with carpal tunnel syndrome. Note in the bottom pictures that the nerve is enlarged, hypoechoic (darker), and that the fascicular architecture has been lost. From Preston DC, Shapiro BE. *Electromyography and Neuromuscular Disorders.* 4th ed. Philadelphia, PA: Elsevier; 2020.

**QUESTION 21.** The following figure is a short-axis view over the median nerve at the wrist in a patient with symptoms of carpal tunnel syndrome (CTS). What is the large structure to the left of the median nerve?

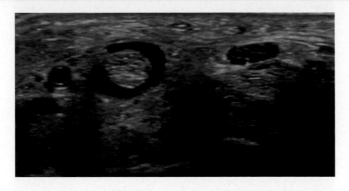

A. An enlarged flexor digitorum superficialis (FDS) muscle
B. A normal median nerve
C. An occluded radial artery
D. A bifid median nerve
E. Tenosynovitis of the flexor carpi radialis (FCR) tendon

**ANSWER:** E. Tenosynovitis of the flexor carpi radialis (FCR) tendon

**COMMENTS AND DISCUSSION**
- The median nerve is seen in the upper right of the image.
- The fascicles are hypoechoic.
- To the left is the highly fibular appearance of the flexor carpi radialis tendon.
- There is an anechoic near-complete ring around that tendon sheath, which also displays posterior acoustic enhancement below.
- This is fluid in the tendon sheath, which is ultrasound evidence of tenosynovitis (Fig. 11.19).
- Ultrasound can assess for associated anomalies and structural lesions (which may be causative), especially:
  - Anomalous muscles
  - Anomalous and congenitally persistent blood vessels
  - Ganglion and synovial cysts, extraneural
  - Ganglion cyst, intraneural (especially for peroneal neuropathy)
  - Tenosynovitis
  - Bone spurs and increased callus
  - Aneurysms
  - Varices
  - Tumors (both benign and malignant)
  - Infiltration (e.g., amyloid)
  - Can also assess muscles for denervation atrophy (Fig. 11.22) and help determine which nerve is likely abnormal, based on the pattern of muscle involvement

 **HIGH-YIELD FACT**

Based on Class II evidence, neuromuscular ultrasound (U/S) of the wrist probably adds value to electrodiagnostic studies when assessing carpal tunnel syndrome (CTS), as it can detect structural abnormalities. If available, neuromuscular U/S should be considered as a screening test for structural abnormalities at the wrist in CTS (Level B).

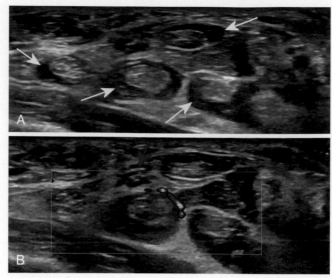

**Fig. 11.19  Tenosynovitis.** (A) Short-axis view of the flexor tendons just proximal to the carpal tunnel. Note that several tendon sheaths are surrounded by tissue with mixed echogenicity (*yellow arrows*), which is synovial hypertrophy. (B) Same image with color Doppler and the *red arrow* pointing to the median nerve. Note the increased vascularity around one of the tendon sheaths. In this case, the tissue surrounding the tendons is synovial hypertrophy. The area that is positive on Doppler indicates active disease. From Preston DC, Shapiro BE. *Electromyography and Neuromuscular Disorders.* 4th ed. Philadelphia, PA: Elsevier; 2020.

**QUESTION 22.** In patients with common peroneal neuropathy and no obvious injury or risk factor, which of the following lesions is most likely to be detected using ultrasound?
- A. Baker's cyst
- B. Popliteal artery aneurysm
- C. Intraneural ganglion
- D. Fracture of the fibular neck
- E. Tendinosis of the biceps femoris

**ANSWER:** C. Intraneural ganglion

**COMMENTS AND DISCUSSION**
- Common peroneal neuropathy at the fibular neck is common with many known risk factors including external compression from habitual leg crossing, immobilization from anesthesia, weight loss, diabetes, and prolonged squatting, among others.
- In addition, the peroneal nerve is susceptible to injury from trauma especially anterior knee dislocation.
- However, if a patient presents with a peroneal neuropathy with no obvious cause or risk factors, ultrasound has demonstrated an intraneural ganglion as the cause in 18% of the cases.

 **HIGH-YIELD FACT**

When patients with peroneal (fibular) neuropathy present without any identifiable risk factors or clear etiology, ultrasound diagnosis reveals that 18% have an intraneural ganglion (a surgically correctable condition).

**QUESTION 23.** Which of the following is a common ultrasound finding in carpal tunnel syndrome?
- A. Increased nerve mobility
- B. Decreased cross-sectional area (CSA)
- C. Wrist/forearm median nerve CSA ratio >1.4
- D. Decreased outlet ratio
- E. Ulnar/median nerve CSA ratio >1.4

**ANSWER:** C. Wrist/forearm median nerve CSA ratio >1.4

## COMMENTS AND DISCUSSION

- In entrapment neuropathies, the CSA of the nerve increases adjacent to the entrapment site along with a decrease of echogenicity and a loss of fascicular structure.
- One sensitive way of detecting an enlarged CSA is to compare a segment of nerve distally or proximally to the nerve adjacent to the entrapment site.
- In carpal tunnel syndrome, a wrist/forearm median nerve cross-sectional area greater than 1.4 is a very sensitive measure for the presence of carpal tunnel syndrome by ultrasound.

**QUESTION 24.** In carpal tunnel syndrome, the median nerve fascicular echogenicity is best described as:
 A. increased when imaged deep to the transverse carpal ligament.
 B. decreased when imaged just proximal to the transverse carpal ligament.
 C. increased in the presence of tenosynovitis.
 D. highly correlated to conduction block.
 E. decreased in the forearm.

**ANSWER:** B. decreased when imaged just proximal to the transverse carpal ligament.

## COMMENTS AND DISCUSSION

- In entrapment neuropathies, nerves swell and become more hypoechoic (darker).
- Thus, in carpal tunnel syndrome, just proximal to the transverse carpal ligament (the entrapment site), the nerve becomes hypoechoic.

**QUESTION 25.** The image below is a long-axis view of the median nerve at the wrist of a patient with carpal tunnel syndrome who underwent carpal tunnel release 2 months ago yet has persistent disabling symptoms. Which of the following is **TRUE**?

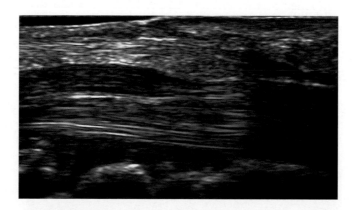

 A. This is a normal finding after surgical carpal tunnel release.
 B. The median nerve is scarred, so no further surgery is indicated.
 C. There is persistent nerve compression, so repeat surgery is indicated to release the nerve.
 D. A stump neuroma is present because the nerve was lacerated.
 E. A neurofibroma was the initial cause of carpal tunnel syndrome symptoms.

**ANSWER:** C. There is persistent nerve compression, so repeat surgery is indicated to release the nerve.

## COMMENTS AND DISCUSSION

- The ultrasound image shows an enlarged and hypoechoic median nerve (on the left), which then narrows in the center of the image.
- The nerve then becomes slightly larger past this constricted point.
- This "hourglass" constriction, also known as a "notch sign," is a finding consistent with ongoing entrapment neuropathy.
- In this case, the nerve was not completely released and repeat surgery is indicated.

**QUESTION 26.** According to evidence-based guidelines regarding the use of neuromuscular ultrasound in carpal tunnel syndrome (CTS), which statement is **CORRECT**?
A. Median nerve cross-sectional area is established as accurate for the diagnosis of CTS.
B. Median nerve echogenicity is established as accurate for the diagnosis of CTS.
C. Median nerve vascularity is established as accurate for the diagnosis of CTS.
D. When CTS is diagnosed by electrodiagnostic studies, additional ultrasound is not indicated.
E. All of the above

**ANSWER:** A. Median nerve cross-sectional area is established as accurate for the diagnosis of CTS.

**COMMENTS AND DISCUSSION**
- The American Association of Neuromuscular and Electrodiagnostic Medicine (AANEM) published evidence-based guidelines regarding the use of neuromuscular ultrasound in carpal tunnel syndrome.
- The most important conclusion was the following: median nerve cross-sectional area is established as accurate for the diagnosis of carpal tunnel syndrome (Level A).

**QUESTION 27.** Which of the following ultrasound parameters is **NOT** commonly used to assess for median mononeuropathy at the wrist?
A. Median nerve cross-sectional area
B. Median nerve wrist-to-forearm ratio
C. Median nerve mobility
D. Median nerve echogenicity
E. Median nerve anisotropy

**ANSWER:** E. Median nerve anisotropy

**COMMENTS AND DISCUSSION**
- When assessing for median neuropathy and other entrapment neuropathies, the cross-sectional area will increase, the cross-sectional area ratio compared to adjacent segments will also increase, mobility will decrease, and echogenicity will become more hypoechoic. Changes in anisotropy are not commonly used to assess for median mononeuropathy.

**QUESTION 28.** The following figure is of a short-axis view over the median nerve at the wrist with the patient extending their fingers. What is the hypoechoic structure marked by the star?

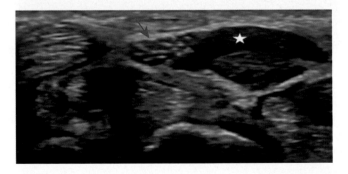

A. Ganglion cyst
B. Lumbrical muscle
C. Flexor digitorum superficialis muscle
D. "Reversed" palmaris longus muscle
E. Thrombosed persistent median artery

**ANSWER:** C. Flexor digitorum superficialis muscle

**COMMENTS AND DISCUSSION**
- The structure marked by the star is hypoechoic, but looking closely it does have some internal echoes.
- One of the tendons of the flexor digitorum sublimis is directly below.
- The structure is intrusion of the flexor digitorum sublimis muscle into the carpal tunnel when the fingers are extended.
- In this case the muscle directly abuts the median nerve (*red arrow*) which is on the left. This is a common anatomic anomaly, which may predispose to carpal tunnel syndrome.

**QUESTION 29.** Which ultrasound finding suggests a schwannoma instead of a neurofibroma?
  A. Positive on color Doppler
  B. Cross-sectional area (CSA) >10 mm$^2$
  C. Eccentric location of the tumor in relationship to the nerve
  D. Internal septations

**ANSWER:** C. Eccentric location of the tumor in relationship to the nerve

**COMMENTS AND DISCUSSION**
- Schwannomas and neurofibromas are both nerve sheath tumors.
- However, the neurofibroma is a tumor of the actual nerve, while a schwannoma is a tumor of the nerve sheath.
- Thus for a neurofibroma, the nerve typically enters the mass at its center and leaves on the opposite side also at its center.
- If the tumor is the eccentric to the nerve, it is more likely to be a schwannoma.

**QUESTION 30.** In trauma, which is **CORRECT** about neuromuscular ultrasound?
  A. Should be delayed a least a week to allow Wallerian degeneration to occur
  B. Can be used to determine if the nerve is in continuity
  C. Is useful in assessing the amount of axonal loss
  D. Ideally used at the same time as electrodiagnostic studies

**ANSWER:** B. Can be used to determine if the nerve is in continuity

**COMMENTS AND DISCUSSION**
- Ultrasound in traumatic nerve lesions
  - Can assess for nerve continuity much earlier than electrodiagnostic studies
    - No need to wait for Wallerian degeneration
    - However, after Wallerian degeneration, electrodiagnostic studies are much better in assessing the degree of axonal loss.
  - Can assess severity and type of injury:
    - Neurotmesis (complete transection):
      - Retraction and laxity of disconnected nerve segments proximally and distally
      - Stump neuroma chronically (Fig. 11.20)
    - Axonotmesis
      - Nerve will remain in continuity.
      - May demonstrate a bulbous focal swelling (neuroma in-continuity)

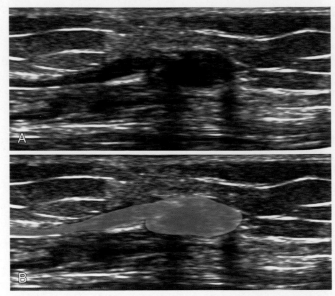

**Fig. 11.20 Stump neuroma.** (A) Superficial radial nerve in the long axis in a patient with a laceration injury to the lateral forearm. (B) Same image with the nerve in *yellow*. When a nerve is transected, it will classically end in a hypoechoic spherical structure, known as a stump neuroma. This occurs because during attempted nerve regrowth, the nerve grows into a disorganized ball of nerve fibers, the stump neuroma. From Preston DC, Shapiro BE. *Electromyography and Neuromuscular Disorders.* 4th ed. Philadelphia, PA: Elsevier; 2020.

**QUESTION 31.** Which of the following are associated with hypertrophic nerves on ultrasound?
  A. Chronic inflammatory demyelinating polyneuropathy (CIDP)
  B. Multifocal motor neuropathy with conduction block (MMNCB)
  C. Charcot-Marie-Tooth (CMT) type 1A
  D. Leprosy
  E. All of the above

**ANSWER:** E. All of the above

**COMMENTS AND DISCUSSION**
- In the evaluation of polyneuropathy, ultrasound is useful in assessing for hypertrophic nerves, which can markedly narrow the differential diagnosis.
- Ultrasound is useful in assessing for diffuse and multifocal nerve hypertrophy.
- Nerve hypertrophy is classically associated with demyelinating polyneuropathy.
- Ultrasound can assess nerve segments that are difficult to evaluate with electrodiagnostic studies, especially
    ◦ Brachial plexus
    ◦ Proximal nerves
- All the disorders listed in the question are associated with nerve hypertrophy on ultrasound.
    ◦ Charcot-Marie-Tooth polyneuropathy, demyelinating types
        • Ultrasound: diffuse and symmetric nerve hypertrophy
    ◦ Acquired inflammatory demyelinating polyneuropathy
        • Ultrasound: multifocal, asymmetric, and often proximal nerve hypertrophy, seen in:
            • Chronic inflammatory demyelinating polyneuropathy (CIDP) (Fig. 11.21)
            • Lewis-Sumner syndrome (LSS)
            • Multifocal motor neuropathy with conduction block (MMNCB)
    ◦ Ultrasound nerve hypertrophy may also be in seen in other conditions, including:
        • Guillain-Barré syndrome
        • Acromegaly
        • Leprosy

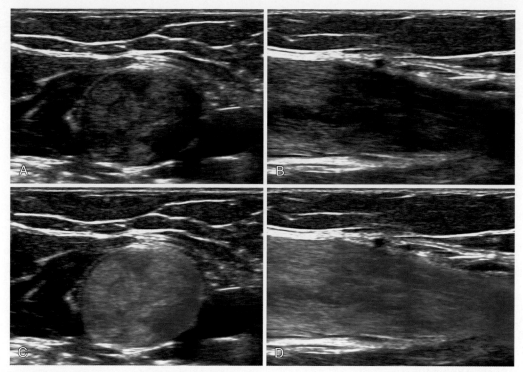

**Fig. 11.21 Massive nerve enlargement in a patient with chronic inflammatory demyelinating polyneuropathy (CIDP).** (A, C) Transverse view of the median nerve in the upper arm showing hyperechoic and hypoechoic fascicles with a cross-sectional area (CSA) of 267 mm². (B, D) Longitudinal view of the median nerve in the upper arm. (C, D) Same images with the nerves colored in *yellow*. The median nerve in the upper arm is one of the optimal locations to assess for hypertrophic nerves in inflammatory neuropathies. From Preston DC, Shapiro BE. *Electromyography and Neuromuscular Disorders*. 4th ed. Philadelphia, PA: Elsevier; 2020.

## ◎ HIGH-YIELD FACT

> Focused study assessing the bilateral median nerves in the forearm, the bilateral median nerves in the arm, and the bilateral trunks of the brachial plexus has a very high sensitivity and specificity of diagnosing CIDP, LSS, and MMNCB, and differentiating them from amyotrophic lateral sclerosis (ALS) and axonal polyneuropathies.

**QUESTION 32.** Which of the following is **MOST SENSITIVE** in assessing for tongue fasciculations?
   A. Clinical exam
   B. Needle EMG: concentric needle
   C. Needle EMG: monopolar needle
   D. Ultrasound
   E. Muscle impedance

**ANSWER:** D. Ultrasound

### COMMENTS AND DISCUSSION

- Role of ultrasound is limited to a few indications in patients with suspected motor neuron disease:
  - To assess for fasciculations
    - Of all techniques, ultrasound has the highest yield for assessment of tongue fasciculations.
    - It has the ability to view superficial and deep limb muscles, as well as visualize a large area of muscle at all times.
    - May allow patients to meet the Awaji criteria for amyotrophic lateral sclerosis (ALS), leading to earlier entry into clinical trials
  - To help exclude a motor demyelinating polyneuropathy, especially multifocal motor neuropathy with conduction block (MMNCB)

## ◎ HIGH-YIELD FACT

Ultrasound is better for assessing fasciculations than the clinical exam and needle electromyography.

**QUESTION 33.** The following are short-axis views of the tibialis anterior and extensor digitorum longus muscles adjacent to the tibia. (left, symptomatic side; right, asymptomatic side.)

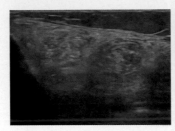 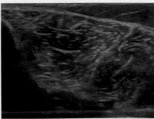

The above is most consistent with:

A. distal myopathy.
B. acute peroneal neuropathy.
C. chronic peroneal neuropathy.
D. S1 radiculopathy.
E. piriformis syndrome.

**ANSWER:** C. chronic peroneal neuropathy.

### COMMENTS AND DISCUSSION

- Role of ultrasound in myopathy is limited to a few indications:
  - May aid in the selection of an appropriate biopsy site
  - Pattern of muscle involvement may limit the differential diagnosis depending on which muscles are normal and which are abnormal (e.g., the involvement of the long finger fingers with relative sparing the flexor carpi ulnaris in inclusion body myositis).
  - To help differentiate denervation atrophy, dystrophy, and myositis:
    - Denervation atrophy
      - Increased muscle echogenicity
      - "Moth-eaten" appearance
      - Muscle atrophy
    - Dystrophy (Fig. 11.22)
      - Increased muscle echogenicity
      - "Ground glass," homogeneous appearance
      - Muscle atrophy
      - Loss of adjacent bone shadows distally due to ultrasound attenuation by increased fat and fibrous tissue
    - Myositis
      - Increased muscle echogenicity
      - "Ground glass," homogeneous appearance
      - Relatively retained bulk (initially)
      - Retained adjacent bone shadows due to edema and inflammation, which do not attenuate the ultrasound signal and the absence of increased fat and fibrous tissue
  - Muscle echogenicity subjectively assessed by the Heckmatt scale:
    - 1: normal
    - 2: increased echogenicity but the bone shadow is well seen
    - 3: increased echogenicity with the bone shadow partially obscured
    - 4: markedly increased echogenicity with the bone shadow completely obliterated

- In comparing the symptomatic versus the asymmetric side on the image:
  - The muscle on the symptomatic side is distinctly abnormal.
  - It is quite hyperechoic.
  - However, it is not homogeneous and has more of a "moth-eaten" appearance.
  - This is the pattern seen with denervation atrophy.
  - In this case the tibialis anterior and extensor digitorum longus muscle are both abnormal compared to the contralateral side.
  - This finding would be expected in a chronic peroneal neuropathy as the muscle atrophy and increased fat and fibrous tissue takes time to develop.

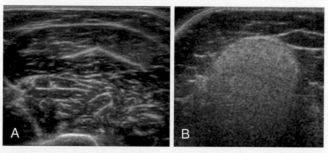

**Fig. 11.22 Muscle in myogenic pathology.** (A) Short-axis view of the biceps in a normal individual. (B) Short-axis view of the biceps in a patient with muscular dystrophy. Note the "ground glass" and homogeneous appearance of muscle in the dystrophy patient.

**QUESTION 34.** What is the classic ultrasound appearance of muscle in an autoimmune myositis?
  A. "Moth-eaten" pattern
  B. Increased muscle echogenicity with loss of bone shadows distally
  C. Increased muscle echogenicity with retained bone shadows distally
  D. Increased subcutaneous edema
  E. Loss of fascial planes

**ANSWER:** B. Increased muscle echogenicity with loss of bone shadows distally

**COMMENTS AND DISCUSSION**
- Denervation atrophy results in a heterogeneous "moth-eaten" pattern
- Dystrophy results in increased muscle echogenicity with loss of bone shadows distally (due to ultrasound attenuation from fat and fibrous tissue).
- Myositis has a pattern of increased muscle echogenicity with retained bone shadows distally.
- Typically, subcutaneous tissue and fascia are normal in myositis.

**QUESTION 35.** The following figure is a view between the seventh and eight ribs. The *arrow* is pointing to:

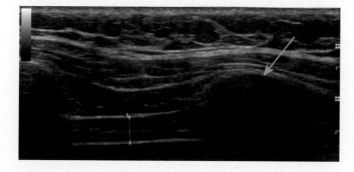

  A. skin.
  B. intercostal muscles.
  C. rib.
  D. diaphragm.
  E. serratus anterior.

**ANSWER:** C. rib.

## COMMENTS AND DISCUSSION

- The green arrow is pointing to the rib. There is a prominent posterior acoustic shadowing below as is commonly seen in bone.
- Ultrasound of the diaphragm (Fig. 11.23)
  - Ultrasound is useful to assess diaphragmatic function in cases of suspected neuromuscular causes of respiratory insufficiency.
  - Ultrasound technique to assess echogenicity, thickness, and a thickening ratio
    - Patient in the supine position
    - Standard linear probe placed over the anterior axillary line along the inferior costal margin between the eighth and ninth ribs, or the seventh and eighth ribs
    - The intercostal muscles are visualized between the ribs.
    - The diaphragm lies below with hyperechoic borders, which represent the parietal pleura and peritoneum membranes.
    - On the right, the liver acts as the "acoustic" window as the spleen does on the left.

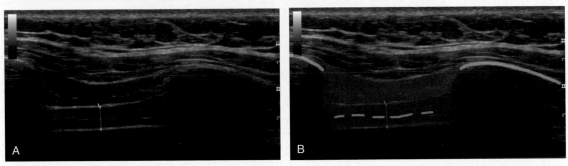

**Fig. 11.23 A Normal diaphragm on ultrasound. Sagittal oblique view across the interspace between the seventh and eighth ribs at the anterior axillary line.** (A) Native image. (B) Same image with the diaphragm in *red*, intercostal muscles in *purple*, and bone echoes of the two ribs in *green*. The diaphragm typically has a hyperechoic border, both superiorly and inferiorly. In many patients, there may be a thin piece of hyperechoic connective tissue running in the center of the diaphragm *(light blue)*. Adapted from Preston DC, Shapiro BE. *Electromyography and Neuromuscular Disorders*, 4th Edition. Philadelphia, PA: Elsevier.

- The diaphragm is assessed for:
  - Echogenicity
  - Thickness at end expiration
    - Normal thickness is >2 mm.
    - Any thickness below this, especially when associated with increased echogenicity, indicates atrophy and dysfunction of the diaphragm.
  - Thickness at the end inspiration during deep breathing
    - A "thickening ratio" percentage can then be calculated =

$$\frac{\text{thickness end inspiration} - \text{thickness end expiration}}{\text{thickness end expiration}} \times 100$$

    - Normal diaphragm thickens in size >20% during end inspiration compared to end expiration

**QUESTION 36.** Which hemidiaphragm is easier to visualize in normal individuals?
  A. Right
  B. Left
  C. No difference between left and right sides

**ANSWER:** A. Right

## COMMENTS AND DISCUSSION

- Ultrasound cannot see well through air.
- It needs an acoustic window to visualize the diaphragm.
- On the right, the liver serves that purpose as does the spleen on the left.
- Because the liver is much larger, it is easier to get a good acoustic window on the right as opposed to the left.

**QUESTION 37.** Which is the optimal probe used to measure diaphragm thickness and the thickening ratio?
A. 15-MHz linear probe
B. 18-MHz hockey stick probe
C. 6-MHz curvilinear probe

**ANSWER:** A. 15-MHz linear probe

**COMMENTS AND DISCUSSION**
- To visualize the diaphragm from the surface: it is only 2–3 mm from the surface and thus a high-frequency linear probe in the range of 15–18 MHz is preferable.
- The hockey stick probe could be used but would likely not be large enough to span the two ribs. A standard linear probe is optimal.

**QUESTION 38.** What is the best location to view the diaphragm between two ribs using the ultrasound?
A. Anterior axillary line
B. Midaxillary line
C. Posterior axillary line
D. Midclavicular line
E. Subxiphoid

**ANSWER:** A. Anterior axillary line.

**COMMENTS AND DISCUSSION**
- Although the diaphragm can be viewed from multiple different locations, the optimal location is the anterior axillary line along the costal margin, which allows views of the diaphragm between the seventh and eighth ribs or the eighth and ninth ribs.

**QUESTION 39.** What is a normal diaphragm thickness at the end of expiration?
A. >1 mm
B. >2 mm
C. >5 mm
D. >10 mm
E. >1 cm

**ANSWER:** B. >2 mm

**COMMENTS AND DISCUSSION**
- Normal diaphragm thickness at the end of expiration is >2 mm.
- Any thickness smaller than this especially when associated with increased echogenicity is consistent with diaphragmatic dysfunction.

**QUESTION 40.** What is a normal thickening ratio of the diaphragm comparing end inspiration to end expiration?
A. >10%
B. >20%
C. >50%
D. >100%

**ANSWER:** B. >20%

**COMMENTS AND DISCUSSION**
- Like all muscles, the diaphragm thickens with contraction.
- One can calculate a thickening ratio by measuring the thickness at the end of inspiration compared to the end of expiration.
- To calculate a percentage, the difference in thickness between end inspiration and end expiration is divided by the end expiration thickness and then multiplied by 100.
- A normal thickening ratio is >20%.

**QUESTION 41.** Which is the optimal probe used to measure diaphragm excursion?
- A. 15-MHz linear probe
- B. 18-MHz hockey stick probe
- C. 6-MHz curvilinear probe

**ANSWER:** C. 6 MHz curvilinear probe

## COMMENTS AND DISCUSSION

- To look for excursion, one needs to visualize the diaphragm behind the liver or spleen (Fig. 11.24).
- It is very deep at that location.
- High frequencies are not able to penetrate to deep structures. Thus a low-frequency probe such as the curvilinear probe is required.
- Ultrasound technique to assess excursion
  - Patient in the supine position
  - Curvilinear probe placed over the right and then left midclavicular line
  - M-mode used
  - Diaphragm excursion recorded posterior to the liver on the right and spleen on the left with deep breathing
  - Normally the diaphragm moves toward the probe during contraction as the diaphragm descends toward the abdomen.
  - If the diaphragm moves away from the probe with inspiration (known as paradoxical movement of the diaphragm), this implies severe diaphragmatic dysfunction.
  - Excursion between inspiration and expiration is measured:
    - Normal >1.9 cm on each side
    - Excursion >2.5 cm definitely excludes any diaphragmatic dysfunction.
    - The left diaphragm normally moves more than the right, but not by more than 50% compared to the right.
    - Movement >50% on the left compared to the right implies some dysfunction on the right.

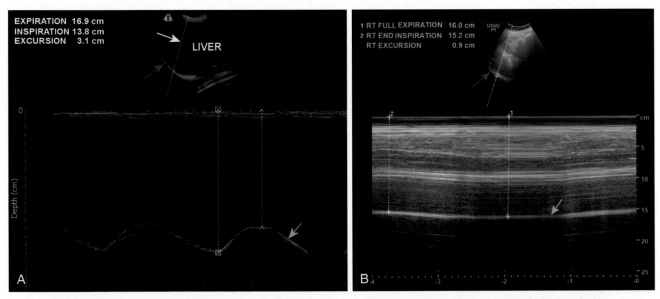

**Fig. 11.24 M-mode and excursion of the diaphragm.** With the probe placed subcostally at the midclavicular line, the posterior diaphragm (*red arrows*) will be seen as a bright line adjacent to the liver. The index line (*yellow arrows*) of the M-mode is placed over this line and the echo (*green arrows*) is then recorded over time on M-mode. The patient performs deep breathing for several cycles. The normal range of excursion between inspiration and expiration is greater than 1.9 cm. (A) Normal patient with an excursion of 3.1 cm. (B) Near-complete paralysis of the diaphragm with minimal excursion of 0.9 cm. From Preston DC, Shapiro BE. *Electromyography and Neuromuscular Disorders.* 4th ed. Philadelphia, PA: Elsevier; 2020.

**QUESTION 42.** Normal diaphragm excursion is normally greater on the left compared to the right.
  A. TRUE
  B. FALSE

**ANSWER:** A. TRUE

**COMMENTS AND DISCUSSION**
- On the right, the liver is below the diaphragm whereas on the left, it is the spleen.
- As the liver is larger and has more mass, the diaphragm normally moves less on the right as compared to the left.

**QUESTION 43.** How would you interpret this M-mode of the right hemidiaphragm?

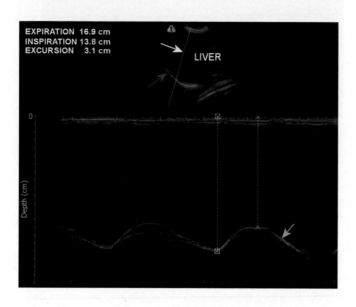

  A. Normal
  B. Reduced motion
  C. Complete phrenic neuropathy
  D. Poor patient cooperation
  E. Paradoxical movement

**ANSWER:** A. Normal

**COMMENTS AND DISCUSSION**
- The image on the top is the standard B-mode with the index line superimposed (*yellow arrow*).
- The bright line of the diaphragm is behind the liver (*red arrow*).
- A single line of amplitude mode information (*yellow arrow*) is recorded over time on the bottom on the screen (M-mode).
- The diaphragm (*green arrow*) normally moves toward the probe during inspiration (the crest of the waveform) and away from the probe (the trough of the waveform).
- Normal diaphragmatic excursion is >1.9 cm. Thus this excursion of 3.1 cm is normal.

**QUESTION 44.** How would you interpret this M-mode of the right hemidiaphragm?

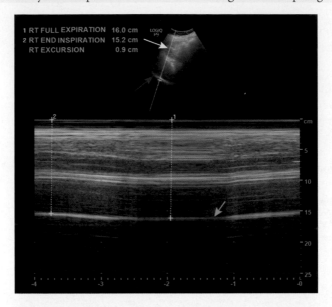

A. Normal
B. Reduced motion
C. Complete phrenic neuropathy
D. Poor patient cooperation
E. Paradoxical movement

**ANSWER:** C. Complete phrenic neuropathy

## COMMENTS AND DISCUSSION

- The image on the top is the standard B-mode with the index line superimposed (*yellow arrow*).
- The bright line of the diaphragm is behind the liver (*red arrow*).
- In the case here the M-mode shows essentially no motion with breathing (*green arrow*).
- The red arrow points at the bright line which is the diaphragm behind the liver.
- This represents complete diaphragmatic dysfunction as would occur in a complete phrenic neuropathy.
- A similar picture could occur with poor patient cooperation, but obviously there would be a limit to how long an individual would be able to hold their breath.
- In paradoxical movement, one sees the diaphragm moving away from the probe during inspiration.
- Ultrasound technique to aid needle electromyography (EMG) of the diaphragm
  ○ Ultrasound can be used to:
    - Identify the diaphragm
    - Measure the distance from the surface to the diaphragm
    - Ensure that lung tissue does not appear during inspiration
    - Guide the needle placement. Note that needle placement can be performed either blindly with the aid of the preceding information or under direct ultrasound guidance.

## SUGGESTED READINGS

Cartwright MS, Hobson-Webb LD, Boon AJ, et al., American Association of Neuromuscular and Electrodiagnostic Medicine. Evidence-based guideline: neuromuscular ultrasound for the diagnosis of carpal tunnel syndrome. *Muscle Nerve.* 2012;287–293.

Preston DC, Shapiro BE. *Electromyography and Neuromuscular Disorders.* 4th ed. Philadelphia, PA: Elsevier; 2020.

Strakowsi JA. *Introduction to Musculoskeletal Ultrasound: Getting started.* New York, NY: Demosmedical; 2015.

Walker F, Cartwright MS. *Neuromuscular Ultrasound.* New York, NY: Elsevier; 2011.

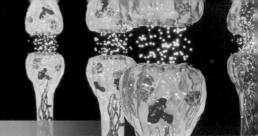

# CHAPTER 12

# Motor Neuron Diseases

## PART 1: PRACTICE TEST

**Q1.** Which of the following motor neuron diseases manifests with upper motor signs **ONLY**?
A. Kennedy disease
B. Amyotrophic lateral sclerosis
C. Progressive muscular atrophy
D. Primary lateral sclerosis
E. Spinal muscular atrophy

**Q2.** A 52-year-old man presents with weakness of the right arm for 6 months, progressing recently into weakness of the left arm and the right leg. Examination shows atrophy of bilateral biceps and triceps with fasciculations of proximal arm and leg muscles bilaterally. There is generalized weakness, grade 3–4, more prominent in the proximal muscles. Sensory examination is normal. Reflexes are brisk (3+) throughout. What electrodiagnostic finding is most likely found in this patient?
A. Prolonged median distal motor latency
B. Ulnar motor conduction block
C. Reduced ulnar sensory nerve action potential (SNAP) amplitude
D. Fibrillation potentials at the lumbar paraspinal muscles
E. Small motor unit action potentials (MUAPs) with normal recruitment

**Q3.** Which of the following patterns of weakness is most likely found in a patient with amyotrophic lateral sclerosis?
A. Weakness of the abductor pollicis brevis with relative sparing of the abductor digiti minimi
B. Weakness of the abductor digiti minimi with relative sparing of the abductor pollicis brevis
C. Weakness of the abductor pollicis brevis with relative sparing of the extensor indicis proprius
D. Weakness of the extensor indicis proprius with relative sparing of the abductor pollicis brevis
E. Weakness of the abductor digiti minimi with relative sparing of the extensor indicis proprius

**Q4.** Which of the following clinical findings help differentiate amyotrophic lateral sclerosis from cervical spinal stenosis?
A. Upper motor neuron signs in the upper extremities
B. Upper motor neuron signs in the lower extremities
C. Lower motor neuron signs in the upper extremities
D. Lower motor neuron signs in the lower extremities
E. Upper and lower motor neuron signs in the upper extremities

**Q5.** Which of the following is **LEAST LIKELY** observed in amyotrophic lateral sclerosis?
A. Cognitive impairment
B. Dyspnea
C. Mood changes
D. Swallowing dysfunction
E. Urinary incontinence

**Q6.** A 47-year-old woman was recently diagnosed with amyotrophic lateral sclerosis. In the past 2 months her husband notes that she laughs inappropriately. At times, she also cries suddenly without any triggers. What is the most effective management in this patient?
A. Quetiapine
B. Quinidine/dextromethorphan
C. Nortriptyline
D. Valproic acid
E. Psychiatric referral

**Q7.** A 50-year-old man developed progressive bilateral upper extremity weakness and atrophy. Sensation was normal. Reflexes were 3+ throughout. Nerve conduction studies showed reduced compound muscle action potential (CMAP) amplitudes in the upper extremities only with normal sensory nerve action potentials (SNAPs) throughout. The needle electromyography (EMG) findings are shown below. Which additional abnormal muscles are needed to fulfill the criteria for definite amyotrophic lateral sclerosis according to the revised El Escorial criteria?

| Muscles | SPONTANEOUS ACTIVITY | MOTOR UNIT ACTION POTENTIALS | | | |
|---|---|---|---|---|---|
| | Fib/PSW | Amp (μV) | Dur (ms) | Polyphasia | Recruitment |
| R Deltoid | 2+ | Large | Long | Mild | Reduced |
| R Biceps | 2+ | Large | Long | Mild | Reduced |
| R Triceps | 3+ | Large | Long | Mild | Reduced |
| R PT | 3+ | Large | Long | Mild | Reduced |
| R FPL | 3+ | Very large | Very long | Moderate | Reduced |
| R EIP | 4+ | Very large | Very long | Moderate | Reduced |
| R C5 PSP | 2+ | N/A | N/A | N/A | N/A |
| R C7 PSP | 3+ | N/A | N/A | N/A | N/A |

*Amp, amplitude; Dur, duration; EIP, extensor indicis proprius; Fib, fibrillation potentials; FPL, flexor pollicis longus; N/A, not applicable; PSW, positive sharp waves; PT, pronator teres; PSP, paraspinal; R, right*

A. Right genioglossus, and left deltoid, biceps, and triceps muscles
B. Left deltoid, biceps, triceps, and T10 and T12 paraspinal muscles
C. Right first dorsal interossei and T10 and T12 paraspinal muscles
D. Right vastus medialis, tibialis anterior, medial gastrocnemius, and T10 and T12 paraspinal muscles
E. Bilateral vastus medialis, tibialis anterior, and medial gastrocnemius muscles

**Q8.** Which of the following statements is **TRUE** regarding the Awaji criteria for the diagnosis of amyotrophic lateral sclerosis (ALS) when compared to the revised El Escorial criteria?
A. Higher sensitivity and specificity
B. Higher sensitivity but no change in specificity
C. Higher specificity but no change in sensitivity
D. Similar sensitivity and specificity
E. Assisting in the early diagnosis of concomitant dementia

**Q9.** Which of the following statements regarding the Awaji revision of the El Escorial criteria of fasciculation potentials in amyotrophic lateral sclerosis (ALS) is **CORRECT**?
A. Fasciculation potentials are required for the diagnosis of ALS.
B. Fasciculation potentials are relevant only when seen without fibrillation potentials.
C. Fasciculation potentials are equivalent to fibrillation potentials when associated with reinnervated motor unit action potentials (MUAPs).
D. Fasciculation potentials are difficult to visualize by ultrasound.
E. Fasciculation potentials are specific for ALS.

**Q10.** Which of the following statements regarding distinguishing features of multifocal motor neuropathy from amyotrophic lateral sclerosis (ALS) is **CORRECT**?
A. >50% amplitude/area reduction of compound muscle action potentials (CMAPs) when distal CMAP is <1mV
B. >50% amplitude/area reduction of CMAPs when distal CMAP is >1 mV
C. Brisk myotatic reflexes are specific findings in ALS
D. Absent sensory nerve action potentials
E. Large-amplitude and long-duration motor unit action potentials

**Q11.** A 56-year-old man develops slowly progressive weakness in the past 5–6 years, with similar symptom observed in his older brother. Examination reveals mild dysarthria, prominent tongue atrophy, as well as fasciculations in his tongue and around his mouth. Symmetrical weakness of proximal muscles (grade 4) is noted in his upper and lower extremities, in addition to diffusely reduced deep tendon reflexes. Sensation is normal. What finding is most likely demonstrated on electrodiagnostic examination?
A. Reduced median sensory nerve action potential (SNAP) amplitude
B. Focal slowing of the median nerve in the forearm
C. Neuromyotonia
D. Normal recruitment
E. Small polyphasic motor unit action potentials (MUAPs)

**Q12.** Which of the following is **LEAST LIKELY** to be seen in Kennedy disease?
A. Myotonia
B. Testicular atrophy
C. Mini-polymyoclonus in the hands
D. Impaired vibration and joint position sense
E. Elevated creatine kinase

**Q13.** In patients with amyotrophic lateral sclerosis, what percentage is familial?
- A. 1%
- B. 5%
- C. 10%
- D. 50%
- E. 30%

**Q14.** What is the most common mutated gene in patients with amyotrophic lateral sclerosis?
- A. *ALS2*
- B. *C9orf72*
- C. *FUS*
- D. *SOD1*
- E. *TARDBP*

**Q15.** A 49-year-old woman presents with behavioral change for 8 months. Her husband describes that she yells at people and sometimes tries to take her clothes off in public. In the past 2 months he also notes that she has difficulty lifting her right arm and walking up steps. Examination shows muscle atrophy in both the proximal and distal upper and lower extremities, along with tongue atrophy and fasciculations. Fasciculations are also observed in her thighs. Deep tendon reflexes are brisk in all extremities. What genetic abnormality is most likely to be found in this patient?
- A. Gene deletion
- B. Gene duplication
- C. Point mutation
- D. Trinucleotide repeat expansion
- E. Hexanucleotide repeat expansion

**Q16.** Which protein accumulation is considered the neuropathological hallmark of amyotrophic lateral sclerosis?
- A. Amyloid
- B. Phosphorylated tau
- C. Progranulin
- D. Synuclein
- E. TAR DNA-binding protein 43 (TDP-43)

**Q17.** Which of the following pathological finding is seen in amyotrophic lateral sclerosis?
- A. Bunina bodies
- B. Hirano bodies
- C. Negri bodies
- D. Pick bodies
- E. Tubulofilamentous inclusions

**Q18.** Which of the following is **CORRECT** regarding gastrostomy in amyotrophic lateral sclerosis?
- A. It may increase survival.
- B. It reduces the risk of aspiration.
- C. It does not improve quality of life.
- D. It should be reserved for cases where forced vital capacity falls below 50%.
- E. It is performed by percutaneous method only.

**Q19.** According to the 1999 American Academy of Neurology (AAN) guideline, noninvasive positive pressure ventilation should be offered to patients with amyotrophic lateral sclerosis when their forced vital capacity (FVC) is less than:
- A. 40%.
- B. 50%.
- C. 60%.
- D. 70%.
- E. 90%.

**Q20.** What is **CORRECT** regarding medical treatment in amyotrophic lateral sclerosis (ALS)?
- A. Riluzole is a free-radical scavenger.
- B. Studies of riluzole demonstrated increased survival by 6 months.
- C. Edaravone is an anti-glutamatergic agent.
- D. Edaravone met the primary end point to improve the Revised ALS Functional Rating Scale (ALSFRS-R) in the initial study.
- E. Both riluzole and edaravone are considered disease-modifying therapies.

**Q21.** Which genetic mutation is responsible for the majority of spinal muscular atrophy (SMA) cases?
- A. Deletion of the *SMN1* gene
- B. Deletion of the *SMN2* gene
- C. Duplication of the *SMN1* gene
- D. Duplication of the *SMN2* gene
- E. Point mutation of the *SMN1* gene

**Q22.** What developmental milestone is never achieved and serves to differentiate spinal muscular atrophy type 1 (SMA1) from spinal muscular atrophy types 2, 3, and 4 (SMA2, SMA3, and SMA4)?
- A. Sitting
- B. Crawling
- C. Standing
- D. Walking
- E. Speaking the first word

**Q23.** What is the mechanism of action of nusinersen?
- A. Inclusion of exon 7 in the *SMN1* gene during alternative splicing
- B. Exclusion of exon 7 in the *SMN1* gene during alternative splicing
- C. Inclusion of exon 7 in the *SMN2* gene during alternative splicing
- D. Exclusion of exon 7 in the *SMN2* gene during alternative splicing
- E. Replacing the *SMN1* gene by a viral vector

**Q24.** What is the most common number of copies of the *SMN2* gene in spinal muscular atrophy type 2 (SMA2)?
A. 1
B. 2
C. 3
D. 4
E. 5

**Q25.** A 6-week-old baby presents with a weak cry, inspiratory stridor, and respiratory distress. Chest X-ray shows diaphragmatic paralysis. In addition, generalized weakness is noted in all four extremities. Genetic testing of the *SMN1* gene is negative. What gene is most likely responsible for this patient's condition?
A. *BSCL2*
B. *DMD*
C. *HSPB1*
D. *IGHMBP2*
E. *SMN2*

**Q26.** Which of the following pathogens does **NOT** cause poliomyelitis (infection of anterior horn cells)?
A. *Borrelia burgdorferi*
B. Non-polio enterovirus
C. Poliovirus
D. West Nile virus

**Q27.** A 23-year-old man presents with weakness of the right hand for 8 months. On examination, there is weakness and atrophy of the right intrinsic hand muscles including the abductor pollicis brevis, abductor digiti minimi, first dorsal interossei, and finger extensors. Sensory examination is unremarkable. Deep tendon reflexes are 1+ in the right biceps, triceps, and brachioradialis. Examination in the other extremities is normal. Which of the following investigations is most useful to confirm the diagnosis?
A. Genetic testing
B. Computerized tomography (CT) angiogram of the neck
C. Creatine kinase
D. Dynamic magnetic resonance imaging (MRI) of the cervical spine with contrast
E. Lumbar puncture

**Q28.** A 64-year-old man presents with proximal muscle weakness in both arms and legs, gait unsteadiness, numbness in both hands and feet, urinary incontinence, and dementia. Examination reveals both upper and lower motor neuron features in both arms and legs. What is the most likely finding on his sural nerve biopsy?
A. Segmental demyelination
B. Onion bulb formation
C. Giant axons
D. Polyglucosan bodies
E. Tomacula

**Q29.** What is the treatment of choice for Brown-Vialetto-Van Laere disease?
A. Vitamin B1
B. Vitamin B2
C. Vitamin B5
D. Vitamin B6
E. Vitamin B12

**Q30.** A 45-year-old man presents with several years history of progressive weakness, imbalance, and tremor. He has a recent history of schizoaffective disorder. His neurological examination shows nystagmus, cerebellar ataxia, generalized weakness, and hyperreflexia. Which blood test is most useful in the diagnosis?
A. Hexosaminidase A enzyme activity
B. Phytanic acid serum level
C. Testosterone serum level
D. Acid-alpha glucosidase enzyme activity
E. Alpha-galactosidase enzyme activity

**Q31.** A 66-year-old man presents with a several-year history of numbness of the left face followed by slurred speech, chewing difficulties, muscle twitches in the limbs, and mild generalized weakness. His neurological examination shows dysarthria, asymmetrical lower facial weakness and sensory loss, weak jaw opening, tongue weakness, and limb fasciculations. His reflexes are brisk in the upper and lower extremities with Babinski signs. Electromyography reveals dissemination of denervation in the bulbar and three spinal segments of the neuraxis with normal sensory nerve action potentials. What is the most likely diagnosis?
A. Muscle-specific tyrosine kinase (MuSK)–positive myasthenia gravis
B. X-linked bulbospinal muscular atrophy (Kennedy disease)
C. Facial onset sensory and motor neuronopathy (FOSMN)
D. Progressive bulbar palsy form of motor neuron disease
E. Chronic inflammatory demyelinating polyneuropathy (CIDP)

# PART 2: QUESTIONS WITH ANSWERS AND DISCUSSION

**QUESTION 1.** Which of the following motor neuron diseases manifests with upper motor signs **ONLY**?
- A. Kennedy disease
- B. Amyotrophic lateral sclerosis
- C. Progressive muscular atrophy
- D. Primary lateral sclerosis
- E. Spinal muscular atrophy

**ANSWER:** D. Primary lateral sclerosis

## COMMENTS AND DISCUSSION

- Motor neuron diseases are a group of disorders that predominantly or exclusively affect motor neurons, including:
  - Lower motor neurons
    - Anterior horn cells in the ventral spinal cord
    - Motor neurons in cranial nerve nuclei, which supply somatic and brachial voluntary muscles (especially cranial nerves V, VII, IX, X, XI, XII)
  - Upper motor neurons
    - Betz cells (pyramidal neurons) in the primary motor cortex
- Symptoms and signs depend on whether lower and/or upper motor neurons are affected.
  - Lower motor neuron (LMN): weakness, muscle atrophy, fasciculations, hypotonia, hyporeflexia
  - Upper motor neuron (UMN): weakness, hyperreflexia, clonus, Babinski sign spasticity
- The prototypic and most common motor neuron disorders are amyotrophic lateral sclerosis (ALS) and spinal muscular atrophy (SMA)
- Kennedy disease, SMA, and progressive muscular atrophy all manifest with pure LMN disease, whereas primary lateral sclerosis has only UMN findings. ALS has both UMN and LMN findings.
- Most motor neuron diseases are neurodegenerative, some are genetic, and some are infectious (Table 12.1). Sporadic forms may be acquired, or caused by known or unknown genetic defects, in which case only one family member manifests clinical symptoms.

**TABLE 12.1** Various forms of motor neuron diseases. Motor neuron diseases can be classified as genetic or acquired, and familial, or sporadic.

| Disorder | ETIOLOGY | | FORM | |
| --- | --- | --- | --- | --- |
| | Genetic | Acquired | Familial | Sporadic |
| Amyotrophic lateral sclerosis | ✓ | ✓ | ✓ (10%) | ✓ (90%) |
| Spinal muscular atrophy | ✓ | | ✓ | ✓ |
| Kennedy disease (X-linked bulbospinal muscular atrophy) | ✓ | | ✓ | ✓ |
| Hirayama disease | ? | ✓ | Very rare | ✓ |
| Adult Tay-Sachs disease | ✓ | | ✓ | ✓ |
| Adult polyglucosan body disease | ✓ | | ✓ | ✓ |
| Poliomyelitis and other infections causing myelitis | | ✓ | | ✓ |
| Riboflavin-responsive motor neuron disorders | ✓ | | ✓ | ✓ |

Of note, the sporadic form may be acquired or genetic, either from known or yet unknown genetic defects. ?, unknown or not clearly established yet.

- ALS has a typical onset in 50s to 70s.
- ALS prevalence is about 4 in 100,000.
- Prognosis is poor. Patients typically die within 3–5 years, but the natural history of the disease may vary with 20% patients living longer than 5 years and 10% more than 10 years.
- Clinical features
  - In the classic form: LMN + UMN features
  - Symptoms often start in one limb (usually distal arm or leg) and spread to others.
  - There are multiple variants of ALS (Table 12.2).

**TABLE 12.2** Amyotrophic lateral sclerosis (ALS): the classic form and its variants.

| MND variant | LMN features | UMN features | Bulbar involvement |
| --- | --- | --- | --- |
| Classic ALS | ++ | ++ | +/- (often) |
| Progressive muscular atrophy (PMA) | ++ | - | +/- (often) |
| Primary lateral sclerosis (PLS) | - | ++ | +/- |
| Progressive bulbar palsy (PBP) | +/- | +/- | +++ |
| Flail arm/flail leg syndrome | + | +/- | - |

*UMN*, upper motor neuron; *LMN*, lower motor neuron; *MND*, motor neuron disease.

- Spine imaging is usually performed to exclude cervical and/or lumbar spinal stenosis, while brain magnetic resonance imaging (MRI) is recommended for bulbar onset or an UMN predominant presentation. In some cases, MRI may reveal Wallerian degeneration of corticobulbar/corticospinal tracts, same as pathological finding (Fig. 12.1). If patients have associated frontotemporal dementia (FTD), atrophy of frontal and temporal regions may be seen on neuroimaging.

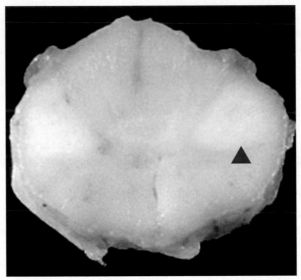

**Fig. 12.1** Gross pathology of amyotrophic lateral sclerosis. A crosssection of the thoracic spinal cord of a patient with amyotrophic lateral sclerosis demonstrates pallor of bilateral corticospinal tracts due to degeneration (red arrowhead). Additionally, there is degeneration of the anterior horn cells in the bilateral ventral gray matter, although this is not evident in gross specimens. From Klatt EC. *Robbins & Cotran Atlas of Pathology*. 4th ed. Elsevier; 2021;19:495-548.e7.

**QUESTION 2.** A 52-year-old man presents with weakness of the right arm for 6 months, progressing recently into weakness of the left arm and the right leg. Examination shows atrophy of bilateral biceps and triceps with fasciculations of proximal arm and leg muscles bilaterally. There is generalized weakness, grade 3–4, more prominent in the proximal muscles. Sensory examination is normal. Reflexes are brisk (3+) throughout. What electrodiagnostic finding is most likely found in this patient?

A. Prolonged median distal motor latency
B. Ulnar motor conduction block
C. Reduced ulnar sensory nerve action potential (SNAP) amplitude
D. Fibrillation potentials at the lumbar paraspinal muscles
E. Small motor unit action potentials (MUAPs) with normal recruitment

**ANSWER:** D. Fibrillation potentials at the lumbar paraspinal muscles

### COMMENTS AND DISCUSSION

- The diagnosis in this patient is amyotrophic lateral sclerosis (ALS). He has lower motor neuron features (muscle atrophy, fasciculations) mixed with upper motor neuron features (hyperreflexia).

- Nerve conduction studies (NCSs) in ALS show:
  - Normal sensory studies (unless there is a coexisting entrapment neuropathy or peripheral polyneuropathy)
  - Motor studies show axonal loss patterns (reduced CMAP amplitudes, normal or slightly prolonged latencies, and normal or slightly slowed velocities) with motor conduction velocities that are at >75% of the lower limit of normal, minimum F-wave latency at <130% of the upper limit of normal, and distal CMAP latency that is <150% of normal.
  - The absence of conduction block, as defined by CMAP area reduction on proximal versus distal stimulation of >50%, or pathologic temporal dispersion, as defined by proximal CMAP duration that is >30% of the distal value. Both are best evaluated when the distal CMAP amplitude is large enough to allow such assessment (usually >1 mV).
- Needle EMG
  - Spontaneous activity: fibrillations (or positive sharp waves) and/or fasciculations, in distal, proximal, and paraspinal muscles
  - Voluntary activity: large motor unit action potentials (MUAPs) with increased duration and reduced recruitment, compatible with chronic neurogenic change
  - In the presence of chronic neurogenic changes, the clinical significance of fasciculation potentials are equivalent to that of both fibrillation potentials and positive sharp waves.
- According to diagnostic criteria, abnormalities need to be present in three of four neuraxis segments (bulbar, cervical, thoracic, lumbosacral).
- In this case, prolonged distal motor latency indicates distal demyelination, and motor conduction block indicates focal demyelination, which are not features of ALS. In addition, small, short-duration MUAPs indicate a myopathic and not a neurogenic process.

**QUESTION 3.** Which of the following patterns of weakness is most likely found in a patient with amyotrophic lateral sclerosis?
  A. Weakness of the abductor pollicis brevis with relative sparing of the abductor digiti minimi
  B. Weakness of the abductor digiti minimi with relative sparing of the abductor pollicis brevis
  C. Weakness of the abductor pollicis brevis with relative sparing of the extensor indicis proprius
  D. Weakness of the extensor indicis proprius with relative sparing of the abductor pollicis brevis
  E. Weakness of the abductor digiti minimi with relative sparing of the extensor indicis proprius

**ANSWER:** A. Weakness of the abductor pollicis brevis with relative sparing of the abductor digiti minimi

## COMMENTS AND DISCUSSION
- In patients with amyotrophic lateral sclerosis (ALS) in whom the hands are affected, there is often a *split hand sign* where the abductor pollicis brevis (APB) and first dorsal interossei (FDI) are more affected than the abductor digiti minimi (ADM).
- This is thought to be related to more T1 contribution to APB and FDI, whereas ADM has more C8. However, why T1-innervated muscles are more affected than C8-innervated muscles remains unknown.

 **HIGH-YIELD FACT**

Split hand sign, characterized by atrophy of thenar eminence/lateral hand (APB and FDI) with relative sparing of hypothenar eminence (ADM), is a feature of ALS.

**QUESTION 4.** Which of the following examination findings help differentiate amyotrophic lateral sclerosis from cervical spinal stenosis?
  A. Upper motor neuron signs in the upper extremities
  B. Upper motor neuron signs in the lower extremities
  C. Lower motor neuron signs in the upper extremities
  D. Lower motor neuron signs in the lower extremities
  E. Upper and lower motor neuron signs in the upper extremities

**ANSWER:** D. Lower motor neuron signs in the lower extremities

## COMMENTS AND DISCUSSION

- In cervical spinal stenosis, there are lower motor neuron features at the level of the lesion (i.e., upper limbs) due to involvement of the anterior horn cells, and upper motor neuron features at the levels below (i.e., lower limbs) due to compression of the pyramidal tract. Thus this may mimic amyotrophic lateral sclerosis (ALS).
- In cervical spinal stenosis, there should not be lower motor neuron features in the lower extremities. The presence of lower motor neuron signs in the lower extremities helps differentiate ALS from cervical spinal stenosis. Nevertheless, if a patient has tandem stenosis (i.e., both cervical and lumbar stenosis), there could also be lower motor neuron signs in the lower extremities.
- In patients with ALS, neuroimaging of the spine should be considered to exclude spinal stenosis, which is potentially treatable.

**QUESTION 5.** Which of the following is **LEAST LIKELY** to be observed in amyotrophic lateral sclerosis?
- A. Cognitive impairment
- B. Dyspnea
- C. Mood changes
- D. Swallowing dysfunction
- E. Urinary incontinence

**ANSWER:** E. Urinary incontinence

## COMMENTS AND DISCUSSION

- About 20% of patients with amyotrophic lateral sclerosis (ALS) have bulbar onset, which portends poor prognosis.
- Bulbar symptoms include dysarthria (spastic and/or flaccid), dysphagia, and sialorrhea (excessive drooling).
- Respiratory difficulty and respiratory failure can ensue due to weakness of respiratory muscles including the diaphragm.
- About 5% of patients with ALS have the frontotemporal dementia (FTD) phenotype, whereas about 15% of FTD patients also have the ALS phenotype.
- Patients may have cognitive or behavioral abnormalities, especially in FTD associated with ALS (FTD-ALS), which are typically due to *C9orf72* mutations. Impaired executive function and disinhibition are the main cognitive features due to frontal lobe involvement. However, ALS not associated with *C9orf72* or overt FTD may also exhibit cognitive or behavioral issues.
- Patients with ALS are not uncommonly overcome by depression and anxiety.
- Patients with ALS typically have no bladder involvement due to sparing of Onuf's nucleus. This nucleus is located in the ventral horn of the sacral spinal cord, and contains lower motor neurons that innervate the striated urethral sphincter and the external anal sphincter.

**QUESTION 6.** A 47-year-old woman was recently diagnosed with amyotrophic lateral sclerosis. In the past 2 months her husband notes that she laughs inappropriately. At times, she also cries suddenly without any triggers. What is the most effective management in this patient?
- A. Quetiapine
- B. Quinidine/dextromethorphan
- C. Nortriptyline
- D. Valproic acid
- E. Psychiatric referral

**ANSWER:** B. Quinidine/dextromethorphan

## COMMENTS AND DISCUSSION

- This patient has pseudobulbar affect (PBA), which is inappropriate laughing and crying. This can be treated with quinidine/dextromethorphan, which was shown to be effective, or selective serotonin reuptake inhibitors (SSRIs).
- Tricyclic antidepressants such as nortriptyline may be useful but not very effective, and valproic acid is not indicated.
- PBA is not due to depression or anxiety, and does not require a psychiatric referral.

◎ **HIGH-YIELD FACT**

Pseudobulbar affect (PBA), inappropriate laughing or crying, can be seen in ALS, and is best treated with dextromethorphan/quinidine or SSRIs.

QUESTION 7. A 50-year-old man developed progressive bilateral upper extremity weakness and atrophy. Sensation was normal. Reflexes were 3+ throughout. Nerve conduction studies showed reduced compound muscle action potential (CMAP) amplitudes in the upper extremities only with normal sensory nerve action potentials (SNAPs) throughout. The needle electromyography (EMG) findings are shown below. Which additional abnormal muscles are needed to fulfill the criteria for definite amyotrophic lateral sclerosis according to the revised El Escorial criteria?

| Muscles | SPONTANEOUS ACTIVITY Fib/PSW | MOTOR UNIT ACTION POTENTIALS Amp (μV) | Dur (ms) | Polyphasia | Recruitment |
|---|---|---|---|---|---|
| R Deltoid | 2+ | Large | Long | Mild | Reduced |
| R Biceps | 2+ | Large | Long | Mild | Reduced |
| R Triceps | 3+ | Large | Long | Mild | Reduced |
| R PT | 3+ | Large | Long | Mild | Reduced |
| R FPL | 3+ | Very large | Very long | Moderate | Reduced |
| R EIP | 4+ | Very large | Very long | Moderate | Reduced |
| R C5 PSP | 2+ | N/A | N/A | N/A | N/A |
| R C7 PSP | 3+ | N/A | N/A | N/A | N/A |

*Amp*, amplitude; *Dur*, duration; *EIP*, extensor indicis proprius; *Fib*, fibrillation potentials; *FPL*, flexor pollicis longus; *N/A*, not applicable; *PSW*, positive sharp waves; *PT*, pronator teres; *PSP*, paraspinal; *R*, right.

A. Right genioglossus, and left deltoid, biceps, and triceps muscles
B. Left deltoid, biceps, triceps, and T10 and T12 paraspinal muscles
C. Right first dorsal interossei and T10 and T12 paraspinal muscles
D. Right vastus medialis, tibialis anterior, medial gastrocnemius, and T10 and T12 paraspinal muscles
E. Bilateral vastus medialis, tibialis anterior, and medial gastrocnemius muscles

**ANSWER:** D. Right vastus medialis, tibialis anterior, medial gastrocnemius, and T10 and T12 paraspinal muscles

## COMMENTS AND DISCUSSION

- The diagnostic criteria of ALS were proposed mainly for research purposes to recruit patients early and with a clear and unambiguous diagnosis.
- In clinical practice, patients may not fulfill all criteria early on.
- Two main criteria: Revised El Escorial (Airlie House) and Awaji criteria
- Both criteria require evidence of denervation and reinnervation in three of four body segments (bulbar, cervical, thoracic, lumbosacral).
- EMG is a crucial tool to confirm lower motor neuron (LMN) involvement in the affected and clinically unaffected regions, as well as to exclude other mimics.
- The main difference between these two criteria is that the Awaji criteria allows the use of fasciculations as evidence of active denervation only when the chronic neurogenic changes are present, whereas the revised El Escorial criteria do not (Table 12.3).
- In this case, needle EMG was performed only in muscles innervated by the cervical cord (region) with evidence of ongoing denervation and chronic reinnervation. For clinically definite ALS as per

**TABLE 12.3** Revised El Escorial criteria for the diagnosis of amyotrophic lateral sclerosis (ALS).

| Diagnostic certainty | Involvement |
|---|---|
| Definite | (UMN + LMN) x 3 |
| Laboratory supported familial ALS | (UMN + LMN) x 1 + confirmed genetic testing |
| Probable | (UMN + LMN) x 2 (some UMN signs must be rostral to LMN signs) |
| Probable (laboratory supported) | LMN by EMG x 2 AND UMN in at least one region of the LMN findings |
| Possible | (UMN + LMN) x 1 OR UMN x 2 or more |
| Suspected | LMN x 2 or more |

x 1, x 2, x 3 refer to 1, 2 or 3 segments of the neuraxis, respectively. Note that all levels of diagnosis require progressive spread of signs of degeneration within or between regions AND lack of electrophysiologic or neuroimaging evidence suggestive of other causes.
*UMN*, upper motor neuron; *LMN*, lower motor neuron.

revised El Escorial criteria, the presence of UMN and LMN signs in three of four regions (brain stem, cervical, thoracic, and lumbosacral) is required. The combination of active and chronic denervation is needed in two more regions, which can be bulbar, thoracic, or lumbosacral. Studying the right vastus medialis and tibialis anterior confirms LMN findings of the lumbosacral regions, whereas studying the T10 and T12 paraspinal muscles confirms LMN findings of the thoracic region.

- Option A has muscles in only the cervical (deltoid, biceps, and triceps) and bulbar (genioglossus) regions. Option B has muscles in only the cervical (deltoid, biceps, triceps) and thoracic (T10 and T12 paraspinal) regions. Option C has muscles in only the cervical (first dorsal interossei) and thoracic (T10 and T12 paraspinal) regions. Option E has muscles in only the lumbosacral regions (vastus medialis, tibialis anterior, medial gastrocnemius).

**QUESTION 8.** Which of the following statements is **TRUE** regarding the Awaji criteria for the diagnosis of amyotrophic lateral sclerosis (ALS) when compared to the revised El Escorial criteria?
   A. Higher sensitivity and specificity
   B. Higher sensitivity but no change in specificity
   C. Higher specificity but no change in sensitivity
   D. Similar sensitivity and specificity
   E. Assisting in the early diagnosis of concomitant dementia

**ANSWER:** B. Higher sensitivity but no change in specificity

**COMMENTS AND DISCUSSION**
- The Awaji criteria differ from the El Escorial ALS criteria in two ways. First, the Awaji criteria allow for a combination of electrodiagnostic and clinical criteria for lower motor neuron signs to determine if a single limb is abnormal. Second, the Awaji criteria permit fasciculation potentials by needle electromyography to be used as evidence of ongoing (active) denervation in a muscle with evidence of neurogenic change.
- The Awaji ALS criteria were proposed to improve the sensitivity and early diagnosis of ALS. Systematic review and meta-analysis of eight studies showed that sensitivity was 81% with the Awaji criteria versus 62% with the El Escorial criteria, whereas the specificities for both sets of criteria were similar at 98%.

**QUESTION 9.** Which of the following statements regarding the Awaji revision of the El Escorial criteria of fasciculation potentials in amyotrophic lateral sclerosis (ALS) is **CORRECT**?
   A. Fasciculation potentials are required for the diagnosis of ALS.
   B. Fasciculation potentials are relevant only when seen without fibrillation potentials.
   C. Fasciculation potentials are equivalent to fibrillation potentials when associated with reinnervated motor unit action potentials (MUAPs).
   D. Fasciculation potentials are difficult to visualize by ultrasound.
   E. Fasciculation potentials are specific for ALS.

**ANSWER:** C. Fasciculation potentials are equivalent to fibrillation potentials when associated with reinnervated MUAPs.

**COMMENTS AND DISCUSSION**
- The Awaji revision of the El Escorial criteria added fasciculation potentials as a diagnostic criterion of active denervation, but only when accompanied by reinnervated MUAPs.
- Fasciculation potentials are not required for diagnosis of ALS, and do not have to be seen with fibrillation potentials.
- Ultrasound detects fasciculations more frequently than electromyography (EMG), particularly in the tongue.
- Fasciculations may be seen in other neuropathies or even in normal patients.

**QUESTION 10.** Which one of the following statements regarding distinguishing features of multifocal motor neuropathy from amyotrophic lateral sclerosis (ALS) is **CORRECT**?
   A. >50% amplitude/area reduction of compound muscle action potentials (CMAPs) when distal CMAP is <1 mV
   B. >50% amplitude/area reduction of CMAPs when distal CMAP is > 1 mV.
   C. Brisk myotatic reflexes are specific findings in ALS
   D. Absent sensory nerve action potentials
   E. Large-amplitude and long-duration motor unit action potentials

**ANSWER:** B. >50% amplitude/area reduction of CMAPs when distal CMAP is >1 mV

## COMMENTS AND DISCUSSION

- Multifocal motor conduction blocks at non-entrapment sites are the hallmark findings of multifocal motor neuropathy.
- Conduction block is confirmed when CMAP amplitude and area decrease >50%, and is considered diagnostic for multifocal motor neuropathy.
- Conduction block is difficult to confirm when the distal CMAP is very low; a distal CMAP lower than 1 mV precludes the confirmation of a block.
- The ALS criteria include the absence of conduction block, as defined by CMAP area reduction on proximal versus distal stimulation of >50%, or pathologic temporal dispersion, as defined by proximal CMAP duration that is >30% of the distal value. Both are best evaluated when the distal CMAP amplitude is large enough (>1 mV) to allow such an assessment.
- The myotatic reflexes may be brisk in multifocal motor neuropathy and, on their own, are not distinguishing features.
- Large-amplitude and long-duration motor unit action potentials are seen in both disorders.
- Absent sensory nerve action potentials exclude both disorders.

**QUESTION 11.** A 56-year-old man develops slowly progressive weakness in the past 5–6 years, with similar symptom observed in his older brother. Examination reveals mild dysarthria, prominent tongue atrophy, as well as fasciculations in his tongue and around his mouth. Symmetrical weakness of proximal muscles (grade 4) is noted in his upper and lower extremities, in addition to diffusely reduced deep tendon reflexes. Sensation is normal. What finding is most likely demonstrated on electrodiagnostic examination?

A. Reduced median sensory nerve action potential (SNAP) amplitude
B. Focal slowing of the median nerve in the forearm
C. Neuromyotonia
D. Normal recruitment
E. Small polyphasic motor unit action potentials (MUAPs)

**ANSWER:** A. Reduced median sensory nerve action potential (SNAP) amplitude

## COMMENTS AND DISCUSSION

- The diagnosis in this patient is Kennedy disease (aka, X-linked bulbospinal muscular atrophy).
- Kennedy disease is inherited as X-linked recessive with lack of male-to-male transmission. Usually males are affected. A daughter of an affected male is an obligatory carrier. Females who carry one allele are usually asymptomatic but can develop symptoms if there is skewed inactivation of the X chromosome.
- Caused by CAG (polyglutamine) repeat expansions in the *AR* gene on the X chromosome encoding for androgen receptor
  - 36-37 repeats: reduced penetrance
  - ≥38 repeats: full penetrance

 **HIGH-YIELD FACT**

> Most trinucleotide repeat expansion disorders are inherited as autosomal dominant, but Kennedy disease is inherited as X-linked.

- Onset is typically in mid-to-late adulthood.
- Clinical features
  - Typical presentation starts with cramps, followed by slowly progressive weakness over decades that affects the proximal muscles symmetrically. Bulbar involvement occurs later, including dysarthria, dysphagia, tongue atrophy, and fasciculations.
  - Perioral fasciculations can be an important diagnostic clue. Patients may have mini-polymyoclonus, which is not specific to Kennedy disease, but also seen in other motor neuron disorders such as amyotrophic lateral sclerosis (ALS), and parkinsonian disorders including multiple system atrophy.
  - Endocrine abnormalities are due to mutations in the androgen receptor gene, manifesting as gynecomastia, testicular atrophy, and infertility.
  - Sensory system is typically spared in motor neuron diseases, although there are some exceptions, most notably with Kennedy disease. These patients may experience sensory symptoms such as impaired vibration and joint position sense, likely due to degeneration of the dorsal root ganglia.
  - The electrodiagnostic findings in Kennedy disease have features similar to those of ALS (i.e., reduced compound muscle action potential [CMAP] amplitudes, fibrillations, fasciculations, large, long-duration

MUAPs with reduced recruitment). In addition, SNAPs are often reduced in Kennedy disease, despite the absence of sensory symptoms or signs.

- In this case, focal slowing of the nerve, indicating focal demyelination, is not a feature of Kennedy disease. In Kennedy disease, the recruitment on voluntary activation is reduced, not normal. Small polyphasic MUAPs indicate myopathic units, which is not a feature of motor neuron diseases. Neuromyotonia is seen in peripheral nerve hyperexcitability syndromes such as Isaacs and Morvan disease.

 **HIGH-YIELD FACT**

Perioral fasciculations can be an important diagnostic clue in Kennedy disease.

 **HIGH-YIELD FACT**

Despite being motor neuron disease, SNAP amplitudes are often reduced in Kennedy disease.

**QUESTION 12.** Which of the following is **LEAST LIKELY** to be seen in Kennedy disease?
- A. Myotonia
- B. Testicular atrophy
- C. Mini-polymyoclonus in the hands
- D. Impaired vibration and joint position sense
- E. Elevated creatine kinase

**ANSWER:** A. Myotonia

**COMMENTS AND DISCUSSION**
- In addition to lower motor neuron weakness, patients with Kennedy disease can have endocrinologic abnormalities such as gynecomastia and testicular atrophy (Fig. 12.2).
- Mini-polymyoclonus in the hands manifesting as fine amplitude trembling movements of fingers can be seen in Kennedy disease, and also occurs in parkinsonian disorders especially multiple system atrophy.
- Electrodiagnostic study in Kennedy disease shows reduced compound muscle action potential (CMAP) amplitudes, the presence of fibrillation potentials, and a neurogenic pattern on needle electromyography (EMG), characterized by large motor unit action potentials (MUAPs) with long duration and reduced recruitment. Sensory nerve action potential (SNAP) amplitudes are often reduced in Kennedy disease, despite it being a motor neuron disorder. However, patients typically do not experience sensory symptoms, although their vibration and joint position sense may be impaired.
- Needle EMG examination of the facial muscles, such as the mentalis muscle, may show grouped repetitive motor unit discharges that occur with mild activation of the facial muscles, which are a highly characteristic feature of Kennedy disease. These discharges are distinguished from myokymic or neuromyotonic discharges, as they occur with mild voluntary contraction rather than spontaneously. Myotonia is not a feature of Kennedy disease.
- Creatine kinase (CK) is often elevated in Kennedy disease, often in the 1000–1500 U/L range. This may lead to misdiagnosis of myopathy.
- Muscle biopsy reveals variability of fiber size with groups of angular atrophic fibers, grouped muscle atrophy, and pyknotic nuclear clumps. Nonspecific myopathic features, including increased central nuclei and necrotic fibers, are also seen, which might also explain the abnormally high Creatine kinase (CK) level.

 **HIGH-YIELD FACT**

Differential diagnoses of mini-polymyoclonus include motor neuron diseases (especially Kennedy disease), and parkinsonian disorders (e.g., multiple system atrophy, Parkinson disease).

 **HIGH-YIELD FACT**

Creatine kinase (CK) can be elevated in motor neuron diseases such as Kennedy disease and ALS, with levels as high as 1000–1500 U/L.

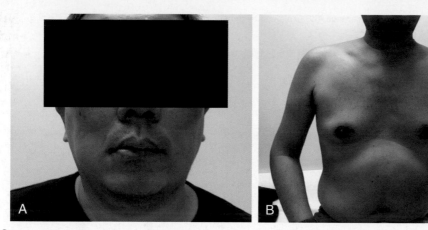

**Fig. 12.2 Kennedy disease.** This man has Kennedy disease with facial asymmetry and weakness (A) and gynecomastia (B). Kennedy disease affects the androgen receptor, resulting in androgen insensitivity and endocrinologic changes including gynecomastia and testicular atrophy (not shown). Courtesy Supoch Tunlayadechanont, MD.

**QUESTION 13.** In patients with amyotrophic lateral sclerosis, what percentage is familial?
- A. 1%
- B. 5%
- C. 10%
- D. 50%
- E. 30%

**ANSWER:** C. 10%

## COMMENTS AND DISCUSSION

- Overall, in patients with amyotrophic lateral sclerosis (ALS), about 10% are familial and the remaining 90% are sporadic. However, genetic mutations may also be identified in some sporadic cases.
- There has been an explosion of gene discovery in ALS in the past decade.
- Among the most important genes are *C9orf72*, *SOD1*, *TARDBP*, and *FUS* (Fig. 12.3).
- Most genes including these four are inherited as autosomal dominant.
  - *SOD1* is the first gene found in ALS. It encodes for *superoxide dismutase 1*, an enzyme important in the breakdown of oxygen free radicals. Notably, TDP-43 inclusions are seen in all forms of genetic ALS, with the exception of those due to *SOD1* mutations.
  - *C9orf72* stands for *chromosome 9 open reading frame 72*. This gene is of great importance, since mutations in this gene are the most common in both familial and sporadic ALS with a known genetic etiology, despite being discovered later. Mutations in this gene involve GGGGCC (hexanucleotide) repeat expansions. It is noteworthy that repeat expansions may not be detected by whole exome sequencing (WES). The typical phenotype associated with *C9orf72* mutations is frontotemporal dementia and amyotrophic lateral sclerosis (FTD-ALS). Besides the clinical features of motor neuron disease, patients also exhibit frontal syndromes, particularly impaired executive function and disinhibition. However, there is significant phenotypic variability, and the phenotypic spectrum of *C9orf72* disease has been expanding. Patients may present with classic ALS, pure motor neuron features, pure cognitive features, or movement disorders such as chorea.
  - *TARDBP* encodes for *TAR DNA-binding protein 43 (TDP-43)*. This gene was discovered based on the fact that TDP-43 is the pathological hallmark in many cases of ALS. However, it is important to note that *TARDBP* mutations are only responsible for a small subset of genetic ALS cases, and not all cases with TDP-43 pathology are due to *TARDBP* mutations.
  - *FUS* encodes for *fused in sarcoma* (FUS) protein, a DNA/RNA binding protein with a role in DNA repair and transcription regulation.
  - Examples of other genes include *CHCHD10*, *CHMP2B*, *UBQLN2*, and *VCP*, among others.

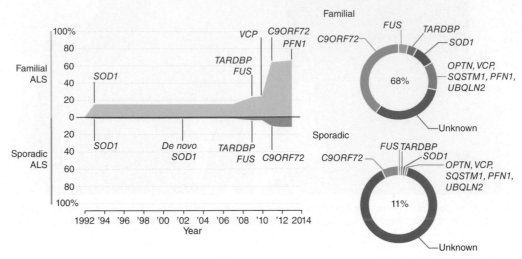

**Fig. 12.3 Genetics of amyotrophic lateral sclerosis (ALS).** The left panel demonstrates gene discoveries in ALS over time. *SOD1* was the first gene discovered. *C9orf72*, discovered later, is the most common gene mutation in both familial ALS and sporadic ALS with identifiable genes, as shown in the right panel. From Renton AE, Chiò A, Traynor BJ. State of play in amyotrophic lateral sclerosis genetics. *Nat Neurosci.* 2014;17(1):17–23.

**QUESTION 14.** What is the most common mutated gene in patients with amyotrophic lateral sclerosis?
A. *ALS2*
B. *C9orf72*
C. *FUS*
D. *SOD1*
E. *TARDBP*

**ANSWER:** B. *C9orf72*

**COMMENTS AND DISCUSSION (see also comments and discussion of Question 13)**
- The most common gene in amyotrophic lateral sclerosis (ALS) is *C9orf72* (Fig. 12.3), despite being one of the most recently discovered genes associated with the disease. Mutations in this gene are the most common in both familial and sporadic cases of ALS with known genetic etiology.
- *SOD1* is the firstly discovered gene in ALS; however, it is much less common than *C9orf72*.
- *FUS, TARDBP*, and *ALS2* are less common than *C9orf72*.

 **HIGH-YIELD FACT**

> The most common genetic mutations in ALS are in the *C9orf72* gene (hexanucleotide GGGGCC repeat expansions), NOT the *SOD1* gene.

**QUESTION 15.** A 49-year-old woman presents with behavioral change for 8 months. Her husband describes that she yells at people and sometimes tries to take her clothes off in public. In the past 2 months he also notes that she has difficulty lifting her right arm and walking up steps. Examination shows muscle atrophy in both the proximal and distal upper and lower extremities, along with tongue atrophy and fasciculations. Fasciculations are also observed in her thighs. Deep tendon reflexes are brisk in all extremities. What genetic abnormality is most likely to be found in this patient?
A. Gene deletion
B. Gene duplication
C. Point mutation
D. Trinucleotide repeat expansion
E. Hexanucleotide repeat expansion

**ANSWER:** E. Hexanucleotide repeat expansion

**COMMENTS AND DISCUSSION (see also comments and discussion of Question 13)**

- The diagnosis in this patient is frontotemporal dementia and amyotrophic lateral sclerosis (FTD-ALS). Frontotemporal dementia often manifests with executive dysfunction and frontal disinhibition, as in this patient. She also has a feature of ALS, a combination of lower and upper motor neuron features. FTD-ALS is due to hexanucleotide (GGGGCC) repeat expansions in the *C9orf72* gene on chromosome 9.
- Patients with ALS may have cognitive or behavioral abnormalities, particularly in case of FTD-ALS, which are often attributed to *C9orf72* mutations. Impaired executive function and disinhibition are the main cognitive features due to frontal lobe involvement. However, ALS cases not associated with *C9orf72* or overt FTD may also have cognitive or behavioral issues.
- 5% of ALS patients have FTD phenotype, whereas about 15% of FTD patients also have the ALS phenotype.

**QUESTION 16.** Which protein accumulation is considered the neuropathological hallmark of amyotrophic lateral sclerosis?
  A. Amyloid
  B. Phosphorylated tau
  C. Progranulin
  D. Synuclein
  E. TAR DNA-binding protein 43 (TDP-43)

**ANSWER:** E. TAR DNA-binding protein 43 (TDP-43)

**COMMENTS AND DISCUSSION**

- TAR DNA-binding protein 43 (TDP-43) accumulation or inclusion is a neuropathological hallmark of amyotrophic lateral sclerosis (ALS). TDP-43 is normally located within the nucleus. In ALS and other neurodegenerative disorders such as Alzheimer disease and frontotemporal dementia, TDP-43 mislocalizes from the nucleus to cytoplasm and forms aggregates or inclusions. How these inclusions contribute to the pathophysiology of ALS remains unclear (Fig. 12.4), but it is one of the active areas of research. TDP-43 inclusions are present in all forms of ALS except those due to *SOD1* mutations.
- Mutations of the *PGRN* gene encoding for progranulin are one of the genetic causes of ALS. However, neuropathologically these cases also have TDP-43 inclusions, not progranulin accumulation. Amyloid and phosphorylated tau accumulation is a hallmark of Alzheimer disease. Synuclein accumulation is seen in Parkinson disease and multiple system atrophy.
- The exact etiology or triggers of motor neuron degeneration in ALS remains unknown.
- Multiple pathologic mechanisms associated with motor neuron degeneration in ALS have been proposed, including
  - Impaired protein homeostasis such as impaired protein degradation by the ubiquitin-proteasome system
  - Increased cellular oxidative stress
  - Mitochondrial dysfunction
  - Impaired DNA repair and impaired RNA processing
  - Impaired vesicular trafficking
  - Neuroinflammation such as microglial activation

 **HIGH-YIELD FACT**

TDP-43 is a neuropathological hallmark in ALS except in ALS due to *SOD1* mutations.

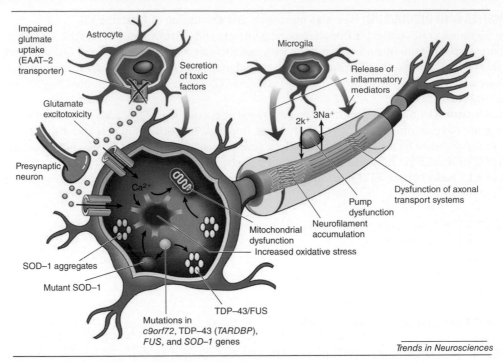

**Fig. 12.4 Pathophysiology of amyotrophic lateral sclerosis (ALS).** Multiple mechanisms have been proposed, including impaired protein homeostasis, increased cellular oxidative stress, mitochondrial dysfunction, impaired axonal transport, and neuroinflammation especially microglial activation, among others. From Vucic S, Rothstein JD, Kiernan MC. Advances in treating amyotrophic lateral sclerosis: Insights from pathophysiological studies. *Trends Neurosci.* 2014;37(8):433–442.

**QUESTION 17.** Which of the following pathological finding is seen in amyotrophic lateral sclerosis?
- A. Bunina bodies
- B. Hirano bodies
- C. Negri bodies
- D. Pick bodies
- E. Tubulofilamentous inclusions

**ANSWER:** A. Bunina bodies

**COMMENTS:**
- In amyotrophic lateral sclerosis (ALS), there is degeneration and loss of the anterior horn cells in the ventral gray matter of the spinal cord.
- In surviving motor neurons, Bunina bodies can be seen as eosinophilic inclusions on hematoxylin and eosin (H&E) staining (Fig. 12.5A). Cytoplasmic TDP-43 inclusions require immunostaining of TDP-43 (Fig. 12.5B). While TDP-43 inclusions have a close relationship with Bunina bodies, they are not identical.
- Hirano bodies are seen in cortical neurons in Alzheimer disease. Negri bodies, eosinophilic inclusions, are seen in rabies, often in Purkinje cells and other neurons. Pick bodies are tau accumulation seen in neurons in patients with the behavioral variant of frontotemporal dementia (bvFTD). Tubulofilamentous inclusions are seen on electron microscopy in patients with inclusion body myositis and oculopharyngeal muscular dystrophy.

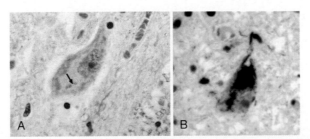

**Fig. 12.5 Neuropathology of amyotrophic lateral sclerosis (ALS).** (A) This hematoxylin and eosin (H&E) staining demonstrates Bunina bodies in the remaining motor neuron as small eosinophilic inclusions. (B) TDP-43 immunostaining reveals TDP-43 inclusions in cytoplasm of the remaining motor neuron within the spinal cord. Normally, TDP-43 is located within the nucleus, but in ALS, there is mislocalization of TDP-43 from nucleus to cytoplasm. From Ellison D, et al. *Neuropathology.* 3rd ed. Elsevier Limited; 2013.

**QUESTION 18.** Which of the following is **CORRECT** regarding gastrostomy in amyotrophic lateral sclerosis?
A. It may increase survival.
B. It reduces the risk of aspiration.
C. It does not improve quality of life.
D. It should be reserved for cases where forced vital capacity falls below 50%.
E. It is performed by percutaneous method only.

**ANSWER:** A. It may increase survival.

**COMMENTS AND DISCUSSION**
- Gastrostomy is considered in patients with amyotrophic lateral sclerosis (ALS) who have poor oral intake or significant weight loss. It may increase survival by 1–4 months and improves quality of life, but it does not reduce the risk of aspiration.
- It should be offered when forced vital capacity (FVC) is greater than 50% of predicted value.
- Although percutaneous endoscopic gastrostomy (PEG) is most commonly performed, other techniques such as radiologically inserted gastrostomy (RIG) and per-oral image-guided gastrostomy are used.

 **HIGH-YIELD FACT**

Gastrostomy in ALS has shown to increase survival by 1–4 months and enhance quality of life, but it does NOT reduce the risk of aspiration.

**QUESTION 19.** According to the 1999 American Academy of Neurology (AAN) guideline, noninvasive positive pressure ventilation should be offered to patients with amyotrophic lateral sclerosis when their forced vital capacity (FVC) is less than:
A. 40%.
B. 50%.
C. 60%.
D. 70%.
E. 90%.

**ANSWER:** B. 50%.

**COMMENTS AND DISCUSSION**
- According to the 1999 American Academy of Neurology (AAN) guideline, non-invasive positive pressure ventilation (NIPPV) should be offered in patients with respiratory symptoms and one of the following:
  - forced vital capacity (FVC) <50% of predicted value
  - maximal static inspiratory pressure (MIP) <60 cmH$_2$O
  - PaCO$_2$ ≥45 mm Hg
  - nocturnal desaturation with an SaO$_2$ <88%.
- However, the European Federation of Neurological Societies (EFNS) guideline recommends NIPPV when FVC is <80% of predicted value.

**QUESTION 20.** What is **CORRECT** regarding medical treatment in amyotrophic lateral sclerosis (ALS)?
A. Riluzole is a free-radical scavenger.
B. Studies of riluzole demonstrated increased survival by 6 months.
C. Edaravone is an anti-glutamatergic agent.
D. Edaravone met the primary end point to improve the Revised ALS Functional Rating Scale (ALSFRS-R) in the initial study.
E. Both riluzole and edaravone are considered disease-modifying therapies.

**ANSWER:** E. Both riluzole and edaravone are considered disease-modifying therapies.

## COMMENTS AND DISCUSSION

- Treatment of ALS is mainly symptomatic and supportive with no curative therapy.
- Multidisciplinary care is proven to be beneficial and improves quality of life.
- Two disease-modifying therapies have modest benefits: riluzole and edaravone. There have been debates regarding the benefits of these medications.
- Riluzole is an antiglutamatergic agent, approved by the U.S. Food and Drug Administration (FDA) in 1995. According to the seminal study in 1994, riluzole 50 μg twice a day taken orally increased 12-month survival by 12% (49% in treatment group versus 37% in placebo group). It was shown to increase survival time by 3 months.
- Edaravone is a free radical scavenger, approved by the U.S. FDA in 2017. It is administered intravenously. This medication initially did not meet the primary end point to improve the Revised ALS Functional Rating Scale (ALSFRS-R). However, in post hoc analysis, it showed a significant decrease in the decline of ALSFRS-R in a small subset of ALS patients who were in the early stages of the disease, within the first 2 years.

**QUESTION 21.** Which genetic mutation is responsible for the majority of spinal muscular atrophy (SMA) cases?
- A. Deletion of the *SMN1* gene
- B. Deletion of the *SMN2* gene
- C. Duplication of the *SMN1* gene
- D. Duplication of the *SMN2* gene
- E. Point mutation of the *SMN1* gene

**ANSWER:** A. Deletion of the *SMN1* gene

## COMMENTS AND DISCUSSION

- Spinal muscular atrophy (SMA) has autosomal recessive inheritance.
- The main responsible gene is the *SMN1* on chromosome 5q13, which encodes the survival motor neuron (SMN) protein essential for the normal function of motor neurons (Fig. 12.6).
- When both alleles of *SMN1* are mutated (deletions in 95% of cases and point mutations in 5%), SMN protein cannot be produced from the *SMN1* gene.
- The upstream *SMN2* gene can produce a small amount of SMN protein. This protein rescues patients from totally absent SMN protein, which would result in severe phenotypes, to having milder phenotypes.
- Due to alternative splicing, exon 7 of the *SMN2* gene is frequently excluded, and the protein produced will be truncated and then degraded (Fig. 12.6). Exon 7 deletion contributes to about 85% of the SMN protein produced by the *SMN2* gene. Thus only 15% of the protein produced from this gene is in full length and able to function. This is important in designing gene therapies for SMA. One strategy is to promote inclusion of the exon 7 during alternative splicing in order to increase the stable form of the SMN protein produced by the *SMN2* gene.
- Thus the number of *SMN2* copies has an inverse correlation with prognosis. The higher number of *SMN2* gene copies the higher the amount of functioning SMN protein, resulting in milder phenotypes of SMA and better prognosis.
- Inclusion of exon 7 in the *SMN2* gene is one of the important strategies in gene therapies of SMA.

---

**CAVEAT**

SMA is due to mutations in the *SMN1* gene, NOT SMA.

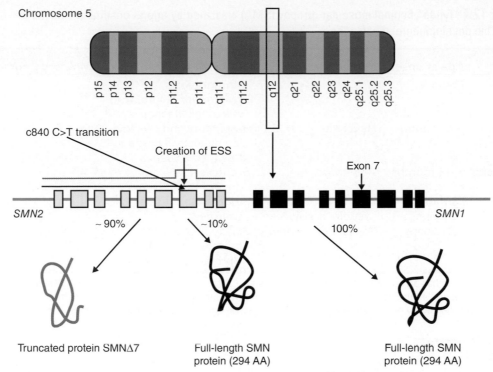

**Fig. 12.6 Production of the survival motor neuron protein by the SMN1 and SMN2 genes.** Normally, the major producer of the survival motor neuron (SMN) protein is the *SMN1* gene (right). In SMA, the *SMN1* gene in both alleles is mutated and cannot produce the SMN protein. The upstream *SMN2* gene can also produce the SMN protein. However, due to exclusion of exon 7 during alternative splicing with creation of an exonic splicing silencer (which promotes exon skipping), 85%–90% of the SMN protein produced from the *SMN2* gene is truncated and then degraded (left, in brown). Only about 10%–15% of the SMN protein produced from the *SMN2* gene is in full length, stable, and can function normally (middle). This small amount of the full-length SMN protein produced from the *SMN2* gene helps convert patients with SMA to milder phenotypes. From Darras BT, et al. Spinal muscular atrophies. In: Darras BT, et al, eds. *Neuromuscular Disorders of Infancy, Childhood, and Adolescence. 2nd ed.* Elsevier; 2015:118)

**QUESTION 22.** What developmental milestone is never achieved and serves to differentiate spinal muscular atrophy type 1 (SMA1) from spinal muscular atrophy types 2, 3, and 4 (SMA2, SMA3, and SMA4)?
A. Sitting
B. Crawling
C. Standing
D. Walking
E. Speaking the first word

**ANSWER:** A. Sitting

**COMMENTS AND DISCUSSION**
- Spinal muscular atrophy (SMA) has a typical onset in childhood.
- Clinical features include lower motor neuron (LMN) weakness, floppy baby, tongue atrophy, tongue fasciculations, bell-shaped abdomen due to use of abdominal rather than chest muscles in respiration, bulbar weakness including swallowing difficulty, and scoliosis, especially in types 1 and 2.
- EMG studies show normal sensory nerve action potentials and reduced amplitudes of compound muscle action potentials, with diffuse active denervation and reinnervation.
- Muscle biopsy is typically not required. If performed, it shows a neurogenic pattern including small or large group muscle fiber atrophy, atrophic fibers, and fiber type grouping.
- SMA is classified into several types based on the age at onset and developmental milestones achieved, which are correlated with the copy number of the *SMN2* gene (Table 12.4).

**TABLE 12.4** Types of spinal muscular atrophy (SMA) classified by age at onset and maximum achievable developmental milestones.

| Type | Age at onset | Motor milestone | Clinical note | *SMN2* copy number |
|------|-------------|-----------------|---------------|---------------------|
| 0 | Prenatal | N/A | Arthrogryposis, respiratory failure, a few-week lifespan | 1 |
| 1 (non-sitters) | 0–6 months | Never sits | Respiratory and swallowing difficulty. Lifespan less than 2 years | 2, 3 |
| 2 (sitters) | 6–18 months | Able to sit | Scoliosis. Lifespan greater than 2 years | 3, 4 |
| 3 | 18 months–21 years | Able to walk but may require assistance | Progressive muscle weakness | 3, 4 |
| 4 | >21 years | Walks independently | Slowly progressive muscle weakness. Normal life expectancy | 4 or more |

Of note, type 1 also has an eponym, Werdnig-Hoffman disease. Type 3 has an eponym, Kugelberg-Welander disease. Type 4 is also called "adult SMA." Type 3 is subdivided into two subtypes, 3a and 3b, based on the age at onset. Type 3a is characterized by onset before the age of 3 years, while type 3b is characterized by onset after 3 years of age.

---

**MNEMONIC**

SMA type 1 – never sits (independently)
SMA type 2 – never walks (independently)
SMA type 3 – able to walk independently at some point

---

**MNEMONIC**

The number of *SMN2* gene copies can be estimated by adding 1 to the number of SMA type. For example, most SMA type 2 patients have 2+1=3 copies of the *SMN2* gene.
However, there is variability and the number of *SMN2* gene copies can differ among patients.

---

**QUESTION 23.** What is the mechanism of action of nusinersen?
  A. Inclusion of exon 7 in the *SMN1* gene during alternative splicing
  B. Exclusion of exon 7 in the *SMN1* gene during alternative splicing
  C. Inclusion of exon 7 in the *SMN2* gene during alternative splicing
  D. Exclusion of exon 7 in the *SMN2* gene during alternative splicing
  E. Replacing the *SMN1* gene by a viral vector

**ANSWER:** C. Inclusion of exon 7 in the *SMN2* gene during alternative splicing

**COMMENTS AND DISCUSSION**
- The *SMN2* gene can produce the survival motor neuron (SMN) protein in a smaller amount, compared to the *SMN1* gene. In spinal muscular atrophy (SMA), where the *SMN1* gene cannot produce the SMN protein, the SMN protein produced by the *SMN2* gene can help convert more severe phenotypes to milder ones. However, ~85% of the SMN protein translated from the *SMN2* gene is unstable and degraded, due to a lack of exon 7 during alternative splicing. Therefore, normally only 15% of the SMN protein produced by the *SMN2* gene is functional.
- Gene therapy in SMA is a remarkable milestone in the treatment of neuromuscular disorders.
- As of March 2023, there are three medications approved by U.S. Food and Drug Administration (FDA) (Table 12.5 and Fig. 12.7).
  ○ Nusinersen is an antisense oligonucleotide (ASO) that binds to the *SMN2* gene and promotes inclusion of exon 7 during alternative splicing. This results in increase in the stable form of the survival motor neuron (SMN) protein.
  ○ Risdiplam is a small molecule that also promotes inclusion of exon 7 during alternative splicing.
  ○ Onasemnogene Abeparvovec-xioi has a mechanism of action different from nusinersen and risdiplam. It is an AAV9-delivered *SMN1* gene replacement. It works by replacing the mutated *SMN1* gene instead of targeting the *SMN2* gene.

- There are still questions regarding which medication should be selected as the first-line treatment, and whether combining these medications would be effective.
- Symptomatic therapies and a multidisciplinary approach, including physical therapy and rehabilitation, nutritional, and pulmonary management, are also important.
- Given the availability of gene therapies, early diagnosis and treatment even before patients become symptomatic are key to success. Therefore, newborn screening is currently available in several U.S. states.

**TABLE 12.5** Summary of approved gene therapies for spinal muscular atrophy.

| | Nusinersen | Onasemnogene Abeparvovec-xioi | Risdiplam |
|---|---|---|---|
| US FDA approval year | 2016 | 2019 | 2020 |
| Type of medication | Antisense oligonucleotide | AAV9-delivered *SMN1* gene replacement | Small molecule, pyridazine derivative |
| Mechanism of action | Binding to a specific intronic sequence downstream to exon 7, which promotes inclusion of exon 7 during splicing of the *SMN2* gene and translation of full-length SMN protein | Delivering *SMN1* gene by an AAV9 viral vector | Promoting inclusion of exon 7 during splicing of the *SMN2* gene |
| Pivotal trial | ENDEAR NURTURE EMBRACE (SMA2, SMA3) | STR1VE-US START (long-term follow up) | FIREFISH SUNFISH |
| Route of administration | Intrathecal | Intravenous | Oral |
| Dosing | 4 loading doses: q 14 days x 3 doses, then q 30 days | Single dose (weight-based) | Daily |
| Indication | All SMA types | All SMA patients <2 years of age | All SMA types ≥2 months of age |
| Side effect | Well-tolerated. However, complications can occur from repeated lumbar puncture. | Elevated liver enzymes including AST, ALT; thrombocytosis | In SMA1, upper respiratory tract infection, pneumonia, cough, vomiting. In SMA2 and SMA3, fever, diarrhea, rash |

*AAV9*, Adeno-associated virus serotype 9; *ALT*, alanine aminotransferase; *AST*, aspartate aminotransferase; *q*, every; *SMN1*, the survival motor neuron 1 gene; *SMN2*, the survival motor neuron 2 gene; *SMA*, spinal muscular atrophy; *SMA1*, spinal muscular atrophy type 1; *SMA2*, spinal muscular atrophy type 2; *SMA3*, spinal muscular atrophy type 3; *US FDA*, The United States Food and Drug Administration

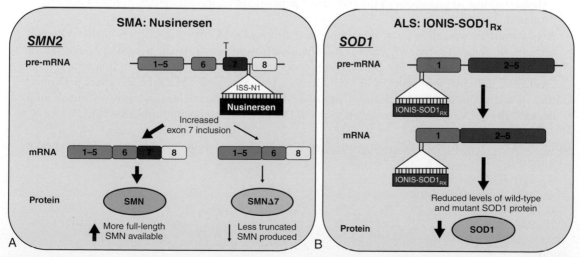

**Fig. 12.7 Mechanism of gene therapies in spinal muscular atrophy (SMA).** (A) Nusinersen and risdiplam work by promoting inclusion of exon 7 during alternative splicing, thereby increasing the full-length survival motor neuron (SMN) protein. (B) Onasemnogene Abeparvovec-xioi is an *SMN1* gene replacement by using an AAV9 viral vector. From Tosolini AP, Sleigh JN. Motor Neuron Gene Therapy: Lessons from Spinal Muscular Atrophy for Amyotrophic Lateral Sclerosis. *Front Mol Neurosci.* 2017 Dec 7;10:405.

**QUESTION 24.** What is the most common number of copies of the *SMN2* gene in spinal muscular atrophy type 2 (SMA2)?
A. 1
B. 2
C. 3
D. 4
E. 5

**ANSWER:** C. 3

**COMMENTS AND DISCUSSION**
- The *SMN2* gene is downstream to the *SMN1* gene. It can produce a small amount of the survival motor neuron (SMN) protein that helps convert more severe phenotypes to milder ones.
- The number of *SMN2* gene copies has an inverse relationship with the severity of spinal muscular atrophy (SMA). In SMA type 0 (SMA0), there is only one copy of the *SMN2* gene. In SMA1 and SMA2, most patients have two and three copies of the *SMN2* gene, respectively. In SMA3, about half of patients have three copies, and the remaining have four copies (and thus a less-severe phenotype or SMA3b). One way to remember is that the number of the *SMN2* copies can be roughly guessed by adding 1 to the number of SMA type. For example, SMA2 would have $2+1=3$ copies of the *SMN2* gene.

**QUESTION 25.** A 6-week-old baby presents with a weak cry, inspiratory stridor, and respiratory distress. Chest X-ray shows diaphragmatic paralysis. In addition, generalized weakness is noted in all four extremities. Genetic testing of the *SMN1* gene is negative. What gene is most likely responsible for this patient's condition?
A. *BSCL2*
B. *DMD*
C. *HSPB1*
D. *IGHMBP2*
E. *SMN2*

**ANSWER:** D. *IGHMBP2*

**COMMENT AND DISCUSSION**
- The diagnosis in this patient is spinal muscular atrophy with respiratory distress (SMARD). The clinical presentation includes lower motor neuron weakness, respiratory distress due to weakness of respiratory muscles and diaphragmatic paralysis, with typical onset in infancy. Babies can have a weak cry and inspiratory stridor, and the autonomic nervous system can also be affected, resulting in excessive sweating, cardiac arrhythmia, constipation, urinary incontinence, and pain insensitivity. SMARD1 is due to mutations in the *IGHMBP2* gene encoding immunoglobulin micro-binding protein 2.
- *BSCL2* mutations result in distal spinal muscular atrophy (SMA) type 5b, which is allelic to hereditary spastic paraplegia type 17. Patients have hand amyotrophy and spastic paraparesis, a condition known as Silver syndrome. The *DMD* gene encodes dystrophin, and mutations in this gene result in Duchenne muscular dystrophy. *HSPB1* mutations are seen in distal SMA type 2b, where patients initially present with distal leg weakness that progresses to the proximal legs and arms within about a decade. The *SMN2* gene is downstream to the *SMN1* gene, which is responsible for SMA.

**QUESTION 26.** Which of the following pathogens does **NOT** cause poliomyelitis (infection of anterior horn cells)?
A. *Borrelia burgdorferi*
B. Non-polio enterovirus
C. Poliovirus
D. West Nile virus

**ANSWER:** A. *Borrelia burgdorferi*

## COMMENTS AND DISCUSSION

- The term "poliomyelitis" refers to infection or inflammation of the anterior horn cells from, which can be caused by any pathogens, not just poliovirus. In addition to poliovirus, other viruses such as West Nile virus (resulting in West Nile poliomyelitis) and enteroviruses D68 and A71 can also cause poliomyelitis.
- *Borrelia burgdorferi* causes Lyme disease, which can present with variety of symptoms including skin rash, cognitive changes, facial palsy, polyradiculopathy, and sensory neuropathy. However, Lyme disease does not cause anterior horn cell loss.
- Poliovirus belongs to the genus Enterovirus and in the family Picornaviridae.
  - Transmission is via fecal-oral route. The incubation period before development of paralysis is about 1–3 weeks.
  - Patients present with acute flaccid paralysis. The urinary bladder can be involved in up to 30% of patients.
  - Poliomyelitis caused by poliovirus infection is very rare in the era of polio vaccine. However, there have been scant reports of vaccine-associated paralytic poliomyelitis (VAPP) after administration of oral polio vaccine (OPV), which is a live-attenuated vaccine. The inactivated polio vaccine (IPV) carries less risk of VAPP and is currently used in the United States.
- West Nile virus is a mosquito-borne flavivirus.
  - West Nile virus infeciton is more prevalent during summer, with a higher incidence in the central and western regions of the United States.
  - In addition to encephalitis and meningitis, West Nile virus can result in poliomyelitis.
- Acute flaccid myelitis can also be caused by non-polio enteroviruses.
  - There were outbreaks of acute flaccid myelitis in the United States from enterovirus D68 and enterovirus A71.
- Post-polio syndrome is a specific syndrome of slowly progressive lower motor neuron weakness that typically occurs several decades after the initial poliovirus infection, often in late adulthood or the elderly. The diagnosis is primarily based on clinical evaluation, as electrodiagnostic studies cannot distinguish stable poliomyelitis from post polio syndrome. The pathophysiology of this syndrome is not yet fully understood, but is believed to result from a reduced number of motor neurons superimposed on the normal aging process and loss of some motor neurons due to the initial poliovirus infection.

**QUESTION 27.** A 23-year-old man presents with weakness of the right hand for 8 months. On examination, there is weakness and atrophy of the right intrinsic hand muscles including the abductor pollicis brevis, abductor digiti minimi, first dorsal interossei, and finger extensors. Sensory examination is unremarkable. Deep tendon reflexes are 1+ in the right biceps, triceps, and brachioradialis. Examination in the other extremities is normal. Which of the following investigations is most useful to confirm the diagnosis?

A. Genetic testing
B. Computerized tomography (CT) angiogram of the neck
C. Creatine kinase
D. Dynamic magnetic resonance imaging (MRI) of the cervical spine with contrast
E. Lumbar puncture

**ANSWER:** D. Dynamic magnetic resonance imaging (MRI) of the cervical spine with contrast

## COMMENTS AND DISCUSSION

- The diagnosis in this patient is Hirayama disease (aka, monomelic amyotrophy).
- Hirayama disease typically has an onset is in late adolescence or young adulthood, and is more common in Asian and Indian populations.
- In Hirayama disease, lower motor neuron weakness (and atrophy) typically involves only one limb, most commonly in the hand or C7, C8, and T1-innervated muscles with sparing of C5 to C6 innervated muscles (Fig. 12.8). The progression is insidious. There is no sensory involvement.
- Investigations of Hirayama disease
  - Electrodiagnosis study shows low compound muscle action potential (CMAP) amplitudes typically recorded over C8/T1-innervated muscles (innervated by the median and ulnar nerves) and a neurogenic pattern on needle electromyography (EMG). Sensory nerve action potentials (SNAPs) are normal.
  - Neuroimaging should be specifically requested as "dynamic flexion cervical spine MRI with contrast," since routine MRI of the cervical spine may not be useful. In the neck flexion position, there is

gadolinium enhancement posterior to the dura, representing engorgement of the spinal venous plexus (Fig. 12.9). In addition, a T2 hyperintense signal at the bilateral ventral gray horns (representing anterior horn cells) can be seen, resulting in a "snake-eye" or "owl-eye" appearance. This is not specific for Hirayama disease, and can also be seen in other disorders affecting the anterior horn cells such as poliomyelitis and spinal cord infarction.

  o CT angiography of the neck and lumbar puncture are not useful in confirming the diagnosis of Hirayama disease.

  o Creatine kinase level is usually normal.

- The etiology remains unclear but is likely acquired with no clear genetic basis. Intermittent ischemia from compression of the dura posteriorly, especially when flexing the neck, has been proposed.

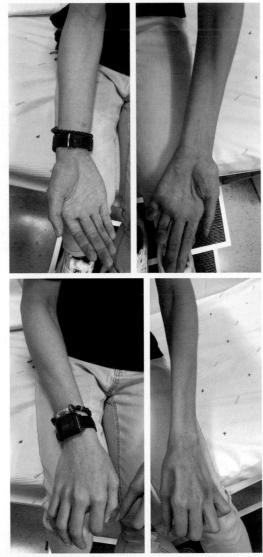

**Fig. 12.8 Hirayama disease.** This figure illustrates a man with Hirayama disease (monomelic amyotrophy) showing prominent atrophy of the intrinsic muscles of the left hand including thenar and hypothenar muscles, as well as forearm muscles. Courtesy Supoch Tunlayadechanont, MD.

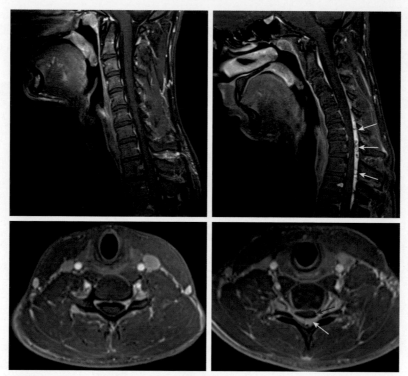

**Fig. 12.9 Magnetic resonance imaging (MRI) with dynamic flexion of the cervical spine in monomelic amyotrophy.** Fat-saturated gadolinium-enhanced MRI scans. *Left,* Neck straight. *Right,* Neck flexed. *Top,* Midsagittal view. *Bottom,* Axial view. Note that with neck flexion, there is gadolinium enhancement posterior to the dura from C4 to T2 *(yellow arrows),* representing venous engorgement as the posterior dura moves forward against the spinal cord. On the axial images, note the similar gadolinium enhancement *(yellow arrow)* and the atrophy of the spinal cord *(red arrow).* (From Preston DC, Shapiro BE. *Electromyography and Neuromuscular Disorders, 4th ed.* Philadelphia: Elsevier; 2020.)

**QUESTION 28.** A 64-year-old man presents with proximal muscle weakness in both arms and legs, gait unsteadiness, numbness in both hands and feet, urinary incontinence, and dementia. Examination reveals both upper and lower motor neuron features in both arms and legs. What is the most likely finding on his sural nerve biopsy?

A. Segmental demyelination
B. Onion bulb formation
C. Giant axons
D. Polyglucosan bodies
E. Tomacula

**ANSWER:** D. Polyglucosan bodies

**COMMENTS AND DISCUSSION**

- The diagnosis in this patient is adult polyglucosan body disease.
  - Adult polyglucosan body disease is an autosomal recessive disorder caused by mutations in the *GBE1* gene which encodes for glycogen branching enzyme.
  - Accumulation of polyglucosan body is a pathological hallmark (Fig. 12.10), found in peripheral nerves, in addition to the central nervous system. The structure of the polyglucosan body is similar to that of Lafora body and corpora amylacea.
  - The clinical presentation includes a combination of upper motor neuron (UMN) and lower motor neuron (LMN) dysfunction, which is similar to amyotrophic lateral sclerosis (ALS). In addition, patients have urinary incontinence, sensorimotor polyneuropathy, and dementia.
  - Brain magnetic resonance imaging (MRI) may show T2/FLAIR (fluid-attenuated inversion recovery) hyperintensity in the periventricular white matter (Fig. 12.10).
- In adult polyglucosan body disease, sensorimotor polyneuropathy in adult polyglucosan body disease is an axonal process. Therefore, segmental demyelination and onion bulb formation, which represent repetitive demyelination and remyelination, should not also be expected in this condition.
- Giant axons are a characteristic finding in giant axonal neuropathy due to mutations in the *GAN* gene encoding for gigaxonin. In addition, giant axons can also be seen in *n*-hexane-induced neuropathy.

- Tomacula, focal areas of sausage-shaped swellings of the myelin sheath, are a pathological hallmark of hereditary neuropathy with liability to pressure palsy (HNPP). Hence, HNPP is also referred to as tomaculous neuropathy. This disorder is causesd by deletion of the *PMP22* gene which encodes for the peripheral myelin protein.

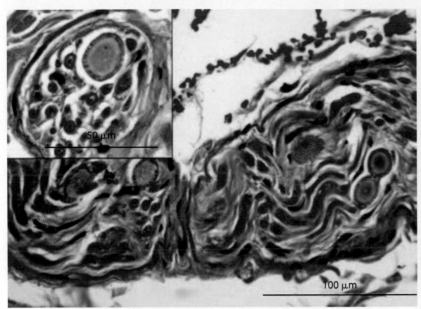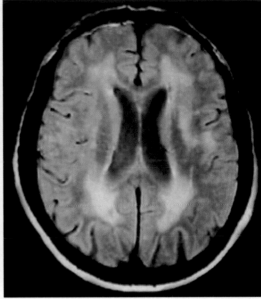

**Fig. 12.10  Adult polyglucosan body disease (APBD).** *Left,* longitudinal and transverse sections *(upper left corner)* of the nerve in a patient with APBD reveals polyglucosan bodies within the axons. *Right,* magnetic resonance imaging of the brain demonstrates periventricular white matter changes on the fluid-attenuated inversion recovery (FLAIR) sequence. From Preston DC, Shapiro BE. *Electromyography and Neuromuscular Disorders,* 4th ed. Philadelphia: Elsevier; 2020.)

**QUESTION 29.** What is the treatment of choice for Brown-Vialetto-Van Laere disease?
  A. Vitamin B1
  B. Vitamin B2
  C. Vitamin B5
  D. Vitamin B6
  E. Vitamin B12

**ANSWER:** B. Vitamin B2

**COMMENTS AND DISCUSSION**
- Brown-Vialetto-Van Laere syndrome (BVVLS) is a riboflavin (vitamin B2)–responsive motor neuron disorder.
- It is autosomal recessive, due to mutations in the genes that have roles in riboflavin transport.
- Fazio-Londe disease is also in the same spectrum but without sensorineural hearing loss.
- The onset of BVVLS is typically in infancy or childhood but patients can also present later in life.
- Clinical features of BVVLS include progressive bulbar palsy involving the facial and extraocular muscles and bilateral sensorineural hearing loss. Later on, patients may develop both upper and lower motor neuron features, cerebellar signs, and respiratory muscle weakness.
- The treatment of BVVLS is riboflavin (vitamin B2) supplementation, along with supportive and symptomatic treatment.

**QUESTION 30.** A 45-year-old man presents with several-years history of progressive weakness, imbalance, and tremor. He has a recent history of schizoaffective disorder. His neurological examination shows nystagmus, cerebellar ataxia, generalized weakness, and hyperreflexia. Which blood test is most useful in the diagnosis?
  A. Hexosaminidase A enzyme activity
  B. Phytanic acid serum level
  C. Testosterone serum level
  D. Acid alpha-glucosidase enzyme activity
  E. Alpha-galactosidase enzyme activity

**ANSWER:** A. Hexosaminidase A enzyme activity

## COMMENTS AND DISCUSSION

- This patient has late-onset Tay-Sachs disease.
- Late-onset Tay-Sachs disease is an autosomal recessive disorder, due to mutations in the *HEXA* gene encoding for hexosaminidase A.
- Hexosaminidase A is a lysosomal enzyme important in ganglioside degradation (Fig. 12.11).
- Hexosaminidase A deficiency results in accumulation of GM2 ganglioside, referred to as GM2 gangliosidosis.
- This disorder is more common in Ashkenazi Jewish, French Canadian, and Cajun populations.
- Late-onset Tay-Sachs disease typically presents with lower motor neuron weakness initially in the lower extremities, upper motor neuron features, cerebellar ataxia, and psychiatric features
- The quadriceps and triceps are often involved.
- Electrodiagnostic studies show reduced compound muscle action potential (CMAP) amplitude on nerve conduction study, and fibrillations, fasciculations, with neurogenic pattern (large, long-duration motor unit action potentials [MUAPs] with reduced recruitment) on needle electromyography (EMG). Complex repetitive discharges (CRDs) are common. Sensory nerve action potential (SNAP) amplitudes may be low.
- Diagnosis can be confirmed by genetic testing or hexosaminidase A enzyme level testing in serum, leukocytes, or fibroblasts.
- Phytanic acid accumulates in Refsum disease, an autosomal recessive disease characterized by retinitis pigmentosa, peripheral neuropathy, cerebellar ataxia, and elevated cerebrospinal fluid (CSF) protein. Acid-alpha glucosidase enzyme activity is reduced in Pompe disease, characterized by early respiratory failure, proximal weakness, and myotonic discharges on needle EMG. Alpha-galactosidase enzyme activity is reduced in leukocytes in Fabry disease, characterized by sensory neuropathy with painful episodes, renal failure, myocardial infarction, stroke, trunk angiokeratomas, and slowed conduction velocities. Testosterone serum level is reduced in Kennedy disease.

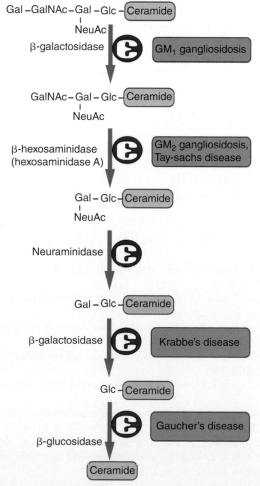

**Fig. 12.11** Ganglioside degradation pathway. Ganglioside GM2 is converted to ganglioside GM3 by the enzyme hexosaminidase. Deficiency in this enzyme results in Tay-Sachs disease. From Baynes JW, Dominicazk MH. *Medical Biochemistry. 5th ed.* Elsevier; 2019.

**QUESTION 31.**  A 66-year-old man presents with a several-year history of numbness of the left face followed by slurred speech, chewing difficulties, muscle twitches in the limbs, and mild generalized weakness. His neurological examination shows dysarthria, asymmetrical lower facial weakness and sensory loss, weak jaw opening, tongue weakness, and limb fasciculations. His reflexes are brisk in the upper and lower extremities with Babinski sign. Electromyography reveals dissemination of denervation in the bulbar and three spinal segments of the neuraxis with normal sensory nerve action potentials. What is the most likely diagnosis?

A.  Muscle-specific tyrosine kinase (MuSK)–positive myasthenia gravis
B.  X-linked bulbospinal muscular atrophy (Kennedy disease)
C.  Facial-onset sensory and motor neuronopathy (FOSMN)
D.  Progressive bulbar palsy form of motor neuron disease
E.  Chronic inflammatory demyelinating polyneuropathy (CIDP)

**ANSWER:** C. Facial-onset sensory and motor neuronopathy (FOSMN)

**COMMENTS AND DISCUSSION**

- Facial-onset sensory and motor neuronopathy (FOSMN) is a rare, slowly-progressive bulbar-onset disorder. It is characterized by facial and perioral sensory symptoms, followed by descending lower motor neuron findings.
- CK enzyme may be modestly elevated.
- Imaging may reveal atrophy of the midcervical cord. Electromyography (EMG) and nerve conduction studies show sensory and motor abnormalities, often in a cranial to caudal gradient of severity. Blink reflexes are commonly absent.
- The underlying etiology of FOSMN is unclear. An underlying inflammatory basis or a neurodegenerative etiology are both speculated.
- MuSK-positive myasthenia gravis should not have sensory loss and denervation in spinal segments. Chronic inflammatory demyelinating polyneuropathy (CIDP) should have areflexia and Kennedy disease does not have upper motor signs or facial sensory loss. The progressive bulbar palsy form of motor neuron disease does not have facial sensory loss.

## SUGGESTED READINGS

Baek WS, Desai NP. ALS: pitfalls in the diagnosis. *Pract Neurol.* 2007;7:74-81.

Brooks BR, Miller RG, Swash M, Munsat TL. El Escorial revisited: Revised criteria for the diagnosis of amyotrophic lateral sclerosis. *Amyotroph Lateral Scler Other Motor Neuron Disord.* 2000;1(5):293-299.

Boonyapisit K. Poliomyelitis and post-poliomyelitis syndrome. In: Katirji B, Kaminski HJ, Ruff RL, eds. *Neuromuscular Disorders in Clinical Practice.* 2nd ed. New York: Springer; 2014:383-393.

Bosch AM, Stroek K, Abeling NG, Waterham HR, Ijlst L, Wanders RJ. The Brown-Vialetto-Van Laere and Fazio Londe syndrome revisited: natural history, genetics, treatment and future perspectives. *Orphanet J Rare Dis.* 2012;7:83.

Nalini A, Gourie-Devi M, Thennarasu K, Ramalingaiah AH. Monomelic amyotrophy: clinical profile and natural history of 279 cases seen over 35 years (1976–2010). *Amyotroph Lateral Scler Frontotemporal Degener.* 2014;15:457-465.

Costa J, Swash M, de Carvalho M. Awaji criteria for the diagnosis of amyotrophic lateral sclerosis: a systematic review. *Arch Neurol.* 2012;69(11):1410.

De Carvalho M, Dengler R, Eisen A, et al. Electrodiagnostic criteria for diagnosis of ALS. *Clin Neurophysiol.* 2008;119:497-503.

de Carvalho MD, Swash M. Awaji diagnostic algorithm increases sensitivity of El Escorial criteria for ALS diagnosis. *Amyotroph Lateral Scler.* 2009;10:53-57.

Fratta P, Nirmalananthan N, Masset L, et al. Correlation of clinical and molecular features in spinal bulbar muscular atrophy. *Neurology.* 2014;82:2077-2084.

Gray F, Gherardi R, Marshall A, Janota I, Poirier J. Adult polyglucosan body disease (APBD). *J Neuropathol Exp Neurol.* 1988;47:459-474.

Katzberg HD, Benatar M. Enteral tube feeding for amyotrophic lateral sclerosis/motor neuron disease. *Cochrane Database Syst Rev.* 2011;1:CD004030.

Kolb SJ, Kissel JT. Spinal muscular atrophy: a timely review. *Arch Neurol.* 2011;68:979-984.

Kuwabara S, Sonoo M, Komori T, et al. Dissociated small hand muscle atrophy in amyotrophic lateral sclerosis: frequency, extent, and specificity. *Muscle Nerve.* 2008;37:426-430.

Lebl DR, Hughes A, Cammisa FP, O'Leary PF. Cervical spondylotic myelopathy: pathophysiology, clinical presentation, and treatment. *HSS J.* 2011;7(2):170-178.

Mathisa S, Goizetc C, Soulagesa A, Vallate JM, Le Massona G. Genetics of amyotrophic lateral sclerosis: a review. *J Neurol Sci.* 2019;399:217-226.

Nalini A, Gourie-Devi M, Thennarasu K, Ramalingaiah AH. Monomelic amyotrophy: clinical profile and natural history of 279 cases seen over 35 years (1976-2010). *Amyotroph Lateral Scler Frontotemporal Degener.* 2014;15(5–6):457–465.

Okamoto K, Mizuno Y, Fujita Y. Bunina bodies in amyotrophic lateral sclerosis. *Neuropathology.* 2008;28(2):109-115.

Oskarsson B, Gendron TF, Staff NP. Amyotrophic lateral sclerosis: an update for 2018. *Mayo Clin Proc.* 2018;93(11):1617-1628.

Pioro EP. Current concepts in the pharmacotherapy of pseudobulbar affect. *Drugs.* 2011;71(9):1193-1207.

Preston DC, Shapiro BE. *Electromyography and Neuromuscular Disorders.* 4th ed. Philadelphia: Elsevier; 2020:525-539.

Wilbourn AJ. The "split hand syndrome." *Muscle Nerve.* 2000;23:138.

Wirth B, Karakaya M, Kye MJ, Mendoza-Ferreira N. Twenty-five years of spinal muscular atrophy research: from phenotype to genotype to therapy, and what comes next. *Annu Rev Genomics Hum Genet.* 2020;21:231-261.

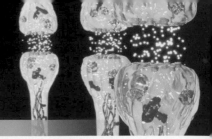

# CHAPTER 13

# Plexus Disorders

**Q1.** The medial antebrachial cutaneous nerve is a branch of the:
A. lateral cord.
B. medial cord.
C. upper trunk.
D. posterior cord.
E. ulnar nerve.

**Q2.** The muscle pair denervated by a lesion of the posterior cord of the brachial plexus is the:
A. rhomboids and infraspinatus.
B. supraspinatus and teres minor.
C. brachioradialis and pronator teres.
D. pronator quadratus and triceps brachii.
E. deltoid and abductor pollicis longus.

**Q3.** A 35-year-old man presents after a motor vehicle accident 2 weeks prior with right upper extremity weakness. He cannot lift his right arm above the shoulder and has numbness at the lateral aspect of the right forearm. Which of the following electrodiagnostic findings is expected in this patient?
A. Reduced right median compound muscle action potential (CMAP) amplitude
B. Reduced right ulnar CMAP amplitude
C. Reduced right musculocutaneous CMAP amplitude
D. Absent right ulnar sensory nerve action potential (SNAP)
E. Absent right medial antebrachial cutaneous SNAP

**Q4.** A 37-year-old man presents after a motor vehicle accident 2 weeks prior with weakness of the right deltoid, biceps, supraspinatus, and infraspinatus. Sensory deficit is present in the lateral forearm. Nerve conduction study shows normal median and ulnar compound muscle action potentials (CMAPs); however, the median sensory nerve action potential (SNAP) recording the index finger is absent, and the radial SNAP is reduced. The ulnar SNAP is preserved. What is the most likely diagnosis?
A. C5 or C6 radiculopathy
B. Upper trunk plexopathy
C. Middle trunk plexopathy
D. Lateral cord plexopathy
E. Median neuropathy

**Q5.** A 42-year-old-man presents after a motor vehicle accident 6 weeks prior with right upper extremity weakness and numbness. You suspect a lateral cord plexopathy based on physical examination. Abnormal electromyography (EMG) findings are expected in which of the following three muscles?
A. Deltoid, rhomboid, and brachioradialis
B. Biceps, serratus anterior, and infraspinatus
C. Rhomboid, serratus anterior, and supraspinatus
D. Deltoid, biceps, and supraspinatus
E. Biceps, brachialis, and pronator teres

**Q6.** A 47-year-old man presents after a motor vehicle accident 2 weeks prior with right upper extremity weakness and numbness. The nerve conduction study is shown below. What is the diagnosis?

| | Latency (ms) | | Amplitude (mV) | | CV (m/s) | |
|---|---|---|---|---|---|---|
| | **R** | **L** | **R** | **L** | **R** | **L** |
| Median, APB (M) | 3.4 | | 7.0 | | | |
| | | | 6.0 | | 56 | |
| Ulnar, ADM (M) | 3.2 | | 8.2 | | | |
| | | | 8.0 | | 56 | |
| | | | 7.0 | | 62 | |
| Median/index (S) | 2.4 | 2.6 | 12 | 20 | 53 | 55 |
| Ulnar (S) | 2.1 | 2.2 | 18 | 20 | 54 | 56 |
| Radial (S) | 2.0 | 1.8 | 8 | 20 | 52 | 66 |
| LABC (S) | 1.5 | 1.9 | 5 | 12 | 56 | 52 |

*ADM*, abductor digiti minimi; *APB*, abductor pollicis brevis; *CV*, conduction velocity; *L*, left; *LABC*, lateral antebrachial cutaneous nerve; *M*, motor; *ms*, millisecond; *m/s*, meter per second; *mV*, millivolt; *R*, right; *S*, sensory

A. Upper trunk plexopathy
B. Lower trunk plexopathy
C. Lateral cord plexopathy
D. Posterior cord plexopathy
E. Medial cord plexopathy

**Q7.** A 23-year-old man sustained a gunshot wound to the right posterior shoulder 2 months prior resulting in weakness of the right triceps, and wrist flexor and extensor muscles. The nerve conduction study shows normal median and ulnar compound muscle action potentials (CMAPs). The median sensory nerve action potential (SNAP) recording the middle finger and radial SNAP recording from the snuffbox are reduced. The median (recording the index finger) and ulnar SNAPs are normal. Needle electromyography (EMG) shows neurogenic changes in the right triceps, pronator teres, and flexor carpi radialis. What is the most likely diagnosis?
A. Upper trunk plexopathy
B. Middle trunk plexopathy
C. Lower trunk plexopathy
D. Lateral cord plexopathy
E. Posterior cord plexopathy

**Q8.** Which of the following helps differentiate C7 radiculopathy from a middle trunk plexopathy?
A. Median sensory nerve action potential (SNAP) (recording the thumb)
B. Median SNAP (recording the middle finger)
C. Ulnar compound muscle action potential (CMAP)
D. Involvement of the pronator teres
E. Involvement of the extensor indicis proprius

**Q9.** A 6-month-old boy has had left arm weakness since birth. Delivery was prolonged and required forceps. At rest, the arm is adducted, elbow extended, and forearm pronated. There is severe weakness and atrophy of biceps and deltoid, whereas the hand moves well. The biceps reflex is absent. The median sensory response is absent on nerve conduction study. The most likely lesion location is at the:
A. musculocutaneous nerve.
B. upper trunk.
C. C5 and C6 nerve roots.
D. lateral cord.
E. axillary nerve.

**Q10.** The first change seen on electrodiagnostic study in a severe axon-loss plexopathy is:
A. fibrillations in the affected muscles.
B. decrease in the sensory amplitudes.
C. decrease in the motor amplitudes.
D. increased polyphasic motor unit action potentials (MUAPs).
E. reduced recruitment in the affected muscles.

**Q11.** A 65-year-old man, who is a heavy smoker, presents with a 4 months history of weakness of all right intrinsic hand muscles, impaired sensation in the fourth and fifth fingers up to the medial forearm, and a right. Horner syndrome. You suspect Pancoast tumor. What is the most likely abnormal electrodiagnostic finding?
A. Reduced musculocutaneous compound muscle action potential (CMAP) amplitude
B. Conduction slowing in the ulnar motor study of less than 70% of the lower normal limit
C. Absent lateral antebrachial cutaneous sensory study
D. Prolonged median motor latency greater than 140% of the upper normal limit
E. Reduced ulnar CMAP amplitude

**The following vignette is for QUESTIONS 12 through 14:**

> A 23-year-old football player develops severe right shoulder pain and weakness of the right arm after being tackled 3 months prior. On examination, he has weakness of the right biceps and numbness at the palmar aspect of the right thumb, index finger, and the lateral side of the right forearm.

**Q12.** Which of the following statements is **CORRECT**?
A. The injury may result from plexus traction.
B. Nerve roots can also be injured.
C. Pain is a common feature.
D. Preserved sensory nerve action potentials (SNAPs) portend poor prognosis.
E. All of the above

**Q13.** Which two cervical roots are most commonly involved with burners or stingers?
A. C3 and C4
B. C4 and C5
C. C5 and C6
D. C6 and C7
E. C7 and T1

**Q14.** Which of the following is the most useful and localizing electrodiagnostic finding in this patient?
A. Median compound muscle action potential (CMAP) amplitude
B. Median sensory nerve action potential (SNAP) amplitude
C. Ulnar CMAP amplitude
D. Ulnar SNAP amplitude
E. Radial CMAP amplitude

**Q15.** A 50-year-old man presents with 1-week history of right shoulder weakness preceded by several days of severe pain in the right shoulder. He has weakness of right arm abduction with a normal hand grip. In addition to the nerve involved in this patient, what two nerves are commonly affected in this disorder?
A. Dorsal scapular and ulnar nerves
B. Dorsal scapular and thoracodorsal nerves
C. Median and radial nerves
D. Anterior and posterior interosseous nerves
E. Long thoracic and thoracodorsal nerves

**Q16.** A 50-year-old man presents with acute onset of severe right arm pain and weakness for 1 week. He had started lifting weights, which he had never done before. On examination, he has weakness of the shoulder girdle muscles including deltoid and spinati. What is the treatment that may improve outcome in this patient?
A. Amitriptyline
B. Gabapentin
C. Ibuprofen
D. Intravenous immunoglobulins
E. Prednisone

**Q17.** Which of the following is a common feature of neuralgic amyotrophy?
A. Bulbar involvement
B. Painless onset
C. Prominent sensory loss on examination
D. Winging of scapula
E. Good response to plasma exchange

**Q18.** The two most useful nerve conduction studies (NCSs) in the evaluation of lower brachial plexopathy are:
A. median and lateral antebrachial sensory NCSs.
B. lateral and medial antebrachial sensory NCSs.
C. ulnar and medial antebrachial sensory NCSs.
D. median and ulnar palmar mixed NCSs.
E. radial and lateral antebrachial sensory NCSs.

**Q19.** A 70-year-old ex-smoker presents with right hand weakness and numbness in the medial forearm for 6 months. Atrophy and weakness of all intrinsic hand muscles are noted on examination, along with right Horner syndrome. What is the next most appropriate step of investigation in this patient?
A. Lumbar puncture
B. Brain magnetic resonance imaging (MRI) with gadolinium
C. C-spine MRI without gadolinium
D. Chest computerized tomography (CT) with contrast
E. Ultrasound of the right median nerve

**Q20.** A 28-year-old woman presents for an evaluation of pain in the left shoulder, aggravated by lifting the arm above the head such as when swimming or washing her hair. Examination reveals atrophy and weakness of the left thenar muscles. Which of the following statements about this disorder is **CORRECT**?
A. The upper trunk of the brachial plexus is usually injured.
B. There is a fibrous band between the cervical rib and the first thoracic rib.
C. The C8 is more preferentially involved than T1 nerve fibers.
D. Horner syndrome is often seen.
E. Abnormal lateral antebrachial sensory response is a key electrodiagnostic finding.

**Q21.** A 61-year-old man presents with weakness of the right intrinsic hand muscles and numbness in the right fourth and fifth fingers for 2 weeks. He underwent a recent coronary artery bypass graft surgery, and noticed these symptoms soon after from the surgery. His nerve conduction studies are shown below.

| | Latency (ms)* | | Amplitude (mV) | | CV (m/s) | |
|---|---|---|---|---|---|---|
| | **R** | **L** | **R** | **L** | **R** | **L** |
| Median, APB (M) | 3.4 | | 5.0 | | | |
| | | | 5.0 | | 56 | |
| Ulnar, ADM (M) | 3.3 | | 4.1 | | | |
| | | | 4.0 | | 56 | |
| | | | 4.0 | | 62 | |
| Radial, EIP (M) | 2.2 | 2.3 | 0.9 | 3.3 | | |
| Median index finger (S) | 2.4 | | 20 | | 53 | |
| Ulnar little finger (S) | NR | 2.1 | NR | 15 | NR | |
| Radial (S) | 2.2 | | 18 | | 52 | |
| MABC (S) | 1.5 | 1.7 | 12 | 11 | 56 | |

*ADM,* abductor digiti minimi; *APB,* abductor pollicis brevis; *CV,* conduction velocity; *EIP,* extensor indicis proprius; *L,* left; *M,* motor; *MABC,* medial antebrachial cutaneous nerve; *ms,* millisecond; *m/s,* meter per second; *mV,* millivolt; *NR,* no response; *R,* right; *S,* sensory

On needle electromyography (EMG), active denervation and reduced recruitment are seen in the right abductor digiti minimi (ADM), first dorsal interosseous (FDI), flexor pollicis longus (FPL), and extensor indicis proprius (EIP) muscles. Where is the most likely location of the lesion in this patient?

A. Right ulnar mononeuropathy
B. Right medial cord brachial plexopathy
C. Right lower trunk brachial plexopathy
D. Right extraspinal C8 anterior ramus
E. Right intraspinal C8 nerve root

**Q22.** A 53-year-old man with history of nasopharyngeal carcinoma status post-surgery, chemotherapy, and radiation 10 years prior presents with worsening weakness of the right arm for 6 months and occasional muscle twitching in the area of the biceps muscle. Examination reveals wasting of the right deltoid, supraspinatus, infraspinatus, and biceps muscles, with reduced sensation in the lateral forearm. You suspect radiation plexopathy. Which of the following findings on needle EMG is most specific for this condition?

A. Myotonic discharges
B. Fasciculation potentials
C. Myokymic discharges
D. Cramp discharges
E. Neuromyotonic discharges

**The following vignette is for QUESTIONS 23 through 25:**

A 55-year-old woman is admitted to the hospital for pulmonary embolism and treated with low-molecular-weight heparin. Two days after the admission, she cannot lift her left leg off the bed, and also complains of numbness at the left anteromedial thigh down to the medial calf. Examination demonstrates weakness of the left hip flexion, hip adduction, and knee extension.

**Q23.** What is the next appropriate step of investigation?
A. Nerve conduction study and needle electromyography
B. Ultrasound of the left femoral artery
C. Computerized tomography (CT) of the abdomen and pelvis
D. Magnetic resonance imaging (MRI) of the lumbosacral spine with gadolinium
E. Biopsy of the rectus femoris muscle

**Q24.** Four weeks later, there is no clinical improvement. Which of the following muscles is expected to show evidence of active denervation on needle electromyography?
A. Adductor longus
B. Semitendinosus
C. Short head of biceps femoris
D. Tibialis posterior
E. Gluteus medius

**Q25.** Nerve conduction studies are also performed, and the results are shown below. Which additional electrodiagnostic studies would be the most useful in this patient?

| | Latency (ms) | | Amplitude (mV) | | CV (m/s) | |
|---|---|---|---|---|---|---|
| | **R** | **L** | **R** | **L** | **R** | **L** |
| Superficial peroneal (S) | 1.9 | 1.9 | 12 | 13.6 | 68 | 52 |
| Sural (S) | 2.0 | 2.0 | 8.0 | 7.4 | 66 | 61 |
| Tibial, AH (M) | 2.7 | 2.8 | 11.3 | 15.1 | | |
| | | | 9.0 | 13.0 | 41 | 40 |
| Peroneal, EDB (M) | 3.4 | 3.0 | 4.8 | 5.0 | | |
| | | | 4.6 | 4.9 | 60 | 56 |
| | | | 4.6 | 4.7 | 57 | 58 |

*AH,* abductor hallucis; *CV,* conduction velocity; *EDB,* extensor digitorum brevis; *L,* left; *M,* motor; *ms,* millisecond; *m/s,* meter per second; *mV,* millivolt; *R,* right; *S,* sensory

A. Saphenous sensory nerve action potentials (SNAPs)
B. Lateral cutaneous nerve of thigh SNAPs
C. Plantar mixed nerve studies
D. H reflexes
E. Tibial F waves

**The following vignette is for QUESTIONS 26 and 27:**

> A 62-year-old woman with diabetes mellitus and hypertension developed severe pain in the left thigh 1 week ago. A few days later, she also has buckling of the knee. On examination, there is weakness of left hip flexion and knee extension. Ankle dorsiflexion and knee flexion are normal. No sensory deficit is noted.

**Q26.** Which of the following is most likely associated with her diagnosis?
  A. Type 1 diabetes mellitus
  B. Retroperitoneal hematoma
  C. Hand weakness
  D. Thyroid disorder
  E. Weight loss

**Q27.** Which statement is **CORRECT** regarding the treatment in this patient?
  A. Prednisone may decrease the severity of pain.
  B. Intravenous immunoglobulin (IVIG) has consistent benefits in motor function improvement.
  C. Plasma exchange is often required.
  D. Long-term immunosuppressive therapy is required.
  E. Physical therapy should be avoided because it increases nerve inflammation.

**Q28.** A 20-year-old 5-foot-tall (152 cm) woman delivered her first child 2 weeks prior. The birth weight of her baby is 8.6 pounds (3.9 kg). One day later, she has numbness of the right lateral leg and weakness (Medical Research Council [MRC] grade 1/5) of right ankle dorsiflexion, inversion, and eversion, but normal plantar flexion. Hip abduction and hip internal rotation are also weak (MRC grade 4/5). On nerve conduction study, the right superficial peroneal sensory nerve action potential (SNAP) is absent. What is the **MOST LIKELY** diagnosis?
  A. Right peroneal neuropathy
  B. Right tibial neuropathy
  C. Right sciatic neuropathy
  D. Right lumbosacral plexopathy
  E. Right L5 radiculopathy

**The following vignette is for QUESTIONS 29 and 30:**

> A 67-year-old man presents with a right foot drop for 2 months. He has difficulty walking and has frequent tripping of the right foot. Numbness in the right lateral calf and the dorsum of the right foot is noted.

**Q29.** Weakness of which of the following movements is key to differentiate L5 radiculopathy from peroneal neuropathy?
  A. Ankle dorsiflexion
  B. Ankle plantar flexion
  C. Ankle inversion
  D. Ankle eversion
  E. Knee extension

**Q30.** Which electrodiagnostic finding is key to confirm L5 radiculopathy and help exclude a lower lumbosacral plexopathy?
  A. Reduced peroneal compound muscle action potential (CMAP) amplitude recording the tibialis anterior
  B. Reduced peroneal CMAP amplitude recording the extensor digitorum brevis
  C. Reduced tibial CMAP amplitude
  D. Preserved superficial peroneal sensory nerve action potential (SNAP)
  E. Absent saphenous SNAP

**Q31.** Which electrodiagnostic finding below is key to confirm a lower lumbosacral plexopathy and exclude an S1 radiculopathy?
  A. Reduced peroneal compound muscle action potential (CMAP) amplitude recording of the tibialis anterior
  B. Reduced peroneal CMAP amplitude recording the extensor digitorum brevis
  C. Reduced tibial CMAP amplitude
  D. Preserved superficial peroneal sensory nerve action potential (SNAP)
  E. Absent sural SNAP

---

## PART 2   QUESTIONS WITH ANSWERS AND DISCUSSION

**QUESTION 1.** The medial antebrachial cutaneous nerve is a branch of the:
  A. lateral cord.
  B. medial cord.
  C. upper trunk.
  D. posterior cord.
  E. ulnar nerve.

**ANSWER:** B. medial cord

## COMMENTS AND DISCUSSION

- The brachial plexus is formed by the anterior (ventral) rami of the C5–T1 spinal nerves, and comprises, from proximal to distal, all the trunks, divisions. and cords (Fig. 13.1).
- Main root component of the trunks of the brachial plexus
  - Upper trunk: C5–6
  - Middle trunk: C7
  - Lower trunk: C8–T1
- Anatomic variation
  - Pre-fixed brachial plexus: C4–C7
  - Post-fixed brachial plexus: C6–T2
- The medial antebrachial cutaneous (MAC or MABC) nerve and medial brachial cutaneous (MBC) nerve arise from the medial cord. The MABC supplies cutaneous sensation to the medial forearm, and the MBC to the medial arm. Thus, medial cord or lower trunk lesions, which are more proximal than the take-off of the MABC, result in sensory impairment in the medial forearm and reduced MABC sensory nerve action potential (SNAP) on electrodiagnostic study (Fig. 13.2).
- Lateral antebrachial cutaneous nerve (LAC or LABC) is a terminal branch of the musculocutaneous nerve that comes off the lateral cord of the brachial plexus. The LABC supplies cutaneous sensation to the lateral forearm. Thus lateral cord or upper trunk lesions, which are proximal to the take-off of musculocutaneous nerve, result in sensory impairment in the lateral forearm, and reduced LABC SNAPs on electrodiagnostic study (Fig. 13.2).

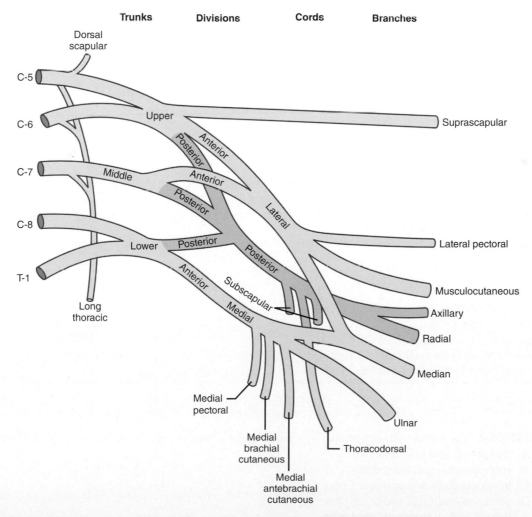

**Fig. 13.1 The anatomy of the brachial plexus.** The brachial plexus comprises three trunks (upper, middle, and lower), six divisions (three anterior and three posterior), and three cords (lateral, medial, and posterior), as well as its terminal branches. From Hollinshead WH. *Anatomy for Surgeons, Volume 2: The Back and Limbs.* New York: Harper & Row; 1969.

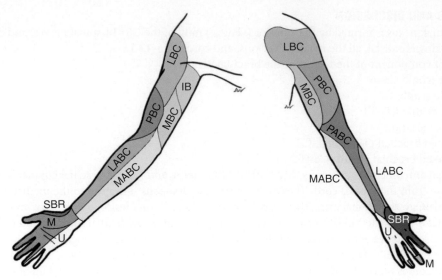

**Fig. 13.2 The skin areas that are supplied by the upper limb terminal cutaneous nerves** (*M*, median; *U*, ulnar; *SBR*, superficial branch of radial; *MABC*, medial antebrachial cutaneous; *LABC*, lateral antebrachial cutaneous; *MBC*, medial brachial cutaneous; *PABC*, posterior antebrachial cutaneous; *PBC*, posterior brachial cutaneous; *LBC*, lateral brachial cutaneous; *IB*, intercostal branch). The medial antebrachial cutaneous nerve (MABC, or MAC) supplies the medial forearm, whereas the lateral antebrachial cutaneous nerve (LABC, or LAC) supplies the lateral forearm. Courtesy of Stephen H. Colbert, MD, Columbia, MO.

- Dorsal scapular nerve (C4–C5) and long thoracic nerve (C5–C7) arise directly from the roots soon after exiting the intervertebral foramina. Thus involvement of one of these nerves indicates that the lesion is proximal to the trunks of the brachial plexus and, most likely, at the root level.
- Suprascapular nerve arises from the upper trunk. Thus involvement of this nerve indicates that the lesion is either an isolated suprascapular neuropathy, upper trunk plexopathy, or C5–6 radiculopathy.
- Involvement of the radial and axillary nerves occurs with lesions of the posterior cord.

## ◎ HIGH-YIELD FACT

Cutaneous nerves in the forearm
**Medial** forearm – **Medial** antebrachial cutaneous nerve (MABC or MAC) – abnormal in **medial cord** and **lower** trunk lesions
**Lateral** forearm – **Lateral** antebrachial cutaneous nerve (LABC or LAC) – abnormal in **lateral cord** and **upper** trunk lesions
**Posterior** forearm – **Posterior** antebrachial cutaneous nerve – abnormal in high radial nerve lesions

## MNEMONIC

Upper trunk is derived from C5–6 roots
Middle trunk is derived from C7 root
Lower trunk is derived from C8–T1 roots

**QUESTION 2.** The muscle pair denervated by a lesion of the posterior cord of the brachial plexus is the:
   A. rhomboids and infraspinatus.
   B. supraspinatus and teres minor.
   C. brachioradialis and pronator teres.
   D. pronator quadratus and triceps brachii.
   E. deltoid and abductor pollicis longus.

**ANSWER:** E. deltoid and abductor pollicis longus.

**COMMENTS AND DISCUSSION**

- The clinical and electrodiagnostic findings in *posterior cord brachial plexus lesions* are:
  - Motor involvement
    - The nerves that derive from the posterior cord are the upper and lower subscapular, thoracodorsal, and the terminal branches of the posterior cord, which are axillary and radial nerves.
    - There is often involvement of the axillary nerve (deltoid, teres minor), radial nerve (brachioradialis, triceps, wrist and finger extensors), and thoracodorsal nerve (latissimus dorsi).
    - Radial compound muscle action potential (CMAP) (recording the extensor indicis proprius [EIP] or extensor digitorum communis [EDC]) and axillary CMAP (recording the deltoid), if performed on nerve conduction studies, are abnormal.
    - Needle examination of the involved muscles is abnormal.
    - In a patient with weakness of radial-innervated muscle (abductor pollicis longus), involvement of the deltoid (axillary nerve) indicates the location to be higher at the posterior cord.
  - Sensory involvement
    - Impaired sensation in the axillary and radial distributions including the lateral shoulder (axillary nerve), posterior arm and forearm, as well as the radial dorsal hand (superficial radial nerve)
    - Only superficial radial sensory nerve action potential (SNAP) is abnormal on routine nerve conduction studies. Median and ulnar SNAPs are spared.
  - Deep tendon reflexes
    - Brachioradialis and triceps reflex are depressed or absent.

 **HIGH-YIELD FACT**

Latissimus dorsi is supplied by the thoracodorsal nerve and is abnormal in a posterior cord lesion.

 **HIGH-YIELD FACT**

Involvement of the axillary nerve (innervating the deltoid and teres minor muscles) is one key to differentiate a posterior cord lesion from a pure radial nerve lesion.

- In this scenario, the deltoid is innervated by the axillary nerve through the posterior cord.
- The abductor pollicis longus is innervated by the posterior interosseous nerve from the radial nerve and the posterior cord.
- The rhomboids are innervated by the dorsal scapular nerve directly from the C5 nerve root (and partially C4).
- The infraspinatus is innervated by the suprascapular nerve directly from the upper trunk.
- The teres minor is innervated by the axillary nerve from the posterior cord.
- The brachioradialis and triceps are innervated by the radial nerve from the posterior cord.
- The pronator quadratus is innervated by the anterior interosseous nerve from the median nerve and the medial cord.

**QUESTION 3.** A 35-year-old man presents after a motor vehicle accident 2 weeks prior with right upper extremity weakness. He cannot lift his right arm above the shoulder and has numbness at the lateral aspect of the right forearm. Which of the following electrodiagnostic findings is expected in this patient?
A. Reduced right median compound muscle action potential (CMAP) amplitude
B. Reduced right ulnar CMAP amplitude
C. Reduced right musculocutaneous CMAP amplitude
D. Absent right ulnar sensory nerve action potential (SNAP)
E. Absent right medial antebrachial cutaneous SNAP

**ANSWER:** C. Reduced right musculocutaneous CMAP amplitude

## COMMENTS AND DISCUSSION

- This patient most likely has an upper trunk brachial plexopathy. Inability to lift the right arm above the shoulder is likely due to weakness of the deltoid and/or the supraspinatus, which are supplied by the C5–6 nerve roots and the upper trunk of the brachial plexus. The sensation at the lateral aspect of the right forearm is in the distribution of the C6 dermatome and the lateral antebrachial cutaneous nerve (LABC), which is a branch of the musculocutaneous nerve.
- The clinical and electrodiagnostic findings in *upper trunk brachial plexus lesions* are:
  - Motor involvement
    - Suprascapular nerve (supraspinatus and infraspinatus), musculocutaneous nerve (biceps), axillary nerve (deltoid), and radial nerve that supplies C5–6 innervated muscles (brachioradialis) are affected. Pronator teres and flexor carpi radialis (C6–7 median-innervated) and triceps (C6-7-8 radial-innervated) may also be affected.
    - CMAPs of the median and ulnar nerves are all normal. It is very important to note that median and ulnar CMAPs on routine nerve conduction studies (NCSs) assess C8–T1 nerve roots, which travel through the lower trunk and the medial cord of the brachial plexus. Therefore, both are normal in upper trunk lesions.
    - Additional motor NCSs of the musculocutaneous and axillary nerves, which are not routinely performed, demonstrate low-amplitude CMAPs.
    - Needle examination is very important in distinguishing upper trunk from lateral cord plexopathies.
      - In upper trunk lesions, there are abnormalities in the involved muscles mentioned above (i.e., supraspinatus, infraspinatus, biceps, and deltoid).
      - Examination of the deltoid, brachioradialis, and suprascapular muscles are crucial to differentiate between upper trunk and lateral cord lesions. Abnormalities of the deltoid and/or brachioradialis on needle examination indicate an upper trunk, rather than lateral cord, lesion, since the innervation to both of these travels through the posterior cord. In addition, examination of suprascapular-innervated muscles (supraspinatus and/or infraspinatus) shows abnormalities in the upper trunk, but not in lateral cord lesions.
  - Sensory involvement
    - Sensory impairment of the thumb, index, lateral hand, lateral forearm, and lateral arm.
    - Abnormal SNAPs are key findings to differentiate from root lesions. In root lesions (radiculopathy), which are preganglionic, SNAPs are normal despite sensory impairment on examination.
    - Note that it takes at least 5–11 days for Wallerian degeneration to cause changes in SNAP amplitudes. Therefore, timing needs to be taken into consideration. Hence, it is important to recall that normal SNAPs may occur in (1) hyperacute plexus lesions where Wallerian degeneration has not yet taken place, (2) proximal demyelinating plexus lesions, and (3) preganglionic root lesions.
    - LABC SNAP is key to indicate that the lesion is at the lateral cord or upper trunk levels, **not** at the median or radial nerve.
    - Median SNAP recording the index finger (C6) and the superficial radial SNAP (C6) on routine NCSs are low in amplitude or absent. However, the ulnar SNAP (C8, lower trunk, medial cord) is spared.
  - Deep tendon reflexes
    - Impaired (reduced or absent) at biceps and brachioradialis, but triceps reflex (C6, C7, C8) is spared or only partially affected.
- In this case, a reduced right musculocutaneous CMAP amplitude is expected, since the musculocutaneous nerve comes off the upper trunk. In addition, the right LABC SNAP amplitude, **not** the medial antebrachial cutaneous nerve (MABC) which comes off the lower trunk, should also be reduced. Median and ulnar CMAPs should be normal, since the intrinsic hand muscles are supplied by the median and the ulnar nerves, which receive innervation from the C8–T1 nerve roots, lower trunk, and medial cord of the brachial plexus. The ulnar SNAP would be affected in lesions of the lower trunk and medial cord of the brachial plexus.

## ◎ HIGH-YIELD FACT

SNAPs are key to differentiate between root and plexus lesions. They are preserved in the former but abnormal in the latter.

**HIGH-YIELD FACT**

Deltoid is useful to differentiate between upper trunk and lateral cord lesions, since this muscle is preserved in the latter.

 **HIGH-YIELD FACT**

Normal SNAPs occur in:
1. Preganglionic lesions (e.g., root, spinal cord, or central lesions)
2. Hyperacute axonal plexus lesions before Wallerian degeneration has occurred
3. Proximal purely demyelinating plexus lesions

**QUESTION 4.** A 37-year-old man presents after a motor vehicle accident 2 weeks prior with right deltoid, biceps, supraspinatus, and infraspinatus. Sensory deficit is present in the lateral forearm. Nerve conduction study shows normal median and ulnar compound muscle action potentials (CMAPs); however, the median sensory nerve action potential (SNAP) recording the index finger is absent, and the radial SNAP is reduced. The ulnar SNAP is preserved. What is the **MOST LIKELY** diagnosis?
   A. C5 or C6 radiculopathy
   B. Upper trunk plexopathy
   C. Middle trunk plexopathy
   D. Lateral cord plexopathy
   E. Median neuropathy

**ANSWER:** B. Upper trunk plexopathy

**COMMENTS AND DISCUSSION (see also comments and discussion from Question 3)**
- The clinical and electrodiagnostic findings described in the question are compatible with an upper trunk lesion.
- Weakness of the right deltoid, biceps, supraspinatus, and infraspinatus indicates impairment of the C5–6 nerve roots or the upper trunk of the brachial plexus. The lesion cannot be at the lateral cord of the brachial plexus, since the deltoid muscle innervated by the axillary nerve via the upper trunk and posterior cord, and the supraspinatus and infraspinatus muscles innervated by the suprascapular nerve via the upper trunk and proximal to the lateral cord are affected. Sensory impairment in the lateral forearm is attributed to the lateral antebrachial cutaneous nerve, which comes off the musculocutaneous nerve, the terminal branch of the lateral cord of the brachial plexus.
- In upper trunk lesions (C5–6 nerve root fibers), the median and ulnar CMAPs (C8–T1 nerve root component, lower trunk, medial cord) are normal. Regarding sensory studies in upper trunk lesions, the median SNAP recording index finger and/or thumb (upper trunk, lateral cord) is absent, and the radial SNAP (upper and middle trunk, posterior cord) is reduced, whereas the ulnar SNAP (lower trunk, medial cord) is preserved.
- If this patient's injury was due to root avulsions, all SNAPs would be normal as the lesion is preganglionic.
- If this case was a middle trunk plexopathy, nerve fibers traveling from the C7 nerve root would be prominently affected. Thus the median and ulnar CMAPs, as well as the median SNAP recording the index finger, would be normal.
- In a lateral cord plexopathy, the deltoid muscle innervated by the axillary nerve via the upper trunk and posterior cord, and the supraspinatus and infraspinatus muscles innervated by the suprascapular nerve via the upper trunk and proximal to the lateral cord, should be normal.
- The motor and sensory involvement in this patient is not in the median nerve distribution.

**QUESTION 5.** A 42-year-old-man presents after a motor vehicle accident 6 weeks prior with right upper extremity weakness and numbness. You suspect a lateral cord plexopathy based on physical examination. Abnormal electromyography (EMG) findings are expected in which of the following three muscles?

A. Deltoid, rhomboid, and brachioradialis
B. Biceps, serratus anterior, and infraspinatus
C. Rhomboid, serratus anterior, and supraspinatus
D. Deltoid, biceps, and supraspinatus
E. Biceps, brachialis, and pronator teres

**ANSWER:** E. Biceps, brachialis, and pronator teres

## COMMENTS AND DISCUSSION

- The clinical and electrodiagnostic findings in a *lateral cord brachial plexus lesion* are:
  o Motor involvement
    - Musculocutaneous nerve (biceps and brachialis); C6–7 portion of the median nerve (pronator teres and flexor carpi radialis).
    - In contrast to upper trunk lesions, the suprascapular nerve (supraspinatus and infraspinatus), axillary nerve (deltoid), and C5–6 portion of radial nerve (brachioradialis) are spared. The rhomboid muscles are supplied by the dorsal scapular nerve, which comes off the C5 nerve root proximal to the upper trunk. The brachioradialis muscle is supplied by the radial nerve through the posterior cord (not the lateral cord), upper trunk, and C5–6 nerve roots. The serratus anterior is supplied by the long thoracic nerve, which comes off directly from the C5–7 nerve roots.
    - Median and ulnar compound muscle action potentials (CMAPs) are normal.
    - Needle examination shows abnormalities in the involved muscles mentioned above (i.e., biceps, brachialis, pronator teres, and flexor carpi radialis).
    - Needle examination of supraspinatus, infraspinatus, deltoid, and brachioradialis are normal. This helps differentiate between a lateral cord and an upper trunk lesion.
  o Sensory involvement
    - Because the lateral cord supplies all sensory fibers to the musculocutaneous and median nerves, sensation will be abnormal in the median nerve and lateral antebrachial cutaneous (LABC) nerve territories.
    - LABC and median SNAPs are abnormal, whereas the radial and ulnar SNAPs are spared.
  o Deep tendon reflexes
    - Biceps reflex is depressed or absent.
- In this case, the musculocutaneous nerve arises from the lateral cord to supply the biceps and brachialis muscles. In addition, the lateral cord also contributes to the median nerve, specifically the C6–7 contribution to the median nerve. Pronator teres (C6–7) is supplied by the median nerve component that receives a contribution from the lateral cord, which arises from the upper (C6) and middle (C7) trunks.
- The following muscles are preserved in lateral cord lesions:
  o The supraspinatus and infraspinatus muscles are supplied by the suprascapular nerve, which comes off the upper trunk, proximal to the lateral cord.
  o The rhomboid muscles are supplied by the dorsal scapular nerve, which comes off the C4–5 nerve roots proximal to the upper trunk.
  o The brachioradialis muscle is supplied by the radial nerve through the posterior cord (not the lateral cord), upper trunk, and C5–6 nerve roots.
  o The deltoid is supplied by the axillary nerve through the posterior cord (not the lateral cord), upper trunk, and C5–6 nerve roots.
  o The serratus anterior is supplied by the long thoracic nerve, which comes off directly from C5–7 nerve roots.

**QUESTION 6.** A 47-year-old man presents after a motor vehicle accident 2 weeks prior with right upper extremity weakness and numbness. The nerve conduction study is shown below. What is the diagnosis?

| | Latency (ms) | | Amplitude (mV) | | CV (m/s) | |
|---|---|---|---|---|---|---|
| | R | L | R | L | R | L |
| Median, APB (M) | 3.4 | | 7.0 | | | |
| | | | 6.0 | | 56 | |
| Ulnar, ADM (M) | 3.2 | | 8.2 | | | |
| | | | 8.0 | | 56 | |
| | | | 7.0 | | 62 | |
| Median/index (S) | 2.4 | 2.6 | 12 | 20 | 53 | 55 |
| Ulnar (S) | 2.1 | 2.2 | 18 | 20 | 54 | 56 |
| Radial (S) | 2.0 | 1.8 | 8 | 20 | 52 | 66 |
| LABC (S) | 1.5 | 1.9 | 5 | 12 | 56 | 52 |

*ADM*, abductor digiti minimi; *APB*, abductor pollicis brevis; *CV*, conduction velocity; *LABC*, lateral antebrachial cutaneous nerve; *L*, left; *M*, motor; *R*, right; *S*, sensory; *ms*, millisecond; *m/s*, meter per second; *mV*, millivolt

A. Upper trunk plexopathy
B. Lower trunk plexopathy
C. Lateral cord plexopathy
D. Posterior cord plexopathy
E. Medial cord plexopathy

**ANSWER:** A. Upper trunk plexopathy

**COMMENTS AND DISCUSSION (see also comments and discussion from Questions 4 and 5)**
- The routine sensory studies demonstrate reduced median, lateral antebrachial cutaneous (LABC), and radial sensory nerve action potential (SNAP) amplitudes but a preserved ulnar SNAP amplitude. Note the value of comparing the SNAPs between both sides.
- The motor studies demonstrate normal median and ulnar motor responses.
- Putting all findings together, the lesion is placed at the upper trunk of the brachial plexus.
  - In a lateral cord lesion, the radial SNAP should be normal, since the sensory fibers of the radial nerve (from the snuffbox) travel through the posterior cord to the upper trunk, and thus are affected in the upper trunk but not in lateral cord lesions.
  - In a posterior cord lesion, the radial SNAP is abnormal, whereas the median and ulnar SNAPs and the median and ulnar compound muscle action potentials (CMAPs) should be preserved, since these fibers travel through the medial cord (except fibers for median SNAPs which travel through the lateral cord). The radial sensory fibers (from the snuffbox) travel through the radial nerve and the posterior cord before going to the upper trunk.
  - In medial cord or lower trunk lesions, the median and ulnar CMAPs, as well as the ulnar SNAP are abnormal, whereas the median and radial SNAPs should be preserved. In addition, abnormal medial antebrachial cutaneous (MABC) SNAP (not tested in this patient) is useful in localizing a lesion to the medial cord or the lower trunk.

**QUESTION 7.** A 23-year-old man sustained a gunshot wound to the right posterior shoulder 2 months prior resulting in weakness of the right triceps, and wrist flexor and extensor muscles. The nerve conduction study shows normal median and ulnar compound muscle action potentials (CMAPs). The median sensory nerve action potential (SNAP) recording the middle finger and radial SNAP recording from the snuffbox are reduced. The median (recording the index finger) and ulnar SNAPs are normal. Needle electromyography (EMG) shows neurogenic changes in the right triceps, pronator teres, and flexor carpi radialis. What is the **MOST LIKELY** diagnosis?
A. Upper trunk plexopathy
B. Middle trunk plexopathy
C. Lower trunk plexopathy
D. Lateral cord plexopathy
E. Posterior cord plexopathy

**ANSWER:** B. Middle trunk plexopathy

**COMMENTS AND DISCUSSION**
- The clinical and electrodiagnostic findings in *middle trunk brachial plexus lesions* are:
  - Motor involvement
    - C7 median-innervated muscles (flexor carpi radialis, pronator teres); C7 radial-innervated muscles (triceps)
    - Routine median and ulnar CMAPs are normal, since they evaluate the lower plexus lesion. C7/middle trunk-innervated muscles are not examined in routine motor studies unless radial motor nerve conduction studies (NCSs) are done.
    - Needle examination shows abnormalities in the involved muscles above.
  - Sensory involvement
    - Sensory impairment of the middle finger (C7), and possibly also index (C6 +/− C7) and ring fingers (C8 +/− C7)
    - Median SNAP recording the middle finger is low in amplitude or absent.
    - Median SNAP recording the index finger and radial SNAP recording from the snuffbox may also be low or absent.
    - Abnormal median SNAP recording the middle finger is crucial, as this differentiates middle trunk lesions from C7 root lesions. In C7 lesions, which are preganglionic lesions, the SNAP would be normal.
  - Deep tendon reflexes
    - The triceps reflex is depressed or absent.
- In this case, weakness and/or denervation of the right triceps (C6–7–8) along with the pronator teres (C6–7) and flexor carpi radialis (C6–7) indicate an abnormality in the distribution of C6–7 or the upper or middle trunk of the brachial plexus. Triceps are supplied by the radial nerve, which originates from the posterior cord, whereas the pronator teres and flexor carpi radialis are supplied by the lateral cord component of the median nerve. Therefore, abnormalities in these muscles cannot be localized to only one cord.
- Abnormal median SNAP (recording the middle finger) and radial SNAP, along with normal median SNAP (recording the index fingers and thumb) and ulnar SNAP, as well as normal median and ulnar CMAPs, indicate a middle trunk lesion, not of the upper or the lower trunk.
- C7 radiculopathy is excluded, since the radial SNAP and median SNAP (recording the middle finger) should be normal in a preganglionic lesion (i.e., radiculopathy).

 **HIGH-YIELD FACT**

> Abnormal median SNAP recording the middle finger is useful to differentiate between middle trunk and C7 root lesions. It is preserved in root lesions.

**QUESTION 8.** Which of the following helps differentiate C7 radiculopathy from a middle trunk plexopathy?
- A. Median sensory nerve action potential (SNAP) (recording the thumb)
- B. Median SNAP (recording the middle finger)
- C. Ulnar compound muscle action potential (CMAP)
- D. Involvement of the pronator teres
- E. Involvement of the extensor indicis proprius

**ANSWER:** B. Median SNAP (recording the middle finger)

**COMMENTS AND DISCUSSION (see also comments and discussion from Question 7)**
- Sensory innervation of the middle finger is via the median nerve, lateral cord, middle trunk, and C7 nerve root. In contrast, median SNAP (recording the thumb) receives fibers form the lateral cord, upper trunk (not the middle trunk), and the C6 nerve root.
- Median SNAP (recording the middle finger) is normal in C7 radiculopathy, a preganglionic lesion, but abnormal in middle trunk plexopathy.
- Ulnar CMAP has innervation via the medial cord, lower trunk, and C8 nerve root, and is, therefore, preserved in both C7 radiculopathy and middle trunk plexopathy.

- Pronator teres receives motor supply from the median nerve, lateral cord, upper and middle trunk, and C6–7 nerve roots. Thus it is affected in both C7 radiculopathy and middle trunk plexopathy.
- The extensor indicis proprius receives motor supply from the radial nerve, posterior cord, middle and lower trunks, and the C7 and C8 nerve roots, and hence may be affected in both C7 radiculopathy and middle trunk plexopathy.

**QUESTION 9.** A 6-month-old boy has had left arm weakness since birth. Delivery was prolonged and required forceps. At rest, the arm is adducted, elbow extended, and forearm pronated. There is severe weakness and atrophy of biceps and deltoid, whereas the hand moves well. The biceps reflex is absent. The median sensory response is absent on nerve conduction study. The most likely lesion location is at the:

A. musculocutaneous nerve.
B. upper trunk.
C. C5 and C6 nerve roots.
D. lateral cord.
E. axillary nerve.

**ANSWER:** B. upper trunk.

### COMMENTS AND DISCUSSION

- This infant has brachial plexopathy from birth trauma ("obstetric brachial plexopathy"; Fig. 13.3).
    - Risk factors are difficult delivery and shoulder dystocia
    - There are two main types.
        - *Erb-Duchenne palsy* (aka Erb palsy)
            - Upper trunk brachial plexopathy
            - Due to traction injuries from stretch between the shoulder and neck, similar to the Burner syndrome in contact sports
            - Clinical features: weakness of the muscles supplied by the suprascapular, musculocutaneous, and axillary nerves, as well as C5–6 portion of the radial nerve
                - Weakness of supraspinatus and deltoid → weakness of shoulder abduction
                - Weakness of musculocutaneous nerve → weakness of elbow flexion and forearm supination
                - Weakness of infraspinatus → weakness of external rotation of the shoulder
                - Thus, Erb palsy will result in shoulder adduction, elbow extension, forearm pronation, and internal rotation of the shoulder.
            - This results in a characteristic "waiter's tip" posture.

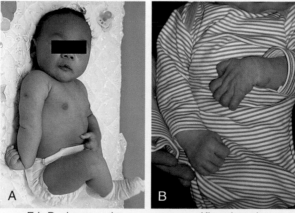

Erb-Duchenne palsy          Klumpke palsy

**Fig. 13.3 Brachial plexopathy from birth trauma.** (A) Erb-Duchenne palsy. This is due to injuries to the upper trunk of the brachial plexus. The weakness of involved muscles results in shoulder adduction, elbow extension, forearm pronation, and internal rotation of the shoulder, giving a feature of "waiter's tip" posture. (B) Klumpke palsy. This is due to injuries to the lower trunk of the brachial plexus. There is mainly weakness of the intrinsic hand muscles with preservation of the proximal muscles, giving a feature of claw hand. From (A) Heise CO, Martins R, Siqueira M. Arq. Neuro-Psiquiatr., 2015 73(9):803–8. (B), Buchanan EP, Richardson R, Tse R. *J Hand Surg Am.* 2013 Aug;38(8):1567-70.

- *Klumpke palsy*
  - Lower trunk brachial plexopathy
  - Due to traction injuries when the arm is pulled upward
  - Clinical features: weakness of C8/T1 median-, ulnar-, and radial-innervated muscles. These are mainly intrinsic hand muscles.
    - Weakness of these muscles results in a "claw hand."
- This infant has an Erb palsy. The lesion is not at the musculocutaneous nerve, axillary nerve, or at the C5 and C6 roots, since the median sensory response is absent. Lateral cord lesions would not result in weakness of the deltoid, which is innervated by the axillary nerve through the posterior cord.

 **HIGH-YIELD FACT**

Erb-Duchenne palsy – Upper trunk lesion – Waiter's tip posture
Klumpke palsy – Lower trunk lesion

**QUESTION 10.** The first change seen on electrodiagnostic study in a severe axon-loss plexopathy is:
A. fibrillations in the affected muscles.
B. decrease in the sensory amplitudes.
C. decrease in the motor amplitudes.
D. increased polyphasic motor unit action potentials (MUAPs).
E. reduced recruitment in the affected muscles.

**ANSWER:** E. reduced recruitment in the affected muscles.

**COMMENTS AND DISCUSSION**
- Immediately after axonal injury, there is reduced recruitment on needle electromyography (EMG) in weak muscles.
- However, the distal nerve remains excitable until Wallerian degeneration occurs.
  - The distal CMAP remains normal for 1 to 2 days after injury, giving rise to a pattern of conduction block on nerve conduction study (NCS) that mimics the one seen with segmental demyelination. The motor amplitude then decreases between day 3 and 6.
  - The distal SNAP remains normal for 5 to 6 days and then decreases rapidly to reach its nadir in 10 to 11 days.
- Fibrillation potentials start appearing approximately 10 to 14 days later in muscles very close to the site of injury. In the following weeks, more distal muscles will show fibrillation potentials as well.
- Reinnervation, starting with polyphasic MUAPS, follows denervation and generally takes many weeks to months after nerve injury.

**QUESTION 11.** A 65-year-old man, who is a heavy smoker, presents with a 4 months history of weakness of all right intrinsic hand muscles, impaired sensation in the fourth and fifth fingers up to the medial forearm, and a right Horner syndrome. You suspect Pancoast tumor. What is the most likely abnormal electrodiagnostic finding?
A. Reduced musculocutaneous compound muscle action potential (CMAP) amplitude
B. Conduction slowing in the ulnar motor study of less than 70% of the lower normal limit
C. Absent lateral antebrachial cutaneous sensory study
D. Prolonged median motor latency greater than 140% of the upper normal limit
E. Reduced ulnar CMAP amplitude

**ANSWER:** E. Reduced ulnar CMAP amplitude

**COMMENTS AND DISCUSSION**

- Pancoast or apical lung tumors usually affect the lower trunk of the brachial plexus.
- The clinical and electrodiagnostic findings in *lower trunk brachial plexus lesions* are:
  - Motor involvement
    - C8/T1-innervated muscles, supplied by the median, ulnar, and radial nerves. All intrinsic hand muscles are involved. Examples (not intended to be a complete list) include:
      - C8/T1 median-innervated muscles: abductor pollicis brevis (APB) and flexor pollicis longus (FPL)
      - C8/T1 ulnar-innervated muscles: abductor digiti minimi (ADM) and first dorsal interossei (FDI)
      - C8/T1 radial-innervated muscles: extensor indicis proprius (EIP)
    - Median and ulnar CMAPs are low in amplitude or absent.
    - Needle examination shows abnormalities in the involved muscles mentioned above, and is crucial to differentiate between the lower trunk and medial cord lesions. Examples of these muscles include EIP, extensor digitorum communis (EDC), and extensor pollicis longus (EPL). These muscles are abnormal in lower trunk lesions, but spared in medial cord lesions, since they are innervated by the posterior cord.
  - Sensory involvement
    - Sensory impairment of the ring and little fingers, medial hand, medial forearm, and medial arm.
    - Ulnar SNAP is low in amplitude or absent. However, median SNAP is normal.
    - Abnormal ulnar SNAP differentiates the lower trunk lesion from a C8/T1 root lesion. In the latter, SNAP would be spared.
    - It is notable that the combination of abnormal ulnar and median CMAPs, abnormal ulnar SNAP, but preserved median SNAP indicates the lower trunk or medial cord lesion.
    - MABC SNAP is key to indicate that the lesion is more proximal at the medial cord or lower trunk levels, **not** at the median, ulnar, or radial nerves.
    - Often, a lower trunk lesion may be confused with an ulnar nerve lesion. Thus examination of the MABC is very important to differentiate between these two.
  - Deep tendon reflexes
    - There are no abnormalities in deep tendon reflexes.
- In this case, atrophy and weakness of all intrinsic hand muscles, along with impaired sensation in the fourth and fifth fingers (C8 dermatome) up to the medial forearm (T1 dermatome) indicate involvement of the C8–T1 nerve roots or the lower trunk of the brachial plexus.
- Horner syndrome manifesting as miosis, ptosis, and anhidrosis, also supports the C8-T1 nerve root or lower trunk lesion. Horner syndrome is more likely to be present in neoplastic invasion of the brachial plexus and can helps distinguish this condition from radiation plexopathy in patients who have recieved prior radiation therapy.
- In lower trunk plexopathy, median, ulnar, and radial CMAP amplitudes are reduced. In addition, the medial antebrachial cutaneous nerve, which comes off the medial cord, is abnormal in lower trunk lesions.
- The lateral antebrachial cutaneous nerve comes off the musculocutaneous nerve. Thus, musculocutaneous CMAP and lateral antebrachial cutaneuos (LABC) SNAP amplitudes would be abnormal in an upper trunk or lateral cord lesion, but not in a lower trunk lesion.
- In lower trunk plexopathy from a Pancoast tumor, the pathology is an axonal process, not demyelination. Therefore, there is reduced CMAP amplitudes, rather than significant slowing.
- Prolonged median motor latency would indicate distal demyelination, and conduction slowing in the ulnar motor study would be consistent with focal slowing. However, this patient has a more proximal lesion at the lower trunk, and the pathology is most likely an axonal process, not demyelination.

## ◎ HIGH-YIELD FACT

Abnormal ulnar CMAP and SNAP + Abnormal median CMAP + Preserved median SNAP = Lower trunk or medial cord lesion.

**HIGH-YIELD FACT**

> Needle EMG of C7–8/radial-innervated muscles (e.g., EIP) is useful to differentiate between lower trunk and medial cord lesions. These muscles would be abnormal in lower trunk but not medial cord lesions.

**The following vignette is for QUESTIONS 12 through 14:**

> A 23-year-old football player develops severe right shoulder pain and weakness of the right arm after being tackled 3 months prior. On examination, he has weakness of the right biceps and numbness at the palmar aspect of the right thumb, index finger, and the lateral side of the right forearm.

**QUESTION 12.** Which of the following statements is **CORRECT?**
  A. The injury may result from plexus traction.
  B. Nerve roots can also be injured.
  C. Pain is a common feature.
  D. Preserved sensory nerve action potentials (SNAPs) portend poor prognosis.
  E. All of the above

**ANSWER:** E. All of the above

**COMMENTS AND DISCUSSION**
- This patient has sustained a traumatic injury to the brachial plexus, nerve roots, or both.
- Traumatic brachial plexopathy is the most common cause of brachial plexopathy.
- Traction injuries or stretching of the brachial plexus typically results in upper trunk brachial plexopathy.
- Nerve root avulsion results from separation of the roots from the spinal cord and carries poor prognosis.
- Electrodiagnostic studies are useful to differentiate a nerve root avulsion from a brachial plexus lesion:
  ○ In pure root avulsion, SNAPs are preserved, since the lesion is preganglionic.
  ○ In brachial plexopathy, SNAPs are abnormal after Wallerian degeneration occurs, since the lesion is post-ganglionic.
  ○ However, SNAPs can also be abnormal if a root avulsion occurs in combination with a brachial plexopathy.
- During contact sports such as football, traction injuries and stretching of the lateral neck between the head and shoulder areas result in upper trunk brachial plexopathy or nerve root avulsion, or both. This entity is also called as "burner or stinger syndrome." Patients typically have pain in the thumb, index, and lateral aspect of the forearm, which are the cutaneous areas innervated by the upper trunk.

 **HIGH-YIELD FACT**

> SNAPs are useful to differentiate a root avulsion from a traumatic plexus lesion. They are preserved in the former but abnormal in the latter once Wallerian degeneration occurs.

**QUESTION 13.** Which two cervical roots are most commonly involved with burners or stingers?
  A. C3 and C4
  B. C4 and C5
  C. C5 and C6
  D. C6 and C7
  E. C7 and T1

**ANSWER:** C. C5 and C6

**COMMENTS AND DISCUSSION (see also comments and discussion from Question 12)**
- *Burner syndrome* (aka stinger syndrome) is a traumatic brachial plexopathy due to a traction injury, typically from contact sports (e.g., football).

- During the injury there is depression of the shoulder and lateral flexion of the neck to the contralateral side, leading to traction, compression, or a direct blow to the upper roots of the brachial plexus.
- This typically results in upper trunk brachial plexopathy and/or C5 and C6 root injury.

**QUESTION 14.** Which of the following is the most useful and localizing electrodiagnostic finding in this patient?
   A. Median compound muscle action potential (CMAP) amplitude
   B. Median sensory nerve action potential (SNAP) amplitude
   C. Ulnar CMAP amplitude
   D. Ulnar SNAP amplitude
   E. Radial CMAP amplitude

**ANSWER:** B. Median sensory nerve action potential (SNAP) amplitude

**COMMENTS AND DISCUSSION (see also comments and discussions from Questions 12 and 13)**
- The main differential diagnoses in this patient are upper trunk brachial plexopathy and C5–6 nerve root avulsion.
- To differentiate between these two, median SNAP is very useful. Median SNAP amplitude is reduced in the upper trunk plexopathy but preserved in nerve root avulsion, in which the lesion is preganglionic.
- Median CMAP, ulnar CMAP, and ulnar SNAP would be abnormal in lower trunk or C8–T1 root lesions.
- Radial CMAP would be abnormal in C7–8 root, middle/lower trunk, or posterior cord lesions.

**QUESTION 15.** A 50-year-old man presents with 1-week history of right shoulder weakness preceded by several days of severe pain in the right shoulder. He has weakness of right arm abduction with a normal hand grip. In addition to the nerve involved in this patient, what two nerves are commonly affected in this disorder?
   A. Dorsal scapular and ulnar nerves
   B. Dorsal scapular and thoracodorsal nerves
   C. Median and radial nerves
   D. Anterior and posterior interosseous nerves
   E. Long thoracic and thoracodorsal nerves

**ANSWER:** D. Anterior and posterior interosseous nerves

**COMMENTS AND DISCUSSION**
- The diagnosis in this patient is most likely *neuralgic amyotrophy* (aka brachial plexitis or Parsonage-Turner syndrome).
- This patient's weakness of right shoulder abduction may be due to involvement of the supraspinatus muscle (innervated by the suprascapular nerve) and/or the deltoid muscle (innovated by the axillary nerve). The supraspinatus muscle primarily abducts the shoulder in the first 15 degrees, and further abduction beyond this degree is mainly the function of the deltoid muscle.
- The term brachial plexitis may be misleading, since this entity indeed tends to involve one or more individual nerves, rather than the brachial plexus itself.
- Lumbosacral plexitis is a rare counterpart of brachial plexitis that involves the leg.
- Classic clinical scenario: antecedent upper respiratory tract infection or other viral infections, trauma or vaccination → (days to weeks later) severe pain in the shoulder → (about 1–2 weeks after the onset of pain) once pain subsides, weakness becomes apparent and often more prominent
- Clinical features
  o It is important to note that neuralgic amyotrophy tends to affect individual nerves, mostly motor nerves and motor branches, rather than typical brachial plexus distributions. Therefore, the diagnosis may be missed.
  o Predilection for these predominantly motor nerves (in order of frequency)
    - Suprascapular nerve → weakness of the supraspinatus and infraspinatus muscles
    - Long thoracic nerve → weakness of the serratus anterior muscle → medial winging of scapula
    - Anterior interosseous (AIN) nerve → AIN syndrome → weakness of the flexor pollicis longus (FPL), flexor digitorum profundus digits 2, 3 (FDP2, 3), and pronator quadratus (PQ). Due to weakness of FPL and FDP 2, 3, patient is unable to perform an "OK sign."

- Axillary nerve
- Musculocutaneous nerve
- Posterior interosseous nerve
- Radial nerve
- Phrenic nerve
  - Predilection to these individual motor branches
    - Motor branch to the brachialis
    - Motor branch to the pronator teres
    - Motor branch to the supraspinatus
    - Motor branch to the triceps
    - Motor branch to the flexor pollicis longus
    - Motor branch to the flexor digitorum profundus 2, 3 (FDP2, 3)

## ◎ HIGH-YIELD FACT

Neuralgic amyotrophy has a predilection for individual, mostly motor nerves or individual motor branches. Common nerves are the suprascapular, long thoracic, anterior interosseous (AIN), axillary, musculocutaneous, posterior interosseous (PIN), radial, and phrenic nerves.

- Thus, in cases presenting with involvement of these individual nerves and motor branches, it is important to keep neuralgic amyotrophy at the differential diagnosis.
- In fact, the actual lesion sites are not often at these individual nerves, but rather in the fascicular component within the parent nerves, which are located proximally near or at the brachial plexus.
- Pathophysiology
  - Thought to be immune-mediated, given frequent history of prior viral infection or vaccination
  - Nerve swelling and fascicular entwinement (torsion of the nerve) can be visualized on ultrasound.
- Investigations
  - Electrodiagnostic studies to demonstrate involvement of brachial plexus, individual nerves, or motor branches as mentioned above
  - Ultrasound to demonstrate
    - Nerve swelling with or without constriction
    - Fascicular entwinement
    - Denervation atrophy of muscles supplied by the individual nerves
- Treatment
  - Mainly supportive and symptomatic therapies including pain control
  - Steroids may have a role in cases of severe pain
    - In one observational study by van Eijk and colleagues, patients receiving oral prednisone (60 mg/day in the first 7 days with tapering doses in the next 6 days) in the acute phase had shorter time to initial pain relief, compared to the historical controls who did not receive oral steroids (12.5 versus 20.5 days).
  - Immunotherapies such as intravenous immunoglobulin remain controversial.
- Hereditary neuralgic amyotrophy
  - Genetic disorder, in contrast to immune-mediated process in classic neuralgic amyotrophy
  - Autosomal dominant, due to mutations in the *SEPT9* gene
  - When to suspect hereditary neuralgic amyotrophy?
    - Recurrent brachial plexopathy, either on the ipsilateral or contralateral side
    - Onset in childhood or adolescence
    - Severe brachial plexopathy

## MNEMONIC

Hereditary neuralgic amyotrophy is due to mutations in the *SEPT9* gene.
SEPTember is the 9th month of the year, thus *SEPT9*.

##  HIGH-YIELD FACT

Think about hereditary neuralgic amyotrophy when encountering recurrent brachial plexopathy.

**QUESTION 16.** A 50-year-old man presents with acute onset of severe right arm pain and weakness for 1 week. He had started lifting weights, which he had never done before. On examination, he has weakness of the shoulder girdle muscles including deltoid and spinati. What is the treatment that may improve outcome in this patient?
  A. Amitriptyline
  B. Gabapentin
  C. Ibuprofen
  D. Intravenous immunoglobulins
  E. Prednisone

**ANSWER:** E. Prednisone

**COMMENTS AND DISCUSSION (see also comments and discussion from Question 15)**
- The diagnosis in this patient is neuralgic amyotrophy (aka brachial plexitis). Severe shoulder pain followed by muscle weakness, which becomes more apparent later, is a classic presentation of this disorder. Heavy exercise (e.g., weightlifting as in this case), can be one of the possible triggering events, in addition to viral illnesses or vaccination, that may precede the onset of the symptoms.
- Treatment of neuralgic amyotrophy remains supportive and symptomatic in most cases.
  - In patients with severe pain, there may be a role of steroids. In one observational study by van Eijk et al., patients receiving oral prednisone (60 mg/day in the first 7 days with tapering doses in the next 6 days) in the acute phase had shorter time to initial pain relief, 12.5 versus 20.5 days, compared to the control group.
  - Short-term opioid analgesia may be needed. Amitriptyline, gabapentin, and ibuprofen may be used if pain persists, but are unlikely to control severe pain in the acute stage.
  - The role of intravenous immunoglobulin, plasmapheresis, and other immunosuppressive therapies remains controversial.

**QUESTION 17.** Which of the following is a common feature of neuralgic amyotrophy?
  A. Bulbar involvement
  B. Painless onset
  C. Prominent sensory loss on examination
  D. Winging of scapula
  E. Good response to plasma exchange

**ANSWER:** D. Winging of scapula

**COMMENTS AND DISCUSSION (see also comments and discussion from Questions 15 and 16)**
- Classic clinical features of neuralgic amyotrophy include severe shoulder pain followed by weakness of the shoulder girdle, and often winging of the scapula due to the frequent involvement of the long thoracic nerve.
- Of interest, although pain is severe and refractory to analgesics, patients often have minimal or only mild sensory impairment on sensory examination. Prominent sensory loss on examination is uncommon, though patients can have paresthesia or sensory complaints.
- Treatment with intravenous immunoglobulin and plasma exchange remains controversial. There is no bulbar involvement.

**QUESTION 18.** The two most useful nerve conduction studies (NCSs) in the evaluation of lower brachial plexopathy are:
A. median and lateral antebrachial sensory NCSs.
B. lateral and medial antebrachial sensory NCSs.
C. ulnar and medial antebrachial sensory NCSs.
D. median and ulnar palmar mixed NCSs.
E. radial and lateral antebrachial sensory NCSs.

**ANSWER:** C. ulnar and medial antebrachial sensory NCS.

**COMMENTS AND DISCUSSION**
- The ulnar and medial antebrachial sensory nerves originate from the medial cord, which in turn originates from the lower trunk.
- The median sensory fibers originate from the lateral cord and upper/middle trunks.
- The radial sensory fibers originate from the posterior cord and upper and middle trunks.
- The lateral antebrachial sensory fibers originate from the lateral cord and upper trunk.
- The palmar mixed studies evaluate slowing at the wrist and have no role here.

**QUESTION 19.** A 70-year-old ex-smoker presents with right hand weakness and numbness in the medial forearm for 6 months. Atrophy and weakness of all intrinsic hand muscles are noted on examination, along with right Horner syndrome. What is the next most appropriate step of investigation in this patient?
A. Lumbar puncture
B. Brain magnetic resonance imaging (MRI) with gadolinium
C. C-spine MRI without gadolinium
D. Chest computerized tomography (CT) with contrast
E. Ultrasound of the right median nerve

**ANSWER:** D. Chest computerized tomography (CT) with contrast

**COMMENTS AND DISCUSSION**
- This patient most likely has a *neoplastic brachial plexopathy* manifesting as a lower trunk brachial plexopathy from neoplastic invasion of an apical lung tumor or Pancoast syndrome.
- There are multiple mechanisms in which neoplasm can cause brachial plexopathy.
  - Local invasion. For example, Pancoast tumor can directly invade the lower trunk of the brachial plexus.
  - Compression from a mass lesion. For example, metastatic lesion(s) to the lymph node(s) can compress the brachial plexus.
  - Infiltration. Main examples include hematologic malignancies such as leukemia or lymphoma, but also some solid tumors.
- Pain is a prominent feature that can help differentiate brachial plexopathy related to neoplasm from radiation plexopathy, which is typically painless.
- In addition, the presence of Horner syndrome favors a neoplastic brachial plexopathy, rather than radiation plexopathy. Horner syndrome is due to the involvement of inferior sympathetic ganglion or T1 nerve root. However, the absence of Horner syndrome does not exclude a neoplastic brachial plexopathy.
- Atrophy and weakness of all intrinsic hand muscles indicate involvement of the lower trunk of the brachial plexus.
- SNAPs are important to differentiate plexus from root lesions, since both may be invaded by cancer. SNAPs are abnormal in plexus lesions but spared in root lesions.
- In this patient, the next most appropriate step is a CT scan of the chest with contrast for evaluation of a possible tumor. Lumbar puncture is unlikely to yield diagnostic results, especially in the case of lower trunk brachial plexopathy, where the lesion is outside the central nervous system and beyond the proximal nerve roots. MRI of the brain or the cervical spine may be indicated later to assess for metastatic disease, but it is not necessary initially. Ultrasound of the median nerve would not be useful.

**QUESTION 20.** A 28-year-old woman presents for an evaluation of pain in the left shoulder, aggravated by lifting the arm above the head such as when swimming or washing her hair. Examination reveals atrophy and weakness of the left thenar muscles. Which of the following statements about this disorder is **CORRECT**?

A. The upper trunk of the brachial plexus is usually injured.
B. There is a fibrous band between the cervical rib and the first thoracic rib.
C. The C8 is more preferentially involved than T1 nerve fibers.
D. Horner syndrome is often seen.
E. Abnormal lateral antebrachial sensory response is a key electrodiagnostic finding.

**ANSWER:** B. There is a fibrous band between cervical rib and the first thoracic rib.

**COMMENTS AND DISCUSSION**

- The diagnosis in this case is *neurogenic thoracic outlet syndrome* (nTOS)
- Neurogenic thoracic outlet syndrome (aka true neurogenic thoracic outlet syndrome) is different from vascular thoracic outlet syndrome, which is caused by impingement of the subclavian and axillary vessels, or disputed TOS when there is only pain with no neurological or vascular deficits or findings.
- Many cases of cervical radiculopathy or ulnar entrapment may be misdiagnosed as nTOS.
- Pathophysiology
  - Compression by a fibrous band running from a rudimentary cervical rib to the first thoracic rib (Fig. 13.4)

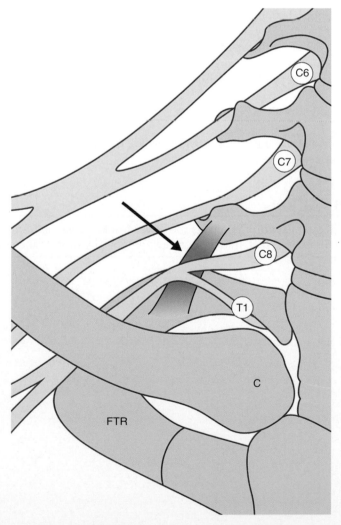

**Fig. 13.4 Neurogenic thoracic outlet syndrome.** This figure demonstrates compression of the lower trunk of the brachial plexus by the fibrous band running from a rudimentary cervical rib to the first thoracic rib. Adapted from Levin KH, Wilbourn AJ, Maggiano HJ. Cervical rib and median sternotomy-related brachial plexopathies: A reassessment. *Neurology.* 1998;50:1407–1413.

- ○ The lower trunk of the brachial plexus is compressed.
  - ○ Preferential involvement of T1 > C8 fibers, since the compression is from below, closer to where the T1 fibers are located
- Clinical features
  - ○ Weakness of C8/T1 median-, ulnar-, and radial-innervated muscles
  - ○ Given that there is a predilection for T1 fibers, thenar muscles (mostly T1-innervated) are more affected than hypothenar muscles (mostly C8-innervated). For example, the abductor pollicis brevis (APB) and first dorsal interosseous (FDI) muscles are more affected than the abductor digiti minimi (ADM). This can result in "split-hand," similar to what is seen in amyotrophic lateral sclerosis (ALS).
  - ○ Sensory impairment in the areas affected by the lower trunk lesion, including the ring and little fingers, medial hand, medial forearm, and medial arm
- Investigations
  - ○ Nerve conduction studies often demonstrate a classic pattern in true nTOS, due to the preferential involvement of T1 fibers (in order of frequency).
    - Absent or very low-amplitude medial antebrachial cutaneous (MABC) sensory nerve action potential (SNAP)
    - Low-amplitude median compound muscle action potential (CMAP)
    - Low- or borderline-amplitude ulnar SNAP
    - Low- or borderline-amplitude ulnar CMAP
  - ○ Needle electromyography (EMG) showed reduced recruitment of large reinnervated motor unit action potentials (MUAPs), with more prominent changes in muscles innervated by T1 than C8, and only a limited amount of fibrillation potentials.
  - ○ Plain radiographs may demonstrate a rudimentary cervical rib. However, clinical correlation is necessary, since a rudimentary cervical rib can also be present in asymptomatic individuals.
- In this case, a sensory study of the MABC, not the lateral antebrachial cutaneous nerve, is usually often reduced or absent due to involvement of the lower trunk. Unlike lower trunk plexopathy from neoplastic invasion, Horner syndrome is usually absent in nTOS.
- Treatment
  - ○ Supportive and symptomatic
  - ○ Physical therapy
  - ○ In cases with severe deficits or pain refractory to medical treatment, surgery of a rudimentary cervical rib should be considered.

## ◎ HIGH-YIELD FACT

Neurogenic thoracic outlet syndrome affects the lower trunk. However, T1 fibers are typically more affected than C8 fibers. Thus, thenar muscles are typically more affected.

**QUESTION 21.** A 61-year-old man presents with weakness of the right intrinsic hand muscles and numbness in the right fourth and fifth fingers for 2 weeks. He underwent a recent coronary artery bypass graft surgery, and noticed these symptoms soon after surgery. His nerve conduction studies are shown below.

| | Latency (ms) | | Amplitude (mV) | | CV (m/s) | |
|---|---|---|---|---|---|---|
| | *R* | *L* | *R* | *L* | *R* | *L* |
| Median, APB (M) | 3.4 | | 5.0 | | | |
| | | | 5.0 | | 56 | |
| Ulnar, ADM (M) | 3.3 | | 4.1 | | | |
| | | | 4.0 | | 56 | |
| | | | 4.0 | | 62 | |
| Radial, EIP (M) | 2.2 | 2.3 | 0.9 | 3.3 | | |
| Median index finger (S) | 2.4 | | 20 | | 53 | |
| Ulnar little finger (S) | NR | 2.1 | NR | 15 | NR | |
| Radial (S) | 2.2 | | 18 | | 52 | |
| MABC (S) | 1.5 | 1.7 | 12 | 11 | 56 | |

*ADM*, abductor digiti minimi; *APB*, abductor pollicis brevis; *CV*, conduction velocity; *EIP*, extensor indicis proprius; *L*, left; *M*, motor; *MABC*, medial antebrachial cutaneous nerve; *ms*, millisecond; *m/s*, meter per second; *mV*, millivolt; *NR*, no response; *R*, right; *S*, sensory

On needle electromyography (EMG), active denervation and reduced recruitment are seen in the right abductor digiti minimi (ADM), first dorsal interosseous (FDI), flexor pollicis longus (FPL), and extensor indicis proprius (EIP) muscles. Where is the **MOST LIKELY** location of the lesion in this patient?
- A. Right ulnar mononeuropathy
- B. Right medial cord brachial plexopathy
- C. Right lower trunk brachial plexopathy
- D. Right extraspinal C8 anterior ramus
- E. Right intraspinal C8 nerve root

**ANSWER:** D. Right extraspinal C8 anterior ramus

**COMMENTS AND DISCUSSION**
- This patient developed weakness in the right intrinsic hand muscles and numbness of the fourth and fifth fingers. Based on the symptoms, the differential diagnoses include right ulnar neuropathy, lower brachial plexopathy, and C8 radiculopathy.
- Intraspinal root lesion is excluded, given the absent ulnar sensory nerve action potential (SNAP). In addition, reduced radial compound muscle action potential (CMAP) amplitude and abnormalities seen on needle electromyography (EMG) in C8-innervated muscles beyond the ulnar nerve distribution exclude an isolated lesion of the ulnar nerve.
- Normal medial antebrachial cutaneous nerve (MABC) excludes the possibility of a complete lesion at the medial cord or the lower trunk of the brachial plexus.
- This patient has a *postoperative brachial plexopathy* from traction from a median sternotomy for coronary artery bypass graft surgery. This affects the C8 anterior primary ramus, which is also a part of lower brachial plexus but proximal to the lower trunk proper.
- Possible mechanisms:
  - Compression of the first rib on the C8 anterior primary ramus.
  - Fracture of the first rib at the costotransverse articulation with penetration of the lower trunk. If the edge of the fractured rib is angled upward, it is likely to damage C8 nerve fibers and spare T1 nerve fibers as they remain below the first rib at this level (Fig. 13.5).
- Often painful
- Often affects the lower trunk or medial cord, especially the C8 fibers
- Often misdiagnosed as ulnar neuropathy at the elbow.
- Demonstration of the motor and sensory involvement beyond the ulnar nerve territory is crucial. Weakness of the C8/T1 median- and/or radial-innervated muscles indicates that this is not a pure

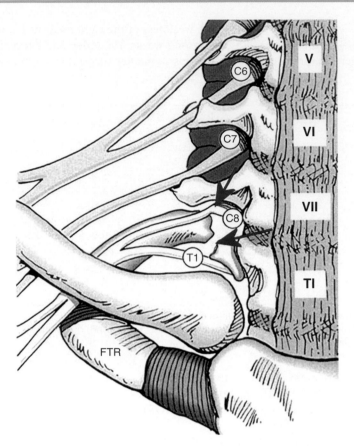

**Fig. 13.5 Post-median sternotomy brachial plexopathy.** This figure illustrates the anatomical relationship between the C8 nerve root (*blue arrow*) and fracture of the first rib (*red arrow*) near the costotransverse articulation in a patient who has undergone median sternotomy. *FTR*, first thoracic rib. Adapted from Levin KH, Wilbourn AJ, Maggiano HJ. Cervical rib and median sternotomy-related brachial plexopathies: A reassessment. *Neurology.* 1998;50:1407–1413.

ulnar nerve lesion. If the MABC SNAP is abnormal, it indicates a lesion of the medial cord or lower trunk. Then, these two locations can be differentiated by motor nerve conduction study (NCS) or needle EMG of C8/radial-innervated muscles such as the extensor indicis proprius (EIP), which would be abnormal in the lower trunk lesion, but not the medial cord lesion.

- If the lesion site is at the C8 anterior primary ramus (before it forms the lower trunk), as seen often with post-median sternotomy, the MABC SNAP will be spared. However, if the lesion had been at the lower trunk, the MABC would have been abnormal. In post-operative brachial plexopathy affecting the C8 anterior primary ramus, motor studies recording the intrinsic hand muscles show predominant abnormalities in muscles with more C8 contribution such as the abductor digiti minimi (ADM) and EIP, whereas muscles with more T1 contribution such as the abductor pollicis brevis (APB) may be relatively spared.
- Pathology of post-operative brachial plexopathy is mostly demyelination, which carries good prognosis, although a significant degree of axonal loss may occur. Treatment is mainly supportive and symptomatic.

**QUESTION 22.** A 53-year-old man with history of nasopharyngeal carcinoma status post-surgery, chemotherapy, and radiation 10 years prior presents with worsening weakness of the right arm for 6 months and occasional muscle twitching in the area of the biceps muscle. Examination reveals wasting of the right deltoid, supraspinatus, infraspinatus, and biceps muscles, with reduced sensation in the lateral forearm. You suspect radiation plexopathy. Which of the following findings on needle EMG is most specific for this condition?
A. Myotonic discharges
B. Fasciculation potentials
C. Myokymic discharges
D. Cramp discharges
E. Neuromyotonic discharges

**ANSWER:** C. Myokymic discharges

**COMMENTS AND DISCUSSION**
- *Radiation brachial plexopathy* is often included in the differential diagnosis of brachial plexopathy in a patient with history of cancer who has undergone radiation therapy.
- This is a delayed phenomenon typically occurring several years after radiation.
- Radiation brachial plexopathy is typically painless, as opposed to brachial plexopathy due to neoplasm, which is typically painful. In addition, Horner syndrome is usually absent in radiation plexopathy (Table 13.1).
- It is important to note that myokymic discharges on needle electromyography (EMG) are highly suggestive of radiation brachial plexopathy, rather than brachial plexopathy related to neoplasm. This may also be seen clinically as worm-like movements of affected muscles.
- This patient likely has radiation brachial plexopathy. Wasting of the deltoid, supraspinatus, infraspinatus, and biceps muscles, as well as reduced sensation in the area supplied by the lateral antebrachial cutaneous nerve indicate upper trunk involvement.
- Myotonic discharges do not occur with radiation plexopathy, whereas fasciculation potentials and cramp discharges may be seen but are not specific for this diagnosis. Rarely some neuromyotonic discharges have been seen in radiation plexopathy.

 **HIGH-YIELD FACT**

Radiation plexopathy – painless
Neoplastic plexopathy – painful

 **HIGH-YIELD FACT**

Myokymic discharges are highly suggestive of radiation brachial and lumbosacral plexopathy. In addition to radiation, myokymia is seen in hypocalcemic tetany, brain stem lesions such as multiple sclerosis, and Guillain-Barré syndrome.

**TABLE 13.1** Differentiating features between brachial plexopathy related to neoplasm versus radiation

|  | Neoplastic plexopathy | Radiation plexopathy |
| --- | --- | --- |
| Onset | Variable | Delayed (several years) after radiation |
| Pain | Painful | Painless |
| Horner syndrome | May be present | Absent |
| Myokymia | Absent | Often present |

**The following vignette is for QUESTIONS 23 through 25:**

A 55-year-old woman is admitted to the hospital for pulmonary embolism and treated with low-molecular-weight heparin. Two days after the admission, she cannot lift her left leg off the bed, and also complains of numbness at the left anteromedial thigh down to the medial calf. Examination demonstrates weakness of the left hip flexion, hip adduction, and knee extension.

**QUESTION 23.** What is the next appropriate step of investigation?
  A. Nerve conduction study and needle electromyography
  B. Ultrasound of the left femoral artery
  C. Computerized tomography (CT) of the abdomen and pelvis
  D. Magnetic resonance imaging (MRI) of the lumbosacral spine with gadolinium
  E. Biopsy of the rectus femoris muscle

**ANSWER:** C. Computerized tomography (CT) of the abdomen and pelvis

### COMMENTS AND DISCUSSION

- This patient most likely has a retroperitoneal hematoma compressing the upper lumbar plexus.
- The lumbosacral plexus is derived from anterior (ventral) rami of the L1–S3 roots.
- The lumbosacral plexus comprises the upper lumbar plexus (L1–L4) and the lower lumbosacral plexus (L4–S3) (Fig. 13.6).
- The upper lumbar plexus has two main divisions derived from the L2–L4 roots
  - Anterior division
    - Forms the obturator nerve
    - Motor supply—thigh adductors (adductor longus, adductor brevis, adductor magnus, and gracilis)
    - Sensory supply—small area in the medial thigh
  - Posterior division
    - Forms the femoral nerve
    - Motor supply—iliopsoas (hip flexion), quadriceps (knee extension), pectineus, and sartorius
    - Sensory supply—medial calf (saphenous nerve) and anterior and medial thigh (intermediate and medial cutaneous nerve of thigh)
  - Other branches of the upper lumbar plexus that are direct extensions from the nerve roots
    - Iliohypogastric nerve (L1)
    - Ilioinguinal nerve (L1)
    - Genitofemoral nerves (L1–2)
    - Lateral cutaneous nerve of thigh (L2–3)
      - Pure sensory nerve
      - Supplies cutaneous sensation to the lateral thigh
      - Entrapment of this nerve causes "meralgia paresthetica"
        - Painful paresthesia in the skin area over the lateral thigh
        - Risk factors—obesity, pregnancy, wearing tight garments or belts, diabetes
        - Common entrapment site of the lateral cutaneous nerve of thigh is the inguinal ligament. This nerve passes under the inguinal ligament usually within 2 cm of the anterior superior iliac spine (ASIS), but this can be variable.

---

**MNEMONIC**

Divisions of the upper lumbar plexus are reversed from the location of the supplied muscles.
Femoral nerve supplies the quadriceps, which are more anterior → posterior division.
Obturator nerve supplies the thigh adductors, which are more posterior → anterior division.

---

- Retroperitoneal hematoma predominantly involves the upper lumbar plexus.
- Risk factors for retroperitoneal hematoma include pelvic surgery, anticoagulation use, femoral vessel catheterization, and hemophilia.
- Traction injury during pelvic surgery usually involves the femoral nerve, mainly, but may include the upper lumbar plexus.

---

 ### HIGH-YIELD FACT

Entrapment of:
- Lateral cutaneous nerve of thigh → meralgia paresthetica
- Superficial radial nerve → cheiralgia paresthetica

---

 ### HIGH-YIELD FACT

Cutaneous supply of the thigh
Medial and intermediate cutaneous nerves of thigh – Femoral nerve
Lateral cutaneous nerve of thigh – Direct extension of L2–3 roots
Posterior cutaneous nerve of thigh – Sacral plexus

- It is important to demonstrate involvement of both the femoral and obturator nerves to confirm that the lesion is at the lumbar plexus, rather than the femoral nerve alone.
- In this patient, weakness of the left hip flexion (iliopsoas muscle) and knee extension (quadriceps) indicate an abnormality in the femoral nerve distribution or the posterior division of the upper lumbar plexus. The femoral nerve supplies sensation to the anteromedial thigh down to the medial calf via the intermediate and medial cutaneous nerves of the thigh, and the saphenous nerve.
- However, because this patient also has weakness of the hip adductors, which are supplied by the obturator nerve from the anterior division of the upper lumbar plexus, involvement in both femoral and obturator distributions suggest the anatomic localization at the upper lumbar plexus.
- CT of the abdomen and pelvis is the investigation of choice to detect blood in the retroperitoneal area.
- Nerve conduction study and needle electromyography can be useful to localize the lesion, but it is too soon to detect abnormalities on these studies. Because it takes time for Wallerian degeneration to occur, sensory nerve action potentials begin to decrease at day 5 and are not completed until day 11. Motor nerve conductions start to degenerate at day 3 and are not completed until day 6. It takes several weeks before fibrillation potentials occur on needle electromyography.
- If the CT scan fails to show an abnormality, then MRI of the lumbosacral spine would be indicated to exclude a structural lesion at the root level.
- Ultrasound of the left femoral artery would likely not be useful in this clinical scenario.

**QUESTION 24.** Four weeks later, there is no clinical improvement. Which of the following muscles is expected to show evidence of active denervation on needle electromyography?
A. Adductor longus
B. Semitendinosus
C. Short head of biceps femoris
D. Tibialis posterior
E. Gluteus medius

**ANSWER:** A. Adductor longus

**COMMENTS AND DISCUSSION**
- The clinical and electrodiagnostic findings in an *upper lumbar plexus lesion* are:
  - Motor involvement
    - Weakness of the muscles supplied by the femoral nerve (iliopsoas and quadriceps) and the obturator nerve (hip adductors)
    - Involvement of the muscles supplied by the obturator nerve are key to differentiate an upper lumbar plexus lesion from a pure femoral nerve lesion.
    - Tibial and peroneal compound muscle action potentials (CMAPs) are normal, since these nerves are from the lower lumbosacral plexus, and thus are not involved in upper lumbar plexus, lesions.
    - Femoral CMAP is low in amplitude when the lesion is axonal and normal when the lesion is purely demyelinating.
    - Needle examination shows abnormalities in the muscles supplied by the femoral and obturator nerves.
  - Sensory involvement
    - Sensory impairment may be found in the medial, anterior, and lateral thigh, as well as the medial calf.
    - Saphenous sensory nerve action potential (SNAP) is low in amplitude or absent.
  - Deep tendon reflex
    - Quadriceps reflex is absent or depressed.

 **HIGH-YIELD FACT**

Thigh adductors (supplied by the obturator nerve) are useful to differentiate the upper lumbar plexus from femoral nerve lesions. They are involved in the former but preserved in the latter.

- In this patient, evidence of active denervation (i.e., fibrillation potentials and/or positive sharp waves) takes several weeks before it can be seen on needle electromyography.
- In this case where the lesion is at the upper lumbar plexus, muscles supplied by the femoral nerve (from the posterior division of the upper lumbar plexus) and the obturator nerve (from the anterior division of the upper lumbar plexus) are affected. Adductor longus, which is supplied by the obturator nerve, would be abnormal.
- Semitendinosus (supplied by the tibial portion of the sciatic nerve, **L5**–S1; bolded text indicating the predominant nerve root), short head of biceps femoris (supplied by the peroneal portion of the sciatic nerve, L5–**S1**), tibialis posterior (supplied by the tibial nerve, **L5**–S1), and gluteus medius (supplied by the superior gluteal nerve which comes off the lumbosacral trunk, L4-**L5**-S1) are not affected in upper lumbar plexus lesions.

**QUESTION 25.** Nerve conduction studies are also performed, and the results are shown below. Which additional electrodiagnostic studies would be the most useful in this patient?

|  | Latency (ms) | | Amplitude (mV) | | CV (m/s) | |
| --- | --- | --- | --- | --- | --- | --- |
|  | R | L | R | L | R | L |
| Superficial peroneal (S) | 1.9 | 1.9 | 12 | 13.6 | 68 | 52 |
| Sural (S) | 2.0 | 2.0 | 8.0 | 7.4 | 66 | 61 |
| Tibial, AH (M) | 2.7 | 2.8 | 11.3 | 15.1 | | |
|  | | | 9.0 | 13.0 | 41 | 40 |
| Peroneal, EDB (M) | 3.4 | 3.0 | 4.8 | 5.0 | | |
|  | | | 4.6 | 4.9 | 60 | 56 |
|  | | | 4.6 | 4.7 | 57 | 58 |

*AH*, abductor hallucis; *CV*, conduction velocity; *EDB*, extensor digitorum brevis; *L*, left; *M*, motor; *ms*, millisecond; *m/s*, meter per second; *mV*, millivolt; *R*, right; *S*, sensory

A. Saphenous sensory nerve action potentials (SNAPs)
B. Lateral cutaneous nerve of thigh SNAPs
C. Plantar mixed nerve studies
D. H reflexes
E. Tibial F waves

**ANSWER:** A. Saphenous sensory nerve action potentials (SNAPs)

**COMMENTS AND DISCUSSION**
- In this patient with an upper lumbar plexus lesion, the nerve conduction study (NCS) is normal, as all these routine NCSs assess nerves derived from the lower lumbosacral plexus.
- Low-amplitude or absent saphenous SNAP on the affected side would be the most helpful study to confirm a postganglionic lesion at the level of the femoral nerve or lumbar plexus, and to exclude a root lesion.
- The sensory study of the lateral cutaneous nerve of thigh is abnormal in meralgia paresthetica, which is not consistent with this patient's clinical presentation.
- The plantar mixed studies are useful to assess for distal tibial neuropathy (i.e., tarsal tunnel syndrome), or when a mild sensory, peripheral polyneuropathy is suspected.
- H reflex measures the integrity of the monosynaptic reflex traveling via the Ia sensory fibers of the tibial nerve at the popliteal fossa to the S1 nerve root, and motor fibers back to the tibial nerve supplying the soleus muscle. The H reflex is normal in upper lumbar plexopathies.
- Tibial F-waves may be abnormal when there is involvement of the tibial nerve or the S1 motor nerve root, and hence is not useful in this case.

**The following vignette is for QUESTIONS 26 and 27:**

A 62-year-old woman with diabetes mellitus and hypertension develops severe pain in the left thigh 1 week ago. A few days later, she also has buckling of the knee. On examination, there is weakness of left hip flexion and knee extension. Ankle dorsiflexion and knee flexion are normal. No sensory deficit is noted.

**QUESTION 26.** Which of the following is **MOST LIKELY** associated with her diagnosis?
A. Type 1 diabetes mellitus
B. Retroperitoneal hematoma
C. Hand weakness
D. Thyroid disorder
E. Weight loss

**ANSWER:** E. Weight loss

**COMMENTS AND DISCUSSION**
- This patient has *diabetic amyotrophy*, aka Bruns-Garland syndrome, diabetic lumbosacral radiculoplexopathy.
- Clinical scenario
  ○ Diabetic amyotrophy typically occurs in individuals with type 2 diabetes who are fairly well controlled and is often associated with recent weight loss.
  ○ Prominent pain in the thigh or pelvis for about 1 to 2 months → after the pain subsides, weakness and muscle wasting become more prominent.
- Diabetic amyotrophy predominantly involves the upper lumbar plexus. Thus muscles in the thigh that are primarily supplied by the L2-L4 nerve roots, the upper lumbar plexus or the femoral and obturator nerves are affected. Less frequently, muscles innervated by the L5 root are also affected.
- Of interest, as the name implies ("radiculoplexopathy"), there is also involvement of nerve roots.
- Pathophysiology
  ○ There is pathological evidence showing microinfarcts of the lumbar plexus and nerve roots due to microvasculitis.
- Diabetic amyotrophy presents with clinical and electrophysiologic findings consistent with those of an upper lumbar plexus, with concomitant root involvement.
  ○ In general, sensory nerve action potentials (SNAPs) are spared in root lesions, which are preganglionic. However, in diabetic amyotrophy, there is a combination of root and plexus involvement. Therefore, SNAPs are often low in amplitude or absent. In addition, these patients often have some distal diabetic polyneuropathy at baseline.
  ○ Needle examination shows abnormalities in muscles supplied by the upper lumbar plexus, as well as the paraspinal muscles, since there is also root involvement.
- In this patient, a retroperitoneal hematoma, which often involves the upper lumbar plexus, is unlikely in the absence of anticoagulation or other bleeding risk factors. In addition, hand weakness and thyroid disorders are not related to her clinical symptoms.
- Treatment
  ○ Mainly supportive and symptomatic (e.g., pain control and physical therapy)
  ○ Immunotherapies such as intravenous methylprednisolone and intravenous immunoglobulin are used by some but remain controversial.
  ○ Recovery is slow and, in severe cases, often incomplete.

## ◎ HIGH-YIELD FACT

In diabetic amyotrophy, there is involvement of not only the lumbosacral plexus, but also the nerve roots, hence the name "diabetic lumbosacral radiculoplexopathy."

**QUESTION 27.** Which statement is **CORRECT** regarding the treatment in this patient?
A. Prednisone may decrease the severity of pain.
B. Intravenous immunoglobulin (IVIG) has consistent benefits in motor function improvement.
C. Plasma exchange is often required.
D. Long-term immunosuppressive therapy is required.
E. Physical therapy should be avoided because it increases nerve inflammation.

**ANSWER:** A. Prednisone may decrease severity of pain.

## COMMENTS AND DISCUSSION

- Treatment of diabetic amyotrophy is mainly supportive and symptomatic.
- Given the evidence of microvasculitis on pathologic studies of the nerves, immunotherapies including steroids, IVIG, as well as plasma exchange have been used. However, the results of IVIG and plasma exchange are inconsistent, and these therapies are not routinely employed in current clinical practice. Randomized controlled studies are required to evaluate the role of these therapies.
- Intravenous methylprednisolone was found to be beneficial in improving pain in one open-label study. Thus it may be considered in cases with severe pain. However, it should be used with caution due to the risk of steroid-induced hyperglycemia. Although there may be a role of corticosteroids in pain reduction, further prospective randomized controlled studies are needed to assess their efficacy. Long-term immunosuppressive therapies are not typically recommended for treatment of diabetic amyotrophy.
- With supportive and symptomatic therapies, muscle weakness in diabetic amyotrophy may take several months or years to resolve. Physical therapy can have a role in maintaining muscle strength and improving function. There is no evidence that physical therapy increases nerve inflammation in diabetic amyotrophy.

**QUESTION 28.** A 20-year-old 5-foot-tall (152 cm) woman delivered her first child 2 weeks prior. The birth weight of her baby is 8.6 pounds (3.9 kg). One day later, she has numbness of the right lateral leg and weakness (Medical Research Council [MRC] grade 1/5) of right ankle dorsiflexion, inversion, and eversion, but normal plantar flexion. Hip abduction and hip internal rotation are also weak (MRC grade 4/5). On nerve conduction study, the right superficial peroneal sensory nerve action potential (SNAP) is absent. What is the **MOST LIKELY** diagnosis?

A. Right peroneal neuropathy
B. Right tibial neuropathy
C. Right sciatic neuropathy
D. Right lumbosacral plexopathy
E. Right L5 radiculopathy

**ANSWER:** D. Right lumbosacral plexopathy

## COMMENTS AND DISCUSSION

- This is a case of *intrapartum lumbosacral plexopathy* or "maternal obstetrical palsy," caused by compression by the fetal head on the lumbosacral trunk during labor (Fig. 13.6).
- *Anatomy of the lower lumbosacral plexus.* From the lower lumbosacral plexus, the sciatic nerve and other nerves originate Fig. 13.7:
  - Sciatic nerve
    - Two divisions—peroneal division (lateral) and tibial division (medial). These two divisions run together in the thigh.
    - Motor supply—knee flexors (hamstrings, which include semimembranosus, semitendinosus, short and long heads of biceps femoris)

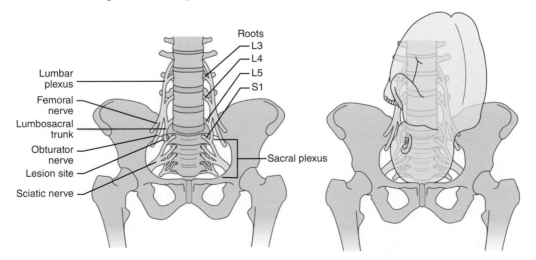

**Fig. 13.6 Intrapartum lumbosacral plexopathy.** In intrapartum lumbosacral plexopathy, patients usually present with foot drop, mimicking peroneal neuropathy. In fact, the pathology is at the lumbosacral trunk, not the peroneal nerve per se, which is compressed by the fetal head against the maternal pelvis. From Katirji B, Wilbourn AJ, Scarberry SL, et al. Intrapartum maternal lumbosacral plexopathy: Foot drop during labor due to lumbosacral trunk lesion. *Muscle Nerve.* 2002;26:340–347.

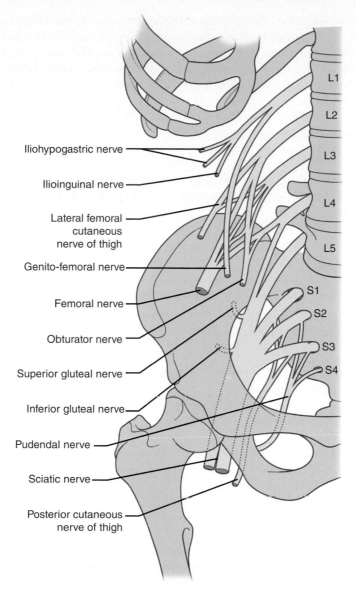

**Fig. 13.7 Lumbosacral plexus.** The lumbosacral plexus comprises the upper lumbar plexus (L1–4) and the lower lumbosacral plexus (L5–S3). From Mayo Clinic and Mayo Foundation. *Clinical Examinations in Neurology.* Philadelphia: WB Saunders; 1956.

- Sensory supply—lower leg below the knee except for the medial calf (which is supplied by saphenous nerve)
- At the popliteal fossa, divides into the common peroneal and tibial nerves
  - Superior gluteal nerve (L4–**L5**–S1, mainly L5)
    - Supplies the tensor fascia latae (hip internal rotation), gluteus minimus, and gluteus medius (hip abduction and internal rotation)
  - Inferior gluteal nerve (L5–**S1**–S2, mainly S1)
    - Comes off more distally, near or just distal to where the trunk already joins the S1 root
    - Supplies the gluteus maximus (hip extension)
- L4–L5 component of the lower lumbosacral plexus is known as the *lumbosacral trunk (or cord)*. It descends over the ala of the sacrum adjacent to bone and is unprotected by a muscle (Fig. 13.7).
- The clinical and electrodiagnostic findings in the *lower lumbosacral plexus lesion* are:
  - Motor involvement
    - Weakness of the muscles supplied by the sciatic nerve (hamstrings) and tibial and peroneal nerves. Muscles supplied by the superior gluteal nerve (gluteus medius and tensor fascia latae) and the inferior gluteal nerve (gluteus maximus) may also be affected.
    - Both peroneal and tibial compound muscle action potentials (CMAPs) are low in amplitude or absent.

- Needle examination shows abnormalities in the involved muscles mentioned in the preceding text.
- It is important to examine the hamstrings and muscles supplied by the superior and/or inferior gluteal nerves. Involvement of the hamstrings indicates that the lesion is at or above the sciatic nerve. Involvement of the tensor fascia latae, gluteus medius, and/or gluteus maximus indicates that the lesion is at the level of lower lumbosacral plexus or more proximal.
  - ○ Sensory involvement
    - Sensory impairment in the posterior thigh (supplied by the posterior cutaneous nerve of thigh), lateral and posterior calf, and entire foot.
    - Both superficial peroneal and sural sensory nerve action potentials (SNAPs) are low in amplitude or absent.
    - Abnormal SNAPs are useful to differentiate lower lumbosacral plexus lesions from multiple root or cauda equina lesions. SNAPs would be normal in root or spinal cord lesions, which are preganglionic.
  - ○ Deep tendon reflex
    - Ankle reflex is absent or reduced.

## ◎ HIGH-YIELD FACT

> Hamstrings are involved with a lesion at or proximal to the sciatic nerve.
>
> Tensor fascia latae, gluteus medius, and gluteus maximus are involved with a lesion at or proximal to the lumbosacral plexus, including the lumbosacral trunk.

- *Intrapartum lumbosacral plexopathy.* The onset of intrapartum lumbosacral plexopathy is immediately or within a few days after childbirth.
- Risk factors—low maternal height (less than 5 feet), small pelvis or large newborn resulting in cephalopelvic disproportion and a prolonged or difficult labor.
- Pathophysiology
  - ○ Fetal head compresses on the lumbosacral trunk against the pelvis.
  - ○ Fibers that are destined to be the peroneal division of the sciatic nerve lie posteriorly and are more susceptible to compression against the pelvis.
  - ○ The superior gluteal nerve is also commonly affected.
- Lesion site is the lumbosacral trunk, which comprises mainly fibers from the L4–5 nerve roots destined for the gluteal and sciatic nerves.
- Patients typically present with foot drop. This can be misdiagnosed as a peroneal nerve lesion. However, in intrapartum lumbosacral plexopathy, the deficits are beyond the peroneal nerve distribution, and it is crucial to demonstrate these both clinically and electrophysiologically.
- Clinical and electrodiagnostic features
  - ○ Weakness in peroneal nerve distribution → foot drop
  - ○ Weakness in superior gluteal nerve distribution → weakness of hip internal rotation (tensor fascia latae and gluteus medius) and hip abduction (gluteus medius)
  - ○ Sensory impairment is mainly in the L4–5 dermatomes, but may also involve the sole of foot, posterior calf, and thigh (S1)
  - ○ To differentiate a lumbosacral trunk lesion from a peroneal nerve lesion, electrodiagnostic studies, especially needle electromyography, can be very useful. Abnormalities of the gluteus medius, gluteus maximus, and tensor fascia latae muscles confirm that the lesion is beyond the peroneal nerve distribution.
- Diagnosis can be made clinically and electrophysiologically. Neuroimaging is typically not required.
- Treatment is conservative. Most cases are demyelinating and typically recover in 2 to 3 months.
- In this patient, there is severe weakness of muscles supplied by the peroneal nerve (ankle dorsiflexion and eversion) and the tibial nerve (ankle inversion), as well as weakness of muscles supplied by the superior gluteal nerve (hip abduction by the gluteus medius, hip internal rotation by the tensor fascia latae). In addition, there is sensory impairment in the lateral calf, which is within the L5 dermatomal area. Taken together, these findings suggest a lesion at the L5-nerve root or the lumbosacral trunk.
- Given the foot drop and numbness at the lateral leg, the lesion is often considered to be a peroneal palsy. However, the involvement is beyond the distribution supplied by the peroneal nerve alone. The tibial L5-innervated muscles as well as the muscles supplied by the superior and inferior gluteal nerves are also involved. Thus the lesion has to be above the peroneal nerve, at least at the level of the lumbosacral trunk.
- The abnormal superficial peroneal SNAP does not support an L5 root lesion, which is preganglionic.
- In summary, with all the findings, the lesion can be placed at the right lumbosacral trunk.

**HIGH-YIELD FACT**

In postpartum foot drop, the lesion site is at the lumbosacral trunk, not the peroneal nerve. It is important to perform a clinical and electrophysiologic examination of the tensor fascial latae and/or gluteus medius, as these muscles are affected in lumbosacral trunk lesions but preserved in peroneal nerve lesions.

**The following vignette is for QUESTIONS 29 and 30:**

A 67-year-old man presents with a right foot drop for 2 months. He has difficulty walking and has frequent tripping of the right foot. Numbness in the right lateral calf and the dorsum of the right foot is noted.

**QUESTION 29.** Weakness of which of the following movements is key to differentiate L5 radiculopathy from peroneal neuropathy?
   A. Ankle dorsiflexion
   B. Ankle plantar flexion
   C. Ankle inversion
   D. Ankle eversion
   E. Knee extension

**ANSWER:** C. Ankle inversion

**COMMENTS AND DISCUSSION**
- Both L5 radiculopathy and peroneal neuropathy may present with foot drop due to weakness of the tibialis anterior, which mediates ankle dorsiflexion. In addition, in both L5 radiculopathy and peroneal neuropathy, patients may also have weakness of ankle eversion (due to weakness of peroneus longus and peroneus brevis).
- However, in L5 radiculopathy, there is involvement beyond the peroneal nerve territory as muscles supplied by the tibial (L5) nerve are also affected. This includes the tibialis posterior (ankle inversion) and the flexor digitorum longus (toe flexion). These muscles are preserved in peroneal neuropathy.
- Ankle plantar flexion (tibial nerve, S1 root) and knee extension (femoral nerve, L2–4 roots) are preserved in both L5 radiculopathy and peroneal neuropathy.

**MNEMONIC**

L5 **in**cludes ankle **in**version deficit.

**QUESTION 30.** Which electrodiagnostic finding is key to confirm L5 radiculopathy and help exclude a lower lumbosacral plexopathy?
   A. Reduced peroneal compound muscle action potential (CMAP) amplitude recording of the tibialis anterior
   B. Reduced peroneal CMAP amplitude recording the extensor digitorum brevis
   C. Reduced tibial CMAP amplitude
   D. Preserved superficial peroneal sensory nerve action potential (SNAP)
   E. Absent saphenous SNAP

**ANSWER:** D. Preserved superficial peroneal sensory nerve action potential (SNAP)

**COMMENTS AND DISCUSSION**
- Both L5 radiculopathy and lumbosacral plexopathy may cause numbness of the lateral calf and the dorsum of the foot. In radiculopathy, the area of numbness may not be well demarcated, given the overlap of dermatomes. This is in contrast to well-demarcated areas of sensory loss when the lesion involves a peripheral nerve.

- Despite sensory impairment clinically, L5 radiculopathy would have a preserved superficial peroneal SNAP on electrodiagnostic studies, since the lesion is preganglionic. In lumbosacral plexopathy involving the peroneal nerve fibers, superficial peroneal SNAP would be expected to be abnormal in axonal lesions.
- Peroneal compound muscle action potentials (CMAPs) recording the tibialis anterior or extensor digitorum brevis muscle are abnormal in both L5 radiculopathy and lumbosacral plexopathy. Tibial CMAP recording the abductor hallucis brevis muscle should be preserved in both the lumbosacral trunk and L5 radiculopathy, since this muscle is innervated by tibial nerve fibers from the S1 nerve root. An abnormal or absent saphenous SNAP indicates femoral nerve or upper lumbar plexus involvement and would be normal in both L5 radiculopathy and lower lumbosacral plexopathy.

**QUESTION 31.** Which electrodiagnostic finding below is key to confirm a lower lumbosacral plexopathy and exclude an S1 radiculopathy?
   A. Reduced peroneal compound muscle action potential (CMAP) amplitude recording of the tibialis anterior
   B. Reduced peroneal CMAP amplitude recording the extensor digitorum brevis
   C. Reduced tibial CMAP amplitude
   D. Preserved superficial peroneal sensory nerve action potential (SNAP)
   E. Absent sural SNAP

**ANSWER:** E. Absent sural SNAP

**COMMENTS AND DISCUSSION**
- Sural SNAP is abnormal in sciatic neuropathy and lower lumbosacral plexopathy but should be preserved in S1 radiculopathy.
- Superficial peroneal SNAP assesses the superficial peroneal nerve, common peroneal nerve, and peroneal division of the sciatic nerve, along with the L5 fibers that travel through the lower lumbosacral plexus. However, it would not be useful in assessing S1 fibers that run in the lumbosacral plexus, sciatic nerve, and tibial nerve.
- Tibial CMAP amplitudes could be low in either S1 radiculopathy or lower lumbosacral plexopathy. **Typical lesion sites in plexus disorders are summarized in Table 13.2 and Fig. 13.8.**

**TABLE 13.2**  Summary of typical lesion sites in plexus disorders

| Disorder | Typical lesion site |
| --- | --- |
| **Disorders of the brachial plexus** | |
| Erb-Duchenne palsy | Upper trunk |
| Klumpke palsy | Lower trunk |
| Neuralgic amyotrophy | Individual nerves* |
| Neoplastic brachial plexopathy | Lower trunk/pan-plexus |
| Radiation brachial plexopathy | Any parts |
| Neurogenic thoracic outlet syndrome | Anterior rami of the lower trunk (T1 > C8) |
| Post-sternotomy plexopathy | Anterior rami of the lower trunk (C8 > T1) |
| **Disorders of the lumbosacral plexus** | |
| Traumatic plexopathy | Upper lumbar plexus |
| Neoplastic lumbosacral plexopathy | Any parts |
| Radiation lumbosacral plexopathy | Any parts |
| Diabetic amyotrophy | Upper lumbar plexus + lumbar roots |
| Postpartum plexopathy | Lumbosacral trunk |

*Examples include the suprascapular, long thoracic, anterior interosseous, axillary, musculocutaneous, posterior interosseous, radial, and phrenic nerves.

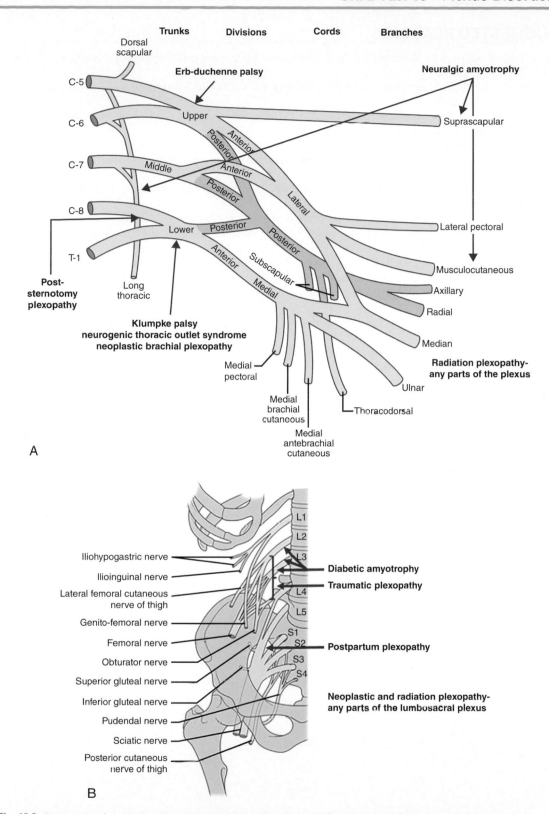

**Fig. 13.8 Summary of typical lesion sites in plexus disorders.** (A) Brachial plexus. Note that neuralgic amyotrophy tends to involve individual nerves coming off the plexus, rather than the plexus nerve itself. (B) Lumbosacral plexus. Note that diabetic amyotrophy (aka diabetic lumbosacral radiculoplexopathy) involves both the upper lumbar plexus and the lumbar nerve roots. Adapted from (A) Hollinshead WH. Anatomy for Surgeons, Volume 2: The Back and Limbs. New York: Harper & Row; 1969, (B) Mayo Clinic and Mayo Foundation. Clinical Examinations in Neurology. Philadelphia: WB Saunders; 1956.

## SUGGESTED READINGS

Dyck PJ, Norell JE, Dyck PJ. Methylprednisolone may improve lumbosacral radiculoplexus neuropathy. *Can J Neurol Sci.* 2001;28(3):224-227.

Ferrante MA. Brachial plexopathies. *Continuum (Minneap Minn).* 2014;20(5 Peripheral Nervous System Disorders):1323-1342.

Ferrante MA. Plexopathy in cancer. In: Stubblefield M, O'Dell M, eds. *Cancer Rehabilitation: Principles & Practice.* New York: Demos Medical Publishing; 2009:567-589.

Katirji B. Peroneal neuropathy. *Neurol Clin.* 1999;17(3):567-591.

Katirji B, Wilbourn AJ, Scarberry SL, et al. Intrapartum maternal lumbosacral plexopathy. *Muscle Nerve.* 2002; 26:340-347.

Katirji B. *Electromyography in Clinical Practice: A Case Study Approach.* 3rd ed. New York: Oxford University Press; 2018:65-83, 150-166.

Laughlin RS, Dyck PJB. Diabetic radiculoplexus neuropathies. *Handb Clin Neurol.* 2014;126:45-69.

Levin KH, Wilbourn AJ, Maggiano HJ. Cervical rib and median sternotomy-related brachial plexopathies: a reassessment. *Neurology.* 1998;50:1407-1413.

Parmer SS, Carpenter JP, Fairman RM, Velazquez OC, Mitchell ME. Femoral neuropathy following retroperitoneal hemorrhage: case series and review of the literature. *Ann Vasc Surg.* 2006;20(4):536-540.

Preston DC, Shapiro BE. *Electromyography and Neuromuscular Disorders.* 4th ed. Philadelphia: Elsevier; 2021: 441-458, 622-640.

Simmons Z. Electrodiagnosis of brachial plexopathies and proximal upper extremity neuropathies. *Phys Med Rehabil Clin N Am.* 2013;24(1):13-32.

Tsao BE, Ferrante MA, Wilbourn AJ, Shields RW. Electrodiagnostic features of true neurogenic thoracic outlet syndrome. *Muscle Nerve.* 2014;49:724-727.

van Alfen N. Clinical and pathophysiological concepts of neuralgic amyotrophy. *Nat Rev Neurol.* 2011;7:315-322.

van Alfen N, van Engelen BG. The clinical spectrum of neuralgic amyotrophy in 246 cases. *Brain.* 2006;129:438-450.

van Eijk JJ, van Alfen N, Berrevoets M, et al. Evaluation of prednisolone treatment in the acute phase of neuralgic amyotrophy: an observational study. *J Neurol Neurosurg Psychiatry.* 2009;80(10):1120-1124.

Weinberg J, Rokito S, Silber JS. Etiology, treatment, and prevention of athletic "stingers." *Clin Sports Med.* 2003; 22:493-500.

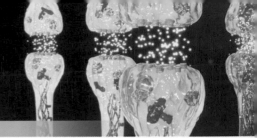

# CHAPTER 14

# Acquired Neuropathies

## PART 1 | PRACTICE TEST

**Q1.** Which of the following pathophysiological mechanisms of peripheral neuropathies is a predictor for good prognosis?
A. Axonal interruption
B. Segmental demyelination
C. Dorsal ganglionopathy
D. Motor neuronopathy
E. Wallerian degeneration

**Q2.** Peripheral polyneuropathy due to axonal degeneration does **NOT** usually manifest as:
A. dying-back polyneuropathy.
B. length-dependent polyneuropathy.
C. distal polyneuropathy.
D. proximal polyneuropathy.
E. stocking and glove polyneuropathy.

**Q3.** Loss of which of the following nerve fibers manifests as sensory impairment to light touch?
A. Unmyelinated C fibers
B. Large and small myelinated fibers
C. Aδ fibers.
D. Aα and Aβ fibers
E. Large or small myelinated fibers

**Q4.** A Which of the following neurological findings is most suggestive of large fiber sensory polyneuropathy is?
A. Hyperalgesia
B. Pseudoathetosis
C. Loss of hair
D. Allodynia
E. Dystrophic nail changes

**Q5.** What is the most useful diagnostic study for assessing large fiber dorsal ganglionopathy?
A. Thermoregulatory sweat testing
B. Sensory nerve conduction studies
C. Quantitative sudomotor axon reflex test (QSART)
D. Quantitative sensory testing
E. Skin biopsy with analysis of intraepidermal nerve fiber density

**Q6.** Which of the following clinical features characterizes small fiber neuropathy?
A. Areflexia
B. Distal hypohidrosis
C. Distal weakness
D. Sensory ataxia
E. Loss of position sense

**Q7.** Mononeuropathy multiplex presenting exclusively with axonal loss is characteristic of which of the following disorders?
A. Multifocal motor neuropathy
B. Lewis-Sumner syndrome
C. Vasculitic neuropathy
D. Multiple entrapment/compressive neuropathies
E. Hereditary neuropathy with liability to pressure palsies

**Q8.** Which primary process is characterized by disruption of the axon and myelin sheath with preservation of **ALL** supporting tissue?
A. Neurapraxia
B. Axonotmesis
C. Neurotmesis
D. First-degree nerve injury
E. Third-degree nerve injury

**Q9.** Which of the following changes does **NOT** occur after axonal transection?
A. The axonal caliber of the proximal stump becomes smaller.
B. Nerve cell body shows signs of chromatolysis.
C. Regeneration from the proximal stump proceeds at a rate of 2–3 cm/day.
D. Myelin of the distal segment disintegrates.
E. Denervated muscles reinnervate through sprouting of intact axons.

**Q10.** Significant dysautonomia is **LEAST** likely to be associated with which of the following conditions?
A. Guillain–Barré syndrome
B. Porphyria
C. Chronic inflammatory demyelinating polyneuropathy
D. Diabetes mellitus
E. AL Amyloidosis

**Q11.** Which of the following peripheral polyneuropathies is **LEAST** likely to involve the facial nerve?
A. Guillain–Barré syndrome
B. Lyme disease
C. Sarcoidosis
D. Chronic inflammatory demyelinating polyneuropathy
E. Tangier disease

**The following vignette is for QUESTIONS 12 through 14.**

A 65-year-old woman developed winging of the scapula after undergoing a scalene lymph node biopsy (see the following figure; note that the patient is trying to abduct the right shoulder).

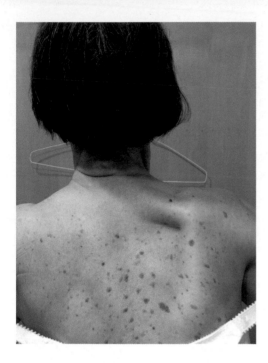

**Q12.** What is the **MOST** likely injured nerve in this patient?
A. Axillary nerve
B. Dorsal scapular nerve
C. Long thoracic nerve
D. Spinal accessory nerve
E. Suprascapular nerve

**Q13.** Which of the following muscles should be spared in this patient despite being innervated by the involved nerve?
A. Upper trapezius
B. Serratus anterior
C. Sternocleidomastoid
D. Levator scapulae
E. Rhomboids

**Q14.** What is **CORRECT** about the expected pattern of scapular winging in this patient?
A. Medial
B. Mild at rest
C. Accentuated by shoulder forward flexion
D. Not associated with sagging of the shoulder
E. Associated with a visible levator scapulae muscle

**Q15.** Which of the following is **CORRECT** regarding the palmar cutaneous sensory branch of the median nerve?
A. It is involved in median nerve entrapment at the carpal tunnel.
B. It innervates the skin over the thenar eminence.
C. It is normal in median nerve lesions in forearm.
D. It is a branch of the median nerve distal to the carpal tunnel.
E. It innervates the entire thumb.

**Q16.** A 25-year-old man is awakened at night with numbness in the right hand. Which of the following electrodiagnostic tests is the most sensitive for detecting mild carpal tunnel syndrome (CTS)?
A. Antidromic median sensory latency (wrist to index)
B. Comparison of mixed median palmar to ulnar palmar latencies
C. Orthodromic median sensory latency (index to wrist)
D. Median motor distal latency recording the abductor pollicis brevis
E. Fibrillation potentials in the abductor pollicis brevis

**Q17.** Which of the following clinical features is expected in a patient with a lesion of the anterior interosseous nerve?
A. Inability to flex the thumb and index finger
B. Inability to abduct the thumb
C. Numbness at base of the thumb
D. Inability to flex the little and ring fingers
E. Numbness in the anterior forearm

**Q18.** Cubital tunnel syndrome refers to entrapment of which of the following?
A. Ulnar nerve at the ligament of Struthers
B. Ulnar nerve at the humeral-ulnar aponeurosis
C. Ulnar nerve at the retrocondylar groove
D. Ulnar nerve at the Guyon canal
E. Median nerve at the elbow

**Q19.** Which of the following signs is **NOT** seen in ulnar neuropathy at the elbow?
A. Tinel sign
B. Froment sign
C. Phalen sign
D. Benedict sign
E. Wartenberg sign

**Q20.** The inching technique is most useful in localizing the site of:
A. a conduction block in a chronic axonal neuropathy.
B. entrapment in ulnar neuropathy at the wrist.
C. nerve injury in an axon-loss plexopathy.
D. axonal loss in radiculopathy.
E. a conduction block in sciatic nerve lesion.

**Q21.** Which of the following statements is **FALSE** regarding Martin-Gruber anastomosis?
  A. It occurs in 20 to 40% of the population.
  B. It consists of a communicating branch from the ulnar to the median nerve.
  C. It consists of nerve fibers destined for the first dorsal interosseous, abductor digiti minimi, and/or adductor pollicis.
  D. It often manifests with an apparent ulnar nerve conduction block in the forearm.
  E. It may be associated with a higher median compound muscle action potential (CMAP) amplitude at the elbow compared to the wrist.

**Q22.** In a median-to-ulnar crossover in the forearm, which of the following findings would be observed?
  A. Conduction block along the median nerve in the forearm recording from the abductor pollicis brevis (APB)
  B. Slowing of ulnar conduction velocity in the forearm
  C. Conduction block along the ulnar nerve in the forearm recording from the abductor digiti minimi (ADM)
  D. Slowing of the median conduction velocity in the forearm.
  E. Higher ulnar compound muscle action potential (CMAP) amplitude at the elbow compared to the wrist

**Q23.** Which of the following statements is **FALSE** regarding ulnar motor conduction study, recording the first dorsal interosseous muscle, compared to recording hypothenar muscles?
  A. It increases the yield of finding ulnar focal slowing or conduction block.
  B. It helps to detect ulnar nerve lesions at the wrist or palm.
  C. It is more likely to show findings of a Martin-Gruber anastomosis.
  D. It often yields higher compound muscle action potential (CMAP) amplitude in amyotrophic lateral sclerosis.
  E. It is more suitable for the inching technique across the wrist.

**Q24.** Which of the following conditions does **NOT** result in a low motor amplitude of the ulnar nerve when stimulating at the wrist and recording from the hypothenar muscles?
  A. Amyotrophic lateral sclerosis
  B. Lambert-Eaton myasthenic syndrome
  C. Martin-Gruber anastomosis
  D. Peripheral polyneuropathy
  E. Ulnar neuropathy

**Q25.** Which of the following findings is seen in a "Saturday night palsy" that presents as pure neurapraxia?
  A. Low amplitude radial sensory nerve action potential (SNAP)
  B. Radial motor conduction block between the axilla and above the spiral groove
  C. Fibrillations in the extensor carpi radialis longus muscle
  D. Normal distal radial compound muscle action potential (CMAP) stimulating the elbow
  E. Fibrillations in the brachioradialis muscle

**Q26.** A 55-year-old man presents with a right foot drop and numbness of the dorsum of the foot. Weakness of which of the following actions excludes a common peroneal neuropathy?
  A. Ankle dorsiflexion
  B. Ankle eversion
  C. Large toe extension
  D. Ankle inversion
  E. Small toe extension

**Q27.** Spontaneous non-traumatic peroneal neuropathy is now recognized to commonly occur after compression of the nerve by which of the following?
  A. Lipoma
  B. Intraneural ganglion cyst
  C. Giant cell tumor
  D. Osteochondroma
  E. Pseudoaneurysm

**Q28.** Rapid-onset foot drop due to peroneal neuropathy is often painful when related to which of the following?
  A. Weight loss
  B. Intraneural ganglion
  C. Habitual leg crossing
  D. Diabetes mellitus
  E. Prolonged hospitalization

**Q29.** Which of the following electrodiagnostic findings is **LEAST** likely encountered in a peroneal nerve lesion across the fibular neck?
  A. Conduction block across the fibular neck when recording from the extensor digitorum brevis (EDB)
  B. Low-amplitude peroneal compound muscle action potential (CMAP) recording from the tibialis anterior
  C. Fibrillation potentials in the tibialis anterior
  D. Prolonged peroneal distal latency recording from the EDB
  E. Decreased recruitment of the extensor hallucis

**The following vignette is for QUESTIONS 30 and 31.**

> A 25-year-old woman noted severe weakness of the right thigh soon after successfully completing a long vaginal delivery. On examination, she had severe weakness of the quadriceps, absent knee reflex, and sensory loss in the anterior thigh and medial leg. Thigh adduction and hip flexion were normal.

**Q30.** The clinical findings in this patient are likely the result of which of the following conditions?
A. Femoral nerve lesion at the inguinal ligament
B. Upper lumbar plexus lesion
C. Obturator nerve lesion
D. Femoral nerve lesion in the pelvis
E. Upper lumbar radiculopathy

**Q31.** Electrodiagnostic studies done 4 weeks later showed fibrillation potentials and only one voluntary motor unit action potential in the quadriceps. The thigh adductors and iliacus were normal. The femoral compound muscle action potential (CMAP) amplitude was normal. Which of the following can be implied from these findings?
A. Severe axon-loss femoral neuropathy with poor prognosis
B. Severe axon-loss lumbar plexopathy with poor prognosis
C. Upper lumbar radiculopathy with good prognosis
D. Predominantly demyelinating femoral neuropathy with good prognosis
E. Upper lumbar radiculopathy with poor prognosis

**Q32.** What is the most common subtype of Guillain–Barré syndrome in North America?
A. Acute inflammatory demyelinating polyneuropathy
B. Acute ataxic neuropathy
C. Acute motor axonal neuropathy
D. Acute pandysautonomia
E. Acute motor sensory axonal neuropathy

**Q33.** In a patient with ascending weakness, which of the following would cast doubt on a diagnosis of Guillain–Barré syndrome?
A. Mild sensory symptoms
B. Bifacial weakness
C. Autonomic dysfunction
D. Respiratory failure
E. Cerebrospinal fluid (CSF) pleocytosis >50 cells/μL

**Q34.** A 42-year-old man presents with rapidly progressive generalized weakness over 2 weeks. There are no sensory symptoms or findings. Cerebrospinal fluid reveals an elevated protein and a normal cell count. Nerve conduction studies show low-amplitude motor responses. Distal latencies, conduction velocities, and F waves are normal. There are no conduction blocks. Sensory nerve conduction responses are normal. Which of the following statements is **FALSE**?
A. This clinical picture is more common in Asia than in North America.
B. This patient likely has positive anti-ganglioside antibodies.
C. Prognosis for recovery in this patient is uniformly very poor.
D. This patient likely has a recent *Campylobacter jejuni* infection.
E. This patient may have had a preceding diarrheal illness.

**Q35.** What is the **MOST** specific electrodiagnostic finding in Guillain–Barré syndrome?
A. Reduced recruitment of motor unit action potentials (MUAPs)
B. Low compound muscle action potential (CMAP) amplitudes
C. Normal sural with reduced amplitude hand sensory nerve action potentials (SNAPs)
D. Conduction block of the median nerve in the forearm
E. Mild slowing of distal and F-wave latencies

**Q36.** Which of the following electrodiagnostic findings is **LEAST** helpful in suggesting the diagnosis of Guillain–Barré syndrome during the first few weeks of illness?
A. Reduced or absent sensory nerve action potentials (SNAPs) in the hand with a normal sural SNAP
B. Delayed, impersistent, or absent F waves
C. Absent tibial H reflexes
D. Multiple or complex A waves
E. (Sural + radial SNAPs)/(median + ulnar SNAPs) ratio <1

**Q37.** Which treatment option has the strongest evidence to support its use in Guillain-Barré syndrome?
A. Plasma exchange followed by intravenous immunoglobulin (IVIG)
B. Plasma exchange or IVIG
C. IVIG followed by plasma exchange
D. Intravenous (IV) methylprednisolone combined with IVIG
E. Oral corticosteroids combined with plasma exchange

**Q38.** Which of the following care or treatment options should be avoided in a patient who is admitted to the hospital for acute paraparesis and is diagnosed with Guillain–Barré syndrome?
A. Deep vein thrombosis prophylaxis
B. Oral corticosteroids
C. Plasma exchange
D. Cardiac monitoring
E. Respiratory monitoring

**Q39.** Which of the following variables carries a poor prognosis in Guillain–Barré syndrome?
A. Young age
B. Preceding upper respiratory infection
C. Severe muscle weakness
D. Rapid progression resulting in respiratory failure
E. Hypernatremia

**Q40.** In patients with Guillain–Barré syndrome, when should the diagnosis of acute-onset chronic inflammatory demyelinating polyneuropathy (CIDP) be suspected?
A. Relapses occur within the first month after onset.
B. Relapses occur less than twice during the first 2 months.
C. The acute event is preceded by a gastrointestinal viral illness.
D. Electrodiagnostic studies show prominent demyelination many months later.
E. Symptoms progress and reach a nadir in 4 weeks.

**Q41.** Which of the following acquired peripheral polyneuropathies is typically **NOT** associated with demyelination?
A. HIV infection
B. Vitamin B12 deficiency
C. Immunoglobulin M (IgM) neuropathy
D. Osteosclerotic myeloma
E. Multifocal motor neuropathy

**Q42.** Erroneous diagnosis of chronic inflammatory demyelinating polyneuropathy (CIDP) is usually caused by which of the following findings?
A. Conduction block at non-entrapment sites
B. Significant slowing of conduction velocities
C. Sural sensory sparing pattern
D. Significant elevation of cerebrospinal fluid (CSF) protein.
E. Subjective perception of treatment benefit

**Q43.** A 45-year-old woman with chronic inflammatory demyelinating polyneuropathy (CIDP) initially responded to intravenous immunoglobulin (IVIG) 2 g/kg divided over 5 days, but worsened two months later. What is the next best treatment?
A. Azathioprine
B. Prednisone
C. Plasmapheresis
D. Maintenance IVIG
E. Cyclophosphamide

**Q44.** Which of the following features characterizes the Lewis-Sumner variant of chronic inflammatory demyelinating polyneuropathy (CIDP)?
A. Axon-loss multiple mononeuropathies
B. Multifocal nerve conduction blocks and slowing
C. Pure motor manifestations
D. Poor response to corticosteroids
E. Normal cerebrospinal fluid (CSF) protein

**Q45.** Monoclonal gammopathy of unknown significance (MGUS) may be associated with peripheral polyneuropathy. Which paraprotein is most likely associated with a demyelinating polyneuropathy?
A. IgA
B. IgD
C. IgG
D. IgM
E. IgE

**Q46.** A 65-year-old man presents with a 2-year history of leg numbness and poor balance. His examination reveals sensory ataxia with a symmetrical predominantly sensory polyneuropathy. Electrophysiological studies show symmetrical and markedly uniform slowing of distal latencies, more than conduction velocities, without conduction blocks. Which of the following is **NOT** associated with this disorder?
A. IgM monoclonal protein
B. Excellent response to immunomodulation
C. Myelin-associated glycoprotein antibodies
D. Loss of reflexes
E. Neuropathic tremor

**Q47.** Which of the following does **NOT** occur in multifocal motor neuropathy?
A. Rare cranial nerve involvement
B. Preservation of tendon reflexes
C. Lack of muscle atrophy
D. Good response to corticosteroids
E. Conduction blocks at non-entrapment sites

**Q48.** A 65-year-old woman with an acquired demyelinating polyneuropathy did not respond to intravenous immunoglobulin (IVIG). Upon further testing, she was found to have an immunoglobulin A (IgA) lambda monoclonal gammopathy and a sclerotic bony lesion in the right femur. Which blood test is likely to be abnormal in this patient?
A. Myelin-associated glycoprotein (MAG) antibodies
B. Vascular endothelial growth factor (VEGF)
B. Ganglioside M1 (GM1) antibodies
C. Ganglioside Q1b (GQ1b) antibodies
E. Jo-1 antibodies

**Q49.** Which of the following types of diabetic neuropathy is most often slowly progressive?
A. Oculomotor neuropathy
B. Lumbosacral radiculoplexopathy
C. Distal symmetrical polyneuropathy
D. Facial neuropathy
E. Thoracic radiculopathy

**Q50.** Which of the following is **NOT** associated with paraneoplastic sensory neuronopathy?
A. Small cell lung cancer
B. Limbic encephalitis
C. Elevated anti-Hu (ANNA-1) antibodies
D. Absent sensory nerve action potentials
E. Elevated anti-Ri (ANNA-2) antibodies

**The following answer options are for QUESTIONS 51 through 55**

> Match the given skin or foot changes with the appropriate disorder with neuropathy.
> A. Thallium poisoning
> B. POEMS syndrome
> C. Charcot-Marie-Tooth disease
> D. Leprosy
> E. Vasculitis or cryoglobulinemia

**Q51.** Pes cavus

**Q52.** Hyperpigmentation or hypertrichosis

**Q53.** Purpuric leg skin eruptions

**Q54.** Transverse nail bands

**Q55.** Hypopigmentation

**Q56.** Which of the following agents may trigger an immune-mediated demyelinating neuropathy?
A. Paclitaxel
B. Phenytoin
C. Infliximab
D. Vincristine
E. Metronidazole

**Q57.** Which of the following conditions has **NOT** been reported to be triggered by immune checkpoint inhibitors, which are used to treat cancer patients?
A. Myasthenia gravis
B. Motor neuron disease
C. Myocarditis
D. Guillain–Barré syndrome
E. Myositi.

**Q58.** Which of the following vitamins, when ingested in toxic amount, causes sensory neuronopathy?
A. Vitamin B12
B. Vitamin E
C. Vitamin A
D. Vitamin B6
E. Vitamin K

---

## PART 2 | QUESTIONS WITH ANSWERS AND DISCUSSION

**QUESTION 1.** Which of the following pathophysiological mechanisms of peripheral neuropathies is a predictor for good prognosis?
A. Axonal interruption
B. Segmental demyelination
C. Dorsal ganglionopathy
D. Motor neuronopathy
E. Wallerian degeneration

**ANSWER:** B. Segmental demyelination

### COMMENTS AND DISCUSSION

- Metabolic, toxic, nutritional, immune, or hereditary factors may damage the peripheral nerves.
- The pathological reactions of peripheral nerves to various insults include one of the following:
  - *Wallerian degeneration*, which is the response to axonal interruption caused by compression, traction, laceration, thermal, chemical, or ischemic nerve injury. This results in distal degeneration of axons and their myelin sheaths.
  - *Axonal degeneration or axonopathy*, which afflicts the longest axons first and proceeds proximally, producing a neurological deficit with a distal to proximal gradient.
  - *Neuronopathy*, which is the result of neuronal (perikaryal) degeneration and may involve the dorsal ganglia (i.e., dorsal ganglionopathy) or anterior horn cell (i.e., motor neuronopathy or motor neuron disease).
  - *Segmental demyelination or myelinopathy*, which is the response to insult on the myelin sheath, Schwann cell, or both. This nerve insult results in dysfunction of nerves, carries the best prognosis among all other pathological processes and has a good potential for treatment and reversal.

**HIGH-YIELD FACT**

Segmental demyelination has the greatest potential for recovery in contrast to neuronopathy, Wallerian degeneration, and axonal degeneration.

**QUESTION 2.** Peripheral polyneuropathy due to axonal degeneration does **NOT** usually manifest as:
  A. dying-back polyneuropathy.
  B. length-dependent polyneuropathy.
  C. distal polyneuropathy.
  D. proximal polyneuropathy.
  E. stocking and glove polyneuropathy.

**ANSWER:** D. proximal polyneuropathy.

## COMMENTS AND DISCUSSION

- Axonal degeneration (or axonopathy), the most common pathological reaction of the peripheral nerve, signifies distal axonal breakdown and is caused by structural derangements within neurons/axons or vascular compromise leading to ischemia. Systemic metabolic disorders, toxin exposure, vasculitis, and some inherited neuropathies are the usual causes of axonal degeneration.
- Axonal polyneuropathy starts at the most distal part of the nerve fiber and progresses toward the neuronal cell body. Hence, it is often referred to as a *dying-back or length-dependent polyneuropathy.*
- It results in a distal not a proximal polyneuropathy. The selective length-dependent vulnerability of distal axons could result from failure of the perikaryon to synthesize enzymes or structural proteins, from alterations in axonal transport, or from regional disturbances of energy metabolism.
- Clinically, dying-back polyneuropathy presents with symmetrical distal loss of sensory and motor function in the lower extremities that extends proximally in a graded manner. The result is sensory loss in a stocking-like pattern, distal muscle weakness and atrophy, and loss of distal limb myotatic reflexes. As the polyneuropathy ascends, it causes hand weakness and atrophy, and a glove-like sensory loss (hence the term *stocking-and-glove sensory loss*).
  - By the time sensory disturbances of the longest nerves in the body (lower limbs) have reached the level of the knees, sensory manifestations are usually noted in the distribution of the second-longest nerves (upper limbs) at the tips of the fingers.
  - When sensory impairment reaches the mid-thigh, involvement of the third-longest nerves, the anterior intercostal and lumbar segmental nerves, gives rise to a tent-shaped area of hypoesthesia on the anterior chest and abdomen. Hoarseness due to involvement of the recurrent laryngeal nerves may occur at this stage also.

**QUESTION 3.** Loss of which of the following nerve fibers manifests as sensory impairment to light touch?
  A. Unmyelinated C fibers
  B. Large and small myelinated fibers
  C. Aδ fibers
  D. Aα and Aβ fibers
  E. Large or small myelinated fibers

**ANSWER:** E. Large or small myelinated fibers

## COMMENTS AND DISCUSSION

- Loss of sensation in peripheral polyneuropathies often involves all sensory modalities.
- However, the impairment may be restricted to selective sensory modalities in many situations, which makes it possible to correlate the type of sensory loss with the diameter of affected afferent fibers (see Fig. 2.3 and Table 2.2).
  - Pain and temperature sensation are mediated by unmyelinated C and small myelinated Aδ fibers.
  - Vibratory sense, proprioception, and the afferent limb of the tendon reflex are mediated by large myelinated Aα and Aβ fibers.
  - Light touch is mediated by *both* large and small myelinated fibers.

**QUESTION 4.** Which of the following neurological findings is most suggestive of large fiber sensory polyneuropathy?
A. Hyperalgesia
B. Pseudoathetosis
C. Loss of hair
D. Allodynia
E. Dystrophic nail changes

**ANSWER:** B. Pseudoathetosis

### COMMENTS AND DISCUSSION

- Sensory polyneuropathy preferentially affecting *large fibers* is characterized by areflexia, sensory ataxia, and loss of joint position and vibration sense (see Table 2.2). Loss of joint position may also manifest as *pseudoathetosis* (involuntary sinuous movements of fingers and hands when the arms are outstretched and the eyes are closed) and/or a *Romberg sign* (disproportionate loss of balance with eyes closed compared with eyes open).
- Sensory polyneuropathy preferentially affecting *small fibers* is characterized by a predominant decrease, in pain and temperature sensation, along with spontaneous burning pain, painful dysesthesias, and dystrophic changes in the skin and hair, such as hair loss or brittle nails. There is preservation of tendon reflexes, balance, and motor strength.
  - *Hyperalgesia* is an increased pain response to noxious stimuli.
  - *Allodynia* is the sensation of pain elicited by non-noxious stimuli (e.g., from contact with clothing, bed sheets, or air flow).

**QUESTION 5.** What is the most useful diagnostic study for assessing large fiber dorsal ganglionopathy?
A. Thermoregulatory sweat testing
B. Sensory nerve conduction studies
C. Quantitative sudomotor axon reflex test (QSART)
D. Quantitative sensory testing
E. Skin biopsy with analysis of intraepidermal nerve fiber density

**ANSWER:** B. Sensory nerve conduction studies

### COMMENTS AND DISCUSSION

- Routine sensory nerve conduction studies assess only large myelinated sensory fibers and are best for assessing large fiber axonopathy and dorsal ganglionopathy.
- Because sweating is mediated by unmyelinated sympathetic cholinergic fibers, the quantitative sudomotor axon reflex test (QSART, see Fig. 9.2) is a highly specific and sensitive method for confirming small nerve fiber damage.
- Thermoregulatory sweat testing (TST, see Fig. 9.3) also assesses sweating that is mediated by unmyelinated sympathetic cholinergic fibers but is less specific than QSART in distinguishing central versus peripheral causation of anhidrosis.
- Skin biopsy with analysis of intraepidermal nerve fiber density is very helpful in confirming the unmyelinated nerve fiber loss.
- Quantitative sensory testing assessing both vibratory and thermal detection thresholds is a useful addition to bedside sensory examination in controlled clinical trials. Its use in routine clinical practice remains limited because the test is still subjective, time consuming, and requires full patient cooperation.

## ◎ HIGH-YIELD FACT

Sensory nerve conduction studies assess large sensory fibers, whereas quantitative sudomotor axon reflex test (QSART), thermoregulatory sweat testing (TST), and skin biopsy with analysis of intraepidermal nerve fiber density assess small fiber sensory fibers.

**QUESTION 6.** Which of the following clinical features characterizes small fiber neuropathy?
- A. Areflexia
- B. Distal hypohidrosis
- C. Distal weakness
- D. Sensory ataxia
- E. Loss of position sense

**ANSWER:** B. Distal hypohidrosis

## COMMENTS AND DISCUSSION
- Small fiber neuropathy is characterized by loss of unmyelinated fibers resulting in sensory symptoms (paresthesia, hypoesthesia, allodynia) and autonomic symptoms (reduced or excessive sweating, constipation or diarrhea, impotence, micturition disturbances, dry eyes and/or mouth, postural hypotension).
- Muscle strength, reflexes, and proprioception remain intact.

**QUESTION 7.** Mononeuropathy multiplex presenting exclusively with axonal loss is characteristic of which of the following disorders?
- A. Multifocal motor neuropathy
- B. Lewis-Sumner syndrome
- C. Vasculitic neuropathy
- D. Multiple entrapment/compressive neuropathies
- E. Hereditary neuropathy with liability to pressure palsies

**ANSWER:** C. Vasculitic neuropathy

## COMMENTS AND DISCUSSION
- In multiple mononeuropathics (mononeuropathy multiplex), the neurological findings point to simultaneous or sequential damage to two or more peripheral nerves.
- Confluent multiple mononeuropathies, such as with involvement of the peroneal and tibial nerves or the median and ulnar nerves, may result in asymmetrical motor weakness and sensory loss, mimicking an asymmetrical peripheral polyneuropathy. In some cases, this may also simulate a length-dependent symmetrical peripheral polyneuropathy.
- Electrodiagnostic studies ascertain whether the primary pathological process is axonal degeneration or segmental demyelination. Approximately two-thirds of patients with multiple mononeuropathies display a picture of axonal damage.
  - Axonal mononeuropathy multiplex is often caused by ischemia; other less common causes are infectious, granulomatous, or neoplastic infiltration. This is usually seen with:
    - Vasculitis (systemic, non-systemic)
    - Diabetes mellitus
    - Sarcoidosis
    - Leprosy
    - Human immunodeficiency virus 1 (HIV-1) infection
  - Demyelinating mononeuropathy multiplex manifests with multifocal demyelination or motor conduction blocks, or both, as seen in:
    - Multifocal motor neuropathy
    - Lewis-Sumner syndrome (multifocal acquired demyelinating sensory and motor neuropathy [MADSAM])
    - Multiple entrapment or compressive neuropathies
    - Hereditary neuropathy with liability to pressure palsies (HNPP)

**QUESTION 8.** Which primary process is characterized by disruption of the axon and myelin sheath with preservation of **ALL** supporting tissue?
A. Neurapraxia
B. Axonotmesis
C. Neurotmesis
D. First-degree nerve injury
E. Third-degree nerve injury

**ANSWER:** B. Axonotmesis

## COMMENTS AND DISCUSSION
- Peripheral nerve injury is classified based on Seddon's or Sunderland's classifications (Fig. 14.1).
   o *Neurapraxia (first-degree nerve injury).* This results in alteration in myelin, leading to segmental block of conduction without Wallerian degeneration. The nerve can still conduct distally but not across the lesion resulting in conduction block. There are no or little changes in the muscles and recovery is usually complete following remyelination within 1–3 months.
   o *Axonotmesis (second-degree nerve injury).* The axons are focally damaged resulting in secondary Wallerian degeneration distal to the site of injury. There is little or no disruption of the supporting structures (endoneurium, perineurium, and epineurium). These lesions have a fair prognosis, since axonal regeneration is well-guided by the intact endoneurial tubes.

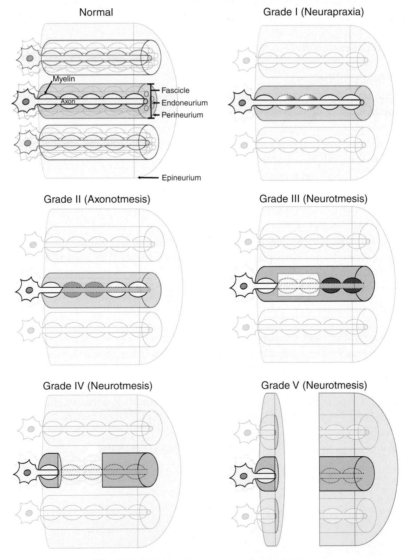

**Fig. 14.1** Classification of peripheral nerve injuries.

- *Neurotmesis.* Here the nerve is either completely severed or seriously disorganized by scar tissue, such that spontaneous regeneration is often not possible. Sunderland subdivided this into three further subtypes, depending on what component of the surrounding nerve stroma is affected:
  - *Third-degree nerve injury,* in which the axons, Schwann cell tubes, and endoneurium are damaged leaving the perineurium and epineurium intact. These lesions have poor prognosis and may require surgical intervention, since axonal regeneration is often misdirected and may lead to neuroma formation.
  - *Fourth-degree nerve injury,* where the perineurium is also disrupted, but the epineurium is intact. These lesions have very poor prognosis and surgery is often required.
  - *Fifth-degree nerve injury,* the most severe type of nerve injury manifesting as complete disruption of the nerve with all supporting structures. The nerve is transected, resulting in loss of continuity between its proximal and distal stumps. These lesions have no chance for improvement without surgical repair.

##  HIGH-YIELD FACT

Neurapraxia is also known as first-degree nerve injury and manifests electrophysiologically as a conduction block.

**QUESTION 9.** Which of the following changes does **NOT** occur after axonal transection?
A. The axonal caliber of the proximal stump becomes smaller.
B. Nerve cell body shows signs of chromatolysis.
C. Regeneration from the proximal stump proceeds at a rate of 2–3 cm/day.
D. Myelin of the distal segment disintegrates.
E. Denervated muscles reinnervate through sprouting of intact axons.

**ANSWER:** C. Regeneration from the proximal stump proceeds at a rate of 2–3 cm/day.

### COMMENTS AND DISCUSSION

- Axonal transection (axotomy) initiates proximal and distal changes (Fig. 14.2):
  - *Proximal changes* include:
    - Morphological changes of the neuronal cell body including the dissolution of the Nissl bodies *(chromatolysis)*
    - Narrowing of the proximal axonal caliber
  - *Distal changes* include:
    - Wallerian degeneration, which results in disintegration of axon and myelin and is completed within 2 weeks. Within a few days, macrophages are recruited into the injury site to digest debris.

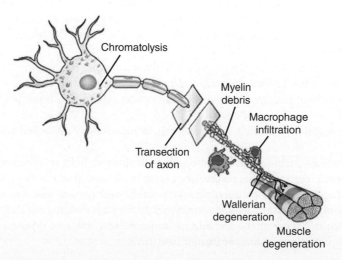

**Fig. 14.2.** Wallerian degeneration following axotomy. From Jankovic J, Newman N, Maziotta J, Pomeroy SL, eds. *Bradley & Daroff's Neurology in Clinical Practice: Vol 1.* 8th ed. Philadelphia: Elsevier/Saunders; 2022.

- Proximal to distal regeneration from the proximal stump, which begins as early as 24 hours following transection but proceeds very slowly at a maximal rate of 2–3 mm/day (often 1 mm/day) and is often incomplete.
- Sprouting of axons from intact nearby motor units, which will ultimately connect to denervated muscle fibers. Evidence of this change on needle EMG including nascent units and satellite potentials is seen after 1 month following axonal injury.

**QUESTION 10.** Significant dysautonomia is **LEAST** likely to be associated with which of the following conditions?
A. Guillain-Barré syndrome
B. Porphyria
C. Chronic inflammatory demyelinating polyneuropathy
D. Diabetes mellitus
E. AL Amyloidosis

**ANSWER:** C. Chronic inflammatory demyelinating polyneuropathy

**COMMENTS AND DISCUSSION**
- Autonomic dysfunction of clinical importance is seen in association with specific acute (e.g., Guillain–Barré syndrome) or chronic (e.g., amyloidosis, porphyria, and diabetes) sensorimotor polyneuropathies. Chronic inflammatory demyelinating polyneuropathy is rarely associated with dysautonomia.
- Autonomic neuropathy usually correlates with the severity of somatic neuropathy. Rarely an autonomic neuropathy may be the exclusive manifestation of a peripheral nerve disorder without somatic nerve involvement.
- The spectrum of autonomic involvement ranges from subclinical functional impairment of cardiovascular reflexes and sudomotor function to severe cardiovascular, gastrointestinal, or genitourinary dysfunction.
- Orthostatic hypotension, resting tachycardia, or diminished heart-rate response to respiration are the hallmarks of cardiac and vasomotor autonomic neuropathy.
  - Orthostatic hypotension occurs mainly because of failure of the sympathetic nervous system to increase systemic vascular resistance in the erect posture and impairment of compensatory cardiac acceleration.
  - Vagal denervation of the heart results in a high resting pulse rate and loss of sinus arrhythmia. This probably explains the increased incidence of painless or silent myocardial infarction in diabetic patients with autonomic neuropathy.
- Gastrointestinal motility abnormalities involving the esophagus, stomach, gallbladder, or bowel may occur. Delayed gastric emptying, usually of solids, leads to nausea, early satiety, and postprandial bloating. Constipation due to colonic hypomotility is more common than diarrhea, which tends to be explosive and paroxysmal. Fecal incontinence may also occur.
- Impaired bladder sensation is usually the first symptom of urinary autonomic dysfunction. Bladder atony leads to prolonged intervals between voiding, gradually increasing urinary retention, and finally overflow incontinence.
- Impotence in men is common in patients with chronic autonomic neuropathy such as diabetes and amyloidosis. It is often the first manifestation of autonomic neuropathy in men with diabetes, occurring in more than 60% of patients. Autonomic dysfunction involves both erectile failure and retrograde ejaculation.
- Sudomotor abnormalities result in distal anhidrosis, compensatory facial and truncal sweating, and heat intolerance.
- Pupillary abnormalities include constricted pupils with sluggish light reaction, which occurs in 20% of unselected diabetic patients. This results from early involvement of the sympathetic nerves that dilate the iris and an imbalance between parasympathetic and sympathetic function.
- A blunted autonomic response to hypoglycemia in patients with diabetic autonomic neuropathy produces an inadequate sympathetic and adrenal response and hence an unawareness of hypoglycemia that may seriously complicate intensive insulin treatment.

**QUESTION 11.** Which of the following peripheral polyneuropathies is **LEAST** likely to involve the facial nerve?

A. Guillain–Barré syndrome
B. Lyme disease
C. Sarcoidosis
D. Chronic inflammatory demyelinating polyneuropathy
E. Tangier disease

**ANSWER:** D. Chronic inflammatory demyelinating polyneuropathy

### COMMENTS AND DISCUSSION

- Cranial nerve involvement occurs in 50% to 75% of cases of patients with Guillain–Barré syndrome. Facial palsy, usually bilateral, occurs in at least 50% of patients.
- Chronic inflammatory demyelinating polyneuropathy is characterized by proximal and distal muscle weakness, areflexia or hyporeflexia, and sensory loss. Less common manifestations are postural tremor, enlargement of peripheral nerves, optic disc edema, facial or bulbar weakness, respiratory failure, and autonomic dysfunction.
- In Lyme disease, a distinctive early neurological syndrome follows the pathognomonic dartboard-like skin lesion (*erythema migrans or erythema chronicum migrans*) in ~15% of patients. This consists of facial palsy (often bilateral), radiculoneuropathy, and lymphocytic meningitis.
- In neurosarcoidosis, cranial neuropathies, particularly facial nerve palsy, are the most common neurological manifestations occurring in three-fourths of patients. Other less common peripheral nerve involvement includes multiple mononeuropathies, truncal sensory mononeuropathies, cauda equina syndrome, chronic symmetrical sensorimotor polyneuropathy, or acute polyradiculoneuropathy resembling Guillain–Barré syndrome.
- Tangier disease is an autosomal recessive disorder characterized by severe deficiency of plasma high-density lipoprotein (HDL), resulting in the deposition of cholesterol esters in many tissues, including the reticuloendothelial system (leading to enlarged yellow-orange tonsils) and peripheral nerves. In adolescence or adult life, approximately half of affected patients develop one of the following two distinct neuropathic syndromes:
  - A progressive symmetrical neuropathy mimicking syringomyelia. This manifests with dissociated loss of pain and temperature sensation in the face, arms, and upper trunk, combined with muscle wasting and weakness in the face and arms.
  - Relapsing multifocal mononeuropathies involving multiple nerves in the cranial, truncal, or appendicular regions.

### The following vignette is for QUESTIONS 12 through 14.

A 65-year-old woman developed winging of the scapula after undergoing a scalene lymph node biopsy (see the following figure; note that the patient is trying to abduct the right shoulder).

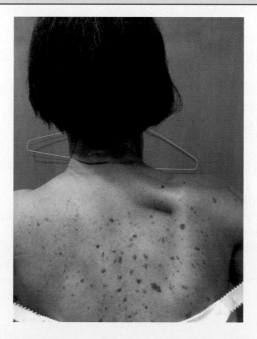

**QUESTION 12.** What is the **MOST** likely injured nerve in this patient?
- A. Axillary nerve
- B. Dorsal scapular nerve
- C. Long thoracic nerve
- D. Spinal accessory nerve
- E. Suprascapular nerve

**ANSWER:** D. Spinal accessory nerve

**COMMENTS AND DISCUSSION**
- This patient has a spinal accessory neuropathy. Surgical interventions involving the neck, namely, in the posterior cervical triangle such as scalene lymph node biopsy, may injure the spinal accessory nerve.
- The serratus anterior (innervated by the long thoracic nerve), trapezius (innervated by the spinal accessory nerve), and rhomboid/levator scapulae (innervated by the dorsal scapular nerve) muscles are the main scapular fixators.
- The axillary nerve innervates the deltoid and teres minor, while the suprascapular nerve innervates the supraspinatus and infraspinatus muscles. Despite being located in the scapular region, these muscles have minimal roles in fixating the scapula to the thoracic cavity.

**QUESTION 13.** Which of the following muscles should be spared in this patient despite being innervated by the involved nerve?
- A. Upper trapezius
- B. Serratus anterior
- C. Sternocleidomastoid
- D. Levator scapulae
- E. Rhomboids

**ANSWER:** C. Sternocleidomastoid

**COMMENTS AND DISCUSSION**
- The spinal accessory nerve is unique among the cranial nerves in having neurons originating in the cervical spinal cord. Therefore, it is the only cranial nerve that both enters and exits the skull. The nerve has a spinal and cranial portion: the spinal portion arises from the gray matter of cervical spinal levels C1 to C5 and enters the skull through the foramen magnum; the cranial portion originates from the dorsolateral surface of the medulla oblongata. The nerve ultimately exits the skull, along with the vagus and glossopharyngeal nerves and jugular vein from the jugular foramen.
- The spinal accessory nerve provides motor innervation to two muscles: the trapezius and sternocleidomastoid. During a scalene lymph node biopsy, only the branch of the spinal accessory nerve that supplies the trapezius muscle passes through this surgical area. Therefore, iaotrogenic injury to the spinal accessory nerve in the context of cervical lymph node biopsy typically spares sternocleidomastoid muscles.

**QUESTION 14.** What is **CORRECT** about the expected pattern of scapular winging in this patient?
- A. Medial
- B. Mild at rest
- C. Accentuated by shoulder forward flexion
- D. Not associated with sagging of the shoulder
- E. Associated with a visible levator scapulae muscle

**ANSWER:** E. Associated with a visible levator scapulae muscle

**COMMENTS AND DISCUSSION**
- Scapular winging refers to translocation of the scapula from its normal position. This may be apparent at rest or accentuated or improved by certain shoulder movements.
- Unilateral winging is most often caused by weakness of the trapezius (Fig. 14.3) or serratus anterior (Fig. 14.4) muscles, usually due to isolated mononeuropathies of the spinal accessory or long thoracic nerves, respectively. Isolated dorsal scapular mononeuropathy, leading to weakness of the rhomboid or levator scapulae muscle, is extremely rare. Bilateral scapular winging from isolated mononeuropathies

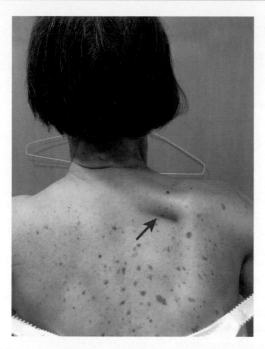

**Fig. 14.3 Scapular winging in this patient with spinal accessory neuropathy and trapezius weakness.** The patient is trying to abduct the right shoulder. Note the lateral translocation of the scapula and prominent levator scapulae *(red arrow)*.

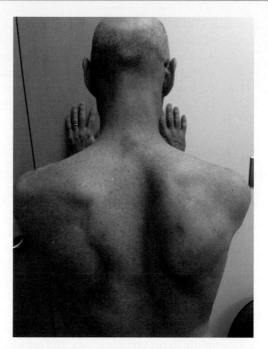

**Fig. 14.4 Scapular winging in another patient with long thoracic neuropathy and serratus anterior weakness.** Note the medial dislocation of the scapula aggravated by protraction (pushing) against resistance.

is unusual. Bilateral scapular winging is usually caused by diffuse weakness of the scapular fixators from generalized neuromuscular diseases, such as facioscapulohumeral muscular dystrophy.

- Patients with unilateral scapular winging often present with shoulder weakness, pain, or both. Shoulder weakness is in all planes of movement but is appreciated primarily with tasks requiring shoulder abduction or forward flexion. The pain is usually deep and poorly localized to the shoulder and scapula. It is often exacerbated by activity and improved following rest.
- Scapular weakness due to trapezius weakness is lateral and prominent at rest with prominent sagging of the shoulder and a visible levator scapulae muscle (which is usually covered by the trapezius). The winging is accentuated by shoulder abduction. This could be distinguished easily from weakness of the serratus anterior (Fig. 14.3, Table 14.1 and see Fig. 1.6).

**TABLE 14.1** Differential features of scapular winging due to trapezius or serratus anterior weakness.

| Muscle | Trapezius weakness | Serratus anterior weakness |
|---|---|---|
| *Innervation* | *Spinal accessory nerve* | *Long thoracic nerve* |
| Scapular winging at rest | Prominent | Mild |
| Shoulder sagging at rest | Obvious | Subtle |
| Levator scapulae at rest | Prominent (with chronic weakness only) | Not visible |
| Relation to midline at rest | Lateral translocation | Medial translocation |
| Winging is accentuated by | Shoulder abduction | Shoulder forward flexion or protraction (pushing) against resistance |

**QUESTION 15.** Which of the following is **CORRECT** regarding the palmar cutaneous sensory branch of the median nerve?
  A. It is involved in median nerve entrapment at the carpal tunnel.
  B. It innervates the skin over the thenar eminence.
  C. It is normal in median nerve lesions in forearm.
  D. It is a branch of the median nerve distal to the carpal tunnel.
  E. It innervates the entire thumb.

**ANSWER:** B. It innervates the skin over the thenar eminence.

### COMMENTS AND DISCUSSION
- The median nerve runs into the forearm between the two heads of the pronator teres (see Fig. 1.2). It then gives off branches to the pronator teres, flexor carpi radialis, flexor digitorum sublimis, and palmaris longus muscles, as well as the anterior interosseous nerve.
- The median nerve then enters the wrist through the carpal tunnel, formed by the carpal bones and the transverse carpal ligament. Before reaching the wrist, the median nerve gives off the palmar cutaneous sensory branch, which runs subcutaneously (not through the carpal tunnel) to innervate the skin over the thenar eminence. Distal to the carpal tunnel, the median nerve divides into motor and sensory divisions. The motor division innervates the first and second lumbricals and most muscles of the thenar eminence including the opponens pollicis, abductor pollicis brevis, and superficial head of the flexor pollicis brevis. The sensory fibers of the median nerve innervate the skin of the thumb, index, middle, and lateral half of the ring fingers.

**QUESTION 16.** A 25-year-old man is awakened at night with numbness in the right hand. Which of the following electrodiagnostic tests is the most sensitive for detecting mild carpal tunnel syndrome (CTS)?
  A. Antidromic median sensory latency (wrist to index)
  B. Comparison of mixed median palmar to ulnar palmar latencies
  C. Orthodromic median sensory latency (index to wrist)
  D. Median motor distal latency recording the abductor pollicis brevis
  E. Fibrillation potentials in the abductor pollicis brevis

**ANSWER:** B. Comparison of mixed median palmar to ulnar palmar latencies

### COMMENTS AND DISCUSSION
- Routine nerve conduction studies used in the diagnosis of carpal tunnel syndrome (CTS) are the:
  o Median motor nerve conduction study
  o Median sensory nerve conduction study (orthodromic or antidromic)
- It is now recognized that median motor and median sensory distal latencies are not sufficiently sensitive in the diagnosis of CTS. Reliance on only on these measurements will fail to detect a significant number (up to one-third) of patients with mild CTS.
- More sensitive tests are now utilized, which increases the sensitivity of electrodiagnostic studies to about 90% to 95% of patients with CTS.
- *Internal comparison nerve conduction studies* are very common (Fig. 14.5). These studies rely on comparing the median distal latency to the distal latency of a neighboring nerve. This often includes the ulnar nerve or radial nerve of the same hand.
  o Comparison of orthodromic median to ulnar palmar mixed latencies (Fig. 14.6A, A1, and A2)
  o Comparison of antidromic median to ulnar sensory latencies recording the ring finger (Fig. 14.6B, B1, and B2)
  o Comparison of median to ulnar motor latencies recording the second lumbrical and second interosseous, respectively (Fig. 14.6C, C1, and C2)
  o Comparison of antidromic median to radial sensory latencies recording the thumb (Fig. 14.6D, D1, and D2)
- *Segmental nerve conduction studies or the inching technique* (antidromic) may also be used.
  o The rationale is that the slow-conducting segment of the median nerve in CTS is typically very short. If this short segment is included in a longer nerve segment, such as the wrist-to-index segment, a mild abnormality may become "diluted" by the normal conduction in the rest of the nerve. As a result, the overall conduction time (i.e., latency) may remain within normal limits in mild and early cases of CTS.
  o Hence, measuring the conduction time of short segments (usually 1-cm increments) of the median nerve across the carpal tunnel is a more sensitive, but time-consuming, study.

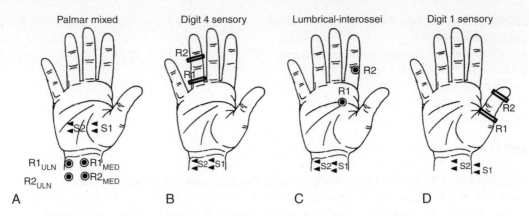

**Fig. 14.5 Comparison studies in the diagnosis of carpal tunnel syndrome.** *S,* stimulation site; *R1 and R2,* active and reference recording sites, respectively. From Katirji B, Kaminski HJ, Preston DC et al., eds. *Neuromuscular Disorders in Clinical Practice.* Boston: Butterworth-Heinemann; 2002.

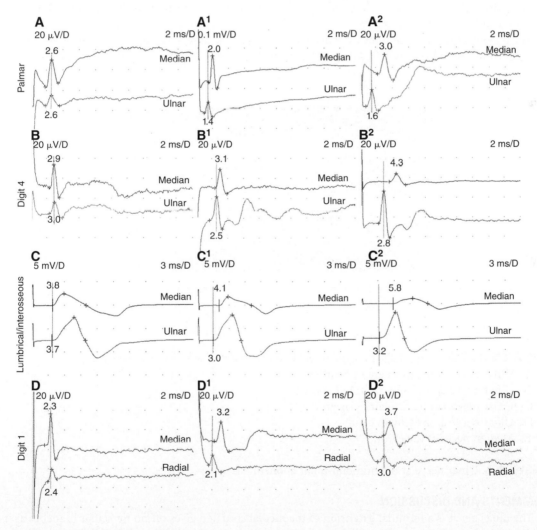

**Fig. 14.6 Comparison studies in the diagnosis of carpal tunnel syndrome.** The numbers shown are in ms and represent peak latencies.

-Palmar mixed study: (A) normal, (A1) mildly abnormal, and (A2) markedly abnormal.

-Median-ulnar sensory study to ring finger: (B) normal, (B1) mildly abnormal, and (B2) markedly abnormal.

-Second lumbrical/interosseous (median-ulnar) motor study: (C) normal, (C1) mildly abnormal, and (C2) markedly abnormal.

-Median-radial sensory study to thumb: (D) normal,

(D1) mildly abnormal, and (D2) markedly abnormal. From Katirji B. *Electromyography in Clinical Practice: A Case Study Approach.* 3rd ed. New York: Oxford University Press; 2018.

**QUESTION 17.** Which of the following clinical features is expected in a patient with a lesion of the anterior interosseous nerve?
  A.  Inability to flex the thumb and index finger
  B.  Inabiliity to abduct the thumb
  C.  Numbness at base of the thumb
  D.  Inability to flex the little and ring fingers
  E.  Numbness in the anterior forearm

**ANSWER:** A. Inability to flex the thumb and index finger

**COMMENTS AND DISCUSSION (see also comments and discussion from Question 16)**
  •  The anterior interosseous nerve is the largest branch of the median nerve and is a pure motor nerve.
  •  It arises from the median nerve distal to motor branches in the upper forearm and innervates the flexor pollicis longus, pronator quadratus, and the median part of the flexor digitorum profundus muscles of the index and middle fingers.
  •  The patient is unable to flex the distal phalanges of the thumb and index finger, making it impossible to form a circle with those fingers (*pinch or OK sign*; Fig. 14.7 and see Fig. 1.3).
  •  The patient should be able to abduct the thumb, since the abductor pollicis brevis is innervated by the main trunk of the median nerve.
  •  The patient should be able to flex the distal phalanges of the little and ring fingers, since the flexor digitorum profundus muscles to the little and ring fingers are innervated by the ulnar nerve.

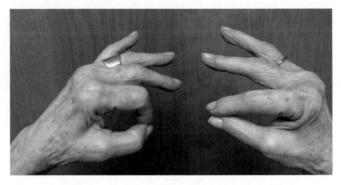

**Fig. 14.7**  The OK sign in a patient with right anterior interosseous neuropathy.

**QUESTION 18.**  Cubital tunnel syndrome refers to entrapment of which of the following?
  A.  Ulnar nerve at the ligament of Struthers
  B.  Ulnar nerve at the humeral-ulnar aponeurosis
  C.  Ulnar nerve at the retrocondylar groove
  D.  Ulnar nerve at the Guyon canal
  E.  Median nerve at the elbow

**ANSWER:** B. Ulnar nerve at the humeral-ulnar aponeurosis

**COMMENTS AND DISCUSSION**
  •  The ulnar nerve is a terminal extension of the medial cord and gives off no muscular branches as it descends through the medial arm.
  •  At the elbow, the nerve enters the *ulnar or retrocondylar groove* formed between the medial epicondyle and the olecranon process. Slightly distal to the groove in the proximal forearm, the ulnar nerve travels under the tendinous arch of the two heads of the flexor carpi ulnaris muscle, known as the *humeral-ulnar aponeurosis or cubital tunnel.*
  •  Muscular branches are then given off to the flexor carpi ulnaris and the medial division (fourth and fifth digits) of the flexor digitorum profundus (see Fig. 1.4).

- Slightly proximal to the wrist, the dorsal ulnar cutaneous sensory branch and palmar cutaneous sensory branch exit to supply sensation to the dorsal medial hand/dorsal fifth and medial fourth digits and proximal medial palm, respectively.
- The ulnar nerve enters the wrist through Guyon canal to supply sensation to the volar fifth and medial fourth digits. It also innervates the hypothenar muscles, the palmar and dorsal interossei, the third and fourth lumbricals, the adductor pollicis, and the deep head of the flexor pollicis brevis.
- Cubital tunnel syndrome is properly used to indicate compression of the ulnar nerve under the humeral-ulnar aponeurosis.
- The ligament of Struthers is a tendinous band stretching between a bony spur on the medial humerus (just cephalad to the medial epicondyle) and the medial humeral epicondyle. Rarely the median nerve is entrapped by this ligament, resulting in pain and paresthesia in the median digits exacerbated by supination of the forearm and extension of the elbow. Weakness of the pronator teres and other median-innervated muscles and sensory loss in a median distribution may occur.

**QUESTION 19.** Which of the following signs is **NOT** seen in ulnar neuropathy at the elbow?
A. Tinel sign
B. Froment sign
C. Phalen sign
D. Benedict sign
E. Wartenberg sign

**ANSWER:** C. Phalen sign

**COMMENTS AND DISCUSSION**
- Tinel sign is elicited by tapping over an injured or entrapped peripheral nerve such as the ulnar nerve at the elbow or the median nerve at the wrist. This elicits paresthesia in the sensory distribution of the nerve.
- Froment sign is evident when attempting to pinch an object or piece of paper. To compensate for intrinsic ulnar hand weakness, the long flexors to the thumb and index finger (innervated by the median nerve) are used to pinch, creating a flexed posture of the thumb and index finger (Fig. 14.8).

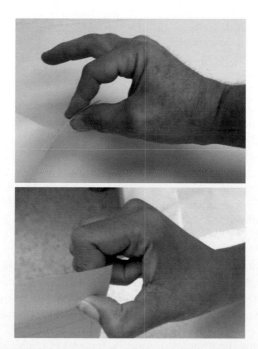

**Fig. 14.8 Froment sign.** This is evident when a patient attempts to pinch an object or piece of paper. The long flexors to the thumb and index finger (innervated by the median nerve) are used to pinch, to compensate for intrinsic ulnar hand weakness. From Preston DC, Shapiro BE. *Electromyography and Neuromuscular Disorders: Clinical-electrophysiologic-ultrasound Correlations.* 4th ed. Elsevier; 2021.

- Benedict sign (aka, Benediction posture or ulnar clawing) manifests as clawing of the ring and little fingers with the metacarpophalangeal joints hyperextended and the proximal and distal interphalangeal joints flexed, due to weakness of the third and fourth lumbricals (Fig. 14.9).
- Wartenberg sign manifests as abduction of the little finger due to weakness of the third palmar interosseous muscle. Patients may report that their little finger gets caught when they try to put their hand in the pocket (Fig. 14.10).
- Phalen maneuver is a highly sensitive and specific sign in carpal tunnel syndrome. Paresthesia in the hand is provoked by holding the wrist in a flexed position.

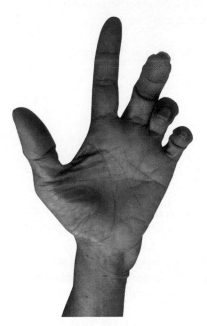

**Fig. 14.9 Benedict sign (aka, Benediction posture or ulnar clawing).** This figure demonstrates clawing of the little and ring fingers with the metacarpophalangeal joints hyperextended and the proximal and distal interphalangeal joints flexed due to weakness of the third and fourth lumbricals.

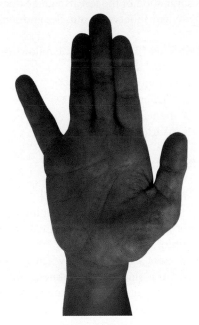

**Fig. 14.10 Wartenberg sign in a patient with left ulnar neuropathy.** There is abduction of the left little finger due to weakness of the third palmar interosseous muscle.

**QUESTION 20.** The inching technique is most useful in localizing the site of:
- A. a conduction block in a chronic axonal neuropathy.
- B. entrapment in ulnar neuropathy at the wrist.
- C. nerve injury in an axon-loss plexopathy.
- D. axonal loss in radiculopathy.
- E. a conduction block in sciatic nerve lesion.

**ANSWER:** B. entrapment in ulnar neuropathy at the wrist.

**COMMENTS AND DISCUSSION**
- Routine nerve conduction studies are often sufficient to localize the site of the lesion in entrapment neuropathies.
- However, during the evaluation of a focal nerve lesion, inclusion of the unaffected segments in conduction velocity calculation dilutes the effect of slowing at the injured site and decreases the sensitivity of the test. Therefore, incremental stimulation across the shorter segment helps localize an abnormality that might otherwise escape detection.
- More-precise localization requires moving the stimulus in short increments (1–2 cm) along the course of the nerve while keeping the recording site constant.
- This procedure is often labeled short-segment incremental stimulation (SSIS) or "inching."

- The analysis of the waveform usually focuses on sudden changes in latency values or an abrupt drop in amplitude.
- The inching technique is particularly useful in assessing patients with carpal tunnel syndrome, ulnar neuropathies at the elbow or wrist, or peroneal neuropathy at the fibular neck. For example, with stimulation of a normal median nerve in 1-cm increments across the wrist, the latency changes ~0.16 to 0.21 ms/cm from the mid-palm to distal forearm. A sharply localized latency increase across a 1-cm segment indicates a focal abnormality of the median nerve.
- The inching technique is not useful in axon-loss lesions, since they are not associated with focal slowing or conduction block.
- The inching technique cannot be done in radiculopathy or sciatic nerve lesion, since these nerve segments are not accessible to nerve conduction studies.

## ◎ HIGH-YIELD FACT

> The inching technique or short-segment incremental segmental stimulation (SSIS) is useful in detecting focal slowing (latency shift) or conduction block in median neuropathy at the wrist, ulnar neuropathy at the elbow or wrist, or peroneal neuropathy at the fibular neck.

**QUESTION 21.** Which of the following statements is **FALSE** regarding Martin-Gruber anastomosis?
- A. It occurs in 20% to 40% of the population.
- B. It consists of a communicating branch from the ulnar to the median nerve.
- C. It consists of nerve fibers destined for the first dorsal interosseous, abductor digiti minimi, and/or adductor pollicis.
- D. It often manifests with an apparent ulnar nerve conduction block in the forearm.
- E. It may be associated with a higher median compound muscle action potential (CMAP) amplitude at the elbow compared to the wrist.

**ANSWER:** B. It consists of a communicating branch from the ulnar to the median nerve.

### COMMENTS AND DISCUSSION
- Martin-Gruber anastomosis (aka, median-to-ulnar crossover) is a normal anatomic variant resulting in a crossover of median to ulnar motor fibers in the forearm, typically between 3 and 10 cm distal to the medial epicondyle (see Fig. 8.1).
- Martin-Gruber anastomosis is present in 20% to 40% of the population.
- It is typically recognized as a drop in amplitude and area between wrist and below-elbow stimulations on routine ulnar motor studies, mimicking a true conduction block in the forearm. Rarely the conduction block is across the elbow when crossing fibers are very proximal, leading to a drop in amplitude and area between the below-elbow and above-elbow stimulation sites.
- When Martin-Gruber crossover fibers terminate in the ulnar thenar eminence (including the adductor pollicis), a higher amplitude is seen when stimulating the median nerve at the antecubital fossa as compared to the median nerve at the wrist.

**QUESTION 22.** In a median-to-ulnar crossover in the forearm, which of the following findings would be observed?
- A. Conduction block along the median nerve in the forearm recording from the abductor pollicis brevis (APB)
- B. Slowing of ulnar conduction velocity in the forearm
- C. Conduction block along the ulnar nerve in the forearm recording from the abductor digiti minimi (ADM)
- D. Slowing of the median conduction velocity in the forearm
- E. Higher ulnar compound muscle action potential (CMAP) amplitude at the elbow compared to the wrist

**ANSWER:** C. Conduction block along the ulnar nerve in the forearm recording from the abductor digiti minimi (ADM)

**COMMENTS AND DISCUSSION (see also comments and discussion from Question 21)**

- Martin-Gruber anastomosis is often recognized as a drop in amplitude and area of between-wrist and below-elbow stimulations on routine ulnar motor studies that mimics a true conduction block in the forearm. Stimulating the median nerve in the antecubital fossa while keeping the recording at the ulnar muscles (such as ADM) will result in a compound muscle action potential (CMAP) that equals the CMAP difference across the pseudo-conduction block.
- Conduction block in the forearm does not occur along the median nerve recording from the APB with a CMAP when stimulating the ulnar nerve at the elbow.
- Higher median (not ulnar) CMAP amplitude at the elbow compared to the wrist may occur with Martin-Gruber anastomosis.
- Slowing of ulnar or median conduction velocities in the forearm does not occur with Martin-Gruber anastomosis.

**QUESTION 23.** Which of the following statements is **FALSE** regarding ulnar motor conduction study, recording the first dorsal interosseous muscle, compared to recording hypothenar muscles?
  A. It increases the yield of finding ulnar focal slowing or conduction block.
  B. It helps to detect ulnar nerve lesions at the wrist or palm.
  C. It is more likely to show findings of a Martin-Gruber anastomosis.
  D. It often yields higher compound muscle action potential (CMAP) amplitude in amyotrophic lateral sclerosis.
  E. It is more suitable for the inching technique across the wrist.

**ANSWER:** D. It often yields higher compound muscle action potential (CMAP) amplitude in amyotrophic lateral sclerosis.

**COMMENTS AND DISCUSSION**

- In an ulnar motor conduction study, recording the first dorsal interosseous muscle in addition to recording the abductor digiti minimi muscle, increases the yield of focal slowing or conduction block at the elbow.
- Recording the first dorsal interosseous muscle is extremely helpful in assessing patients with possible ulnar neuropathy at the wrist or palm. In contrast, recording the hypothenar muscles may miss lesions at Guyon canal or in the palm.
- Recording the first dorsal interosseous muscle is also more suitable for the inching technique across the wrist, since it is less susceptible to stimulation artifact and assesses the deep palmar branch of the ulnar nerve.
- Martin-Gruber anastomosis, manifesting as a pseudo-conduction block in the forearm, is more commonly seen in ulnar nerve conduction study recording of the first dorsal interosseous than of the hypothenar muscles.
- Atrophy and low CMAP amplitudes often affect the lateral hand more than the medial hand in patients with amyotrophic lateral sclerosis (ALS), a phenomenon named "*Split hand syndrome*". Hence, an ulnar motor conduction study, recording the first dorsal interosseous muscle, and a median motor conduction study, recording abductor pollicis brevis, often have low CMAP amplitudes comparing to the ulnar motor conduction study, recording the hypothenar muscles.

**QUESTION 24.** Which of the following conditions does **NOT** result in a low motor amplitude of the ulnar nerve when stimulating at the wrist and recording from the hypothenar muscles?
  A. Amyotrophic lateral sclerosis
  B. Lambert-Eaton myasthenic syndrome
  C. Martin-Gruber anastomosis
  D. Peripheral polyneuropathy
  E. Ulnar neuropathy

**ANSWER:** C. Martin-Gruber anastomosis

**COMMENTS AND DISCUSSION (see also comments and discussion from Questions 22 and 23)**
- Martin-Gruber anastomosis is a median-to-ulnar crossover in the forearm.
- Ulnar nerve conduction studies, recording from the hypothenar muscles, show a normal compound muscle action potential (CMAP) amplitude of the ulnar nerve stimulating at the wrist with a drop in amplitude and area between wrist and below-elbow stimulations mimicking a true conduction block in the forearm.
- In amyotrophic lateral sclerosis, peripheral polyneuropathy, and ulnar neuropathy, there is often axonal loss. Therefore, CMAP amplitude of the ulnar nerve stimulating at the wrist may be low.
- In Lambert-Eaton myasthenic syndrome there is a presynaptic blockage resulting in many muscle fibers not reaching thresholds at their neuromuscular junctions. Consequently, CMAP amplitudes are usually diffusely low, including the ulnar nerve stimulating at the wrist.

**QUESTION 25.** Which of the following findings is seen in a "Saturday night palsy" that presents as pure neurapraxia?
- A. Low amplitude radial sensory nerve action potential (SNAP)
- B. Radial motor conduction block between the axilla and above the spiral groove
- C. Fibrillations in the extensor carpi radialis longus muscle
- D. Normal distal radial compound muscle action potential (CMAP) stimulating elbow
- E. Fibrillations in the brachioradialis muscle

**ANSWER:** D. Normal distal radial compound muscle action potential (CMAP) stimulating the elbow

**COMMENTS AND DISCUSSION**
- The radial nerve passes medial to the humerus and then travels obliquely behind the humerus and through the spiral groove, a shallow groove formed deep to the lateral head of the triceps muscle.
- Before entering the spiral groove in the mid-arm, the radial nerve innervates the triceps and the anconeus muscles and gives off three sensory branches: the posterior cutaneous nerve of the arm (which innervates a strip of skin overlying the triceps muscle), the lower lateral cutaneous nerve of the arm (which innervates the lateral half of the arm), and the posterior cutaneous nerve of the forearm (which innervates the skin of the extensor surface of the forearm).
- In the anterior compartment of the arm, the radial nerve, lying lateral to the humerus, innervates the brachioradialis and the extensor carpi radialis longus (see Fig. 1.5).
- The radial nerve passes anterior to the lateral epicondyle and innervates the extensor carpi radialis brevis and supinator. It then divides into its terminal branches, the superficial radial and posterior interosseous nerves.
- The posterior interosseous nerve, a terminal pure motor branch, passes under the proximal edge of the supinator muscle (*arcade of Frohse*), travels in the forearm, and innervates all the remaining wrist and finger extensors. The superficial radial nerve is a terminal pure sensory nerve and innervates the skin of the proximal two-thirds of the extensor surfaces of the thumb, index, and middle fingers, and half of the ring finger, along with the corresponding dorsum of the hand.
- *Saturday night palsy* and *honeymoon palsy* are due to compression of the radial nerve at the spiral groove of the humerus during drunken sleep or from the weight of a sleeping partner's head, respectively. The radial nerve may also be injured in the arm following fractures of the humerus.
- In pure neurapraxia (first-degree nerve injury), the distal CMAP stimulating at the elbow is normal and there are no fibrillation potentials in affected muscles, including the brachioradialis and extensor carpi radialis longus. There is conduction block in the arm across the spiral groove, since the lesion is purely segmental demyelinating. Radial SNAP is also normal.

**QUESTION 26.** A 55-year-old man presents with a right foot drop and numbness of the dorsum of the foot. Weakness of which of the following actions excludes a common peroneal neuropathy?
- A. Ankle dorsiflexion
- B. Ankle eversion
- C. Large toe extension
- D. Ankle inversion
- E. Small toe extension

**ANSWER:** D. Ankle inversion

**COMMENTS AND DISCUSSION**
- The sciatic nerve is composed of two distinct nerves, the common peroneal and tibial nerves, which share a common sheath from the pelvis to the popliteal fossa. The tibial nerve component innervates all the hamstring muscles except the short head of the biceps femoris, which is innervated by the common peroneal nerve component (see Fig. 1.9).
- The peroneal nerve was renamed the fibular nerve by the Federative Committee on Anatomical Terminology, owing to confusion between the terms peroneal and perineal nerves.
- Soon after the sciatic nerve divides close to the popliteal fossa, the common peroneal nerve gives off the lateral cutaneous nerve of the calf, which innervates the skin over the upper third of the lateral aspect of the leg. The common peroneal nerve then winds around the fibular neck and divides into its terminal branches, the deep and superficial peroneal nerves. The deep peroneal nerve traverses the lateral and then anterior leg compartments and innervates the tibialis anterior, extensor hallucis longus, peroneus tertius, and extensor digitorum longus. It then divides close to the ankle joint to innervate the extensor digitorum brevis and the skin of the web space between the first and second toes (see Fig. 1.10). The superficial peroneal nerve innervates the peroneus longus and brevis and the skin of the lower two-thirds of the lateral aspect of the leg and the dorsum of the foot (except for the first web space).
- A common peroneal nerve lesion leads to weakness of ankle and toe dorsiflexion and ankle eversion. Ankle inversion (L5/tibial nerve) and plantar flexion (S1/tibial neve) remain intact. Sensory impairment is found over the lateral aspect of the lower two-thirds of the leg and the dorsum of the foot.

**QUESTION 27.** Spontaneous non-traumatic peroneal neuropathy is now recognized to commonly occur after compression of the nerve by which of the following?
- A. Lipoma.
- B. Intraneural ganglion cyst
- C. Fiant cell tumor
- D. Osteochondroma
- E. Pseudoaneurysm

**ANSWER:** B. Intraneural ganglion cyst

**COMMENTS AND DISCUSSION**
- Intraneural ganglion is an increasingly recognized cause of peroneal neuropathy. Up to half of patients without a clear cause of peroneal mononeuropathy across the peroneal head have intraneural ganglia.
- These are mucinous cysts, which originate from the superior tibiofibular joint after disruption of its capsule, allowing dissection of the synovial fluid along the articular branch of the peroneal nerve reaching the epineurium of the nerve.
- A giant cell tumor, osteochondroma, schwannoma, lipoma, or pseudoaneurysm are rare causes of peroneal neuropathy.

**QUESTION 28.** Rapid-onset foot drop due to peroneal neuropathy is often painful when related to which of the following?
- A. Weight loss
- B. Intraneural ganglion
- C. Habitual leg crossing
- D. Diabetes mellitus
- E. Prolonged hospitalization

**ANSWER:** B. Intraneural ganglion

**COMMENTS AND DISCUSSION**
- Intraoperative compression due to improper positioning or padding during anesthesia is the leading cause of acute common peroneal neuropathy at the fibular neck.
- Weight loss with habitual leg crossing, prolonged hospitalization, and diabetes mellitus are common precipitating causes of peroneal neuropathy across the fibular neck.

- Peroneal neuropathy due to intraneural ganglion is often associated with significant knee pain, neuropathic pain, and fluctuating foot weakness, which distinguishes them from other compressive neuropathies.
- Devices may compress the peroneal nerve including casts, orthoses, pneumatic compression, antithrombotic stockings, stirrups, and bandages. Peroneal nerve stretch injury may result from an acute forceful foot inversion or prolonged squatting (strawberry pickers' palsy). Fibular fracture, knee dislocation, and lacerations also account for a significant number of cases. In addition, arthroscopic knee surgery and lateral meniscus repair may injure the peroneal nerve.

 **HIGH-YIELD FACT**

> An intraneural peroneal nerve ganglion should be suspected when a spontaneous non-traumatic peroneal nerve lesion presents with significant knee pain, neuropathic pain, or fluctuating foot weakness.

**QUESTION 29.** Which of the following electrodiagnostic findings is **LEAST** likely encountered in a peroneal nerve lesion across the fibular neck?
- A. Conduction block across the fibular neck when recording from the extensor digitorum brevis (EDB)
- B. Low-amplitude peroneal compound muscle action potential (CMAP) recording from the tibialis anterior
- C. Fibrillation potentials in the tibialis anterior
- D. Prolonged peroneal distal latency recording of the EDB
- E. Decreased recruitment of the extensor hallucis

**ANSWER:** D. Prolonged peroneal distal latency recording from the EDB

**COMMENTS AND DISCUSSION**
- Electrodiagnostic studies are useful for localizing lesions and may provide clues to the underlying cause and a guide to prognosis.
- Important strategies for use in patients with a suspected peroneal neuropathy:
  - Peroneal motor study recording the tibialis anterior is most important because the tibialis anterior is the principal ankle dorsiflexor muscle.
  - Peroneal motor study recording the EDB is also useful, but this muscle may be atrophic, particularly in older patients.
  - Superficial peroneal sensory nerve action potential (SNAP)
  - Establishing whether the disorder is demyelinating or axonal and prognosticating the outcome of foot drop are more pertinent while recording the tibialis anterior rather than the EDB. The latter, when low in amplitude due to age or shoe trauma, may result in an erroneous conclusion that the peroneal lesion is axonal or severe. Obtaining bilateral studies for comparison purposes is very useful for estimating the extent of axonal loss by comparing the distal peroneal CMAPs and SNAPs.
  - On needle electromyography (EMG), two deep peroneal-innervated muscles at least (such as the tibialis anterior, extensor hallucis, extensor digitorum longus, and extensor digitorum brevis) and one superficial peroneal-innervated muscle (such as the peroneus longus) should be sampled. In "pure" axonal peroneal lesions, which are non-localizable by nerve conduction study, sampling the short head of the biceps femoris is required for localization and to rule out a high peroneal lesion (sciatic neuropathy affecting the peroneal nerve component, predominantly or exclusively).
- In peroneal nerve lesions, motor nerve conduction studies may demonstrate focal conduction block across the fibular head consistent with segmental demyelination. Axon-loss lesions reveal diffusely low or absent peroneal motor and sensory amplitudes. Mixed lesions exhibit elements of both.
- In peroneal nerve lesions across the fibular head, needle EMG demonstrates denervation in deep peroneal-innervated muscles such as the tibialis anterior, extensor hallucis longus, and extensor digitorum longus and brevis. Superficial peroneal-innervated muscles such as the peroneus longus are often involved less severely and sometimes totally spared, implying a selective deep peroneal nerve lesion. The short head of the biceps femoris, other L5 root-innervated muscles, such as the tibialis posterior, flexor digitorum longus, tensor fascia lata and gluteus medius, and the lower lumbar paraspinal muscles are normal.

**The following vignette is for QUESTIONS 30 and 31.**

> A 25-year-old woman noted severe weakness of the right thigh soon after successfully completing a long vaginal delivery. On examination, she had severe weakness of the quadriceps, absent knee jerk, and sensory loss in the anterior thigh and medial leg. Thigh adduction and hip flexion were normal.

**QUESTION 30.** The clinical findings in this patient are likely the result of which of the following conditions?
  A. Femoral nerve lesion at the inguinal ligament
  B. Upper lumbar plexus lesion
  C. Obturator nerve lesion
  D. Femoral nerve lesion in the pelvis
  E. Upper lumbar radiculopathy

**ANSWER:** A. Femoral nerve lesion at the inguinal ligament

**COMMENTS AND DISCUSSION**
- The femoral nerve innervates the psoas muscle in the pelvis and then passes within the iliacus compartment and innervates the iliacus muscle via a motor branch that originates 4 to 5 cm before the nerve crosses underneath the inguinal ligament (see Fig. 1.7).
- In the anterior thigh, the femoral nerve innervates the quadriceps and sartorius muscles and the skin of the anterior thigh and gives off the saphenous sensory nerve, which innervates the skin of the medial surface of the knee and medial leg.
- The majority of femoral nerve lesions are iatrogenic.
  - During pelvic surgery such as abdominal hysterectomy or renal transplantation, the femoral nerve may become compressed between the self-retaining retractors and the pelvic wall.
  - Following anticoagulant therapy or femoral vessel catheterization, acute retroperitoneal or iliacus hematoma may form and compress the femoral nerve (in some cases, the entire lumbar plexus). Spontaneous retroperitoneal hematoma may also occur in individuals with hemophilia, patients with blood dyscrasias, or following a ruptured abdominal aortic aneurysm.
  - During total hip replacement, particularly during anterior or anterior-lateral approaches, surgical revisions, and complicated reconstructions, femoral nerve injury may occur, although it is less common than sciatic nerve lesions.
  - During lithotomy positioning, which is used for vaginal delivery, vaginal hysterectomy, and prostatectomy, the femoral nerve may become kinked at the inguinal ligament, particularly when the leg is held in extreme hip flexion and external rotation for prolonged periods.
- This patient has a femoral nerve lesion at the inguinal ligament, not in the pelvis, as evidenced by sparing of hip flexion. Upper lumbar plexopathy/radiculopathy and an obturator nerve lesion are excluded, since thigh adduction and hip flexion are normal.

 **HIGH-YIELD FACT**

> A femoral nerve lesion in the pelvis results in denervation of the iliacus, whereas a lesion at the inguinal ligament spares the iliacus.

**QUESTION 31.** Electrodiagnostic studies done 4 weeks later showed prominent fibrillation and only one voluntary motor unit action potential in the quadriceps. The thigh adductors and iliacus were normal. The femoral compound muscle action potential (CMAP) amplitude was normal. Which of the following can be implied from these findings?
  A. Severe axon-loss femoral neuropathy with poor prognosis
  B. Severe axon-loss lumbar plexopathy with poor prognosis
  C. Upper lumbar radiculopathy with good prognosis
  D. Predominantly demyelinating femoral neuropathy with good prognosis
  E. Upper lumbar radiculopathy with poor prognosis

**ANSWER:** D. Predominantly demyelinating femoral neuropathy with good prognosis

## COMMENTS AND DISCUSSION

- Electrodiagnostic studies have both diagnostic and prognostic value.
- The femoral CMAP amplitude and/or area is crucial in these situations, since it is the most useful quantitative measure of the extent of femoral motor axonal loss.
  - The femoral nerve could be stimulated at the groin only; therefore, lesions at the inguinal ligament or pelvis cannot be bracketed by two stimulation sites as done in many more distal peripheral nerve motor conduction studies.
  - Femoral nerve stimulation at the groin is usually distal to the site of the lesion and allows evaluation of a distal CMAP only. Hence, interpretation should take into account the timing of the acute incident and the stage of Wallerian degeneration: the CMAP amplitude starts declining after 1–2 days and reaches its nadir in 4–5 days.
  - In this patient, a normal femoral CMAP 4 weeks after acute injury implies that the femoral nerve lesion is mostly demyelinating, with a good prognosis for recovery. This should be completed in 2–3 months when remyelination is complete.
- Needle electromyography (EMG) in femoral neuropathy reveals denervation of the quadriceps muscle. The iliacus muscle is often normal in inguinal lesions but shows denervation in femoral nerve lesions in the pelvis. Needle EMG of the thigh adductor muscles, innervated by the L2, L3, and L4 nerve roots via the obturator nerve, is normal and helps distinguish femoral nerve lesions from an upper lumbar radiculopathy or plexopathy.
- Fibrillation potentials indicate some degree of axonal loss but have a poor quantitative role. Hence, in this patient with normal femoral CMAP, fibrillation potentials imply an axonal loss that is likely minimal and with no effect on prognosis.

##  HIGH-YIELD FACT

A femoral CMAP assesses the extent of axonal loss in femoral nerve lesions when obtained 5–6 days after symptom onset (sufficient time to complete Wallerian degeneration).

**QUESTION 32.** What is the most common subtype of Guillain-Barré syndrome in North America?
- A. Acute inflammatory demyelinating polyneuropathy
- B. Acute ataxic neuropathy
- C. Acute motor axonal neuropathy
- D. Acute pandysautonomia
- E. Acute motor sensory axonal neuropathy

**ANSWER:** A. Acute inflammatory demyelinating polyneuropathy

## COMMENTS AND DISCUSSION

- Inflammatory demyelinating polyneuropathies are acquired immunologically mediated polyneuropathies classified mostly on the basis of their clinical course into two major groups: (1) Guillain–Barré syndrome (GBS) and (2) chronic inflammatory demyelinating polyneuropathy (CIDP).
- Acute inflammatory demyelinating polyneuropathy (AIDP) is the most common form of GBS in Europe and North America. A second, pure motor axonal subtype called acute motor axonal neuropathy (AMAN), first described in northern China, is the common subtype seen in Asia and India. A third axonal immune-mediated subtype of GBS, called acute motor-sensory axonal neuropathy (AMSAN), is much less common and usually very severe with a poor prognosis.
- Acute ataxic neuropathy and acute pandysautonomia are rare GBS variants (Table 14.2).

**TABLE 14.2** Classification of Guillain-Barré syndrome subtypes and variants.

*Common Subtypes*
  Acute inflammatory demyelinating polyradiculoneuropathy (AIDP)
  Acute motor axonal neuropathy (AMAN)
  Acute motorsensory axonal neuropathy (AMSAN)
*Rare Variants*
  Miller-Fisher syndrome
  Ataxic variant (acute ataxic neuropathy)
  Pharyngeal-cervical-brachial variant
  Multiple cranial neuropathy variant
  Facial diplegia with paresthesia
  Paraparetic variant
  Acute pandysautonomia

**HIGH-YIELD FACT**

Among subtypes of Guillain–Barré syndrome, acute inflammatory demyelinating polyneuropathy (AIDP) is the most common in Europe and North America, whereas acute motor axonal neuropathy (AMAN) is more common in Asia.

**QUESTION 33.** In a patient with ascending weakness, which of the following would cast doubt on a diagnosis of Guillain–Barré syndrome?
A. Mild sensory symptoms
B. Bifacial weakness
C. Autonomic dysfunction
D. Respiratory failure
E. Cerebrospinal fluid (CSF) pleocytosis >50 cells/μL

**ANSWER:** E. Cerebrospinal fluid (CSF) pleocytosis >50 cells/μL

**COMMENTS AND DISCUSSION**

- Patients with Guillain–Barré syndrome (GBS) present with variable weakness with or without sensory symptoms, often worse in the hands and fingers. Sensory loss is not a prominent feature and is frequently limited to distal impairment of vibration sense. Moderate-to-severe pain in the extremities or back occurs in about one-third of patients.
- The fairly symmetrical weakness of the lower limbs ascends proximally over hours to several days and may subsequently involve arms, facial and oropharyngeal muscles, and in severe cases, respiratory muscles. Less often, weakness may be descending and begin in the upper limbs or cranial-innervated muscles.
- Hyporeflexia or areflexia is invariably present, except early in the course of the disease (Table 14.3). Intact reflexes in a moderately weak limb should question the diagnosis of GBS.
- Cranial nerve involvement occurs in up to two-thirds of cases with facial weakness, usually bilateral in half of patients.
- The proportion of patients developing respiratory failure and requiring assisted ventilation increases with age and ranges from 9% to 30% in hospital-based series.
- Autonomic dysfunction of various degrees are common and most frequent in patients with severe weakness and respiratory failure.
- The CSF protein is elevated in 90% of cases and is not usually associated with a cellular response (*albuminocytologic dissociation*). In the first week of neurological symptoms, the CSF protein may be normal in up to 50% of patients.
- In about 10% of patients, there is a slight lymphocytic pleocytosis greater than 10 cells/mm. However, significant CSF pleocytosis (>50 cells) should cast doubt on the diagnosis and suggests infectious processes such as HIV or Lyme infection.

**TABLE 14.3** Diagnostic criteria for Guillain-Barré syndrome.

*Features Required for Diagnosis*
    Progressive weakness of both legs and arms
    Areflexia or hyporeflexia
*Clinical Features Supportive of Diagnosis*
    Progression over days to 4 weeks
    Relative symmetry of symptoms and signs (cranial nerves may be an exception)
    Mild sensory symptoms or signs
    Bifacial palsies
    Autonomic dysfunction
    Absence of fever at onset
    Recovery beginning 2–4 weeks after progression ceases
*Laboratory Features Supportive of Diagnosis*
    Elevated cerebrospinal fluid protein with <10 cells/μL
    Electrodiagnostic features of demyelination, with absent, delayed, or impersistent F responses
        often being the most common abnormalities early in the course

**QUESTION 34.** A 42-year-old man presents with rapidly progressive generalized weakness over 2 weeks. There are no sensory symptoms or findings. Cerebrospinal fluid reveals an elevated protein and a normal cell count. Nerve conduction studies show low-amplitude motor responses. Distal latencies, conduction velocities, and F waves are normal. There are no conduction blocks. Sensory nerve conduction responses are normal. Which of the following statements is **FALSE**?

A. This clinical picture is more common in Asia than in North America.
B. This patient likely has positive anti-ganglioside antibodies.
C. Prognosis for recovery in this patient is uniformly very poor.
D. This patient likely has a recent *Campylobacter jejuni* infection.
E. This patient may have had a preceding diarrheal illness.

**ANSWER:** C. Prognosis for recovery in this patient is uniformly very poor.

## COMMENTS AND DISCUSSION

- This patient has a clinical picture of a Guillain–Barré syndrome (GBS) form referred to as acute motor axonal neuropathy (AMAN).
- AMAN is a form of GBS that is more commonly seen in Asia (in contrast to the United States where most patients have demyelinating electrophysiology).
- The majority of patients have anti-ganglioside antibodies (anti-GM1, anti-GM1b, and anti-GD1a).
- The most common identifiable bacterial organism linked to GBS and particularly AMAN is *Campylobacter jejuni*, a curved Gram-negative rod that is a common cause of bacterial enteritis worldwide. Evidence of *C. jejuni* infection from stool cultures or serological tests is present in up to three-fourths of patients with AMAN and up to one-third of patients with all GBS types in the United States and Western Europe. Molecular mimicry between GM1 ganglioside and *C. jejuni* lipo-oligosaccharide is now established as the pathogenic link for this association.
- Although a number of patients will have axonal loss, the pathophysiology appears to be antibodies affecting sodium conductance at the nodes of Ranvier. This can cause distal *conduction failure* producing low-amplitude motor responses (mimicking true axonal loss). Therefore, some patients with AMAN can show rapid improvement following treatment.

**QUESTION 35.** What is the **MOST** specific electrodiagnostic finding in Guillain–Barré syndrome?

A. Reduced recruitment of motor unit action potentials (MUAPs)
B. Low compound muscle action potential (CMAP) amplitudes
C. Normal sural with reduced amplitude hand sensory nerve action potentials (SNAPs)
D. Conduction block of the median nerve in the forearms
E. Mild slowing of distal and F-wave latencies

**ANSWER:** D. Conduction block the of median nerve in the forearm

## COMMENTS AND DISCUSSION

- Conduction block of motor axons, the electrophysiological correlate of clinical weakness due to demyelination, is recognized by a decrease of greater than 50% in CMAP amplitude and area from distal to proximal stimulation in the absence of temporal dispersion (Fig. 14.11).
- Conduction block at non-entrapment sites is highly specific for acquired demyelination, but it occurs in only 15% to 30% of early GBS, depending on the number of nerves and nerve segments studied.
- Patients with weakness that is related primarily to conduction block tend to have a faster and more complete recovery than those with diffusely low motor amplitudes.
- Prolonged distal motor latencies, reduction in distal CMAP amplitudes, significant CMAP dispersion, and slowing of motor conduction velocities are less common and less specific and tend to occur later in the course of the disease.
- Normal sural with reduced-amplitude sensory nerve action potentials in the hand is referred to as the *sural sparing pattern*. It is not as specific as conduction block for acquired demyelination but is a frequent finding in the acute inflammatory demyelinating polyneuropathy (AIDP) subtype of Guillain–Barré syndrome and chronic inflammatory demyelinating polyneuropathy (CIDP).

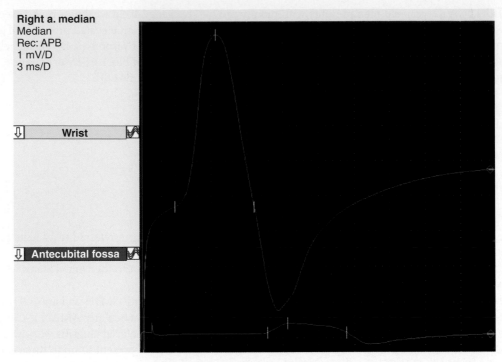

**Right a. median**
Median
Rec: APB
1 mV/D
3 ms/D

Wrist

Antecubital fossa

Fig. 14.11 Conduction block in the forearm in a patient with Guillain-Barré syndrome.

**QUESTION 36.** Which of the following electrodiagnostic findings is **LEAST** helpful in suggesting the diagnosis of Guillain-Barré syndrome during the first few weeks of illness?
A. Reduced or absent sensory nerve action potentials (SNAPs) in the hand with a normal sural SNAP
B. Delayed, impersistent, or absent F waves
C. Absent tibial H reflexes
D. Multiple or complex A waves
E. (Sural + radial SNAPs)/(median + ulnar SNAPs) ratio <1

**ANSWER:** E. (Sural + radial SNAPs)/(median + ulnar SNAPs) ratio <1

**COMMENTS AND DISCUSSION (see also comments and discussion from Question 35)**
- A significant number of patients with Guillain–Barré syndrome (GBS) have normal nerve conduction studies during the first 2 weeks of illness. Electrodiagnostic signs of definite multifocal demyelination (conduction blocks and significant slowing) peak during the third and fourth weeks of illness.
- Although the absence of H reflexes is the most common electrodiagnostic abnormality seen in the first 2 weeks of illness, this finding is least helpful diagnostically because it may be present in elderly as well as in the majority of peripheral polyneuropathies for a variety of causes.
- Apart from conduction blocks and significant slowing, which are diagnostic signs of definite multifocal demyelination, there are several findings that are very helpful and increase the diagnostic power of nerve conduction studies in GBS:
  - *Sural sparing pattern.* Reduced amplitudes or absent sensory nerve action potentials (SNAPs) in the upper extremity combined with normal sural SNAPs is fairly specific for an acquired demyelinating polyneuropathy including GBS and its acute inflammatory demyelinating polyneuropathy (AIDP) subtype, as well as chronic inflammatory demyelinating polyneuropathy (CIDP). This is seen in up to one-half of patients with GBS during the first 2 weeks of the illness.
  - *Absent, delayed, or impersistent F waves.* These findings are common in polyneuropathies but not specific for the demyelinating types. However, abnormal F waves in the presence of normal conduction velocities and distal latencies are more specific, since they suggest proximal acquired demyelination as seen with GBS.
  - *Multiple or complex A (axon) waves.* This is most useful when recorded from several upper limb nerves. A waves may precede or follow, but sometimes replace F waves, and are also commonly

associated with AIDP. The exact pathway of the A wave is unknown in demyelinating polyneuropathies, but it may be generated as a result of ephaptic transmission between two axons with the action potential conducting back down the nerve fiber to the muscle.

- ○ *High sensory ratio [(sural + radial SNAPs)/(median + ulnar SNAPs)].* This is a good substitute for a sural sparing pattern, particularly in elderly patients who have absent sural SNAPs or in patients with pre-existing carpal tunnel syndrome. A high ratio (>1) is fairly specific and distinguishes GBS from other polyneuropathies such as diabetic neuropathies.
- *Sural sparing combined with abnormal F waves* is highly specific (96% specific) for the diagnosis of AIDP and is present in about one-half to two-thirds of patients with AIDP during the first 2 weeks of illness.

 **HIGH-YIELD FACT**

Sural sparing pattern combined with absent/delayed F waves is highly suggestive of Guillain–Barré syndrome.

**QUESTION 37.** Which treatment option has the strongest evidence to support its use in Guillain-Barré syndrome?
  A. Plasma exchange followed by intravenous immunoglobulin (IVIG)
  B. Plasma exchange or IVIG
  C. IVIG followed by plasma exchange
  D. Intravenous (IV) methylprednisolone combined with IVIG
  E. Oral corticosteroids combined with plasma exchange

**ANSWER:** B. Plasma exchange or IVIG

**COMMENTS AND DISCUSSION**
- Therapeutic plasma exchange has been shown to be effective. Six large randomized controlled trials involving more than 600 patients have established the benefit of centrifugal plasma exchange in acute Guillain-Barré syndrome (GBS) by shortening the recovery time. Benefits are best when plasma exchange starts within 2 weeks of symptom onset.
- Plasma exchange and IVIG infusions have been shown to be equally effective. Three randomized trials comparing IVIG with plasma exchange demonstrated the benefit of five daily infusions of immunoglobulin given within the first 2 weeks of the disease.
- There was no advantage of using both together.
- Corticosteroids are not recommended because two randomized controlled trials, one using conventional doses of prednisolone and the other using high-dose IV methylprednisolone, have found no benefit.
- The combination of IVIG with methylprednisolone failed to produce a significant long-term advantage over IVIG alone.

 **HIGH-YIELD FACT**

Plasma exchange and IVIG are equally effective in the treatment of Guillain–Barré syndrome.

**QUESTION 38.** Which of the following care or treatment options should be avoided in a patient who is admitted to the hospital for acute paraparesis and is diagnosed with Guillain-Barré syndrome?
  A. Deep vein thrombosis prophylaxis
  B. Oral corticosteroids
  C. Plasma exchange
  D. Cardiac monitoring
  E. Respiratory monitoring

**ANSWER:** B. Oral corticosteroids

## COMMENTS AND DISCUSSION

- General supportive management is the mainstay of treatment for Guillain–Barré syndrome (GBS). Patients with rapidly worsening acute GBS should be observed in the intensive care unit until the maximum extent of progression has been established.
- The prevention of complications, of which respiratory failure and autonomic dysfunction are the most important, provides the best chance for a favorable outcome.
  - Respiratory and bulbar function, ability to handle secretions, heart rate, and blood pressure should be closely monitored during the progressive phase. Chest physical therapy and frequent oral suctioning aid in preventing atelectasis in patients with impaired cough and sigh.
  - Respiratory failure requiring mechanical ventilation develops in up to 30% of patients with GBS. Predictors of future need for mechanical ventilation include rapid disease progression (onset to admission in <7 days), severity of limb weakness, presence of facial weakness, neck flexor weakness, and bulbar weakness. Hence, patients with one or more of these predictors, evidence of dysautonomia, or signs of respiratory insufficiency should be monitored closely in the intensive care unit until stable or improving.
  - Signs of impending respiratory failure include deterioration in forced vital capacity (FVC) and declining maximal respiratory pressures. Elective intubation for ventilatory assistance should be performed when FVC falls below 12–15 mL/kg. It is essential not to delay intubation until hypercapnia and/or hypoxemia have developed. Doing so increases the likelihood of atelectasis, pneumonia, and other complications.
  - In the event of cardiac arrhythmias or marked fluctuations of blood pressure, continuous electrocardiography and blood pressure monitoring allow early detection of life-threatening situations that require prompt treatment.
- Subcutaneous heparin or low-molecular-weight heparin together with calf compression devices should be ordered routinely in immobilized patients to lower the risks of venous thrombosis and pulmonary embolism.
- Corticosteroids are not recommended because they do not produce significant benefit and may, in fact, be harmful in view of the catabolic state in many patients due to increased metabolic requirements, negative caloric intake, and relative starvation.

**QUESTION 39.** Which of the following variables carries a poor prognosis in Guillain–Barré syndrome?
  A. Young age
  B. Preceding upper respiratory infection
  C. Severe muscle weakness
  D. Rapid progression resulting in respiratory failure
  E. Hypernatremia

**ANSWER:** D. Rapid progression resulting in respiratory failure

## COMMENTS AND DISCUSSION

- Approximately 15% of patients with Guillain–Barré syndrome (GBS) have a mild condition, remain ambulatory, and recover after a few weeks. Conversely, 5% to 20% of patients have a fulminant course and develop flaccid quadriplegia, ventilator dependence, and axonal degeneration, often within 2 days of the onset of symptoms. The recovery is delayed and virtually always incomplete and most have substantial residual motor deficits at 1 year of follow-up.
- Patients with acute motor axonal neuropathy (AMAN) and electrophysiologic evidence of axonal failure have a prognosis that is comparable to that of patients with acute inflammatory demyelinating polyneuropathy (AIDP). This is explained by reversible conduction failure caused by transitory dysfunction at the nodes of Ranvier without secondary axonal degeneration.
- Predictors of poor recovery in GBS include older age (≥60 years), history of preceding diarrheal illness, ventilatory support, rapid progression reaching maximum deficit in less than 7 days, hyponatremia, and low distal CMAP amplitudes (20% of lower limit of normal or less) or unexcitable nerves.
- Syndrome of inappropriate antidiuretic hormone secretion (SIADH), often asymptomatic, is seen in about half of patients with GBS during the course of the illness. SIADH, with its resultant hyponatremia, is an independent predictor of poor outcome in GBS.
- Upper respiratory infection and severity of weakness have no correlation with outcome.

**HIGH-YIELD FACT**

Old age, preceding diarrheal illness, rapid progression of weakness, and respiratory failure are poor prognostic predictors in Guillain–Barré syndrome.

**QUESTION 40.** In patients with Guillain–Barré syndrome, when should the diagnosis of acute-onset chronic inflammatory demyelinating polyneuropathy (CIDP) be suspected?
A. Relapses occur within the first month after onset.
B. Relapses occur less than twice during the first 2 months.
C. The acute event is preceded by a gastrointestinal viral illness.
D. Electrodiagnostic studies show prominent demyelination many months later.
E. Symptoms progress and reach a nadir in 4 weeks.

**ANSWER:** D. Electrodiagnostic studies show prominent demyelination.

**COMMENTS AND DISCUSSION**
- Guillain–Barré syndrome (GBS) and chronic inflammatory demyelinating polyneuropathy (CIDP) are autoimmune inflammatory neuropathies that share several electrophysiological, histological, and autoimmune features.
- Acute-onset CIDP (A-CIDP) refers to CIDP that presents acutely, mimicking GBS, which is then followed by a chronic or relapsing disease compatible with CIDP.
- Treatment-related fluctuations may follow therapy for GBS with plasma exchange or intravenous immunoglobulin (IVIG). One or more episodes of deterioration following the initial improvement or stabilization after treatment may be encountered in 10% to 20% of patients. This may pose practical problems both in terms of treatment and in differentiating these patients from those who are developing A-CIDP.
- Distinguishing between GBS and A-CIDP during the initial phase is difficult. A-CIDP should be considered with:
  ◦ Slow progression and deterioration that continues beyond 8 weeks
  ◦ More than two relapses, particularly when they occur beyond 1 month of the illness
  ◦ Evidence of severe demyelinating changes on electrodiagnostic studies many months after the acute episode

**QUESTION 41.** Which of the following acquired peripheral polyneuropathies is typically **NOT** associate with demyelination?
A. HIV infection
B. Vitamin B12 deficiency
C. Immunoglobulin M (IgM) neuropathy
D. Osteosclerotic myeloma
E. Multifocal motor neuropathy

**ANSWER:** B. Vitamin B12 deficiency

**COMMENTS AND DISCUSSION**
- Acquired demyelinating peripheral polyneuropathies are a heterogeneous group of acquired peripheral nervous system disorders whose common feature is demyelination of peripheral nerves (Table 14.4).
- They include chronic inflammatory demyelinating polyneuropathy (CIDP) and its variants (including CIDP with HIV) and multifocal motor neuropathy, as well as several paraproteinemic neuropathies such as IgM neuropathy and osteosclerotic myeloma.
- CIDP is a heterogeneous group of immune-mediated neuropathies characterized by a relapsing-remitting or a chronically progressive clinical course, typically exceeding 8 weeks, and demyelinating features on electrodiagnostic testing.
- Many similarities and few differences exist between CIDP and acute inflammatory demyelinating polyneuropathy (AIDP), the most common form of Guillain–Barré syndrome (GBS).
  ◦ Both disorders have similar clinical features and involve the spinal roots and peripheral nerves.
  ◦ Both disorders share the cerebrospinal fluid (CSF) albuminocytologic dissociation, nerve conduction features of demyelination, and the pathological findings of multifocal inflammatory demyelination.

**TABLE 14.4** Acquired chronic demyelinating peripheral polyneuropathy.

---

CIDP and its variants
CIDP associated with HIV infection (early phase)
Multifocal motor neuropathy with conduction block
Chronic demyelinating polyneuropathy associated with monoclonal gammopathy
  • IgM neuropathy with or without anti-MAG antibody (DADS neuropathy)
  • POEMS syndrome (osteosclerotic myeloma)
  • Multiple myeloma
  • Waldenström macroglobulinemia
  • Castleman disease
  • Amyloidosis

---

*CIDP*, chronic inflammatory demyelinating polyneuropathy; *DADS* neuropathy, distal acquired symmetrical demyelinating neuropathy; *HIV*, human immunodeficiency virus; *POEMS syndrome*, Polyneuropathy, Organomegaly, Endocrinopathy, Monoclonal gammopathy, and Skin changes syndrome

- ○ Both disorders respond well to IVIG and plasma exchange.
- ○ The major differences between the two conditions are in their time course, prognosis. and response to corticosteroids.
- Vitamin B12 deficiency results in a combined system disease with an axonal predominantly sensory polyneuropathy and a myelopathy.

**QUESTION 42.** Erroneous diagnosis of chronic inflammatory demyelinating polyneuropathy (CIDP) is usually caused by which of the following findings?
A. Conduction block at non-entrapment sites
B. Significant slowing of conduction velocities
C. Sural sensory sparing pattern
D. Significant elevation of cerebrospinal fluid (CSF) protein
E. Subjective perception of treatment benefit

**ANSWER:** E. Subjective perception of treatment benefit

**COMMENTS AND DISCUSSION**
- The diagnosis of chronic inflammatory demyelinating polyneuropathy (CIDP) is supported by electrodiagnostic, ultrasound, CSF, and nerve biopsy findings (Table 14.5).
  - ○ A pattern of nerve conduction changes strongly supports acquired multifocal and non-uniform demyelination. At least three of the following criteria are necessary to fulfill the diagnosis:
    - Reduction in motor conduction velocities in at least two motor nerves (<80% of lower limit of normal [LLN] if CMAP amplitude >80% of LLN, and <70% of LLN if CMAP amplitude <80% of LLN)

**TABLE 14.5** Diagnostic criteria for chronic inflammatory demyelinating polyneuropathy.

---

***Mandatory Clinical Criteria***
  Progressive or relapsing muscle weakness for 2 months or longer
  Symmetrical proximal and distal weakness in upper or lower extremities
  Hyporeflexia or areflexia
***Mandatory Laboratory Criteria***
  Nerve conduction studies with features of demyelination
  Cerebrospinal fluid protein level >45 mg/dL with cell count <10/μL
  Sural nerve biopsy with features of demyelination and remyelination including myelinated
    fiber loss and perivascular inflammation
***Mandatory Exclusion Criteria***
  Evidence of relevant systemic disease or toxic exposure
  Family history of neuropathy
  Nerve biopsy findings incompatible with diagnosis
***Diagnostic Categories***
  Definite: mandatory inclusion and exclusion criteria and all laboratory criteria
  Probable: mandatory inclusion and exclusion criteria and two of three laboratory criteria
  Possible: mandatory inclusion and exclusion criteria and one of three laboratory criteria

---

- Partial conduction block (proximal CMAP amplitude and area <50% of distal in long nerve segments, or proximal CMAP amplitude and area <20%–50% of distal in short nerve segments) or abnormal temporal dispersion in at least one motor nerve at non-entrapment sites
    - Prolonged distal latencies in at least two motor nerves (>125% of upper limit of normal [ULN] if CMAP amplitude >80% of LLN, and >150% of ULN if CMAP amplitude <80% of LLN)
    - Absent F waves or prolonged F-wave latencies in at least two motor nerves (>125% of ULN if CMAP amplitude >80% of LLN, and >150% of ULN if CMAP amplitude <80% of LLN).
  - Neuromuscular ultrasound of peripheral nerves often shows multiple sites of nerve enlargement at non-entrapment sites, increased intra- and inter-nerve size variabilities, and increased nerve vascularization. Enlargement of median nerve segments in the forearm (>10 mm$^2$) and arm (>13 mm$^2$) and in any trunk of the brachial plexus (>8 mm$^2$), is highly specific and sensitive in confirming an acquired demyelinating polyneuropathy including CIDP and its variants and multifocal motor neuropathy. This finding reliably distinguishes them from axonal neuropathies and motor neuron disease.
  - CSF protein values in excess of 45 mg/dL are found in 95% of cases, and levels above 100 mg/dL are common. CSF pleocytosis is rare.
- Erroneous diagnosis of CIDP is often triggered by reliance on the wrong electrophysiologic interpretation of acquired demyelination such as presence of conduction block or slowing of conduction velocity at entrapment sites only; the presence of mild amplitude-dependent slowing in axonal polyneuropathies; inclusion of extremely atypical forms (such as isolated sensory symptoms); and subjective perception of treatment benefit.

 **HIGH-YIELD FACT**

> Common causes of CIDP misdiagnosis include conduction block or slowing of conduction velocity at entrapment sites, and amplitude-dependent slowing of conduction velocity with axonal loss.

**QUESTION 43.** A 45-year-old woman with chronic inflammatory demyelinating polyneuropathy (CIDP) initially responded to intravenous immunoglobulin (IVIG) 2 g/kg divided over 5 days, but worsened two months later. What is the next best treatment?
A. Azathioprine
B. Prednisone
C. Plasmapheresis
D. Maintenance IVIG
E. Cyclophosphamide

**ANSWER:** D. Maintenance IVIG.

**COMMENTS AND DISCUSSION**
- Corticosteroids, plasmapheresis, and immunoglobulin infusion are all effective in CIDP and are the mainstays of treatment. About 50% to 70% of patients respond to each of these treatments. In addition, almost 50% of patients not responding to the first treatment respond to the second therapy.
- The ICE study, a randomized double-blind, placebo-controlled, crossover international trial, resulted in the 2008 US Food and Drug Administration (FDA) approval of IVIG therapy for treatment of CIDP, the first neurological disease to be approved for such a therapy.
  - The study showed that a statistically significant number of patients improved with IVIG compared to placebo, and the time to and probability of relapse was much lower for IVIG versus placebo.
  - The study used an initial IVIG dose of 2 g/kg followed by a maintenance dose of 1 g/kg every 3 weeks.
  - Improvement was seen sometimes as early as the first week of treatment, whereas maximal benefit was reached after several infusions at 2–3 months.
  - Treatment with at least two courses of IVIG administered 3 weeks apart is often required for initial improvement, and continued maintenance therapy is necessary to achieve a maximal therapeutic response.

**QUESTION 44.** Which of the following features characterizes the Lewis-Sumner variant of chronic inflammatory demyelinating polyneuropathy (CIDP)?
A. Axon-loss multiple mononeuropathies
B. Multifocal nerve conduction blocks and slowing
C. Pure motor manifestations
D. Poor response to corticosteroids
E. Normal cerebrospinal fluid (CSF) protein

**ANSWER:** B. Multifocal nerve conduction blocks and slowing

**COMMENTS AND DISCUSSION**

- The Lewis-Sumner syndrome, also described by the acronym *MADSAM* (*multifocal acquired demyelinating sensory and motor neuropathy*), is a multifocal form of CIDP.
- The disorder has a predilection for the upper extremities, with a multifocal distribution of weakness and sensory deficits. Electrophysiological studies demonstrating focal conduction block or severe slowing of nerve conduction distinguishes this multifocal demyelinating neuropathy from the vasculitic axon-loss multiple mononeuropathies.
- Unlike in multifocal motor neuropathy (MMN), patients with the Lewis-Sumner variant of CIDP have clinical and electrophysiological involvement of both motor and sensory nerves, increased cerebrospinal fluid (CSF) protein, and a good response to corticosteroids.

**QUESTION 45.** Monoclonal gammopathy of unknown significance (MGUS) may be associated with peripheral polyneuropathy. Which paraprotein is most likely associated with a demyelinating polyneuropathy?
A. IgA
B. IgD
C. IgG
D. IgM
E. IgE

**ANSWER:** D. IgM

**COMMENTS AND DISCUSSION**

- A monoclonal protein is produced by a single clone of plasma cells and is usually composed of four polypeptides: two identical heavy chains and two light chains. The M protein is named according to the class of heavy chain (IgG, IgM, IgA, IgD, and IgE) and type of light chain, κ (kappa) or λ (lambda).
- In two-thirds of patients with a monoclonal protein, no detectable underlying disease is found, and they are described as having MGUS (monoclonal gammopathy of unknown significance).
- MGUS is present in 1% to 3% of the population, mostly in the elderly.
- Up to one-fourth of patients go on to develop a malignant plasma cell dyscrasia in long-term follow-up with at a rate of 1% per year. Hence, the cumulative risk of progression during one's lifetime is highest in younger patients. A strong predictor of malignant transformation is an increase in serum monoclonal protein concentration.
- Approximately 10% of patients with idiopathic peripheral neuropathy have an associated monoclonal gammopathy, which represents a six-fold increase over the general population of the same age.
- The frequency of monoclonal protein in patients with neuropathy is 60% IgM, 30% IgG, and 10% IgA.
- The most common presentation is a symmetrical sensorimotor polyneuropathy, which may be one of three more common subtypes: CIDP phenotype, distal acquired demyelinating symmetric (DADS) neuropathy, or axonal sensorimotor peripheral polyneuropathy.
- IgM MGUS neuropathy and DADS neuropathy represent a distinct and often homogenous group characterized by slowly progressive sensory ataxic gait. Upper-limb postural tremor can be prominent. Electrodiagnostic studies show slow motor conduction velocities in the demyelinating range, with a predilection for distal demyelination and very prolonged distal motor latencies. Sensory nerve action potentials (SNAPs) are reduced in amplitude or unobtainable. In at least 50% of patients with IgM MGUS neuropathy, the IgM monoclonal protein demonstrates reactivity against myelin-associated glycoprotein (MAG), hence the term anti-MAG neuropathy.
- IgG and IgA often are associated with an axonal polyneuropathy, in contrast to IgM. IgE and IgD are not associated with a polyneuropathy.

**QUESTION 46.** A 65-year-old man presents with a 2-year history of leg numbness and poor balance. His examination reveals sensory ataxia with a symmetrical predominantly sensory polyneuropathy. Electrophysiological studies show symmetrical and markedly uniform slowing of distal latencies, more than conduction velocities, without conduction blocks. Which of the following is **NOT** associated with this disorder?
  A. IgM monoclonal protein
  B. Excellent response to immunomodulation
  C. Myelin-associated glycoprotein antibodies
  D. Loss of reflexes
  E. Neuropathic tremor

**ANSWER:** B. Excellent response to immunomodulation

**COMMENTS AND DISCUSSION (see also comments and discussion from Question 45)**
- Another polyneuropathy that is considered a variant of CIDP is "distal acquired demyelinating symmetric neuropathy," or DADS neuropathy.
- This IgM-associated neuropathy is predominantly sensory and ataxic, and often is demyelinating with distally accentuated slowing of nerve conduction velocities. A neuropathic action tremor is common.
- Electrophysiological studies in DADS neuropathy typically show symmetrical uniform slowing of distal latencies more than proximal conduction velocities (Table 14.6). Additionally, rare conduction blocks may be observed in some cases. The nerve conduction studies may mimic an inherited demyelinating peripheral polyneuropathy such as Charcot-Marie-Tooth disease type 1.
- Nearly two-thirds of these patients have IgM monoclonal gammopathy and at least half of patients with IgM-associated neuropathy have elevated serum antibody titers to myelin-associated glycoprotein (anti-MAG). However, patients with elevated anti-MAG antibody do not all have a detectable IgM paraprotein on immunofixation.
- MAG is a glycoprotein that makes up only 1% of peripheral nerve myelin. It is concentrated in periaxonal Schwann cell membranes, paranodal loops of myelin, and areas of non-compacted myelin, where it serves as a cytoskeletal-associated protein playing a role as an adhesion molecule for interactions between Schwann cells and axons.
- Compared to CIDP, this disorder is relatively resistant to therapy, but may respond favorably to IVIG, cyclophosphamide, or rituximab.

**TABLE 14.6** Distinctive features between chronic inflammatory demyelinating polyneuropathy (CIDP) and distal acquired demyelinating symmetric (DADS) neuropathy with or without elevated anti-myelin-associated-glycoprotein (anti-MAG) antibody.

| Feature | CIDP | DADS neuropathy |
|---|---|---|
| Age | All ages | >50 years |
| Peripheral polyneuropathy | Predominantly motor | Predominantly sensory |
| Clinical deterioration | More rapid | Slow indolent |
| Diffuse slowing | Non-uniform | Uniform |
| Nerve segment slowing | Proximal >distal | Distal > proximal |
| Conduction blocks | Common | Rare |
| Response to therapy | Good | Resistant |

**QUESTION 47.** Which of the following does **NOT** occur in multifocal motor neuropathy?
  A. Rare cranial nerve involvement
  B. Preservation of tendon reflexes
  C. Lack of muscle atrophy
  D. Good response to corticosteroids
  E. Conduction blocks at non-entrapment sites

**ANSWER:** D. Good response to corticosteroids

**COMMENTS AND DISCUSSION**
- Multifocal motor neuropathy (MMN) almost always presents with a progressive, usually distal, asymmetric upper extremity motor weakness in the distribution of a single peripheral nerve, and progressing to affect other nerves.

- There is striking predilection for the upper extremities, and particularly the hands, without upper motor signs. Muscle cramps and fasciculations, particularly after exercise, are common.
- Despite profound weakness, muscle bulk is initially well preserved.
- Cranial nerve involvement is rare.
- Tendon reflexes are depressed or absent but can be normal.
- Electrodiagnostic studies demonstrate persistent focal motor conduction block, defined as more than 50% reduction in amplitude and area in one or more motor nerves at sites not prone to compression.
- The conduction block is confined to motor axons: Sensory conduction are preserved, including along the same nerve segments. This contrasts with Lewis-Sumner syndrome, which is associated with sensory symptoms and abnormal sensory nerve action potentials (SNAPs).
- High titers of IgM anti-GM1 antibodies can be found in 50% to 60% of patients with MMN and conduction block.
- IVIG is the preferred treatment of MMN. Unlike CIDP, prednisone or plasma exchange has little or no benefit.

 **HIGH-YIELD FACT**

> Lewis-Sumner syndrome is distinguished from multifocal motor neuropathy by sensory loss, abnormal SNAPs, and good response to corticosteroids.

**QUESTION 48.** A 65-year-old woman with an acquired demyelinating polyneuropathy did not respond to intravenous immunoglobulin (IVIG). Upon further testing, she was found to have an immunoglobulin A (IgA) lambda monoclonal gammopathy and a sclerotic bony lesion in the right femur. Which blood test is likely to be abnormal in this patient?

A. Myelin-associated glycoprotein (MAG) antibodies
B. Vascular endothelial growth factor (VEGF)
B. Ganglioside M1 (GM1) antibodies
C. Ganglioside Q1b (GQ1b) antibodies
E. Jo-1 antibodies

**ANSWER:** B. Vascular endothelial growth factor (VEGF)

**COMMENTS AND DISCUSSION**

- This patient likely has *POEMS syndrome or Crow-Fukase syndrome.* POEMS is an acronym for polyneuropathy, organomegaly, endocrinopathy, M protein, and skin changes.
  - The initial symptoms in the majority of patients are related to a polyradiculoneuropathy. The polyneuropathy usually begins with sensory changes in the lower limbs followed by sensory ataxia and motor weakness. The clinical course is often slowly progressive but is sometimes more rapidly worsening.
  - The monoclonal protein is usually less than 2 g/dL and may not be detectable using immunofixation in up to 10% of cases. It is virtually always composed of λ light chains associated with IgG or IgA heavy chains.
  - Vascular endothelial growth factor (VEGF) serum level is significantly elevated in POEMS but not in other demyelinating neuropathies. A VEGF level above 200 pg/mL has a sensitivity of 95% and specificity of 68% in the diagnosis of POEMS syndrome.
  - Sclerotic bone lesions, due to plasma cell proliferation, occur as single or multiple plasmacytomas.
- POEMS syndrome should be considered in patients carrying a diagnosis of CIDP who do not respond to standard CIDP therapy, such as IVIG, plasma exchange, or corticosteroids. The clinical and electrophysiological similarities between this condition and CIDP emphasize the need to screen for an occult M protein and sclerotic bone lesions in all adult patients presenting with an acquired demyelinating polyneuropathy by obtaining serum and urine immunofixation, free light chain, VEGF level, and a skeletal survey.
- Criteria are established for POEMS syndrome (Table 14.7). The diagnosis is confirmed when all three major criteria are met along with at least two minor criteria. This has a 100% sensitivity and 100% specificity for diagnosis.

**TABLE 14.7** Diagnostic criteria of POEMS syndrome.

> ***Major Criteria***
>   Polyneuropathy (usually demyelinating)
>   Monoclonal protein (usually IgG or IgA lambda)
>   Elevated serum VEGF
> ***Minor Criteria***
>   Sclerotic bone lesions
>   Organomegaly (hepatomegaly, splenomegaly, or lymphadenopathy)
>   Endocrinopathy (hypogonadism, hyperestrogenemia, or hypoparathyroidism)
>   Polycythemia or thrombocytosis
>   Skin changes (hyperpigmentation, hypertrichosis, thickening, hemangiomas)
>   Leg edema

- Myelin-associated glycoprotein (MAG) antibodies are elevated in two-thirds of patients with IgM-associated neuropathy/DADs neuropathy. Ganglioside M1 (GM1) antibodies are elevated in 50% to 60% of patients with multifocal motor neuropathy, whereas ganglioside Q1b (GQ1b) antibodies are elevated in 90% of patients with the Miller-Fisher syndrome, a variant of GBS. Jo-1 antibodies are elevated in anti-synthetase syndrome.

 **HIGH-YIELD FACT**

> POEMS syndrome should be suspected when a poorly responsive acquired demyelinating polyneuropathy is associated with an IgG or IgA lambda paraproteinemia and elevated serum VEGF.

**QUESTION 49.** Which of the following types of diabetic neuropathy is most often slowly progressive?
  A. Oculomotor neuropathy
  B. Lumbosacral radiculoplexopathy
  C. Distal symmetrical polyneuropathy
  D. Facial neuropathy
  E. Thoracic radiculopathy

**ANSWER:** C. Distal symmetrical polyneuropathy

**COMMENTS AND DISCUSSION**
- Distal symmetrical polyneuropathy is the most common form of diabetic neuropathy, constituting almost three-fourths of all other types of diabetic neuropathies.
- Sensory disturbances have a stocking-glove distribution following a length-dependent pattern. Early sensory manifestations begin in the toes, gradually spreading proximally; when these reach above knee level, the fingers and hands become affected. In more advanced cases, sensation becomes impaired over the anterior chest and abdomen, producing a truncal wedge-shaped area of sensory loss. Most patients will develop only minor motor involvement affecting the distal muscles of the lower extremities.
- The distal symmetrical polyneuropathy may be subclassified further into two major subgroups, depending on the nerve fiber type most involved: large-fiber and small-fiber variants. Although diabetic sensory neuropathy frequently forms a continuous spectrum ranging between these two polar types, selective sensory nerve fiber involvement does occur, giving rise to relatively pure large- or small-fiber-type presentations.
  ○ The large-fiber neuropathy variant presents with painless paresthesia beginning at the toes and feet, impairment of vibration and joint position sense, and diminished muscle stretch reflexes. Early large-fiber involvement is often asymptomatic, but a sensory deficit may be detected by careful examination. In advanced cases, significant ataxia may develop secondary to sensory deafferentation.
  ○ The small-fiber neuropathy frequently presents with pain of a deep, burning, stinging, aching character, often associated with spontaneous shooting pains and allodynia to light touch. Pain and

temperature modalities are impaired, with relative preservation of vibration and joint position sensation and muscle stretch reflexes. The small-fiber variant is often accompanied by autonomic neuropathy.

- In contrast to the distal polyneuropathy, cranial nerve palsies, such as oculomotor and facial neuropathy, thoracic radiculopathy, and lumbosacral radiculoplexopathy, often have an acute/subacute onset and course.

**QUESTION 50.** Which of the following is NOT associated with paraneoplastic sensory neuronopathy?
- A. Small cell lung cancer
- B. Limbic encephalitis
- C. Elevated anti-Hu (ANNA-1) antibodies
- D. Absent sensory nerve action potentials
- E. Elevated anti-Ri (ANNA-2) antibodies

**ANSWER:** E. Elevated anti-Ri (ANNA-2) antibodies

**COMMENTS AND DISCUSSION**
- Paraneoplastic sensory neuronopathy is a distinct progressive, severe sensory neuropathy associated with cancer.
- It is also known as subacute sensory neuronopathy, carcinomatous sensory neuropathy, paraneoplastic sensory ganglionopathy, and malignant inflammatory sensory polyganglioneuropathy.
- It is caused by an autoantibody (anti-Hu or ANNA-1 antibody) directed against a nuclear protein in sensory ganglion cells that is shared by neuronal nuclei and tumors, resulting in an intense inflammatory response in the affected dorsal root ganglia.
- The most common underlying neoplasm is small cell lung cancer (~90%).
- Anti-Hu antibodies have a specificity of 99% and sensitivity of 82% for the detection of cancer.
- Symptoms may develop within days in a fulminant fashion or progress more gradually over months.
    - Numbness, painful paresthesia, and lancinating pain often begin in one limb and progress to involve all four limbs. Upper limbs are usually involved first or almost invariably involved with the progression of the disease. Occasionally, the trunk, face, and scalp are affected in somatotopic regions highly suggestive of neuronopathies.
    - There is global loss of all sensory modalities, with a striking loss of proprioception and inability to localize the limb in space, resulting in sensory ataxia and pseudoathetosis of the upper extremities (Fig. 14.12). Tendon reflexes are globally reduced or absent.

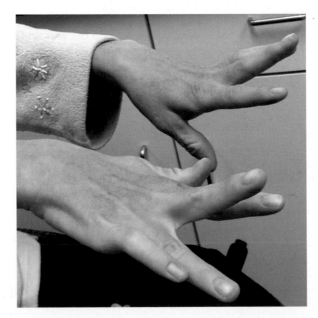

**Fig. 14.12** Pseudoathetosis in a patient with anti-Hu syndrome related to paraneoplastic sensory neuronopathy and small cell lung cancer. Patient is asked to keep hands and fingers at same level while eyes are closed.

- Electrodiagnostic studies show absence of or marked reduction in sensory nerve action potentials (SNAPs). Motor conduction studies are normal with relatively preserved amplitudes of compound muscle action potentials (CMAPs), although the motor conduction velocities may be mildly reduced. Needle electromyography (EMG) is usually normal but may demonstrate minor neurogenic changes.
  - About half of affected patients have symptoms and signs reflecting more widespread involvement of the central and peripheral nervous system including limbic encephalitis, cerebellar degeneration, and autonomic neuronopathy.
- The anti-Ri or ANNA-2 antibody is seen mostly in women with breast cancer and can manifest as opsoclonus-myoclonus syndrome.

**The following answer options are for QUESTIONS 51 through 55.**

Match the given skin or foot changes with the appropriate disorder with neuropathy.
A. Thallium poisoning
B. POEMS syndrome
C. Charcot-Marie-Tooth disease
D. Leprosy
E. Vasculitis or cryoglobulinemia

**QUESTION 51.** Pes cavus
**ANSWER:** C. Charcot-Marie-Tooth disease

**QUESTION 52.** Hyperpigmentation or hypertrichosis
**ANSWER:** B. POEMS syndrome

**QUESTION 53.** Purpuric leg skin eruptions
**ANSWER:** E. Vasculitis or cryoglobulinemia

**QUESTION 54.** Transverse nail bands
**ANSWER:** A. Thallium poisoning

**QUESTION 55.** Hypopigmentation
**ANSWER:** D. Leprosy

**COMMENTS AND DISCUSSION**
- Certain noteworthy skin signs may direct the experienced examiner to a specific diagnosis of an acquired polyneuropathy.
  - Alopecia in thallium poisoning
  - White, transverse nail bands, termed *Mees lines,* in arsenic or thallium intoxications
  - Purpuric skin eruptions of the legs in cryoglobulinemia and some vasculitides
  - Skin hypopigmentation in leprosy
  - Skin hyperpigmentation or hypertrichosis in POEMS (polyneuropathy, organomegaly, endocrinopathy, monoclonal gammopathy, and skin changes) syndrome
- Other skin or skin appendages signs may direct the experienced examiner to a specific diagnosis of an inherited polyneuropathy.
  - Telangiectasias over the abdomen, buttocks, and genitals in Fabry disease
  - Enlarged yellow-orange tonsils in Tangier disease
  - Overriding toes and ichthyosis in Refsum disease
  - Tightly curled hair in giant axonal neuropathy
  - Pes cavus and hammer toes in Charcot-Marie-Tooth (CMT) disease

**QUESTION 56.** Which of the following agents may trigger an immune-mediated demyelinating neuropathy?
A. Paclitaxel
B. Phenytoin
C. Infliximab
D. Vincristine
E. Metronidazole

**ANSWER:** C. Infliximab

**COMMENTS AND DISCUSSION**
- Demyelinating neuropathies may follow the use of tumor necrosis factor alpha antagonists including infliximab, etanercept, and adalimumab. These are used in the treatment of rheumatoid arthritis, ankylosing spondylitis, psoriasis, and Crohn's disease.
- The neuropathies associated with the use of tumor necrosis factor alpha antagonists are often immune-mediated including Guillain–Barré syndrome, Miller-Fisher syndrome, chronic inflammatory demyelinating polyneuropathy, and multifocal motor neuropathy, and may require immunosuppressive treatment.
- Phenytoin may cause a mild and largely reversible or asymptomatic axonal sensorimotor polyneuropathy generally proportional to the duration of phenytoin treatment.
- Vincristine produces a dose-dependent sensorimotor polyneuropathy related to tubulin binding of this drug, which interferes with axonal microtubule assembly, and impair axonal transport.
- The taxanes, paclitaxel and docetaxel, bind to β-tubulin of microtubules, thereby interfering with the dynamic assembly and disassembly of the microtubules. They cause a dose-related sensory ganglionopathy or a sensory and motor neuropathy.
- Metronidazole produces a painful, predominantly axonal sensory polyneuropathy or sensory neuronopathy.

 **HIGH-YIELD FACT**

> Tumor necrosis factor alpha antagonists may trigger Guillain–Barré syndrome, CIDP, and multifocal motor neuropathy.

**QUESTION 57.** Which of the following conditions has **NOT** been reported to be triggered by immune checkpoint inhibitors, which are used to treat cancer patients?
A. Myasthenia gravis
B. Motor neuron disease
C. Myocarditis
D. Guillain-Barré syndrome
E. Myositis

**ANSWER:** B. Motor neuron disease

**COMMENTS AND DISCUSSION**
- The cytotoxic T-lymphocyte–associated antigen 4 (CTLA-4), programmed death 1 (PD-1), and programmed cell death ligand 1 (PD-L1) immune checkpoints play important roles as negative regulators of T-cell activation, prevent autoimmunity, and help tumor cells escape from recognition by the host immune system. Immune checkpoint inhibitors block the immune checkpoint pathways and enhance T-cell immunity. Ipilimumab inhibits CTLA-4 and nivolumab and pembrolizumab inhibit PD-1, whereas atezolizumab, avelumab, and durvalumab inhibit PD-L1.
- Immune checkpoint inhibitors are increasingly used for patients with various cancers including melanoma, non–small cell lung cancer, and urothelial carcinoma, and have shown increased overall survival.
- Immune-related adverse events (irAEs) due to immune checkpoint inhibitors resulting from enhanced immune responses are increasingly recognized as affecting most commonly the skin and gastrointestinal tract. Most are treated with corticosteroids.
- Neurologic irAEs of treatment with immune checkpoint inhibitors include autoimmune encephalitis, transverse myelitis, myositis, myasthenia gravis, and immune polyneuropathies including Guillain–Barré

syndrome and CIDP. Myasthenia gravis and myositis sometimes occur in the same patient, along with myocarditis. However, motor neuron disease has not been described as a complication.

 **HIGH-YIELD FACT**

Immune checkpoint inhibitors may induce autoimmune neuromuscular disorders including myasthenia gravis, myositis, Guillain–Barré syndrome, and CIDP.

**QUESTION 58.** Which of the following vitamins, when ingested in toxic amount, causes sensory neuronopathy?
  A. Vitamin B12
  B. Vitamin E
  C. Vitamin A
  D. Vitamin B6
  E. Vitamin K

**ANSWER:** D. Vitamin B6

### COMMENTS AND DISCUSSION

- Vitamin B6 (pyridoxine) is required for cellular functions and growth. Pyridoxine deficiency and excess cause sensory neuropathy.
- Pregnant and lactating women and elderly individuals are at a greater risk of developing vitamin B6 deficiency. It may also occur in chronic alcoholism, celiac disease, and renal insufficiency with dialysis.
- Pyridoxine deficiency may occur during treatment with isoniazid (INH), hydralazine, or penicillamine. These drugs structurally resemble vitamin B6 and interfere with pyridoxine coenzyme activity. When using these drugs, supplementation with pyridoxine (50–100 mg/day) is recommended.
- Pyridoxine-induced sensory neuronopathy depends on the dose and duration of pyridoxine excess. Pyridoxine at doses greater than 250 mg/day is unsafe but even doses of 50 mg/day for extended duration may be harmful. Painful paresthesia, sensory ataxia, and Lhermitte sign are common features. Nerve conduction studies show low-amplitude or absent sensory nerve action potentials (SNAPs).
- None of the other vitamins, when taken in large doses, are known to cause a neuropathy.

### SUGGESTED READINGS

Albers JW, Kelly Jr JJ. Acquired inflammatory demyelinating polyneuropathies: clinical and electrodiagnostic features. *Muscle Nerve.* 1989;12:435-451.

Allen JA, Lewis RA. CIDP diagnostic pitfalls and perception of treatment benefit. *Neurology.* 2015;85:498-504.

Alshekhlee A, Hachwi RN, Preston DC, Katirji B. New criteria for early electrodiagnosis of acute inflammatory demyelinating polyneuropathy. *Muscle Nerve.* 2005;32:66-72.

Alshekhlee A, Robinson J, Katirji B. Sensory sparing patterns and the sensory ratio in acute inflammatory demyelinating polyneuropathy. *Muscle Nerve.* 2007;35(2):246-250.

Anadani M, Katirji B. Acute-onset chronic inflammatory demyelinating polyneuropathy. An electrodiagnostic study. *Muscle Nerve.* 2015;52:900-905.

Asbury AK, Cornblath DR. Assessment of current diagnostic criteria for Guillain-Barré syndrome. *Ann Neurol.* 1990;27(suppl):S21-S24.

Cornblath DR, Asbury AK, Albers JW, et al. Research criteria for diagnosis of chronic inflammatory demyelinating polyneuropathy (CIDP). *Neurology.* 1991;41:617-618.

Ghavanini AA, Kimpinski K. Revisiting the evidence for neuropathy caused by pyridoxine deficiency and excess. *J Clin Neurom Dis.* 2014;16:25-31.

Gordon PH, Wilbourn AJ. Early electrodiagnostic findings in Guillain-Barré syndrome. *Arch Neurol.* 2001;58:913-917.

Hottinger AF. Neurologic complications of immune checkpoint inhibitors. *Curr Opin Neurol.* 2016;29(6):806-812.

Hughes RAC, Donofrio P, Bril V, et al. Intravenous immune globulin (10% caprylate-chromatography purified) for the treatment of chronic inflammatory demyelinating polyradiculoneuropathy (ICE study): a randomized placebo-controlled trial. *Lancet Neurol.* 2008;7:136-144.

Joint Task Force of the EFNS and the PNS. European Federation of Neurological Societies/Peripheral Nerve Society. Guideline on management of multifocal motor neuropathy. Report of a joint task force of the European Federation of Neurological Societies and the Peripheral Nerve Society. *J Peripher Nerv Syst.* 2006;11:1-8.

Joint Task Force of the EFNS and the PNS. European Federation of Neurological Societies/Peripheral Nerve Society Guideline on management of chronic inflammatory demyelinating polyradiculoneuropathy: report of a joint task force of the European Federation of Neurological Societies and the Peripheral Nerve Society-First Revision. *J Peripher Nerv Syst.* 2010;15:1-9.

Kuntzer T, van Melle G, Regli F. Clinical and prognostic features in unilateral femoral neuropathies. *Muscle Nerve.* 1997;20:205-211.

Kuwabara S, Yuki N, Koga M, et al. IgG anti-GM1 antibody is associated with reversible conduction failure and axonal degeneration in Guillain-Barré syndrome. *Ann Neurol.* 1998;44:202-208.

Li Y, Valent J, Soltanzadeh P, Thakore N, Katirji B. Diagnostic challenges in POEMS syndrome presenting with polyneuropathy: a case series. *J Neurol Sci.* 2017;378:170-174.

Ruts L, Drenthen J, Jacobs BC, van Doorn PA, Dutch GBS Study Group. Distinguishing acute-onset CIDP from fluctuating Guillain-Barré syndrome: a prospective study. *Neurology.* 2010;74(21):1680-1686.

Saifudheen K, Jose J, Gafoor VA, Musthafa M. Guillain-Barre syndrome and SIADH. *Neurology.* 2011;76:701-704.

Stübgen JP. Tumor necrosis factor-alpha antagonists and neuropathy. *Muscle Nerve.* 2008;37:281-292.

Supakornnumporn S, Katirji B. Autoimmune neuromuscular diseases induced by immunomodulating drugs. *J Clin Neuromuscul Dis.* 2018;20(1):28-34.

Suichi T, Misawa S, Sato Y, et al. Proposal of new clinical diagnostic criteria for POEMS syndrome. *J Neurol Neurosurg Psychiatry.* 2019;90:133-137.

Suzuki S, Ishikawa N, Konoeda F, et al. Nivolumab-related myasthenia gravis with myositis and myocarditis in Japan. *Neurology.* 2017;89:1-8.

van Koningsveld R, Steyerberg EW, Hughes RA, Swan AV, van Doorn PA, Jacobs BC. A clinical prognostic scoring system for Guillain-Barre syndrome. *Lancet Neurol.* 2007;6:589-594.

Walgaard C, Lingsma HF, Ruts L, et al. Prediction of respiratory insufficiency in Guillain-Barre Syndrome. *Ann Neurol.* 2010;67:781-787.

Walgaard C, Lingsma HF, Ruts L, et al. Early recognition of poor prognosis in Guillain-Barré syndrome. *Neurology.* 2011;76:968-975.

Young NP, Sorenson EJ, Spinner RJ, et al. Clinical and electrodiagnostic correlates of peroneal intraneural ganglia. *Neurology.* 2009;72:447-452.

Yuki N, Hartung HP. Guillain-Barré syndrome. *N Engl J Med.* 2012;366:2294-2304.

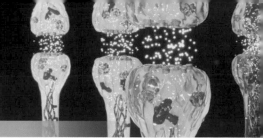

# CHAPTER 15

# Hereditary Neuropathies

## PART 1 | PRACTICE TEST

**Q1.** A 22-year-old woman has long-standing bilateral leg weakness since childhood. Examination reveals high arch feet, shortening of forefeet, and symmetrical atrophy of distal legs. Motor power is grade 4 in both distal lower extremities. There is impairment pinprick sensation, proprioception, and vibration in both feet. Reflexes are reduced at both knees but absent at the ankles. Which of the following tests provides the highest yield for the final diagnosis?
  A.  Genetic testing
  B.  Nerve biopsy
  C.  Muscle biopsy
  D.  Muscle MRI
  E.  Nerve conduction study and needle electromyography

**Q2.** Which of the following genetic mutations is the most common in patients with Charcot-Marie-Tooth disease?
  A.  *PMP22* deletion
  B.  *PMP22* duplication
  C.  *MPZ* mutations
  D.  *GJB1* mutations
  E.  *MFN2* mutations

**The following answer options are for QUESTIONS 3 through 7.**

> *Match the most likely associated genetic mutation with each disease.*
>   A.  *GJB1* mutations
>   B.  *MPZ* mutations
>   C.  *MFN2* mutations
>   D.  *PMP22* deletion
>   E.  *PMP22* duplication

**Q3.** CMT1A
**Q4.** CMT1B
**Q5.** CMT2A
**Q6.** CMT1X
**Q7.** Hereditary neuropathy with liability to pressure palsies (HNPP)

**The following answer options are for QUESTIONS 8 through 13.**

> *Match the mode of inheritance with the disease (each option can be selected more than once).*
>   A.  Autosomal dominant
>   B.  Autosomal recessive
>   C.  X-linked dominant
>   D.  X-linked recessive

**Q8.** CMT1A
**Q9.** CMT1B
**Q10.** CMT2A
**Q11.** CMT1X
**Q12.** CMT4A
**Q13.** Hereditary neuropathy with liability to pressure palsies (HNPP)

**Q14.** Which of the following is **CORRECT** regarding family history in Charcot-Marie-Tooth disease?
  A.  The absence of family history exclude CMT1A since it is autosomal dominant.
  B.  The absence of affected females in the family is a key feature in CMT1X.
  C.  Male-to-male transmission is a feature of CMT1X.
  D.  All children of an affected CMT1X male are an obligatory carrier.
  E.  Consanguinity can be a clue for CMT4A.

**The following answer options are for QUESTIONS 15 through 20.**

> *Match the predominant pathology with the disease (each option can be selected more than once).*
>   A.  Demyelinating process
>   B.  Axonal process
>   C.  Mixed demyelinating and axonal processes

**Q15.** CMT1A
**Q16.** CMT1B
**Q17.** CMT2A
**Q18.** CMT1X
**Q19.** Intermediate CMT
**Q20.** Hereditary neuropathy with liability to pressure palsies (HNPP)

**Q21.** A 7-year-old girl is referred to the electromyography (EMG) lab for evaluation of bilateral leg weakness. Nerve conduction study of the median nerve demonstrates the finding in the following figure. What is the most likely diagnosis?

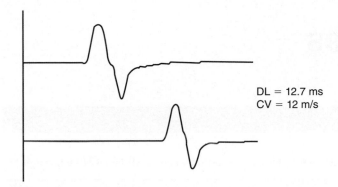

DL = 12.7 ms
CV = 12 m/s

Adapted from Preston DC, Shapiro BE. *Electromyography and Neuromuscular Disorders*, 4th ed. Philadelphia: Elsevier; 2020:34.

A. CMT1A
B. CMT2A
C. Intermediate CMT
D. Hereditary neuropathy with liability to pressure palsies
E. Chronic inflammatory demyelinating polyneuropathy

**Q22.** Which of the following is the electrophysiologic feature that distinguishes the demyelinating types of Charcot-Marie-Tooth disease from immune-mediated acquired demyelinating neuropathies?
A. Conduction block
B. Temporal dispersion
C. Reduction of compound muscle action potential (CMAP) and sensory nerve action potential (SNAP) amplitudes
D. Nerve conduction velocity greater than 35 m/s in the upper extremity
E. Uniform slowing of nerve conduction velocities

**Q23.** An 8-month-old baby boy is referred for congenital hypotonia. There is weakness of all extremities, and the infant has recently developed respiratory difficulty. Reflexes are reduced in all extremities. Nerve conduction study reveals conduction velocity of 10 m/s in all tested nerves in both the upper and lower extremities. There is no conduction block. Which of the following genetic mutations is the most common mutation responsible for the disease in this patient?
A. *GDAP1* mutation
B. *GJB1* mutation
C. *MFN2* mutation
D. *PMP22* duplication
E. *PMP22* deletion

**Q24.** Which of the following is the distinguishing electrophysiologic feature of hereditary neuropathy with liability to pressure palsies (HNPP)?
A. Markedly prolonged distal motor latencies at non-entrapment sites
B. Focal slowing or conduction blocks at common entrapment sites
C. Focal slowing or conduction blocks at non-entrapment sites
D. Uniform or diffuse slowing of nerve conduction velocities
E. Reduced compound muscle action potential (CMAP) amplitudes from both proximal and distal stimulation sites

**Q25.** A 10-year-old boy developed an episode of weakness and numbness of the left face, arm, and leg, as well as dysarthria lasting for 1 hour. The symptoms resolved spontaneously. On examination, pes cavus was noted. He had mild weakness and impaired sensation of all modalities in both distal lower extremities, as well as absent ankle reflexes. Magnetic resonance imaging (MRI) of the brain was unremarkable. You suspected Charcot-Marie-Tooth disease. Which of the following genetic mutations is most likely found in this patient?
A. *GDAP1* mutation
B. *GJB1* mutation
C. *PMP22* deletion
D. *MPZ* mutation
E. *PMP22* duplication

**Q26.** Which of the following Charcot-Marie-Tooth genes has the pathophysiological mechanism that is closely linked to mitochondrial dynamics?
A. GJB1
B. MFN2
C. MPZ
D. PMP22
E. TRPV4

**Q27.** Vocal cord involvement is most likely a manifestation of Charcot-Marie-Tooth disease due to which of the following genes?
A. *GJB1*
B. *MPZ*
C. *MFN2*
D. *PMP22*
E. *TRPV4*

**Q28.** A 20-year-old woman has had recurrent episodes of painless mononeuropathies. At age 18 years, she developed right peroneal neuropathy that resolved after 2 weeks. Six months ago, she developed left carpal tunnel syndrome, which resolved after 2 weeks. Two days ago, she developed numbness of the right ring and little fingers. Examination reveals grade 3/5 weakness of the right abductor digiti minimi, first dorsal interossei, and flexor digitorum profundus of digits 4 and 5. If a nerve biopsy of the affected nerve is performed, which of the following is most likely found?

A. Myelin ovoid
B. Onion bulb formation
C. Segmental demyelination
D. Focal swelling of the myelin sheath
E. Invasion of mixed inflammatory cells into the blood vessel wall

**Q29.** Which of the following features argues against the diagnosis of distal hereditary motor neuropathy (dHMN)?

A. Subtle sensory impairment on examination
B. Marked atrophy of hands and feet
C. Absent ankle reflexes
D. Reduced compound muscle action potential (CMAP) amplitudes on nerve conduction studies
E. Small short-duration polyphasic motor unit action potentials (MUAPs) on needle electromyography (EMG)

**Q30.** A 12-year-old boy has had worsening weakness of both ankles and feet since the age of 8 years. Lately, he has had weakness of both hands and visual difficulties. Examination reveals distal weakness, atrophy, sensory loss, and areflexia. Funduscopic examination reveals bilateral optic atrophy. Brain magnetic resonance imaging (MRI) reveals subcortical white matter hyperintensities on the T2-weighted sequence. Mutation in which of the following genes is most likely found in this patient?

A. *MFN2*
B. *PMP22*
C. *GJB1*
D. *OPA1*
E. *MT-ND1* in the mitochondrial DNA

**The following answer options are for QUESTIONS 31 through 33.**

*Match the nerve biopsy with the gene.*

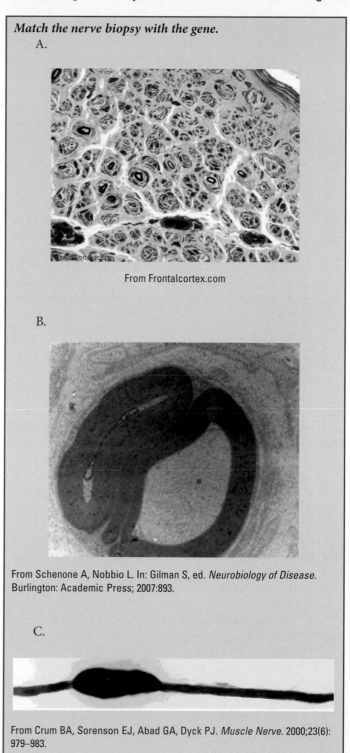

A.

From Frontalcortex.com

B.

From Schenone A, Nobbio L. In: Gilman S, ed. *Neurobiology of Disease.* Burlington: Academic Press; 2007:893.

C.

From Crum BA, Sorenson EJ, Abad GA, Dyck PJ. *Muscle Nerve.* 2000;23(6): 979–983.

**Q31.** *PMP22* duplication
**Q32.** *PMP22* deletion
**Q33.** *MTMR2* mutation

**Q34.** A 25-year-old man has had worsening lancinating pain in his hands and feet since age 14 years. In the past few years he also has weakness of both feet and hands. On examination, there are chronic bilateral foot ulcers, as well as amputation of some fingers and toes. There is loss of pinprick and temperature sensation, as well as proprioception and vibration in the bilateral hands and feet. Motor power is grade 4 in distal lower and upper extremities. What is the **MOST LIKELY** diagnosis in this patient?
A. Charcot-Marie-Tooth disease
B. Distal hereditary motor neuropathy
C. Fabry disease
D. Familial amyloid polyneuropathy
E. Hereditary sensory and autonomic neuropathy

**Q35.** A 29-year-old woman presents with fluctuating episodes of burning sensation in bilateral hands and feet since childhood. On examination, redness and allodynia of the bilateral hands and feet are noted. Which of the following genes are **MOST LIKELY** associated with this condition?
A. *ABCA1*
B. *CLCN1*
C. *GLA*
D. *SCN9A*
E. *TTR*

**Q36.** A 42-year-old woman has had numbness of both hands and feet since age 24. She also has had difficulty speaking and swallowing in the past 5 years. Examination reveals dysarthria and marked limitation of extraocular movements in all directions. Motor power is normal. Sensory examination shows impaired pinprick sensation and markedly impaired proprioception and vibration in both lower extremities. Reflexes are absent in the lower extremities. She walks with a wide-based gait. Which of the following statements is **CORRECT** regarding the disease in this patient?
A. This disorder is due to a mutation in the mitochondrial DNA.
B. This disorder is associated with nuclear DNA depletion.
C. There is a point mutation in the tRNA leucine (tRNA$^{\text{Leu(UUR)}}$) gene.
D. Mutations in the same gene can also cause chronic progressive external ophthalmoplegia (CPEO).
E. Muscle biopsy in this patient does not have ragged-red fibers or cytochrome oxidase (COX)-negative fibers, since there is no weakness on examination.

**Q37.** A 35-year-old man presents for an evaluation of peripheral neuropathy. Oral examination reveals the finding in the figure below. Which of the following is associated with this disease?

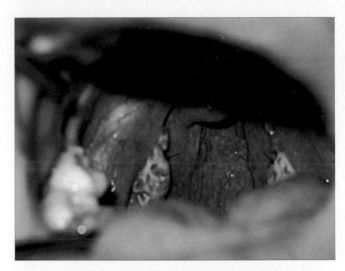

From Puntoni M, Sbrana F, Bigazzi F, et al. *Am J Cardiovasc Drugs.* 2012;12:303–311.

A. Angiokeratoma
B. Dysphagia
C. Leukodystrophy
D. Reduced high-density lipoprotein (HDL) cholesterol
E. Myopathy

**Q38.** Which of the following medications should be avoided in patients with Charcot-Marie-Tooth disease?
A. Cisplatin
B. Nitrofurantoin
C. Paclitaxel
D. Vincristine
E. All of the above

## PART 2 | QUESTIONS WITH ANSWERS AND DISCUSSION

**QUESTION 1.** A 22-year-old woman has long-standing bilateral leg weakness since childhood. Examination reveals high arch feet, shortening of forefeet, and symmetrical atrophy of distal legs. Motor power is grade 4 in both distal lower extremities. There is impairment pinprick sensation, proprioception, and vibration in both feet. Reflexes are reduced at both knees but absent at the ankles. Which of the following tests provides the highest yield for the final diagnosis?

    A. Genetic testing
    B. Nerve biopsy
    C. Muscle biopsy
    D. Muscle MRI
    E. Nerve conduction study and needle electromyography

**ANSWER:** A. Genetic testing

### COMMENTS AND DISCUSSION

- This patient has pes cavus, characterized by high arch feet and shortening of forefeet, which indicates that the neuropathy was present during developmental periods as a child. It is a common finding in Charcot-Marie-Tooth disease (CMT), but also may be seen in other conditions where distal muscle weakness was present during childhood development, including other hereditary neuropathies as well as upper motor neuron disorders (e.g., Friedreich's ataxia and hereditary spastic paraplegia). In addition, this patient has motor and sensory impairment, as well as hyporeflexia, which involved mainly the distal lower extremities.
- History in Charcot-Marie-Tooth disease
  - Age at onset is typically in childhood, although there is variability.
  - Long-standing clumsiness; inability to participate in sports well at school
  - Family history is useful, and can suggest mode of inheritance.
    - However, negative family history does not exclude CMT.
    - Autosomal dominant
      - Multiple generations are affected.
      - However, *de novo* mutations may occur in CMT. In this case, family history can be absent.
    - Autosomal recessive
      - Multiple family members in one generation without affected individuals in other generations
      - There may be consanguinity.
      - In a small family, family history can be absent.
    - X-linked recessive
      - No male-to-male transmission is key, since the X chromosome from the father does not pass along to the son.
      - Females can also be affected due to skewed inactivation of the X chromosome. They typically have milder symptoms and later ages at onset, compared to affected males.

### ◎ HIGH-YIELD FACT

Absence of family history does not exclude CMT, since mutations can be *de novo* or inherited as autosomal recessive.

### ◎ HIGH-YIELD FACT

Females may also be affected in X-linked CMTs due to skewed inactivation of the X chromosome. Affected females typically have milder symptoms and later ages at onset.

- Physical examination in Charcot-Marie-Tooth disease
  - Foot deformities (Fig. 15.1)
    - Pes cavus
      - *Pes Cavus:* High arch foot, shortening of forefoot
      - Indicates that neuropathy was present during the developmental period
      - Not specific to CMT; can be seen in other neuropathies that occur during the developmental period
    - Hammer toes
    - *Cavovarus:* high arch foot and inward turning (varus deformity) of the hindfoot
    - Examination of a patient's shoe can be useful.
  - *Inverted champagne bottle* appearance of the legs
    - Due to greater degree of atrophy in the distal legs
  - Weakness and sensory loss, which mainly affect the distal legs
    - Despite sensory loss on examination, patients with CMT may have only mild or no sensory complaints.
    - Impaired ankle dorsiflexion can result in a steppage gait.
  - Ankle reflex is often absent.
    - If ankle reflex is still preserved when there is weakness of bilateral feet or ankles, the diagnosis of CMT should be questioned.

## ◎ HIGH-YIELD FACT

Pes cavus indicates that neuropathy was present during development in childhood. This is not specific to CMT.

- Action hand tremor
  - *Roussy-Lévy syndrome* is an old terminology describing a phenotype of gait ataxia, areflexia, pes cavus, distal muscle weakness. and hand tremor.
  - Also known as hereditary areflexic dystasia
  - Most cases of Roussy-Lévy syndrome likely have CMT1A
- Electrodiagnostic findings in Charcot-Marie-Tooth disease
  - Demyelinating CMT

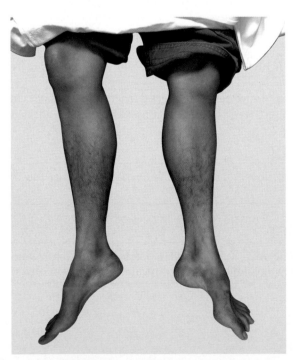

**Fig. 15.1 Feet and legs in Charcot-Marie-Tooth disease (CMT).** This figure demonstrates bilateral pes cavus characterized by high arch feet and shortening of forefeet, as well as inverted champagne bottle appearance of bilateral legs.

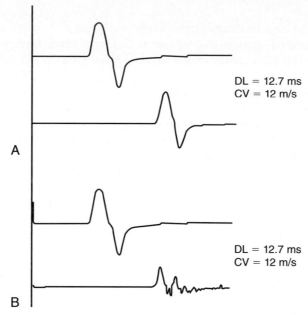

**Fig. 15.2 Electrodiagnostic features of hereditary demyelinating neuropathies (e.g., in demyelinating Charcot-Marie-Tooth disease) in contrast to acquired demyelinating neuropathies.** (A) Diffuse slowing without conduction block or temporal dispersion. This pattern is seen in hereditary demyelinating neuropathies (e.g., demyelinating forms of CMT). (B) Conduction block and temporal dispersion. This pattern is seen in acquired demyelinating neuropathies (e.g., Guillain–Barré syndrome). From Preston DC, Shapiro BE. *Electromyography and Neuromuscular Disorders*, 4th ed. Philadelphia: Elsevier; 2020:34.

- Diffuse or uniform slowing of nerve conduction is a very important feature (Fig. 15.2). This contrasts with acquired demyelination, where focal slowing, conduction block, or temporal dispersion is seen.
- Temporal dispersion is typically not seen in CMT.
- Nerve conduction velocity (NCV) in the forearms is typically less than 38 m/s.
- If compound muscle action potential (CMAP) is very low in amplitude, blink reflex testing can be useful. Blink reflex R1 latency greater than 13 ms is suggestive of demyelinating types of CMT.
  o Axonal CMT
    - Reduced CMAP and sensory nerve action potential (SNAP) amplitudes
    - Mild slowing of NCV can be found, typically greater than 38 m/s in the forearms.
  o Intermediate CMT
    - NCV between 35 and 45 m/s in the forearms.

## ◎ HIGH-YIELD FACT

**Electrodiagnostic features**
In **hereditary** demyelinating neuropathies (e.g., CMT) - **uniform or diffuse** slowing of nerve conduction
In **acquired** demyelinating neuropathies - **focal** slowing, conduction block, or temporal dispersion

- Nerve pathology in Charcot-Marie-Tooth disease (see also comments and discussion from Question 37 in Chapter 10)
  o Demyelinating CMT
    - Onion bulb formation
      - Concentric layers of Schwann cell processes
      - Onion bulb formation is evidence of repetitive demyelination and remyelination.
      - In demyealinating CMT, diffuse onion bulb formation without inflammation is observed, in contrast to multifocal onion bulb formation with inflammation seen in chronic inflammatory demyelinating polyneuropathy (CIDP).
    - Focally folded myelin sheath
      - Found in CMT4B (due to *MTMR2* mutations) and CMT4A (due to *GDAP1* mutations)
      - Can also be seen in CMT1B (due to *MPZ* mutations)

- Axonal CMT
  - Loss of small and large myelinated nerve fibers
  - Evidence of regenerating axons may be seen as clusters of small, myelinated nerve fibers.
- Among all options in this case, genetic testing has the highest yield for the definite diagnosis of CMT.
- There is no unified approach for genetic testing.
- There are at least two approaches to genetic testing for CMT: single gene testing and targeted gene sequencing (gene panels) using next-generation sequencing technology.
- The latter approach has been used increasingly in current clinical practice due to lower costs of next-generation sequencing and cost effectiveness.
- However, it is important to note that duplications (e.g., *PMP22* duplication) and deletions (e.g., *PMP22* deletion in hereditary neuropathy with liability to pressure palsies [HNPP]) can be missed on next-generation sequencing. It is critical to understand the limitation of tests in various laboratories.
- The four most common CMT genes include *PMP22* (duplication), *GJB1*, *MPZ*, and *MFN2*. *PMP22* duplication is the most common, and *GJB1* and *MPZ* mutations are the next most common. Other genes are variable and found much less frequently.
- Thus, the principle is that if clinicians would like to pursue screening genetic testing for CMT first, it may be reasonable to first screen for these three to four genes (*PMP22* duplication, *GJB1*, *MPZ*. and possibly *MFN2*). The specific genetic testing is especially important for *PMP22* duplication, since this can be missed on next-generation sequencing.
- Phenotypes can be useful to suggest which gene screening would give high diagnostic yield. For example,
  - Demyelinating phenotype (NCV <38 m/s): screen for *PMP22* duplication (CMT1A) first; *MFN2* gene testing may not be needed.
  - Axonal phenotype (NCV >38 m/s): screen for *MFN2* (CMT2A), *GJB1* (CMT1X, especially when there is no male-to-male transmission), and *MPZ* first.
  - Intermediate phenotype (NCV 35–45 m/s): screen for *GJB1* (especially if no male-to-male transmission) or *MPZ* first.
  - There are other phenotypic clues that can be useful in identifying a particular genotype, such as the presence of optic neuropathy, sensorineural hearing loss, or subcortical white matter abnormalities.
- After testing these 3–4 genes, searching for other genes may be more cost effective by using next-generation sequencing technology or gene panel testing.
- Nerve biopsy is useful in differentiating the primary demyelinating pathology (e.g., onion bulb formation) from axonal pathology (e.g., axonal loss, myelin ovoids). However, nerve pathology is unlikely to pinpoint the specific type of CMT, and further genetic testing is still required for a definite diagnosis. Nerve conduction study to determine NCV is also useful to differentiate between demyelinating versus axonal versus intermediate CMT. It is less invasive than nerve biopsy, but similarly, it still cannot pinpoint the specific type of CMT.
- Muscle biopsy and muscle MRI are unlikely to be useful in CMT.

**QUESTION 2.** Which of the following genetic mutations is the most common in patients with Charcot-Marie-Tooth disease?
- A. *PMP22* deletion
- B. *PMP22* duplication
- C. *MPZ* mutations
- D. *GJB1* mutations
- E. *MFN2* mutations

**ANSWER:** B. *PMP22* duplication

## COMMENTS AND DISCUSSION
- Charcot-Marie-Tooth disease (CMT), aka hereditary motor sensory neuropathies (HMSNs) is a group of the most common hereditary neuropathies.
- The most common type of CMT is CMT1A. Most of CMT1A cases are due to *PMP22* duplication. The minority of CMT1A can be due to point mutations in the *PMP22* gene.
- PMP22 deletion is associated with hereditary neuropathy with liability to pressure palsies (HNPP). *MPZ* mutations are associated with CMT1B. *GJB1* mutations are associated with CMT1X. *MFN2* mutations are associated with CMT2A.

- Other hereditary neuropathies include:
  - Hereditary sensory autonomic neuropathies (HSANs)
  - Distal hereditary motor neuropathies (dHMNs)
  - Hereditary neuropathies that overlap with other disorders, for example
    - Hereditary spastic paraplegia (HSP)
    - Spinocerebellar ataxia (SCA)
  - Metabolic neuropathies
  - Neuropathies in mitochondrial disorders
- CMT is a heterogeneous group of hereditary neuropathies with a confusing classification and some overlaps.
  - Overlaps within the same category of CMT (i.e., the same gene can be responsible for several types of CMT, called phenotypic variability)
  - Overlaps between different categories (i.e., the same gene can be responsible for several phenotypes: CMT, HSAN, dHMN, or HSP)
- Genotype–phenotype correlation is complex: not a 1:1 relationship
  - One gene can cause many phenotypes.
  - One phenotype can be associated with many genes.
  - Next-generation sequencing has been used increasingly in current clinical practice.
- CMT is classified based on:
  - Inheritance: autosomal dominant, autosomal recessive, X-linked
  - Primary pathology: demyelinating versus axonal
  - Nerve conduction velocity in the forearms:
    - Demyelinating type: <38 m/s
    - Axonal type: >38 m/s
    - Intermediate type: 35–45 m/s
- New classification schemes attempt to use gene names and descriptions (e.g., demyelinating versus axonal versus intermediate, and inheritance), rather than running numbers or letters. However, the nomenclature with designated numbers and letters is still commonly used in clinical practice.
- Commonly used classification scheme (Table 15.1)
  - CMT1: Autosomal dominant, demyelinating
  - CMT2: Autosomal dominant, axonal
  - CMT3
    - Previously known as Déjerine-Sottas syndrome or congenital hypomyelinating neuropathy
    - Very early (infantile onset), severe demyelinating neuropathy
    - Nerve conduction velocity is typically very slow, less <10 m/s
    - CMT3 is no longer used
      - After the gene discoveries, this category has been incorporated into CMT1 (for autosomal dominant genes) and CMT4 (for autosomal recessive genes)
  - CMT4: Autosomal recessive
    - Can be either demyelinating or axonal, but most are demyelinating
    - The classification of autosomal recessive (AR) genes is confusing.
      - Most AR genes are categorized under CMT4.
      - Some AR genes with axonal pathology are incorporated into CMT2.

**TABLE 15.1** Overview of classification of Charcot-Marie-Tooth disease (CMT).

| Type | Inheritance | Primary pathology | NCV (m/s) |
|---|---|---|---|
| CMT1 | Autosomal dominant | Demyelinating | <38 |
| CMT2 | Autosomal dominant | Axonal | >38 |
| CMT4 | Autosomal recessive | Mostly demyelinating | Mostly <38 |
| CMTX | X-linked | Mostly axonal | Mostly >38 |
| Intermediate forms | | | |
| CMTDI | Autosomal dominant | Mixed demyelinating and axonal | 35–45 |
| CMTRI | Autosomal recessive | | |

CMT is classified based on primary pathology and inheritance. Nerve conduction velocities are measured in the upper extremities. Of note, CMT3 (aka Déjerine-Sottas syndrome) is severe infantile-onset demyelinating neuropathy, which is currently incorporated into CMT1.

- Some clinicians do not use CMT4 nomenclature, but rather put AR genes under CMT1 (if pathology is demyelinating process) or CMT2 (if pathology is axonal).
  - However, in this book, CMT4 category is used for AR genes.
  - CMTX: X-linked
    - Can be either demyelinating or axonal, but most are axonal
  - Intermediate forms: main feature is a nerve conduction velocity in the upper extremities between 35 and 45 m/s
    - Can be either autosomal dominant (dominant intermediate Charcot-Marie-Tooth [DI-CMT] or CMTDI disease) or recessive (recessive intermediate Charcot-Marie-Tooth [RI-CMT or CMTRI] disease).
    - Pathology is mixed between axonal and demyelinating processes.

## MNEMONICS

| | | |
|---|---|---|
| Autosomal dominant | → Demyelinating | → CMT1 |
| | → Axonal | → CMT2 |
| Autosomal recessive | | → CMT4 |
| X-linked | | → CMTX |
| | NCS 35-45 m/s | → Intermediate CMT |

**The following answer options are for QUESTIONS 3 through 7.**

*Match the most likely associated genetic mutation with each disease.*
A. *GJB1* mutations
B. *MPZ* mutations
C. *MFN2* mutations
D. *PMP22* deletion
E. *PMP22* duplication

**QUESTION 3.** CMT1A
**ANSWER:** E. *PMP22* duplication

**QUESTION 4.** CMT1B
**ANSWER:** B. *MPZ* mutations

**QUESTION 5.** CMT2A
**ANSWER:** C. *MFN2* mutations

**QUESTION 6.** CMT1X
**ANSWER:** A. *GJB1* mutations

**QUESTION 7.** Hereditary neuropathy with liability to pressure palsies (HNPP)
**ANSWER:** D. *PMP22* deletion

### COMMENTS AND DISCUSSION
- CMT1A
  - Autosomal dominant, demyelinating
  - CMT1A is due to *PMP22* duplication in most cases. Some are *de novo* and family history is often absent. Point mutations can be found in the minority. In contrast, hereditary neuropathy with liability to pressure palsies (HNPP) is due to *PMP22* deletion.
  - It is important to note that next-generation sequencing can miss deletions or duplications.
  - *PMP22* encodes for peripheral myelin protein, which has a key role in the formation and maintenance of compact myelin.
  - CMT1A is the most common form of Charcot-Marie-Tooth disease (CMT). Thus, it is reasonable to screen for *PMP22* duplication first, when CMT is suspected and demyelinating features are seen (e.g., nerve conduction velocity [NCV] <38 m/s in the forearms or uniform slowing).

**HIGH-YIELD FACT**

| | |
|---|---|
| **CMT1A** | **large** gene (*PMP22* duplication) |
| **HNPP** | **small** gene (*PMP22* deletion) |

- CMT1B
  - Autosomal dominant, demyelinating
  - Due to mutations in the *MPZ* gene encoding myelin protein zero
  - In addition to CMT1B, mutations in the *MPZ* gene can also cause an axonal phenotype (CMT2I) and intermediate phenotype (DI-CMTD).
  - Patients may have Adie (tonic) pupil
- CMT2A
  - Autosomal dominant, axonal
  - Due to mutations in the *MFN2* gene encoding mitofusin
  - Mitofusin 2 has an important role in mitochondrial fusion.
  - Patients may have optic atrophy and sensorineural hearing loss, which are features seen in mitochondrial diseases.
  - White matter hyperintensities can be seen on T2-weighted magnetic resonance imaging (MRI) of the brain. Similar features can be seen on CMTX (due to *GJB1* mutations).

**MNEMONICS**

*CMT genes that involve mitochondrial dynamics.*
**MFN2 (CMT2A)** encoding mitoFUSIN 2, which has a role in mitochondrial **FUSION**.
**GDAP1 (CMT4A)** has a role in mitochondrial **FISSION**.

- CMT1X
  - X-linked recessive (no male-to-male transmission)
  - Intermediate phenotype: mixed between demyelinating and axonal features
  - The second most common CMT after CMT1A
  - Affects both men and women, the latter due to skewed inactivation of the X chromosome.
  - Men typically have more severe phenotype, whereas women are less severe with later ages at onset.
  - Due to mutations in the *GJB1* gene encoding gap junction beta 1 (aka connexin 32)
  - Connexin 32 forms a hexamer, is expressed in Schwann cells, and also in oligodendroglia. It has an important role in gap junction formation at the non-compact regions of myelin, including paranodal regions and Schmidt-Lanterman incisures.
  - Patients can have stroke-like episodes, split-hand syndrome, and white matter abnormalities
- Hereditary neuropathy with liability to pressure palsies (HNPP)
  - Typically involves multiple nerves (usually at different timing) at common entrapment sites
  - Electrophysiology shows evidence of demyelinating neuropathy including focal slowing, conduction block, and/or temporal dispersion at common entrapment sites. This contrasts with multifocal motor neuropathy (MMN), which shows these acquired demyelinating features at *non-entrapment sites* such as the median or ulnar nerve in the forearm

 **HIGH-YIELD FACT**

CMT in which **subcortical white matter abnormalities** can be seen include **CMT2A and CMTX**.

- Autosomal dominant
- Responsible gene is the same as CMT1A: *PMP22*. However, in HNPP, there is *PMP22* deletion, in contrast to *PMP22* duplication in CMT1A
- Pathology: tomaculous neuropathy (*tomacula* from Latin meaning sausage) characterized by focal sausage-shaped swelling of myelin, typically seen on teased nerve fiber preparation (see Fig. 10.23)
- Benefits of nerve decompression at entrapment sites in HNPP remain unclear, and this is not routinely recommended.

**HIGH-YIELD FACT**

**Electrophysiology in HNPP versus MMN**
**HNPP** – evidence of demyelination (focal slowing, conduction block, temporal dispersion) at
   **COMMON** entrapment sites
**MMN** – evidence of demyelination (focal slowing, conduction block, temporal dispersion) at
   **UNCOMMON** entrapment sites

## MNEMONICS

**Hereditary neuropathy with liability to PRESSURE palsies (HNPP)** – **Pressure** results in recurrent
entrapment neuropathy.

**The following answer options are for QUESTIONS 8 through 13.**

*Match the mode of inheritance with the disease (each option can be selected more than once).*
   A. Autosomal dominant
   B. Autosomal recessive
   C. X-linked dominant
   D. X-linked recessive

**QUESTION 8.** CMT1A
**ANSWER:** A. Autosomal dominant

**QUESTION 9.** CMT1B
**ANSWER:** A. Autosomal dominant

**QUESTION 10.** CMT2A
**ANSWER:** A. Autosomal dominant

**QUESTION 11.** CMT1X
**ANSWER:** D. X-linked recessive

**QUESTION 12.** CMT4A
**ANSWER:** B. Autosomal recessive

**QUESTION 13.** Hereditary neuropathy with liability to pressure palsies (HNPP)
**ANSWER:** A. Autosomal dominant

**COMMENTS AND DISCUSSION (see also comments and discussion from Question 7 and Table 15.1)**
- CMT4
  - Autosomal recessive; almost all CMT4 are the demyelinating type.
  - Consanguinity can be present.
  - Rare, but has great genetic heterogeneity.
  - Examples include CMT4A (due to *GDAP1* mutations) and CMT4B1 (due to *MTMR2* mutations)
  - *GDAP1* has an important role in mitochondrial fission.
- CMT1 (including CMT1A and CMT1B) and CMT2 are inherited in an autosomal dominant manner.
- CMTX (including CMT1X) has an X-linked inheritance.
- Hereditary neuropathy with liability to pressure palsies (HNPP) has an autosomal dominant inheritance.

**QUESTION 14.** Which of the following is **CORRECT** regarding family history in Charcot-Marie-Tooth
   disease?
   A. The absence of family history exclude CMT1A since it is autosomal dominant.
   B. The absence of affected females in the family is a key feature in CMT1X.
   C. Male-to-male transmission is a feature of CMT1X.
   D. All children of an affected CMT1X male are an obligatory carrier.
   E. Consanguinity can be a clue for CMT4A.

**ANSWER:** E. Consanguinity can be a clue for CMT4A.

**COMMENTS AND DISCUSSION (see also comments and discussion from Question 13)**

- CMT1A is inherited in an autosomal dominant manner. A typical autosomal dominant pedigree shows that multiple family members in multiple generations are affected. However, family history can be absent, since some CMT1A patients have *de novo* mutations.
- CMT1X is inherited in an X-linked manner.
  - The key feature of X-linked inheritance is no male-to-male transmission. The presence of male-to-male transmission would argue against X-linked inheritance, since the X chromosome from the father would not be inherited by the son.
  - X-linked disorders including CMT1X predominantly affect males. However, females may also be symptomatic, due to skewed inactivation of X chromosomes. Affected females typically have a milder severity of symptoms compared to affected males.
  - A daughter of an affected male of CMT1X is an obligatory carrier, since she inherits an X chromosome from her father, which is mutated.
- CMT4A is inherited in an autosomal recessive manner. Consanguinity can be a clue for autosomal recessive diseases including CMT4A. An autosomal recessive pedigree typically shows affected individuals in skipped generations.

**The following answer options are for QUESTIONS 15 through 20.**

> ***Match the predominant pathology with the disease (each option can be selected more than once).***
> A. Demyelinating process
> B. Axonal process
> C. Mixed demyelinating and axonal processes

**QUESTION 15.** CMT1A
**ANSWER:** A. Demyelinating process

**QUESTION 16.** CMT1B
**ANSWER:** A. Demyelinating process

**QUESTION 17.** CMT2A
**ANSWER:** B. Axonal process

**QUESTION 18.** CMT1X
**ANSWER:** C. Mixed demyelinating and axonal processes

**QUESTION 19.** Intermediate CMT
**ANSWER:** C. Mixed demyelinating and axonal processes

**QUESTION 20.** Hereditary neuropathy with liability to pressure palsies (HNPP)
**ANSWER:** A. Demyelinating process

**COMMENTS AND DISCUSSION**

- The primary pathology in CMT1 including CMT1A and CMT1B is demyelination. In CMT2 including CMT2A, the primary pathology is an axonal process. Most CMT4 has demyelination as the primary pathology; however, some have primary axonal pathology. On nerve biopsy, most cases of CMTX including CMT1X have primary axonal pathology despite having nerve conduction velocities (NCVs) typically in the demyelinating range. In intermediate forms of CMT, the primary pathology is mixed between demyelinating and axonal processes.
- Nerve conduction study is useful in the determination of the primary pathology. In demyelinating forms of CMT, NCVs in the forearms are typically less than 38 m/s. In axonal forms of CMT, NCVs are typically greater than 38 m/s. In intermediate forms and in CMTX, NCVs are typically between 35 to 45 m/s.
- In hereditary neuropathy with liability to pressure palsies (HNPP), the primary pathology is demyelination. However, in contrast to CMT1 and other demyelinating forms of CMT, HNPP has focal demyelination at the common entrapment sites. The classic nerve pathology of HNPP is focal myelin swelling at these sites, called tomacula (meaning sausage). Nerve conduction studies in HNPP show focal slowing or conduction block, in contrast to uniform slowing in CMT1 and other demyelinating CMTs.

**QUESTION 21.** A 7-year-old girl is referred to the electromyography (EMG) lab for evaluation of bilateral leg weakness. Nerve conduction study of the median nerve demonstrates the finding in the following figure. What is the **MOST LIKELY** diagnosis?

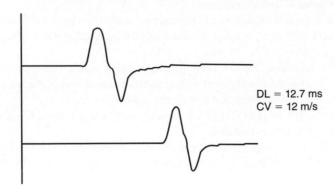

DL = 12.7 ms
CV = 12 m/s

Adapted from Preston DC, Shapiro BE. *Electromyography and Neuromuscular Disorders,* 4th ed. Philadelphia: Elsevier; 2020:34.

   A. CMT1A
   B. CMT2A
   C. Intermediate CMT
   D. Hereditary neuropathy with liability to pressure palsies
   E. Chronic inflammatory demyelinating polyneuropathy

**ANSWER:** A. CMT1A

## COMMENTS AND DISCUSSION

- This nerve conduction study (NCS) demonstrates marked (12 m/s) and uniform slowing of nerve conduction velocity (NCV) of the median nerve. This finding is suggestive of hereditary demyelinating forms of neuropathies including demyelinating forms of Charcot-Marie-Tooth (CMT) disease in which demyelination occurs diffusely resulting in uniform or diffuse slowing. Among all options, CMT1A is a demyelinating form of CMT.
- Although hereditary neuropathy with liability to pressure palsies (HNPP) is also a hereditary demyelinating neuropathy, demyelination occurs focally at common entrapment sites. Therefore, in HNPP, there is focal slowing or conduction block at the common entrapment sites, similar to in acquired neuropathies, instead of diffuse or uniform slowing in demyelinating CMT.
- In acquired demyelinating neuropathies such as acute inflammatory demyelinating polyneuropathy (AIDP) and chronic inflammatory demyelinating polyneuropathy (CIDP), demyelination is multifocal. NCS in acquired demyelinating neuropathies typically demonstrates focal slowing, conduction block, or temporal dispersion, instead of diffuse and uniform slowing in hereditary demyelinating neuropathies.
- CMT2A has a primary axonal pathology. Therefore, uniform and diffuse slowing is not expected. NCSs in axonal CMTs can show reduced compound muscle action potential (CMAP) and sensory nerve action potential (SNAP) amplitudes, as well as NCV greater than 38 m/s.
- Intermediate CMT is a category, which was established later.
  - No consensus definition, but usually this refers to CMT that has an NCV between 35 and 45 m/s
  - It has mixed pathology between demyelination and axonal loss. Marked and uniform slowing as in this case should not be seen.
  - Can be autosomal dominant (designated as DI-CMT or CMTDI) or autosomal recessive (RI-CMT or CMTRI)

**QUESTION 22.** Which of the following is the electrophysiologic feature that distinguishes the demyelinating types of Charcot-Marie-Tooth disease from immune-mediated acquired demyelinating neuropathies?
- A. Conduction block
- B. Temporal dispersion
- C. Reduction of compound muscle action potential (CMAP) and sensory nerve action potential (SNAP) amplitudes
- D. Nerve conduction velocity greater than 35 m/s in the upper extremity
- E. Uniform slowing of nerve conduction velocities

**ANSWER:** E. Uniform slowing of nerve conduction velocities

**COMMENTS AND DISCUSSION**
- In hereditary demyelinating neuropathies such as demyelinating types of CMT, nerve conduction study (NCS) typically shows uniform or diffuse slowing, since demyelination in these disorders occurs diffusely.
- Nerve conduction velocity (NCV) in demyelinating CMT is typically less than 38 m/s in the forearms.
- In contrast, in immune-mediated acquired demyelinating neuropathies, demyelination occurs in a multifocal distribution. Evidence of focal demyelination on NCS includes focal slowing, temporal dispersion, and conduction block.
- Reduction of CMAP and SNAP amplitudes is a feature of axonal loss, rather than demyelination. NCV greater than 35 m/s in the forearm is not in the demyelinating range, and, therefore, suggests a primary axonal process.

**QUESTION 23.** An 8-month-old baby boy is referred for congenital hypotonia. There is weakness of all extremities, and the infant has recently developed respiratory difficulty. Reflexes are reduced in all extremities. Nerve conduction study reveals conduction velocity of 10 m/s in all tested nerves in both the upper and lower extremities. There is no conduction block. Which of the following genetic mutations is the most common mutation responsible for the disease in this patient?
- A. *GDAP1* mutation
- B. *GJB1* mutation
- C. *MFN2* mutation
- D. *PMP22* duplication
- E. *PMP22* deletion

**ANSWER:** D. *PMP22* duplication

**COMMENTS AND DISCUSSION**
- The most likely diagnosis in this baby is Déjerine-Sottas syndrome (DSS), aka CMT3.
- Both DSS and CMT3 are old nomenclature.
- Patients with DSS have various mutations including *PMP22* duplication (most common), *MPZ*, *EGR2*, and *PRX*.
- Thus, DSS is now classified under other CMT categories according to the responsible gene.
- However, the term DSS may still be useful in identifying the severe phenotype of demyelinating CMT forms.
- For example, if this patient has *PMP22* duplication, they would be classified as *severe CMT1A, DSS phenotype*.
- DSS typically presents in an infantile period due to very severe neuropathy. Patients can present with hypotonia, generalized weakness, and respiratory failure. Nerve conduction velocity is in demyelinating range, and typically extremely slow as in this patient (10 m/s or even less).

**QUESTION 24.** Which of the following is the distinguishing electrophysiologic feature of hereditary neuropathy with liability to pressure palsies (HNPP)?
A. Markedly prolonged distal motor latencies at non-entrapment sites
B. Focal slowing or conduction blocks at common entrapment sites
C. Focal slowing or conduction blocks at non-entrapment sites
D. Uniform or diffuse slowing of nerve conduction velocities
E. Reduced compound muscle action potential (CMAP) amplitudes from both proximal and distal stimulation sites

**ANSWER:** B. Focal slowing or conduction blocks at common entrapment sites

**COMMENTS AND DISCUSSION**
- In hereditary neuropathy with liability to pressure palsies (HNPP), there is evidence of focal demyelination characterized by focal myelin swelling (tomacula) at common entrapment sites on nerve pathology. On nerve conduction study, there is focal slowing or conduction block at common entrapment sites such as the ulnar nerve at the elbow, median nerve at the wrist, or peroneal nerve at the fibular neck.
  - This contrasts with uniform or diffuse slowing often seen in other hereditary demyelinating neuropathies such as demyelinating CMT forms.
  - This is also in contrast to acquired demyelinating polyneuropathies such as chronic inflammatory demyelinating polyneuropathy (CIDP) or multifocal motor neuropathy (MMN), where evidence of focal demyelination including focal slowing and conduction blocks typically occurs at non-entrapment sites such as the ulnar or median nerves in the forearm.
- Markedly prolonged distal motor latencies at non-entrapment sites are suggestive of distal demyelination. This can be seen most prominently in anti-myelin–associated glycoprotein (MAG) neuropathy, which classically presents with the distal acquired demyelinating symmetrical (DADS) phenotype.
- Reduced CMAP amplitudes from both proximal and distal stimulation sites are suggestive of primary axonal pathology.

**QUESTION 25.** A 10-year-old boy developed an episode of weakness and numbness of the left face, arm, and leg, as well as dysarthria lasting for 1 hour. The symptoms resolved spontaneously. On examination, pes cavus was noted. He had mild weakness and impaired sensation of all modalities in both distal lower extremities, as well as absent ankle reflexes. Magnetic resonance imaging (MRI) of the brain was unremarkable. You suspected Charcot-Marie-Tooth disease. Which of the following genetic mutations is most likely found in this patient?
A. *GDAP1* mutation
B. *GJB1* mutation
C. *PMP22* deletion
D. *MPZ* mutation
E. *PMP22* duplication

**ANSWER:** B. *GJB1* mutation

**COMMENTS AND DISCUSSION**
- This patient most likely has CMT1X. A stroke-like episode is an important clue in this patient.
- In addition to stroke-like episodes, patients with CMT1X can have split-hand syndrome and white matter abnormalities on brain magnetic resonance imaging (MRI).
- CMT1X is due to mutations in the *GJB1* gene encoding connexin 32 (aka gap junction beta 1 [GJB1]) protein.
- In addition to *GJB1* mutations (CMT1X), subcortical white matter abnormalities are also seen in *MFN2* mutations (CMT2A).

**QUESTION 26.** Which of the following Charcot-Marie-Tooth genes has the pathophysiological mechanism that is closely linked to mitochondrial dynamics?
A. *GJB1*
B. *MFN2*
C. *MPZ*
D. *PMP22*
E. *TRPV4*

**ANSWER:** B. *MFN2*

**COMMENTS AND DISCUSSION**
- The *MFN2* gene, which is responsible for CMT2A, encodes mitofusin 2. This protein has an important role in mitochondrial dynamics, specifically mitochondrial fusion.
- The *GDAP1* gene responsible for CMT4A has an important role in mitochondrial fission.
- Mitochondrial mechanisms are not implicated in the pathogenesis of *GJB1*, *MPZ*, *PMP22*, or *TRPV4* mutations.

**QUESTION 27.** Vocal cord involvement is most likely a manifestation of Charcot-Marie-Tooth disease due to which of the following genes?
A. *GJB1*
B. *MPZ*
C. *MFN2*
D. *PMP22*
E. *TRPV4*

**ANSWER:** E. *TRPV4*

**COMMENTS AND DISCUSSION**
- Vocal cord paralysis is a phenotypic clue that can be seen in some forms of CMT including CMT2C (due to *TRPV4* mutations), CMT4B1 (due to *MTMR2* mutations), and CMT4A (due to *GDAP1* mutations).
- Vocal cord paralysis in not encountered with *GJB1*, *MPZ*, *MFN2*, or *PMP22* mutations.

**QUESTION 28.** A 20-year-old woman has had recurrent episodes of painless mononeuropathies. At age 18 years, she developed right peroneal neuropathy that resolved after 2 weeks. Six months ago, she developed left carpal tunnel syndrome, which resolved after 2 weeks. Two days ago, she developed numbness of the right ring and little fingers. Examination reveals grade 3/5 weakness of the right abductor digiti minimi, first dorsal interossei, and flexor digitorum profundus of digits 4 and 5. If a nerve biopsy of the affected nerve is performed, which of the following is most likely found?
A. Myelin ovoid
B. Onion bulb formation
C. Segmental demyelination
D. Focal swelling of the myelin sheath
E. Invasion of mixed inflammatory cells into the blood vessel wall

**ANSWER:** D. Focal swelling of the myelin sheath

**COMMENTS AND DISCUSSION**
- This patient has recurrent entrapment neuropathy: peroneal neuropathy (likely at the fibular head), carpal tunnel syndrome, and ulnar neuropathy (likely at the elbow). The most likely diagnosis is hereditary neuropathy with liability to pressure palsies (HNPP).
- The characteristic nerve pathology in this disorder is focal swelling of myelin sheath, called tomacula (meaning sausage). HNPP is due to *PMP22* deletion, in contrast to *PMP22* duplication in CMT1A.

- Myelin ovoid is a feature that is suggestive of primary axonal degeneration.
- Onion bulb formation is due to concentric layers of Schwann cell processes, and indicative of repetitive demyelination and remyelination. Diffuse onion bulb formation can be seen in demyelinating CMT such as CMT1A.
- Segmental demyelination is suggestive of acquired demyelination such as acute inflammatory demyelinating polyneuropathy (AIDP) and chronic inflammatory demyelinating polyneuropathy (CIDP).
- Invasion of mixed inflammatory cells into blood vessel walls (or intramural infiltration of inflammatory cells) is a feature of vasculitic neuropathies.

**QUESTION 29.** Which of the following features argues against the diagnosis of distal hereditary motor neuropathy (dHMN)?
A. Subtle sensory impairment on examination
B. Marked atrophy of hands and feet
C. Absent ankle reflexes
D. Reduced compound muscle action potential (CMAP) amplitudes on nerve conduction studies
E. Small short-duration polyphasic motor unit action potentials (MUAPs) on needle electromyography (EMG)

**ANSWER:** E. Small short-duration polyphasic motor unit action potentials (MUAPs) on needle electromyography (EMG)

**COMMENTS AND DISCUSSION**
- Distal hereditary motor neuropathy (dHMN) is a group of hereditary neuropathies that lie within the same spectrum of Charcot-Marie-Tooth disease (CMT).
  ○ Lower motor neuron weakness and atrophy of distal extremities
  ○ Reduced or absent reflexes
  ○ Sensory exam is normal or only minimally abnormal.
  ○ Upper motor neuron features may be present.
  ○ Nerve conduction study demonstrates intact SNAPs and reduced CMAP amplitudes.
  ○ Needle EMG is useful to differentiate between dHMN and distal myopathies
    - In dHMN, there are large, long-duration MUAPs with reduced recruitment.
    - In distal myopathy, there are small, short-duration polyphasic MUAPs with early recruitment.
- There are phenotypic overlaps between dHMN and CMT and hereditary spastic paraparesis.

**QUESTION 30.** A 12-year-old boy has had worsening weakness of both ankles and feet since the age of 8 years. Lately, he has had weakness of both hands and visual difficulties. Examination reveals distal weakness, atrophy, sensory loss, and areflexia. Funduscopic examination reveals bilateral optic atrophy. Brain magnetic resonance imaging (MRI) reveals subcortical white matter hyperintensities on the T2-weighted sequence. Mutation in which of the following genes is most likely found in this patient?
A. *MFN2*
B. *PMP22*
C. *GJB1*
D. *OPA1*
E. *MT-ND1* in the mitochondrial DNA

**ANSWER:** A. *MFN2*

**COMMENTS AND DISCUSSION**
- Among various types of Charcot-Marie-Tooth disease (CMT), optic atrophy is a clue for CMT2A, which is due to *MFN2* mutations. The *MFN2* gene encodes mitofusin 2, which has an important role in mitochondrial dynamics, specifically mitochondrial fusion.
- Patients with CMT2A can have optic atrophy and sensorineural hearing loss, which may be seen in mitochondrial diseases. In addition, patients with CMT2A may have white matter abnormalities on brain magnetic resonance imaging (MRI).
- *PMP22* deletion or duplication is not associated with optic atrophy.
- Mutations in the *OPA1* gene are associated with autosomal dominant optic atrophy. However, peripheral neuropathy is not a feature of this disorder.

- Mutations in the *MT-ND1* gene in the mitochondrial genome are associated with Leber hereditary optic neuropathy (LHON). LHON typically affects young males, and the classic clinical presentation is visual loss due to optic neuropathy, which commonly involves both eyes. Peripheral neuropathy is not a feature of LHON.

**The following answer options are for QUESTIONS 31 through 33.**

*Match the nerve biopsy with the gene.*

A.

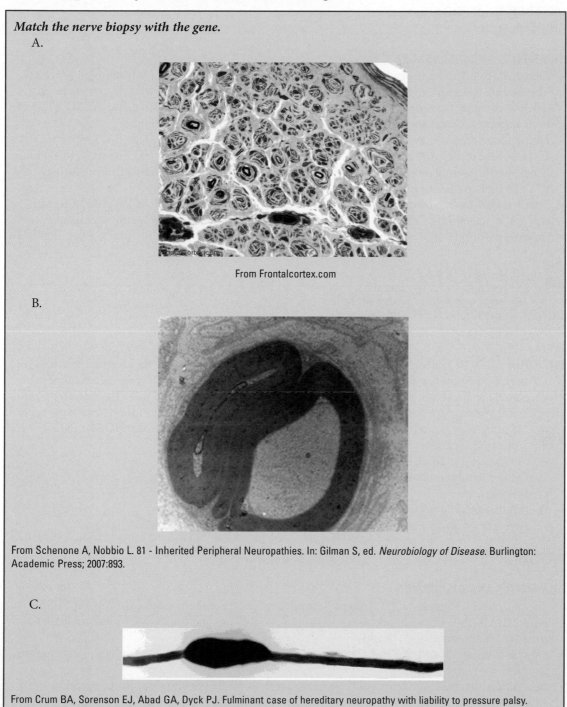

From Frontalcortex.com

B.

From Schenone A, Nobbio L. 81 - Inherited Peripheral Neuropathies. In: Gilman S, ed. *Neurobiology of Disease*. Burlington: Academic Press; 2007:893.

C.

From Crum BA, Sorenson EJ, Abad GA, Dyck PJ. Fulminant case of hereditary neuropathy with liability to pressure palsy. *Muscle Nerve*. 2000;23(6):979–983.

**QUESTION 31.** *PMP22* duplication
**ANSWER:** Figure A.

**QUESTION 32.** *PMP22* deletion
**ANSWER:** Figure C.

**QUESTION 33.** *MTMR2* mutation
**ANSWER:** Figure B.

**COMMENTS AND DISCUSSION**
- Figure A demonstrates onion bulb formation, which is concentric layers of Schwann cell processes. This finding is suggestive of repetitive demyelination and remyelination, which occurs in chronic demyelinating process such as demyelinating forms of Charcot-Marie-Tooth disease (CMT). CMT1A is an autosomal dominant demyelinating CMT caused by *PMP22* duplication.
- Figure B demonstrates focally folded myelin sheath, which can be seen in some CMT forms including CMT4B (due to *MTMR2* mutations) and CMT4A (due to *GDAP1* mutations). However, this finding is not specific to only these two CMT forms, and can also rarely be seen in other forms such as CMT1B (due to *MPZ* mutations).
- Figure C demonstrates focal swelling of myelin sheath, called *tomacula* (from Latin meaning sausage). Tomaculous neuropathy is a characteristic feature of hereditary neuropathy with liability to pressure palsies (HNPP), which is due to *PMP22* deletion.

 **HIGH-YIELD FACT**

| | |
|---|---|
| **CMT1A** | **large** gene (*PMP22* duplication) |
| **HNPP** | **small** gene (*PMP22* deletion) |

**QUESTION 34.** A 25-year-old man has had worsening lancinating pain in his hands and feet since age 14 years. In the past few years, he also has weakness of both feet and hands. On examination, there are chronic bilateral foot ulcers, as well as amputation of some fingers and toes. There is loss of pinprick and temperature sensation, as well as proprioception and vibration in the bilateral hands and feet. Motor power is grade 4 in distal lower and upper extremities. What is the **MOST LIKELY** diagnosis in this patient?
A. Charcot-Marie-Tooth disease
B. Distal hereditary motor neuropathy
C. Fabry disease
D. Familial amyloid polyneuropathy
E. Hereditary sensory and autonomic neuropathy

**ANSWER:** E. Hereditary sensory and autonomic neuropathy

**COMMENTS AND DISCUSSION**
- The most likely diagnosis in this patient is hereditary sensory and autonomic neuropathy (HSAN), especially HSAN1. Chronic foot ulcers and amputation of toes and fingers are important diagnostic clues for HSAN, especially HSAN1.
- Small and unmyelinated (Aδ and C) nerve fibers are predominantly involved, resulting in autonomic features.
- In addition, there is involvement of large nerve fibers, as evident by impaired proprioception and vibration on examination.
- There are various forms of HSAN, but the most common one is HSAN1.
- General clinical features: lancinating leg pain and loss of pain and temperature sensation, resulting in hand or foot ulcers, osteomyelitis, and eventually amputation (Fig. 15.3)
- HSAN1
  ◦ Autosomal dominant, axonal neuropathy
  ◦ Autonomic features may not be prominent
  ◦ Due to *SPTLC1* (HSAN1A) and *SPTLC2* (HSAN1C) mutations, and other genes

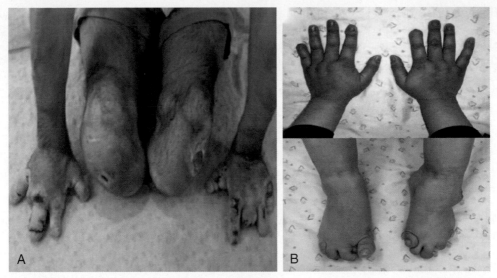

**Fig. 15.3 Hereditary sensory autonomic neuropathy (HSAN).** This figure demonstrates two siblings with HSAN2A due to the *WNK1/HSN2* mutation. HSAN is characterized by loss of pain and temperature sensation resulting in chronic ulcers and amputations in the upper and lower extremities. From Rahmani B, Fekrmandi F, Ahadi K, et al. A novel nonsense mutation in *WNK1/HSN2* associated with sensory neuropathy and limb destruction in four siblings of a large Iranian pedigree. *BMC Neurol.* 2018;18(1):195.

- HSAN2D
  - Autosomal recessive, axonal neuropathy
  - Due to *SCN9A* mutations encoding Nav1.7 voltage-gated sodium channel
  - This gene is also responsible for familial (aka primary) erythromelalgia manifesting as red hands and feet.

**QUESTION 35.** A 29-year-old woman presents with fluctuating episodes of burning sensation in bilateral hands and feet since childhood. On examination, redness and allodynia of the bilateral hands and feet are noted. Which of the following genes is most likely associated with this condition?
  A. *ABCA1*
  B. *CLCN1*
  C. *GLA*
  D. *SCN9A*
  E. *TTR*

**ANSWER:** D. *SCN9A*

**COMMENTS AND DISCUSSION (see also comments and discussion from Question 34)**
- Burning sensation in both hands and feet since childhood suggests a hereditary neuropathy involving small nerve fibers. Redness of bilateral hands and feet on examination, called erythromelalgia, is an important diagnostic clue.
- The diagnosis in this patient is most likely *familial erythromelalgia*, which is due to mutations in the *SCN9A* gene encoding the Nav1.7 voltage-gated sodium channel. Patients with familial erythromelalgia typically present with recurrent episodes of burning sensation in hands and feet, along with erythromelalgia.
- *ABCA1* mutations are associated with Tangier disease. *CLCN1* mutations involving the chloride channel gene are associated with myotonia congenita. Mutations in the *GLA* gene, encoding the alpha-galactosidase enzyme, cause Fabry disease. Mutations in the *TTR* gene is responsible for transthyretin amyloidosis, a type of familial amyloid polyneuropathy.

**QUESTION 36.** A 42-year-old woman has had numbness of both hands and feet since age 24. She also has had difficulty speaking and swallowing in the past 5 years. Examination reveals dysarthria and marked limitation of extraocular movements in all directions. Motor power is normal. Sensory examination shows impaired pinprick sensation and markedly impaired proprioception and vibration in both lower extremities. Reflexes are absent in the lower extremities. She walks with a wide-based gait. Which of the following statements is **CORRECT** regarding the disease in this patient?

A. This disorder is due to a mutation in the mitochondrial DNA.

B. This disorder is associated with nuclear DNA depletion.

C. There is a point mutation in the tRNA leucine (tRNA$^{Leu(UUR)}$) gene.

D. Mutations in the same gene can also cause chronic progressive external ophthalmoplegia (CPEO).

E. Muscle biopsy in this patient does not have ragged-red fibers or cytochrome oxidase (COX)-negative fibers, since there is no weakness on examination.

**ANSWER:** D. Mutations in the same gene can also cause chronic progressive external ophthalmoplegia (CPEO).

**COMMENTS AND DISCUSSION**

- This patient has *sensory ataxic neuropathy, dysarthria, and ophthalmoplegia (SANDO).*
- SANDO is a mitochondrial disorder caused by mutations of the *POLG1* gene, which encodes the gamma subunit of DNA polymerase in the nuclear genome, not in the mitochondrial genome. Mutations in this gene result in mitochondrial DNA depletion. This disorder is inherited in an autosomal recessive manner and does not exhibit mitochondrial inheritance, since it is caused by mutations in the nuclear genome. Despite no apparent weakness or muscle involvement, muscle biopsy of patients with SANDO may show ragged-red fibers and cytochrome C oxidase (COX)–negative fibers, as seen in other mitochondrial myopathies.
- *POLG1* mutations are also associated CPEO. The point mutation (m.3243A>G) in the tRNA leucine (tRNA$^{Leu(UUR)}$) gene in the mitochondrial DNA is associated with mitochondrial encephalomyopathy, lactic acidosis, and stroke-like episodes (MELAS).
- Other inherited neuropathies associated with mitochondrial diseases include:
  - CMT associated with abnormal mitochondrial dynamics
    - Impaired mitochondrial fusion: *MFN2* gene (CMT2A)
    - Impaired mitochondrial fission: *GDAP1* gene (CMT4A)
  - Neuropathy, ataxia, and retinitis pigmentosa (NARP)
    - In the same phenotypic spectrum as maternally-inherited Leigh syndrome (MILS)
    - NARP is due to mitochondrial mutations in the same gene as MILS.

**QUESTION 37.** A 35-year-old man presents for an evaluation of peripheral neuropathy. Oral examination reveals the finding in the figure below. Which of the following is associated with this disease?

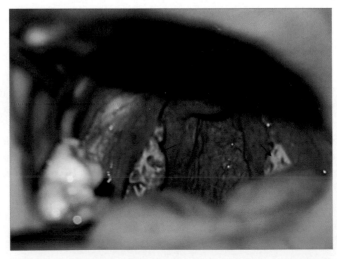

From Puntoni M, Sbrana F, Bigazzi F, et al. Tangier disease. *Am J Cardiovasc Drugs.* 2012;12:303–311.

A. Angiokeratoma
B. Dysphagia
C. Leukodystrophy
D. Reduced high-density lipoprotein (HDL) cholesterol
E. Myopathy

**ANSWER:** D. Reduced high-density lipoprotein (HDL) cholesterol

## COMMENTS AND DISCUSSION

- This figure demonstrates orange-colored tonsils. This finding, along with polyneuropathy is suggestive of *Tangier disease*.
- Dysphagia, myopathy, and leukodystrophy are not features of Tangier disease.
- Angiokeratomas are small dark red papules seen in Fabry disease.
- Metabolic neuropathies are a group of inherited neuropathies caused by an identifiable enzyme deficiency. These include:
  - Tangier disease
    - Peripheral neuropathy with orange-colored tonsils
    - Patients with Tangier disease may have pseudo-syringomyelia characterized by dissociation between pain and temperature impairment, and proprioception and vibration impairment.
    - Due to mutations in the *ABCA1* gene encoding an ATP-binding cassette transporter protein
    - Mutations in this gene results in reduced high-density lipoprotein (HDL) levels.
  - Fabry disease
    - Angiokeratoma corporis diffusum are small dark red papules in the periumbilical region and bathing trunk areas and are highly suggestive of Fabry disease.
    - Brain involvement: stroke, transient ischemic attack, and T1-weighted magnetic resonance imaging (MRI) hyperintensity at the bilateral posterior thalami
    - Renal involvement: renal failure, proteinuria
    - Cardiac involvement: cardiac arrhythmia, left ventricular hypertrophy
    - Peripheral nerve involvement: small fiber neuropathy resulting in acroparesthesia (paresthesia of the hands and feet)
    - X-linked recessive: no male-to-male transmission; females can also be affected due to skewed inactivation of X chromosome, but any symptoms are usually less severe
    - Mutations in the *GLA* gene encoding the alpha-galactosidase enzyme
    - Enzyme replacement therapy is available.
- Leukodystrophies are also associated with peripheral neuropathies.
  - X-linked adrenoleukodystrophy
    - In children, there are posterior-predominant white matter changes.
    - Neuropathies typically occur in an adult form: adrenomyeloneuropathy (AMN).
    - In AMN, there is involvement of both the spinal cord and the peripheral nerves, resulting in a combination of upper and lower motor neuron features.
    - X-linked adrenoleukodystrophy is inherited in an X-linked recessive manner, and can affect both males and females.
    - Due to mutations in the *ABCD1* gene encoding an ATP-binding cassette transporter protein
  - Metachromatic leukodystrophy
    - Variable age at onset; can present in children and adults
    - Brain MRI demonstrates leukodystrophy with sparing of subcortical U-fibers.
    - Peripheral nerve can be involved, resulting in a combination of upper and lower motor neuron features; mainly a demyelinating process
    - Due to mutations of the *ARSA* gene encoding the arylsulfatase A enzyme
  - Krabbe disease (aka globoid cell leukodystrophy)
    - Can be demyelinating or axonal neuropathy
    - Due to mutations in the *GALC* gene encoding the galactocerebrosidase enzyme

**QUESTION 38.**  Which of the following medications should be avoided in patients with Charcot-Marie-Tooth disease?
  A.  Cisplatin
  B.  Nitrofurantoin
  C.  Paclitaxel
  D.  Vincristine
  E.  All of the above

**ANSWER:** E. All of the above

**COMMENTS AND DISCUSSION**
- All of the above medications should be avoided in patients with Charcot-Marie-Tooth disease (CMT), since these are known to be toxic to the peripheral nerves.
- The use of these agents in the setting of CMT can worsen peripheral neuropathy.

**SUGGESTED READING**

Cavallaro T, Tagliapietra M, Fabrizi GM, et al. Hereditary neuropathies: A pathological perspective. *J Peripher Nerv Syst.* 2021;26 Suppl 2:S42–S60.

Frasquet M, Sevilla T. Hereditary motor neuropathies. *Curr Opin Neurol.* 2022;35(5):562–570.

Houlden H, Blake J, Reilly MM. Hereditary sensory neuropathies. *Curr Opin Neurol.* 2004;17(5):569–577.

Klein CJ. Charcot-Marie-Tooth Disease and Other Hereditary Neuropathies. *Continuum (Minneap Minn).* 2020;26(5):1224–1256.

Pisciotta C, Shy ME. Neuropathy. *Handb Clin Neurol.* 2018;148:653–665.

Rajabally YA, Adams D, Latour P, Attarian S. Hereditary and inflammatory neuropathies: a review of reported associations, mimics and misdiagnoses. *J Neurol Neurosurg Psychiatry.* 2016;87(10):1051–1060.

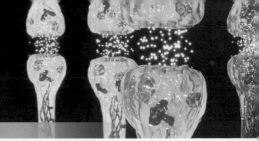

# CHAPTER 16

# Neuromuscular Junction (NMJ) Disorders

## PART 1 | PRACTICE TEST

**Q1.** Which process produces miniature end plate potentials?
A. Influx of $Ca^{2+}$ into the presynaptic nerve terminal
B. Synaptobrevin binding to syntaxin
C. Spontaneous release of acetylcholine (ACh) vesicles into the synaptic cleft
D. Hydrolysis of ACh by acetylcholinesterase
E. Internalization of ACh receptors

**Q2.** Which protein is essential for the exocytosis of synaptic vesicles in the presynaptic nerve terminal?
A. Choline
B. Synaptobrevin
C. Contactin
D. Agrin
E. Lipoprotein receptor–related protein 4

**Q3.** Which protein plays an important role in clustering, organizing, and stabilizing acetylcholine receptors in the postsynaptic membrane?
A. MuSK
B. Syntaxin
C. Contactin
D. Dystroglycan
E. Desmin

**Q4.** Myasthenia gravis (MG) is increasingly recognized as a seropositive disorder. However, which of the following antibodies has not been associated with MG?
A. Antibody to muscle-specific kinase (MuSK)
B. Antibody to agrin
C. Antibody to acetylcholine receptor (AChR)
D. Antibody to P/Q-type voltage-gated calcium channel
E. Antibody to low-density lipoprotein receptor–related protein 4 (LRP4)

**Q5.** A 30-year-old woman presents with weakness in the evening. She has difficulty getting up from the couch after watching a nighttime movie with her husband. She feels normal in the morning. You are considering generalized myasthenia gravis (MG). Which of the following statements is **CORRECT** regarding this disorder?
A. Only T cell–mediated processes initiate the immunologic attack.
B. Acetylcholine receptor (AChR) antibodies are positive in all patients with generalized MG.
C. Muscle-specific kinase (MuSK) antibodies are more commonly positive in older men.
D. Simplification of the postsynaptic membrane is a common pathological finding.
E. All patients with thymoma develop MG.

**Q6.** A 20-year-old woman presents with ptosis and ophthalmoplegia for 2 years. Which of the following symptoms is an **ATYPICAL** presentation for myasthenia gravis?
A. Unilateral ptosis
B. Ophthalmoplegia without diplopia
C. Neck flexor weakness
D. Proximal muscle weakness
E. Facial weakness

**Q7.** The curtain eyelid sign is performed by:
A. manually raising the less-involved eyelid and observing worse ptosis in the contralateral lid.
B. manually raising both eyelids and observing downward movements of both eyes.
C. manually raising the more ptotic eyelid and observing elevation of the contralateral eyelid.
D. demonstrating improvement of ptosis after brief eye closure.
E. manually raising the more ptotic lid, causing increased ptosis on the opposite side.

**Q8.** Which of the following statements is **CORRECT** regarding myasthenia gravis (MG)?
A. Patients with ocular MG usually have fixed symmetric ptosis.
B. Eighty percent of patients with ocular myasthenia have positive acetylcholine receptor (AChR) antibody.
C. Anti-MuSK (muscle-specific kinase) antibody-positive patients usually have isolated ocular symptoms.
D. Thymoma is present in 50% of patients with ocular myasthenia.
E. In purely ocular MG for more than 2 years, there is a 90% likelihood that it remains ocular.

**Q9.** A 35-year-old woman presents with right ptosis and diplopia for 6 months. Initially, she was thought to have a lazy eye; however, she had to change prism glasses three times in the past 6 months. Which of the following statements is **CORRECT** regarding the office edrophonium (Tensilon) test in the diagnosis of myasthenia gravis (MG)?
A. The test is done infrequently, since it is not often available.
B. Atropine injection is required immediately following edrophonium.
C. Cardiac monitoring is required when atropine is not available.
D. The test has a low sensitivity for symptoms restricted to the eyes.
E. Other myopathies and brain stem lesions may have false-positive tests.

**Q10.** A 20-year-old woman is referred for subjective diplopia and mild left ptosis mostly in the evening. There is no clear ophthalmoparesis, ptosis, limb weakness or fatigability on examination. Which of the following test result will confirm the diagnosis of ocular myasthenia?
A. Diplopia improves with the ice pack test.
B. Diplopia improves with edrophonium test.
C. A 5% decremental response is seen on slow repetitive nerve stimulation.
D. Abnormal jitter and blocking are present on single-fiber electromyography.
E. Thymic hyperplasia is present on chest computed tomography.

**Q11.** A 60-year-old woman with acetylcholine receptor (AChR) antibody-positive generalized myasthenia gravis (MG), controlled on prednisone and azathioprine, presents with dysarthria, dysphagia, and respiratory failure requiring intubation. A few days before admission she developed dysuria and fever and received antibiotics. Which of the following statements is **CORRECT**?
A. She may have coexisting anti-MuSK antibodies.
B. Double-seropositive MG patients have a reduced risk of developing a myasthenic crisis.
C. Up to 80% of all MG patients experience at least one episode of a myasthenic crisis.
D. A myasthenic crisis is commonly triggered by infection or medications.
E. The current mortality rate for myasthenic crisis is ~50%.

**Q12.** A 48-year-old woman with generalized myasthenia gravis presents to the emergency department with dysuria and high-grade fever for one day. She is diagnosed with a urinary tract infection. She currently takes prednisone 50 mg daily and azathioprine 100 mg daily. Which of the following antibiotics is most appropriate in this case?
A. Ceftriaxone
B. Ciprofloxacin
C. Azithromycin
D. Amikacin
E. Erythromycin

**Q13.** Which of the following is the **BEST** predictor of respiratory failure in a patient with worsening myasthenia gravis (MG) symptoms?
A. Severe weakness of hip flexors
B. Severe neck flexor muscle weakness
C. Severe facial diplegia
D. Single breath count of 35
E. Complete external ophthalmoplegia

**Q14.** Effective treatments in myasthenic crisis are:
1. intravenous methylprednisolone.
2. intravenous immunoglobulin (IVIG).
3. rituximab.
4. plasma exchange (PLEX).
A. 1 and 2.
B. 1 and 3.
C. 1 and 4.
D. 2 and 3.
E. 2 and 4.

**Q15.** A woman presented with left ptosis and diplopia and was diagnosed with ocular myasthenia. Pyridostigmine up to 90 mg four times a day fails to improve her symptoms. Which of the following treatments is the next most appropriate step?
A. Prednisone
B. Azathioprine
C. Intravenous immunoglobulin (IVIG)
D. Eculizumab
E. Rituximab

**Q16.** Which of the following patients is the best candidate for thymectomy (all have a negative chest computed tomography [CT] for thymoma)?
A. A 25-year-old woman with seronegative ocular myasthenia, controlled with pyridostigmine and prednisone
B. A 30-year-old man with acetylcholine receptor (AChR) antibody-positive generalized myasthenia gravis (MG), currently admitted for myasthenic crisis
C. A 68-year-old woman with muscle-specific kinase (MuSK) antibody–positive MG, well controlled with rituximab
D. A 40-year-old woman with AChR antibody–positive generalized MG, with lingering symptoms
E. A 15-year-old girl with AChR antibody–positive generalized MG, with stable symptoms

**Q17.** Which of the following patients is the best candidate for eculizumab therapy?
- A. A 25-year-old woman with acetylcholine receptor (AChR) antibody-positive ocular MG, well controlled with pyridostigmine
- B. A 30-year-old woman with AChR antibody-positive generalized myasthenia gravis (MG), refractory to prednisone
- C. A 30-year-old woman with muscle-specific kinase (MuSK) antibody-positive MG, refractory to prednisone
- D. A 40-year-old woman with AChR antibody-positive generalized MG, with stable disease
- E. A 70-year-old man with positive-AChR antibody-positive ocular MG, with a contraindication for prednisone

**Q18.** What is the mechanism of action of efgartigimod?
- A. Inhibits cholinesterase in the synaptic cleft
- B. Targets B cells
- C. Reduces immunoglobulin G (IgG) and pathogenic autoantibody levels by reducing IgG recycling
- D. Blocks the formation of the membrane attack complex (MAC)
- E. Increases the expression of anti-inflammatory genes

**Q19.** You recommended thymectomy to your 25-year-old patient with generalized myasthenia gravis (MG) with positive acetylcholine receptor (AChR) antibody. How would you counsel this patient regarding the outcome for thymectomy in non-thymomatous MG?
- A. MG goes into remission immediately after surgery.
- B. Able to discontinue pyridostigmine within 3 months after surgery
- C. Able to discontinue corticosteroid within 3 months after surgery
- D. Able to reduce corticosteroid dose in 6–12 months after surgery
- E. Surgery decreases the risk for progression to malignant thymoma.

**Q20.** A 30-year-old woman presents with flaccid dysarthria and dysphagia for 2 months. Weakness of proximal muscles is graded at 4/5 in both the upper and lower extremities. Anti-MuSK (muscle-specific kinase) antibodies are positive. Which of the following is the most effective treatment in this condition?
- A. Pyridostigmine
- B. Methotrexate
- C. Intravenous immunoglobulin (IVIG)
- D. Rituximab
- E. Eculizumab

**Q21.** A 25-year-old woman with acetylcholine receptor (AChR) antibody-positive generalized myasthenia gravis (MG) for 2 years is in remission, on pyridostigmine 60 mg every 8 hours and prednisolone 10 mg per day. She is planning on getting pregnant. Which of the following medications is **MOST** contraindicated in pregnancy?
- A. Pyridostigmine
- B. Prednisolone
- C. Azathioprine
- D. Mycophenolate mofetil
- E. Intravenous immunglobulin (IVIG)

**Q22.** Which test result is seen in presynaptic neuromuscular junction (NMJ) disorders?
- A. Reduced sensory nerve action potential amplitudes
- B. Slowed motor conduction velocity
- C. Incremental response on slow (low-frequency) repetitive nerve stimulation (RNS)
- D. Incremental response on rapid (high-frequency) RNS
- E. Normal single-fiber electromyography (EMG)

**Q23.** A 50-year-old man presents with proximal muscle weakness for 6 months. Symptoms are worse in the morning and partially improved in the evening. He has no sensory symptoms but he reports dry mouth in the past several months. Examination is notable for weakness of the proximal lower extremities and absnet deep tendon reflexes. Which of the following antibodies is the **MOST LIKELY** to be positive in this patient?
- A. Acetylcholine receptor (AChR) antibodies
- B. Muscle-specific kinase (MuSK) antibodies
- C. Voltage-gated calcium channel antibodies
- D. Voltage-gated potassium channel antibodies
- E. 3-Hydroxy-3-methylglutaryl-CoA reductase antibodies

**Q24.** Which of the following symptoms is commonly seen in Lambert-Eaton myasthenic syndrome:
- A. Dry mouth
- B. Diarrhea
- C. Persistent paresthesia
- D. Heliotrope rash
- E. Calcinosis

**Q25.** With which of the following paraneoplastic syndromes is Lambert-Eaton myasthenic syndrome most commonly associated?
- A. Subacute cerebellar degeneration
- B. Sensory neuronopathy
- C. Opsoclonus-myoclonus syndrome
- D. Limbic encephalitis
- E. Thymomatous myasthenia gravis (MG)

**Q26.** A 45-year-old man presents with proximal leg muscle weakness for 8 months. He recently was diagnosed with small-cell lung cancer. You suspect Lambert-Eaton myasthenic syndrome (LEMS). Which of the following results on repetitive nerve stimulation (RNS) of the abductor pollicis brevis muscle is a typical finding in LEMS?
A. A 20% incremental response on 3-Hz RNS
B. A 20% decremental response on 3-Hz RNS
C. A 20% decremental response on 30-Hz RNS
D. A 20% incremental response on 30-Hz RNS
E. A 5% decremental response on 3-Hz RNS

**Q27.** Which of the following medications is **NOT** a treatment option in LEMS?
A. Fluoxetine
B. 3,4-Diaminopyridine
C. Amifampridine phosphate
D. Pyridostigmine
E. Intravenous immunoglobulin (IVIG)

**Q28.** A 30-year-old woman presents with facial diplegia and bulbar weakness followed by descending generalized weakness in the past 2 days. A day before the event she had a facial injection by her friend for wrinkles. On examination, she was intubated with facial diplegia. She can move her eyes following commands but she cannot move her limbs. Reflexes were absent. What is the most useful investigation?
A. Serum creatine kinase
B. Facial nerve conduction study (NCS) and blink reflexes
C. Needle electromyography (EMG) of proximal muscles
D. 30-Hz repetitive nerve stimulation (RNS)
E. Single-fiber EMG

**Q29.** An 18-year-old man presents with long-standing, slowly progressive, generalized weakness since he was a toddler. Examination showed slow pupillary light responses, scoliosis, and reduced muscle bulk throughout. Neck flexors were graded 3+/5. Motor power was 4+/5 throughout. Reflexes were normal. He had a normal creatine kinase (CK) level, electromyography (EMG), and muscle biopsy. Motor conduction studies did not show repetitive compound muscle action potentials (CMAPs). You suspect a congenital myasthenic syndrome. This patient **MOST LIKELY** has a mutation in which of the following genes?
A. *CHRNE*
B. *RAPSN*
C. *COLQ*
D. *DOK7*
E. *CHAT*

**Q30.** An 18-year-old man is sent to the electromyography (EMG) lab for evaluation of possible seronegative myasthenia gravis (MG). He has bilateral ptosis and generalized weakness. On nerve conduction studies, you observe a small wave following the compound muscle action potential (CMAP) as in the following figure. What is the **MOST LIKELY** diagnosis?
A. Agrin antibody–associated MG
B. Slow-channel congenital myasthenic syndrome
C. Mitochondrial myopathy
D. McArdle disease
E. Myofibrillar myopathy

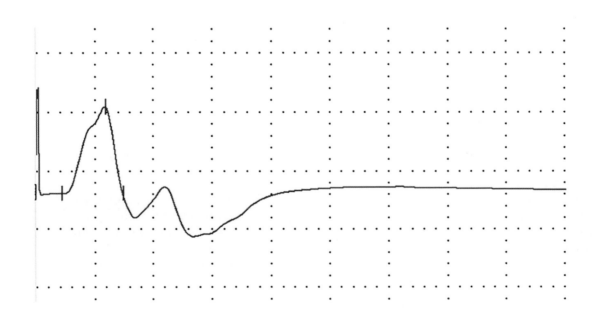

**Q31.** Which two congenital myasthenic syndromes (CMSs) worsen with pyridostigmine?
A. Choline acetyltransferase (*CHAT*) and *RAPSN*-related
B. Slow-channel and *DOK7*-related
C. Fast-channel and slow-channel
D. Acetylcholine receptor deficiency and *CHAT*-related
E. *RAPSN*- and *DOK7*-related

**Q32.** A 42-year-old man had hypotonia, delayed motor milestones, and weakness since birth but without arthrogryposis. He had several episodes of severe weakness with spontaneous improvement for unknown reasons. His older sister also has similar symptoms. On examination, he has a myopathic facies, ptosis, and facial weakness. Weakness is most severe in the shoulder girdle and trunk. Creatine kinase (CK) level was normal. There were mild "myopathic" changes on needle electromyography (EMG) and muscle biopsy. Slow repetitive nerve stimulation (RNS) showed a significant decremental response. Which type of the following congenital myasthenic syndrome (CMS) can mimic the presentation of limb-girdle congenital muscular dystrophy?
A. Choline acetyltransferase deficiency (*CHAT* mutation)
B. Slow-channel
C. Rapsyn deficiency (*RAPSN* mutation)
D. Acetylcholine receptor (AChR) deficiency
E. *DOK7*-related CMS

# PART 2 | QUESTIONS WITH ANSWERS AND DISCUSSION

**QUESTION 1.** Which process produces miniature end plate potentials?
A. Influx of $Ca^{2+}$ into the presynaptic nerve terminal
B. Synaptobrevin binding to syntaxin
C. Spontaneous release of acetylcholine (ACh) vesicles into the synaptic cleft
D. Hydrolysis of ACh by the acetylcholinesterase enzyme
E. Internalization of ACh receptors

**ANSWER:** C. Spontaneous release of acetylcholine (ACh) vesicles into the synaptic cleft

**COMMENTS AND DISCUSSION**
- **Neuromuscular junction (NMJ) physiology**
  - Principal components
    1. Nerve terminal
    2. Synaptic cleft
    3. Postsynaptic membrane
- **Important structures in the NMJ**
  - Nerve terminal contains
    - "Quanta" or discrete units of ACh molecules
    - Choline acetyltransferase needed for ACh synthesis by catalyzing choline and acetate
  - Synaptic cleft contains
    - ACh molecules, released from presynaptic terminal
    - Acetylcholinesterase (AChE)
    - Choline (released by ACh hydrolysis)

- Postsynaptic membrane contains
  - Acetylcholine receptor (AChR)
  - Voltage-gated sodium channels
- **Presynaptic nerve terminal** (Fig. 16.1)
  - Acetylcholine molecules are packed within the vesicles or quanta
  - There are three types of quanta stores.
    - Primary (or immediately available) store: located in the active zone and ready for release
    - Secondary (or mobilization) store: may resupply the primary storage within a few seconds
    - Tertiary (or long-term) store: a reservoir located in the axon and cell body

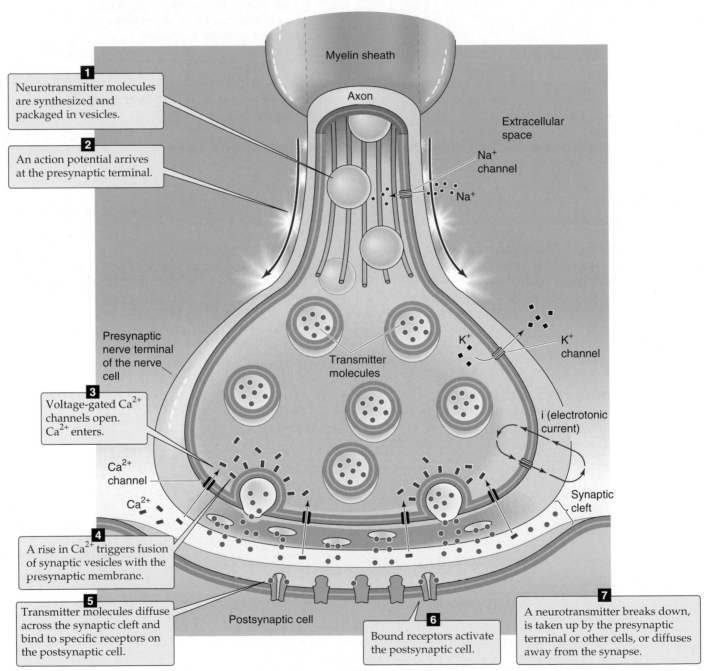

**1** Neurotransmitter molecules are synthesized and packaged in vesicles.

**2** An action potential arrives at the presynaptic terminal.

**3** Voltage-gated Ca²⁺ channels open. Ca²⁺ enters.

**4** A rise in Ca²⁺ triggers fusion of synaptic vesicles with the presynaptic membrane.

**5** Transmitter molecules diffuse across the synaptic cleft and bind to specific receptors on the postsynaptic cell.

**6** Bound receptors activate the postsynaptic cell.

**7** A neurotransmitter breaks down, is taken up by the presynaptic terminal or other cells, or diffuses away from the synapse.

Myelin sheath

Axon

Extracellular space

Na⁺ channel

Na⁺

Presynaptic nerve terminal of the nerve cell

Transmitter molecules

K⁺

K⁺ channel

i (electrotonic current)

Ca²⁺ channel

Ca²⁺

Synaptic cleft

Postsynaptic cell

**Fig. 16.1** A process at the presynaptic nerve terminal in synaptic transmission. From Moczydlowski EG. Synaptic transmission and the neuromuscular junction. In: Boron WF, ed. *Medical Physiology*. 3rd ed. Elsevier; 2017:204–227.e2.

- Spontaneous release of single ACh quanta (leakage) into the synaptic cleft is a normal occurrence → generates miniature end plate potentials (MEPPs)
  - MEPPs do not reach the muscle membrane threshold, so no muscle fiber action potential is generated.
- MEPPs generate end plate noise on needle electromyography (EMG).
- **When a nerve impulse travels to the presynaptic nerve terminal**
  - It activates P/Q type voltage-gated calcium channels (VGCCs) → influx of $Ca^{2+}$
  - Then quanta detach from that cytoskeleton after undergoing conformation changes.
  - Then ACh quanta dock to the presynaptic membrane with the help of several proteins including synaptobrevin, syntaxin, and synaptosome-associated protein of 25 kDa (SNAP-25).
  - This results in vesicular fusion with the membrane.
  - And release of a large amount of ACh molecules into the synaptic cleft
  - Then ACh molecules attach to AChR → large end plate potentials (EPPs) beyond threshold
  - This results in depolarization of the muscle fiber.
  - Then ACh molecules detach from AChR → hydrolyzed by AChE → choline + acetyl
  - Then choline is taken back into presynaptic nerve terminal.
  - Choline is resynthesized to ACh by choline acetyl transferase → packed into the vesicles

**QUESTION 2.** Which protein is essential for the exocytosis of synaptic vesicles in the presynaptic nerve terminal?
  A. Choline
  B. Synaptobrevin
  C. Contactin
  D. Agrin
  E. Lipoprotein receptor–related protein 4

**ANSWER:** B. Synaptobrevin

## COMMENTS AND DISCUSSION

- Exocytosis is a complex process that requires multiple key proteins.
- SNARE proteins are responsible for ACh vesicle docking, priming and fusion
  - SNARE is from **SNA**p and **RE**ceptor.
  - SNAP = soluble NSF attachment protein
  - Important SNARE proteins in exocytosis
    - Synaptobrevin or VAMP (vesicle-associated membrane protein) is in the vesicle membrane.
    - Syntaxin and SNAP-25 (synaptosome-associated protein, 25 kDa) are in the target membrane.
    - Synaptotagmin is a synaptic vesicle protein that has a property of $Ca^{2+}$ sensor for exocytosis.
- **Steps in exocytosis of ACh vesicles** (Fig. 16.2)
  - Mobilizing of ACh vesicles to the presynaptic membrane
    - In the resting state, ACh vesicles anchor to the cytoskeletal structures by synapsin I protein.
    - When depolarization occurs at the presynaptic terminal, the opening of voltage-gated $Ca^{2+}$ channels occurs, followed by a large influx of $Ca^{2+}$ into the nerve terminal.
    - $Ca^{2+}$ ions activate $Ca^{2+}$, or calmodulin-dependent protein kinase, which phosphorylases synpasin I, allowing ACh vesicles to move to the active zone.
  - Docking of ACh vesicles
    - Following mobilization, synaptic vesicles are docked at the active zone with SNARE complex formation.
    - SNAP-25 anchors to the presynaptic membrane.
    - SNAP-25 binds two molecules of syntaxin.
  - v-SNARE (synaptobrevin) binds to SNAP-25 and syntaxin to form a SNARE complex.
  - Exocytosis
    - $Ca^{2+}$ ions bind to synaptotagmin → displace complexin (an enzyme that prevents spontaneous fusion) → triggers fusion → Release of ACh

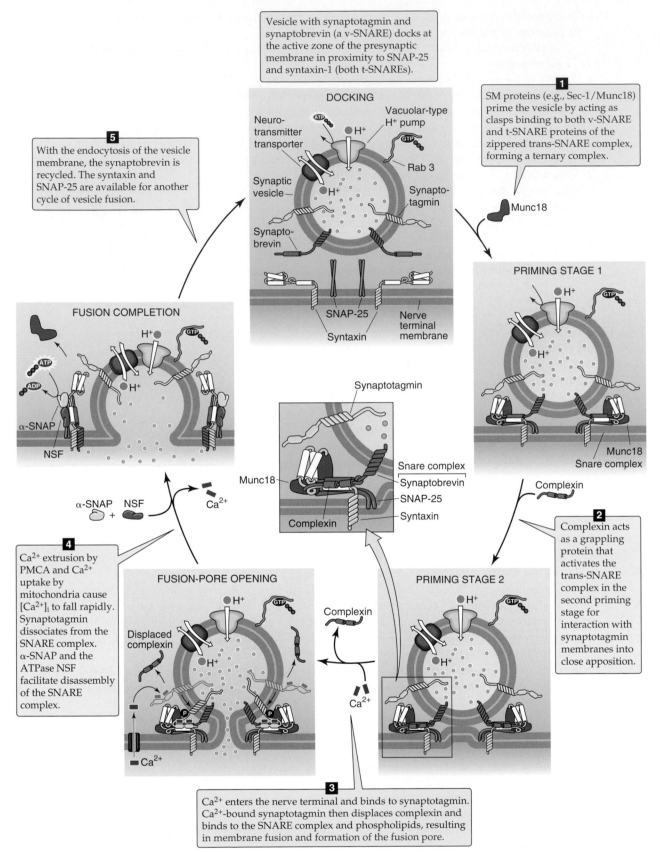

**Fig. 16.2** Exocytosis, fusion, and the cycle of synaptic vesicles. From Moczydlowski EG. *Synaptic transmission and the neuromuscular junction.* In: Boron WF, ed. *Medical Physiology.* 3rd ed. Elsevier; 2017:204–227.e2.

**QUESTION 3.** Which protein plays an important role in clustering, organizing, and stabilizing acetylcholine receptors in the postsynaptic membrane?
A. MuSK
B. Syntaxin
C. Contactin
D. Dystroglycan
E. Desmin

**ANSWER:** A. MuSK

**COMMENTS AND DISCUSSION**

- Junctional folds in the post-synaptic membrane are unique features, which are not present in other synapses.
- Junctional folds increase the postsynaptic surface area to allow a larger number of acetylcholine receptors (AChRs).
- AChRs are located at the top and sides of the folds (Fig. 16.3).

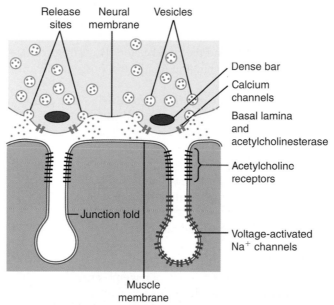

**Fig. 16.3** Junctional folds in the postsynaptic neuromuscular junction. From Khurana I, Khurana A, Kowlgi N. *Textbook of Medical Physiology.* 3rd ed. Elsevier; 2019.

- Voltage-gated sodium channels are abundant at the bottom of the folds for generating action potentials in muscle fibers.
- There are signaling pathways involving multiple proteins from formation, pre-patterning of AChRs in the postsynaptic membrane, to clustering and maintaining of AChRs.
- Five key proteins play significant roles (Fig. 16.4):
  - Agrin
  - Muscle-specific kinase (MuSK)
  - Lipoprotein receptor–related protein 4 (LRP4)
  - DOK-7
  - Rapsyn
- Steps in formation and clustering AChRs within the postsynaptic membrane:
  - Agrin is a large proteoglycan secreted from the presynaptic nerve terminal.
  - After release, agrin binds to LRP4.
  - LRP4 then activates MuSK, causing MuSK phosphorylation.
  - Phosphorylated MuSK creates an active binding site at DOK-7.
  - DOK-7 is phosphorylated by MuSK, which then activates and enhances MuSK phosphorylation and MuSK activity.
  - Full activation of MuSK results in activation of rapsyn.

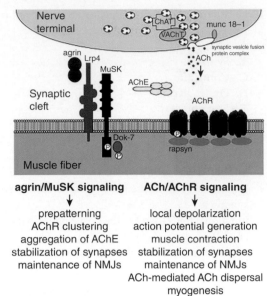

**Fig. 16.4** Postsynaptic signaling pathways to pre-pattern, clustering and maintaining acetylcholine receptors (AChRs). Agrin is released from the presynaptic terminal and then binds to lipoprotein receptor-related protein 4 (LRP4). LRP4 is a co-receptor for agrin and activates muscle-specific kinase (MuSK). Phosphorylated MuSK recruits downstream-of-tyrosin-kinase-7 (DOK-7), an intrinsic activator of MuSK. Full activation of MuSK results in activation of rapsyn, which contributes to the anchoring and clustering of AChRs. ACh, acetylcholine; AChE, acetylcholinesterase; ChAT, choline acetyltransferase; VAChT, vesicular acetylcholine transporter. From Witzemann V, Chevessier F, Pacifici PG, Yampolsky P. The neuromuscular junction: Selective remodeling of synaptic regulators at the nerve/muscle interface. *Mech Dev.* 2013;130(6–8):402–411.

**agrin/MuSK signaling**
↓
prepatterning
AChR clustering
aggregation of AChE
stabilization of synapses
maintenance of NMJs

**ACh/AChR signaling**
↓
local depolarization
action potential generation
muscle contraction
stabilization of synapses
maintenance of NMJs
ACh-mediated ACh dispersal
myogenesis

- Rapsyn is a linker between AChRs and the cytoskeleton (β-dystroglycan).
- Rapsyn induces AChRs clustering by binding AChRs to a postsynaptic cytoskeletal scaffold.

**QUESTION 4.** Myasthenia gravis (MG) is increasingly recognized as a seropositive disorder. However, which of the following antibodies has not been associated with MG?
A. Antibody to muscle-specific kinase (MuSK)
B. Antibody to agrin
C. Antibody to acetylcholine receptor (AChR)
D. Antibody to P/Q-type voltage-gated calcium channel
E. Antibody to low-density lipoprotein receptor–related protein 4 (LRP4)

**ANSWER:** D. Antibody to P/Q-type voltage-gated calcium channel

**COMMENTS AND DISCUSSION**
- In MG, autoantibodies to proteins in the postsynaptic membranes are identified.
- The most common autoantibodies are AChR Ab.
- MuSK Ab can be found in generalized MG with patients who do not have AChR Ab.
- LRP4 Ab and agrin Ab are detected in double-negative (AChR and MuSK) MG patients.
- Antibodies to P/Q-type voltage-gated calcium channel are associated with Lambert-Eaton myasthenic syndrome but not MG.

**QUESTION 5.** A 30-year-old woman presents with weakness in the evening. She has difficulty getting up from the couch after watching a nighttime movie with her husband. She feels normal in the morning. You are considering generalized myasthenia gravis (MG). Which of the following statements is **CORRECT** regarding this disorder?
A. Only T cell–mediated processes initiate the immunologic attack.
B. Acetylcholine receptor (AChR) antibodies are positive in all patients with generalized MG.
C. Muscle-specific kinase (MuSK) antibodies are more commonly positive in older men.
D. Simplification of the postsynaptic membrane is a common pathological finding.
E. All patients with thymoma develop MG.

**ANSWER:** D. Simplification of the postsynaptic membrane is a common pathological finding.

**COMMENTS AND DISCUSSION**
- MG is an autoimmune disease. Both B and T cells have a role in MG immunopathogenesis.
- There are several pathogenic antibodies identified in MG:
  - Acetylcholine receptor antibody (AChR Ab)
    - The most common antibody in MG is AChR Ab, which is found in 85% of patients with generalized MG and 50% of patients with ocular MG.

- AChR Ab is immunoglobulin (IgG) G1 and IgG3 subclasses.
- AChR Ab leads to complement-mediated attack causing:
  - simplification of junctional folds
  - decreased surface area
  - reduced number and density of AChRs
  - increased rate of AChR internalization.
  ○ MuSK antibody (MuSK Ab)
  - MuSK Ab is mainly IgG4 subclass, which lack complement-activating properties.
  - However, MuSK Ab has an effect on postsynaptic differentiation and synaptic function.
  - MuSK Ab blocks the assembly of the agrin-LRP4-MuSK complex, resulting in loss of AChR clustering at the postsynaptic membrane.
  - MuSK Ab can be positive in negative-AChR-Ab generalized MG, varying from 0% to 49% depending on geographic location.
  - Male-to-female ratio is 1:4.
  ○ Other autoantibodies
  - LRP4 Ab are found in 13% of double-negative MG patients.
  - Agrin Ab are also found in 14% of double-negative MG patients.
- Thymus in MG
  ○ Thymoma can be seen in 15% of MG patients.
  ○ Thymic hyperplasia is found in ~65% of AChR-antibody-positive patients with generalized MG.
  ○ Thymoma is very uncommon in patients with MuSK-Ab.
  ○ Only about 50% of patients with thymoma develop MG.

**QUESTION 6.** A 20-year-old woman presents with ptosis and ophthalmoplegia for 2 years. Which of the following symptoms is an **ATYPICAL** presentation for myasthenia gravis?
A. Unilateral ptosis
B. Ophthalmoplegia without diplopia
C. Neck flexor weakness
D. Proximal muscle weakness
E. Facial weakness

**ANSWER:** B. Ophthalmoplegia without diplopia

**COMMENTS AND DISCUSSION**
- The main clinical features of MG are:
  ○ Fluctuating and fatigable weakness
  ○ Worsening following exercise or activity
- Symptoms may involve several muscle groups
  ○ Extraocular muscles causing ptosis (usually asymmetric) and binocular diplopia
  - Diplopia is the most common presenting symptom.
  - Ophthalmoplegia in MG causes diplopia; however, usually this occurs only in late and refractory cases. If patients develop ophthalmoplegia without clinical diplopia, other diagnoses such as mitochondrial myopathy should be considered.
  ○ Bulbar muscles resulting in flaccid dysarthria, dysphagia, and jaw and facial weakness
  ○ Neck flexion or extension, which may cause dropped head
  ○ Limb muscles resulting in proximal and symmetric weakness, and less frequently distal weakness such as wrist extensor weakness
- MuSK antibody-positive MG patients may have atypical presentation that distinguish them from AChR antibody-positive MG patients:
  ○ Neck extensor weakness
  ○ Respiratory muscle weakness
  ○ Severe bulbar weakness
  ○ Fixed facial weakness
  ○ Weakness and/or atrophy of the tongue

**QUESTION 7.** The curtain eyelid sign is performed by:
  A. manually raising the less-involved eyelid and observing worse ptosis in the contralateral lid.
  B. manually raising both eyelids and observing downward movements of both eyes.
  C. manually raising the more ptotic eyelid and observing elevation of the contralateral eyelid.
  D. demonstrating improvement of ptosis after brief eye closure.
  E. manually raising the more ptotic lid, causing increased ptosis on the opposite side.

**ANSWER:** E. manually raising the more ptotic lid, causing increased ptosis on the opposite side

### COMMENTS AND DISCUSSION
- Typical lid signs in myasthenia gravis (MG) include the curtain eyelid sign and Cogan's lid twitch
- *Curtain eyelid sign (enhanced ptosis)*
  o Method: The examiner manually elevates the ptotic lid, or in cases of bilateral but asymmetric presentation, elevates the more ptotic lid. This will result in an increased ptosis on the contralateral eyelid.
  o Explanation
    - Herring's law of reciprocal innervation states that the extraocular muscles receive equal bilateral innervation and a singular signal controls both levator palpebrae.
    - In MG, this sign is most useful when ptosis is unilateral or bilateral but asymmetric. The less-involved lid is open wider at rest (Fig. 16.5A).
    - Both lids receive the same level of innervation and firing is maximal in an attempt to hold the lids open.
    - When the more ptotic lid is manually elevated passively, the compensatory to bilateral lids is reduced and the less ptotic lid drops further (Fig. 16.5B).
    - The manual elevation of the more ptotic lid causes the level of firing to decrease and the previously less ptotic lid suddenly drops.

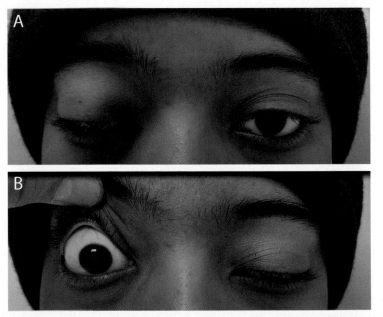

**Fig. 16.5** Curtain eyelid sign. Upper: More ptosis is observed on the right eyelid at rest. Lower: When manually elevating the more ptotic eyelid (right eyelid), increased ptosis of the contralateral side (left eyelid) is observed.

- **Cogan's lid twitch**
  o Method: Ask the patient to look downward for 10-15 seconds or gently close their eyes. Then ask them to look up quickly to the primary position. While the patient is returning to the primary position, observe for twitching of the lids upon upward gaze (the lid quickly comes up, then exhibits a brief twitch downward).

○ Explanation
  • The mechanism is unknown.
  • The twitch is proposed to be related to the initial fatigability of the levator palpebrae muscle, which rapidly recovers after the twitch.
  • It is reported to have 75% sensitivity and 99% specificity for MG.

**QUESTION 8.** Which of the following statements is **CORRECT** regarding myasthenia gravis (MG)?
  A. Patients with ocular myastheni usually have fixed symmetric ptosis.
  B. Eighty percent of patients with ocular myasthenia have positive acetylcholine receptor (AChR) antibody.
  C. Anti-MuSK (muscle-specific kinase) antibody-positive patients usually have isolated ocular symptoms.
  D. Thymoma is present in 50% of patients with ocular myasthenia.
  E. In purely ocular myastheni for more than 2 years, there is a 90% likelihood that it remains ocular.

**ANSWER:** E. In purely ocular myasthenia for more than 2 years, there is a 90% likelihood that it remains ocular.

## COMMENTS AND DISCUSSION
• Clinical presentation of ocular myasthenia
  ○ Symptoms are due only to extraocular muscle weakness, including ptosis, and diplopia with or without ophthalmoparesis.
  ○ Ptosis is usually unilateral.
  ○ The degree of weakness can vary from only mild unilateral ptosis or unilateral single extraocular muscle weakness to complete ophthalmoplegia with bilateral ptosis; however, in cases of bilateral complete ophthalmoplegia, other differential diagnoses (e.g., mitochondrial myopathy) should be considered.

 **KEY POINT**

> Bilateral complete ophthalmoplegia should raise suspicion for mitochondrial myopathy, for example, chronic progressive external ophthalmoplegia (CPEO).

• Antibodies in ocular myasthenia
  ○ AChR antibodies are positive in 50% of ocular myasthenia patients.
  ○ Other antibodies (e.g., MuSK and LRP4 antibodies), are reported to be positive in a small percentage of patients with ocular myasthenia.
• Progression from ocular to generalized MG
  ○ Patients with ocular myasthenia have the potential to transform into generalized MG, ranging from 30%–85%.
  ○ Risk for conversion from ocular myasthenia to generalized MG is high in the following circumstances:
    • Within the first 2 years from onset
    • Patients with positive AChR or MuSK antibodies in serum
    • Presence of abnormal repetitive nerve stimulation (RNS) in the limbs or trapezius muscle (predictable but no strong evidence)
  ○ A study conducted by Grob and colleagues in 2008 found that if the symptoms of MG are confined to the extraocular muscle in the first 2 years, there was a 90% chance that the disorder will not transform to a generalized MG.
• Thymus abnormalities in ocular MG
  ○ All patients should be screened for thymoma.
  ○ Thymoma can be found up to 5% in ocular MG.
  ○ Data on thymectomy for patients with non-thymomatous ocular myasthenia is inconclusive and this is usually not routinely recommended.

**QUESTION 9.** A 35-year-old woman presents with right ptosis and diplopia for 6 months. Initially, she was thought to have a lazy eye; however, she had to change prism glasses three times in the past 6 months. Which of the following statements is **CORRECT** regarding the office edrophonium (Tensilon) test in the diagnosis of myasthenia gravis (MG)?

A. The test is done infrequently, since it is not often available.

B. Atropine injection is required immediately following edrophonium.

C. Cardiac monitoring is required when atropine is not available.

D. The test has a low sensitivity for symptoms restricted to the eyes.

E. Other myopathies and brain stem lesions may have false-positive tests.

**ANSWER:** A. Edrophonium test is done infrequently, since it is not often available.

**COMMENTS AND DISCUSSION**

- Edrophonium (i.e., Tensilon) test is a bedside test for MG.
- Edrophonium is a short-acting acetylcholinesterase inhibitor that is injected intravenously.
- The onset of action is within 10–30 seconds.
- An objective sign (e.g., obvious ptosis or weakness of extraocular muscles) is required to assess the response.
- Should avoid subjective symptoms (e.g., limb weakness) to mimimize bias.
- Cardiac monitoring while performing the test *and* bedside atropine in a syringe (ready to inject) are mandatory.
- Due to the recent limited availability of edrophonium and safety concerns, this test is not widely performed.
- There is no existing good quality study in the accuracy of the edrophonium test. One cohort study reported 92% sensitivity and 97% specificity of the edrophonium test.
- False-positive results in patients with ptosis or extraocular muscle weakness from other causes (such as brain stem lesions and myopathies) may occur but are very rare.

**QUESTION 10.** A 20-year-old woman is referred for subjective diplopia and mild left ptosis mostly in the evening. There is no clear ophthalmoparesis, ptosis, limb weakness or fatigability on examination. Which of the following test results will confirm the diagnosis of ocular myasthenia?

A. Diplopia improves with the ice pack test.

B. Diplopia improves with edrophonium test.

C. A 5% decremental response is seen on slow repetitive nerve stimulation.

D. Abnormal jitter and blocking are present on single-fiber electromyography.

E. Thymic hyperplasia is present on chest computed tomography.

**ANSWER:** D. Abnormal jitter and blocking are present on single-fiber electromyography (EMG).

**COMMENTS AND DISCUSSION**

- Investigations in ocular myasthenia include the ice pack test, edrophonium test (aka Tensilon test), repetitive nerve stimulation, and single-fiber EMG.
- Ice pack test
  - Useful bedside testing
  - Requires objective signs (obvious ptosis or weakness of extraocular muscles) to assess.
  - Should avoid subjective symptoms.
  - Place ice over the symptomatic eye for 2 minutes, and assess for improvement.
- Edrophonium test or (aka Tensilon test)
  - Use intravenous edrophonium, which is a short-acting acetylcholinesterase inhibitor.
  - The onset of action is within 10–30 seconds.
  - Requires objective signs (e.g., obvious ptosis or weakness of extraocular muscles) to assess.
  - Cardiac monitoring while performing the test and bedside atropine in a syringe (ready to inject) are mandatory.
  - Due to recent limited availability of edrophonium and safety concerns, this test is not widely performed.
- Low-frequency (slow) repetitive nerve stimulation (RNS)
  - Can be performed in various muscles (e.g., hypothenar, thenar, trapezius, or orbicularis oculi).
  - A decremental response of 10% or more on RNS is required to be considered positive.
  - RNS has a very low sensitivity (ranging from 10%–39%) in ocular MG but has an 89% specificity.

- Single-fiber EMG (SFEMG, see also comments and discussion in question 6, Chapter 7)
  - Either single-fiber or concentric needles may be used.
  - Normal values depend on the types of needle and tested muscles.
    - SFEMG testing of the frontalis or orbicularis oculi muscle has an 86% to 97% sensitivity.
    - SFEMG specificity ranges from 66% to 98% depending on technical factors, examiner, and quality of study.
    - Blocking of muscle fibers on SFEMG is specific for MG and is always associated with increased jitter.

**QUESTION 11.** A 60-year-old woman with acetylcholine receptor (AChR) antibody-positive generalized myasthenia gravis (MG), controlled on prednisone and azathioprine, presents with dysarthria, dysphagia, and respiratory failure requiring intubation. A few days before admission she developed dysuria and fever and received antibiotics. Which of the following statements is **CORRECT**?
  A. She may have coexisting anti-MuSK antibodies.
  B. Double-seropositive MG patients have a reduced risk of developing a myasthenic crisis.
  C. Up to 80% of all MG patients experience at least one episode of a myasthenic crisis.
  D. Myasthenic crisis is commonly triggered by infection or medications.
  E. The current mortality rate for myasthenic crisis is ~50%.

**ANSWER:** D. Myasthenic crisis is commonly triggered by infection or medications.

**COMMENTS AND DISCUSSION (see also comments and discussion from Question 12)**
- Myasthenic crisis is an exacerbation of MG that affects the bulbar and respiratory muscles, resulting in respiratory failure.
- Myasthenic crisis is a life-threatening condition.
- Fifteen to twenty percent of all patients with MG will have at least one episode of myasthenic crisis.
- Myasthenic crisis usually occurs within the first 2 years of disease onset.
- Due to advances in treatment, ventilatory support and critical care management, mortality rate of myasthenic crisis has decreased dramatically from 40% to less than 5%.
- The most common trigger for myasthenic crisis is infection (30%–40% of all cases).
- Several medications can also trigger myasthenic crisis, especially antibiotics
- Other stressors may also trigger myasthenic crisis
- Noninvasive ventilation (NIV) may be used in myasthenic crisis.
  - NIV can prevent intubation or reintubation.
  - Bilevel positive airway pressure (BiPAP) can be used as NIV in myasthenic crisis.
  - Patients with NIV may need a shorter duration of ventilatory support.
- Respiratory parameters, including forced vital capacity (FVC), should be monitored closely and mechanical ventilation should be considered when:
  - FVC <1 L or <15 mL/kg
  - Negative inspiratory force (NIF) <20 cm $H_2O$ (absolute value)
  - Positive expiratory force (PEF) <40 cm $H_2O$

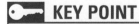 **KEY POINT**

Elective intubation is more favorable compared to emergent intubation.

**QUESTION 12.** A 48-year-old woman with generalized myasthenia gravis presents to the emergency department with dysuria and high-grade fever for one day. She is diagnosed with a urinary tract infection. She currently takes prednisone 50 mg daily and azathioprine 100 mg daily. Which of the following antibiotics is most appropriate in this case?
  A. Ceftriaxone
  B. Ciprofloxacin
  C. Azithromycin
  D. Amikacin
  E. Erythromycin

**ANSWER:** A. Ceftriaxone

**COMMENTS AND DISCUSSION**
- Several medications can trigger myasthenic crisis, especially antibiotics, as shown in Tables 16.1 and 16.2.

 **HIGH-YIELD FACT**

A common pitfall in clinical practice is using several medications that can exacerbate MG and trigger a myasthenic crisis.

**TABLE 16.1** Medication list that can exacerbate myasthenia gravis and trigger myasthenic crisis.

**Medications that should NOT be used in MG**
  Botulinum toxin
  D-penicillamine
  Telithromycin
**Medications that should be AVOIDED in MG**
  Magnesium (intravenous)
  Macrolide antibiotics (e.g., erythromycin, azithromycin, clarithromycin)
  Aminoglycoside antibiotics (e.g., gentamycin, tobramycin, amikacin)
  Fluoroquinolone antibiotics (e.g., ciprofloxacin, levofloxacin, moxifloxacin)
  Corticosteroids (high dose introduced rapidly)
**Medications that can be used with CAUTION if NO alternative is available**
  Immune checkpoint inhibitors (e.g., pembrolizumab, ipilimumab, nivolumab, atezolizumab)
  Procainamide
  Deferoxamine
  Beta-blockers
  Statins
  Chloroquine
  Hydroxychloroquine

**TABLE 16.2** Other stressors that may trigger myasthenic crisis.

Physical stress
Environmental stress
Emotional stress
Infection
Pregnancy
Sleep deprivation
Surgery
Pain
Tapering of immunosuppressive agents

Adapted from Wendell LC, Levine JM. Myasthenic crisis. *Neurohospitalist.* 2011;1(1):16–22.

**QUESTION 13.** Which of the following is the best predictor of respiratory failure in a patient with worsening myasthenia gravis (MG) symptoms?
  A. Severe weakness of hip flexors
  B. Severe neck flexor muscle weakness
  C. Severe facial diplegia
  D. Single breath count of 35
  E. Complete external ophthalmoplegia

**ANSWER:** B. Severe neck flexor muscle weakness

## COMMENTS AND DISCUSSION

- Helpful bedside exams in patients with impending myasthenic crisis include neck flexor testing and single breath count.
- *Neck flexor strength testing*
  - Neck muscle flexor weakness correlates with respiratory muscle weakness and often predicts impending respiratory failure.
- *Single breath count*
  - Instruct the patient to take a deep breath and then count out loud as many numbers as he or she can before needing to take another breath.
  - *Each counted number equals ~100 mL of forced vital capacity (FVC).*
  - Similar to predicted FVC, single breath count depends on age, gender, and height.
  - Most normal individuals can count up to 30 or 50.
  - Single breath count is not useful in patients with dysarthria or underlying lung diseases (e.g., chronic obstructive pulmonary disease [COPD]).
  - If the patient can count to only 10 or less, noninvasive ventilation (NIV) or ventilatory support should be seriously considered.

**QUESTION 14.** Effective treatments in myasthenic crisis are:
1. intravenous methylprednisolone.
2. intravenous immunoglobulin (IVIG).
3. rituximab.
4. plasma exchange (PLEX).
A. 1 and 2.
B. 1 and 3.
C. 1 and 4.
D. 2 and 3.
E. 2 and 4.

**ANSWER:** E. 2 and 4

## COMMENTS AND DISCUSSION

- Effective treatments in myasthenic crisis are IVIG and PLEX.
  - Several retrospective studies suggest that IVIG and PLEX have equal efficacy and similar outcome.
  - However, expert consensus favors PLEX as being superior, with the ability to improve respiratory function more rapidly leading to earlier extubation.

**QUESTION 15.** A woman presented with left ptosis and diplopia and was diagnosed with ocular myasthenia. Pyridostigmine up to 90 mg four times a day fails to improve her symptoms. Which of the following treatments is the next most appropriate step?
A. Prednisone
B. Azathioprine
C. Intravenous immunoglobulin (IVIG)
D. Eculizumab
E. Rituximab

**ANSWER:** A. Prednisone

## COMMENTS AND DISCUSSION

- Treatment of ocular myasthenia can be challenging in clinical practice due to the relatively mild symptoms and the potential side effects of medications.
- Steps in treatment ocular MG are usually:
  - Start pyridostigmine.
  - Start prednisone if pyridostigmine cannot control symptoms.
  - Reduce prednisone dose to 5–10 mg daily and consider maintaining this dose.
  - Consider immunosuppressive agents, only if symptoms relapse on prednisone taper or the patient cannot tolerate prednisone.
  - Thymectomy can rarely be offered if patients are younger than 50 years of age who have positive acetylcholine receptor (AChR) antibodies, are refractory to pyridostigmine and immunosuppressive agents, or have contraindicatoins to immunosuppressive agents.

**QUESTION 16.** Which of the following patients is the best candidate for thymectomy (all have a negative chest computed tomography [CT] for thymoma)?
  A. A 25-year-old woman with seronegative ocular myasthenia, controlled with pyridostigmine and prednisone
  B. A 30-year-old man with acetylcholine receptor (AChR) antibody-positive generalized myasthenia gravis (MG), currently admitted for myasthenic crisis
  C. A 68-year-old woman with muscle-specific kinase (MuSK) antibody–positive MG, well controlled with rituximab
  D. A 40-year-old woman with AChR antibody–positive generalized MG, with lingering symptoms.
  E. A 15-year-old girl with AChR antibody–positive generalized MG, with stable symptoms

**ANSWER:** D. A 40-year-old woman with AChR antibody–positive generalized MG, with lingering symptoms.

**COMMENTS AND DISCUSSION**
- A multicenter, randomized, rater-blinded trial of thymectomy in MG has provided significant evidence that the extended transsternal thymectomy is effective in patients with non-thymomatous AChR antibody–positive generalized MG, between the ages of 18 and 65 years.
- Thymectomy should be considered in:
  ○ All patients with suspected thymoma on chest imaging
  ○ Patients with non-thymomatous MG with:
    - generalized disease and
    - seropositivity for AChR antibodies and
    - aged 18-65 years and
    - persistent symptoms
  ○ Thymectomy should be offered as an elective surgery for patients with a relative stable disease.
  ○ Endoscopic and robotic approaches to thymectomy can be considered, but there are no randomized controlled studies that have specifically addressed this issue their efficacy compared to the extended transsternal thymectomy.

**QUESTION 17.** Which of the following patients is the best candidate for eculizumab therapy?
  A. A 25-year-old woman with acetylcholine receptor (AChR) antibody-positive ocular myasthenia, well controlled with pyridostigmine
  B. A 30-year-old woman with AChR antibody–positive generalized myasthenia gravis (MG), refractory to prednisone
  C. A 30-year-old woman with muscle-specific kinase (MuSK) antibody–positive MG, refractory to prednisone
  D. A 40-year-old woman with AChR antibody–positive generalized MG, with stable disease
  E. A 70-year-old man with positive-AChR antibody–positive ocular myasthenia, with a contraindication for prednisone

**ANSWER:** B. A 30-year-old woman with AChR antibody–positive generalized MG, refractory to prednisone

**COMMENTS AND DISCUSSION**
- Eculizumab is a humanized monoclonal antibody against the terminal C5 complement (Fig. 16.6).
- It prevents the formation of membrane attack complex (MAC) that damages AChRs and the postsynaptic membrane.
- Vaccination against *Neisseria meningitidis* is required at least 2 weeks before starting eculizumab.
- Eculizumab is an effective, US Food and Drug Administration (FDA)–approved and recommended treatment in adults with *refractory AChR antibody–positive generalized MG*. Ravulizumab is a newer recenlty approved agent with similar mechanism of action but a longer half-life.

**QUESTION 18.** What is the mechanism of action of efgartigimod?
  A. Inhibits cholinesterase in the synaptic cleft
  B. Targets B cells
  C. Reduces immunoglobulin G (IgG) and pathogenic autoantibody levels by reducing IgG recycling
  D. Blocks the formation of the membrane attack complex (MAC)
  E. Increases the expression of anti-inflammatory genes

**ANSWER:** C. Reduces IgG and pathogenic autoantibody levels by reducing IgG recycling

**COMMENTS AND DISCUSSION (see also comments and discussion from Question 17)**

- Efgartigimod is a recently FDA-approved treatment for MG.
  - Efgartigimod is a human IgG1 Fc fragment that has high affinity for neonatal Fc receptor (FcRn) (Fig. 16.6).
  - Normally, FcRn prolongs IgG half-life by binding IgGs, preventing them from lysosomal degradation and recycling them back into the circulation.
  - Efgartigimod, due to its high affinity for FcRn, competes with IgG and can block IgG binding to FcRn. As a result, more IgGs are degraded by lysosome, leading to reduced serum IgG and auto-antibody levels.
- Pyridostigmine is a cholinesterase inhibitor that blocks the degradation of acetylcholine in the synaptic cleft, increasing its availability and improving neuromuscular transmission. It is a symptomatic treatment in MG and has no effect on the immune system.
- Eculizumab is a humanized monoclonal antibody against the terminal C5 complement. It prevents the formation of the membrane attack complex (MAC) that damages acetylcholine receptror (AChRs) and the postsynaptic membrane.

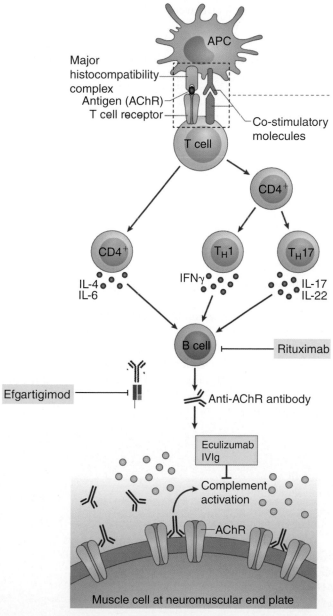

**Fig. 16.6** Mechanism of treatments in myasthenia gravis. *AChR,* acetylcholine receptor; *APC,* antigen-presenting cell; *IL,* interluekin; *IVIG,* intravenous immunoglobulin. Adapted from Dalakas MC. Immunotherapy in MG in the era of biologics. *Nat Rev Neurol.* 2019;15113–124.

**QUESTION 19.** You recommended thymectomy to your 25-year-old patient with generalized myasthenia gravis (MG) with positive acetylcholine receptor (AChR) antibody. How would you counsel this patient regarding the outcome for thymectomy in non-thymomatous MG?
A. MG goes into remission immediately after surgery.
B. Able to discontinue pyridostigmine within 3 months after surgery
C. Able to discontinue corticosteroid within 3 months after surgery
D. Able to reduce corticosteroid dose in 6–12 months after surgery
E. Surgery decreases the risk for progression to malignant thymoma.

**ANSWER:** D. Able to reduce corticosteroid dose in 6–12 months

**COMMENTS AND DISCUSSION**
- The multicenter, randomized, rater-blinded trial of thymectomy in MG in 2016 found that thymectomy was effective in non-thymomatous AChR antibody-positive generalized MG and the efficacy was maintained for 5 years.
  - Thymectomy reduced the weighted average quantitative MG (QMG) score, indicating reduction in symptoms (lower score = milder symptoms).
  - Thymectomy reduced the time-weighted average alternate-day prednisone dose.
  - Both benefits appeared in 6–12 months and were sustained for at least 5 years (duration of trial).

**QUESTION 20.** A 30-year-old woman presents with flaccid dysarthria and dysphagia for 2 months. Weakness of proximal muscles is graded at 4/5 in both the upper and lower extremities. Anti-MuSK (muscle-specific kinase) antibodies are positive. Which of the following is the most effective treatment in this condition?
A. Pyridostigmine
B. Methotrexate
C. Intravenous immunoglobuin (IVIG)
D. Rituximab
E. Eculizumab

**ANSWER:** D. Rituximab

**COMMENTS AND DISCUSSION**
- MuSK antibody-positive MG is usually refractory to the classic treatments for MG.
- Multiple studies and meta-anaylyses have shown that rituximab is an effective treatment in MuSK antibody-positive MG.
- Rituximab is recommended as an early option in patients with positive MuSK antibodies.
- However, in AChR antibody-positive MG, the efficacy of rituximab is uncertain.

**QUESTION 21.** A 25-year-old woman with acetylcholine receptor (AChR) antibody-positive generalized myasthenia gravis (MG) for 2 years is in remission on pyridostigmine 60 mg every 8 hours and prednisolone 10 mg per day. She is planning on getting pregnant. Which of the following medications is **MOST** contraindicated in pregnancy?
A. Pyridostigmine
B. Prednisolone
C. Azathioprine
D. Mycophenolate mofetil
E. Intravenous immunoglobulin (IVIG)

**ANSWER:** D. Mycophenolate mofetil

**COMMENTS AND DISCUSSION**
- Management of MG during pregnancy can be challenging.
  - Worsening of MG symptoms can be seen in the:
    - First trimester
    - First month postpartum
  - During the second and third trimesters, MG is usually better controlled.
- Management of MG during pregnancy is also very challenging, including making decisions about drug choices (Table 16.3).

**TABLE 16.3** Medication for myasthenia gravis MG during pregnancy.

| Medications | Safety concern in pregnancy | Effects on pregnancy | FDA¶ category |
|---|---|---|---|
| Pyridostigmine | Safe during pregnancy | Avoid intravenous form, increased uterine contraction | B |
| Corticosteroid | Safe during pregnancy | Only slightly increased risk of cleft palate (<1%)* | C |
| Azathioprine | In Europe, considered as a nonsteroidal medication of choice in pregnancy | Reported increase rate of prematurity, intrauterine growth retardation, lymphopenia, pancytopenia | D |
| Cyclosporine | Can be used in pregnancy, if benefit > risk | Reported prematurity, intrauterine growth retardation | C |
| Mycophenolate mofetil† | Contraindicated in pregnancy§ | Teratogenic effects High rates of spontaneous abortions | D |
| Methotrexate | Contraindicated in pregnancy | High risk of neural tube defects and anencephaly High rate of abortion | X |
| Cyclophosphamide | Should be avoided in pregnancy | Associated with major congenital malformation (e.g., absent thumbs/great toes/all toes, single coronary artery, etc.) | D |
| Rituximab | Limited data | No report of major fetal malformation | C |
| Eculizumab | Limited data | No report of major fetal malformation AU TGA assigns as category B2‡ | Not assigned |
| Efgartigimod | Limited data | No report of major fetal malformation | Not assigned |

*MG patients who are taking steroids should continue taking them during pregnancy to avoid the risk of exacerbation if they are withdrawn. If MG patients are *not* taking steroids, they can initiate steroid therapy after 12 weeks of gestation when the fetal palate is completely formed, if necessary.
†Women of childbearing age should use *two* forms of contraception while on mycophenolate mofetil.
§If patients who are on mycophenolate mofetil plan for pregnancy, contraception should be continued for at least 6 weeks after discontinuation of this drug.
‡AU TGA: Australian Therapeutic Goods Administration. AU TGA category B2 indicates that the drug has been used by a limited number of pregnant women and women of childbearing age, with no observed increase in the frequency of malformations or other harmful effects on the fetus. Although studies in animals may be lacking, available data suggest no evidence of increased fetal damage.
¶**FDA Category A:** No risk in human studies (studies in pregnant women have not demonstrated a risk to the fetus during the first trimester). **FDA Category B:** No risk in animal studies (there are no adequate studies in humans, but animal studies did not demonstrate a risk to the fetus). **FDA Category C:** Risk cannot be ruled out.

**QUESTION 22.** Which test result is seen in presynaptic neuromuscular junction (NMJ) disorders?
  A. Reduced sensory nerve action potential amplitudes
  B. Slowed motor conduction velocity
  C. Incremental response on slow (low-frequency) repetitive nerve stimulation (RNS)
  D. Incremental response on rapid (high-frequency) RNS
  E. Normal single-fiber electromyography (EMG)

**ANSWER:** D. Incremental response on rapid (high-frequency) RNS

**COMMENTS AND DISCUSSION**
- Reduced safety factor in all neuromuscular junction (NMJ) disorders results in a decremental response with slow (low-frequency) RNS.
- Presynaptic NMJ disorders have an incremental response with rapid (high-frequency) RNS.

- Rapid (high-frequency) RNS
  - Stimulation should be faster than the duration of calcium efflux from the presynaptic nerve terminal (100–200 ms). This results in:
    - Accumulation of calcium
    - Higher number acetylcholine (ACh) quanta released from the presynpatic nerve terminal
    - Higher end plate potentials (EPPs) → more muscle fiber action potentials (MFAPs) generated → incremental response

 **KEY POINT**

> All NMJ disorders → Decremental response with slow (low-frequency) RNS
> Presynaptic NMJ disorders → Incremental response with rapid (high-frequency) RNS

**QUESTION 23.** A 50-year-old man presents with proximal muscle weakness for 6 months. Symptoms are worse in the morning and partially improved in the evening. He has no sensory symptoms, but he reports dry mouth in the past several months. Examination is notable for weakness of the proximal lower extremities and absent deep tendon reflexes. Which of the following antibodies is the **MOST LIKELY** to be positive in this patient?
  A. Acetylcholine receptor (AChR) antibodies
  B. Muscle-specific kinase (MuSK) antibodies
  C. Voltage-gated calcium channel antibodies
  D. Voltage-gated potassium channel antibodies
  E. 3-Hydroxy-3-methylglutaryl-CoA reductase antibodies

**ANSWER:** C. Voltage-gated calcium channel antibodies

**COMMENTS AND DISCUSSION**

- Lambert-Eaton myasthenic syndrome (LEMS) is a presynaptic neuromuscular transmission disorder.
- Antibodies to P/Q-type voltage-gated calcium channels (VGCCs) in the presynaptic nerve terminal result in:
  - Reduced numbers of VGCCs
  - Disorganized transmitter release sites
  - Upregulation of other calcium channels
  - Reduced calcium influx leads to a decrease in the number of ACh quanta released into the synaptic cleft, decreased safety factor, and neuromuscular transmission defect.
- Clinical presentation of LEMS includes:
  - Weakness
    - Lower > upper extremity
    - Proximal > distal
    - Fluctuation; may improve after exercise
    - Often accompanied by generalized fatigue
  - Gait dysfunction (e.g., waddling gait)
  - Areflexia or hyporeflexia
  - Autonomic dysfunction (dry mouth, metallic test, dry eye, orthostatic hypotension, constipation, erectile dysfunction)
  - Ocular, bulbar, and axial weakness is often mild and less common than in MG (Table 16.4).
  - Respiratory failure is rare.
- Voltage-gated potassium channel antibodies are elevated in limbic encephalitis and peripheral nerve hyperexcitability syndromes such as Isaacs and Morvan syndromes.
- 3-Hydroxy-3-methylglutaryl-CoA reductase (HMGCR) antibodies are elevated in statin-induced myositis.

 **HIGH-YIELD FACT**

> Bedside trick in LEMS is facilitation of deep tendon reflexes following isometric contraction of the tested muscles. Areflexia/hyporeflexia → brief exercise → relax → brisker reflexes

**TABLE 16.4** Clinical and laboratory findings in myasthenia gravis (MG) and Lambert-Eaton myasthenic syndrome (LEMS).

| Clinical and laboratory findings | MG | LEMS |
|---|---|---|
| Weakness | Proximal > distal<br>Commonly involves ocular, bulbar, and axial muscles | Proximal > distal<br>Much less commonly involves ocular, bulbar, and axial muscles |
| Fluctuation | Worse with activity or in the evening | Improve with activity or in the evening |
| Autonomic involvement | No | Yes |
| Reflexes | Normal | Areflexia/hyporeflexia |
| Electrodiagnostic studies | | |
| • Low-frequency RNS | Decremental response | Decremental response |
| • High-frequency RNS | Decremental response | Incremental response |
| Antibodies | AChR Ab<br>MuSK Ab<br>Less commonly: LRP4 and agrin Ab | P/Q-type VGCC Ab |
| Tumor association | Thymoma present in 15% of MG especially in AChR Ab-positive MG | ~60% of LEMS have cancer association. Among all associated cancers, 60% is SCLC. |

Ab, antibodies; AChR, acetylcholine receptor; EDX, electrodiagnostic studies; LRP4, lipoprotein receptor–related protein 4; MuSK, muscle-specific kinase; RNS, repetitive nerve stimulation; SCLC, small-cell lung cancer; VGCC, voltage-gated calcium channel.

**QUESTION 24.** Which of the following symptoms is commonly seen in Lambert-Eaton myasthenic syndrome?
A. Dry mouth
B. Diarrhea
C. Persistent paresthesia
D. Heliotrope rash
E. Calcinosis

**ANSWER:** A Dry mouth

**COMMENTS AND DISCUSSION**
- Autonomic dysfunction is seen in LEMS but not in MG.
- Autonomic symptoms that can be seen in LEMS include
  - dry mouth (most common)
  - metallic test
  - dry eye
  - blurred vision
  - abnormal pupillary responses
  - orthostatic hypotension
  - swallowing difficulty
  - early satiety
  - constipation
  - erectile dysfunction
  - bladder dysfunction
- Other clinical findings in LEMS
  - Weakness
    - Lower > upper extremity
    - Proximal > distal
    - Fluctuation; may improve after exercise
    - Patients often complain of generalized fatigue.
  - Paresthesia
  - Gait dysfunction (e.g., waddling gait)
  - Areflexia or hyporeflexia

  ○ Ocular, bulbar, and axial weakness is less common in LEMS, compared to MG, or mild
  ○ Respiratory failure is rare.
- Heliotrope rash and calcinosis are manifestations of dermatomyositis.

**QUESTION 25.** With which of the following paraneoplastic syndromes is Lambert-Eaton myasthenic syndrome most commonly associated?
  A. Subacute cerebellar degeneration
  B. Sensory neuronopathy
  C. Opsoclonus-myoclonus syndrome
  D. Limbic encephalitis
  E. Thymomatous myasthenia gravis (MG)

**ANSWER:** A. Subacute cerebellar degeneration

**COMMENTS AND DISCUSSION**
- LEMS is often associated with tumors, especially small-cell lung cancer (SCLC).
- Antibodies to P/Q-type voltage-gated calcium channels (VGCCs) are detected in 85% to 95% of patients with LEMS.
- Antibodies to P/Q-type VGCCs are also associated with paraneoplastic cerebellar degeneration (PCD), a syndrome that it typically related by the presence of specific autoantibodies, such as anti-Yo, -Hu, or -Ri antibodies.
- Several paraneoplastic neurological syndromes may coexist in the same patient, and LEMS can be associated with the syndrome of subacute cerebellar degeneration.

**QUESTION 26.** A 45-year-old man presents with proximal leg muscle weakness for 8 months. He recently was diagnosed with small-cell lung cancer. You suspect Lambert-Eaton myasthenic syndrome (LEMS). Which of the following results on repetitive nerve stimulation (RNS) of the abductor pollicis brevis muscle is a typical finding in LEMS?
  A. A 20% incremental response on 3-Hz RNS
  B. A 20% decremental response on 3-Hz RNS
  C. A 20% decremental response on 30-Hz RNS
  D. A 20% incremental response on 30-Hz RNS
  E. A 5% decremental response on 3-Hz RNS

**ANSWER:** B. A 20% decremental response on 3-Hz RNS

**COMMENTS AND DISCUSSION**
- Electrodiagnostic studies in LEMS include routine nerve conduction studies, repetitive nerve stimulation (RNS), exercise teesting, and needle EMG.
- Routine nerve conduction studies
  ○ Low compound muscle action potential (CMAP) amplitudes in all motor nerves
  ○ Spared sensory nerve action potentials (SNAPs)
- RNS, which is a test for neuromuscular junction disorder
  ○ Slow (low-frequency) RNS is usually done using 2–3 Hz, whereas rapid (high-frequency) RNS is usually performed using 30–50 Hz.
  ○ In all pre- and postsynaptic neuromuscular junction disorders, there is a >10% decremental response on slow (low-frequency) RNS.
  ○ In presynaptic disorders, there is a >40% incremental response on rapid (high-frequency) RNS.
  ○ In LEMS, a >100% (usually >200%–300%) incremental response on rapid (high-frequency) RNS is seen (Fig. 16.7).
- Exercise testing
  ○ Ten-second tetanic exercise can replace rapid (high-frequency) RNS and is much less painful.
  ○ Baseline CMAP is taken at rest → 10 seconds of maximal isometric exercise → post-exercise CMAP
  ○ Post-exercise CMAP is typically >100% (usually >200%–300%) larger in amplitude than pre-exercise CMAP in LEMS.
- Needle EMG
  ○ Usually normal

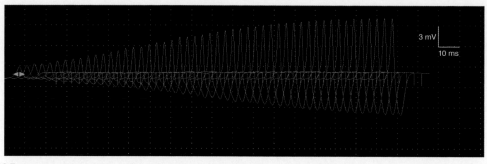

**Fig. 16.7** Incremental response on rapid (high-frequency) repetitive nerve stimulation in a patient with LEMS. In this tracing, 40-Hz RNS was performed while recording the abductor digiti minimi. A marked increment in the CMAP amplitude, demonstrated by a greater than 100% increase from the baseline CMAP amplitude, is noted.

- ○ Motor unit action potentials (MUAPs) may be unstable and/or short in duration and low in amplitude with polyphasia.

 **KEY POINT**

Prominent increment in CMAP amplitudes is seen following either 10 seconds of isometric exercise or rapid (high-frequency) RNS in patients with LEMS.

 **KEY POINT**

Ten seconds of exercise is much LESS painful and more tolerable than rapid RNS.

**QUESTION 27.** Which of the following medications is **NOT** a treatment option in LEMS?
- A. Fluoxetine
- B. 3,4-Diaminopyridine
- C. Amifampridine phosphate
- D. Pyridostigmine
- E. Intravenous immunoglobulin (IVIG)

**ANSWER:** A. Fluoxetine

**COMMENTS AND DISCUSSION**
- Malignancy evaluation is essential in LEMS and, if negative, it should be repeated every 3–6 months for 2 years, since LEMS may precede a diagnosis of cancer.
- Treatment of LEMS consists of:
  - ○ 3,4-Diaminopyridine (3,4-DAP, aka amifampridine) and 3,4-diaminopyridine phosphate (3,4-DAPP, aka amifampridine phosphate)
    - • 3,4-DAPP is the phosphate salt of 3,4-DAP.
    - • Both 3,4-DAP and 3,4-DAPP block calcium-dependent potassium channels in the presynaptic nerve terminal.
    - • This results in prolonged depolarization, leading to prolonged opening of voltage-gated calcium channels (VGCCs) and an increased influx of calcium.
    - • Both 3,4-DAP and 3,4-DAPP serve as symptomatic treatments that improve both weakness and autonomic symptoms.
    - • Side effects include:
      - • Digital and perioral paresthesia
      - • Lower seizure threshold

 **HIGH-YIELD FACT**

3,4-DAP and 3,4-DAPP are FDA-approved treatment for LEMS

 **KEY POINT**

Seizure is an absolute contraindication for amifampridine (3,4-DAP) and amifampridine phosphate (3,4-DAPP).

- Pyridostigmine
  - Augments the benefit of 3,4-DAP and 3,4-DAPP
  - When used alone, does not significantly improve symptoms in LEMS
  - Also increases secretions and improves dry mouth
- IVIG or plasma exchange
  - Can be used in refractory or severe LEMS
- Immunosuppressive agents (e.g., corticosteroids, azathioprine, among others)
  - May be used but few supportive data are available
- Fludrocortisone and/or midodrine
  - Can be used for orthostatic hypotension
- Fluoxetine can be beneficial in treating patients with slow-channel congenital myasthenic syndrome, but it is not effective in treating LEMS.

**QUESTION 28.** A 30-year-old woman presents with facial diplegia and bulbar weakness followed by descending generalized weakness in the past 2 days. A day before the event she had a facial injection by her friend for wrinkles. On examination, she was intubated with facial diplegia. She can move her eyes following commands but she cannot move her limbs. Reflexes were absent. What is the most useful investigation?

A. Serum creatine kinase
B. Facial nerve conduction study (NCS) and blink reflexes
C. Needle electromyography (EMG) of proximal muscles
D. 30-Hz repetitive nerve stimulation (RNS)
E. Single-fiber EMG

**ANSWER:** D. 30-Hz repetitive nerve stimulation (RNS)

**COMMENTS AND DISCUSSION**
- Botulism is caused by the toxin from *Clostridium botulinum*.
- There are several forms of botulism including foodborne botulism, infantile botulism, wound botulism, intestinal botulism, and iatrogenic botulism.
- Botulinum toxin cleaves SNARE proteins, which are essential for acetylcholine (ACh) vesicle fusion and subsequent exocytosis (Fig. 16.8).
- Various subtypes of botulinum toxin subtypes interfere with specific SNARE proteins in the presynaptic nerve terminal (Table 16.5), resulting in blocking of ACh release from muscarinic and nicotinic presynaptic nerve terminals. This can lead to neuromuscular transmission failure at the neuromuscular junction, as well as dysautonomia due to blocking of ACh release from cholinergic nerve fibers in the autonomic nervous system.
- Clinical features of botulism
  - Descending paralysis
  - Blurred vision and diplopia are often the first symptoms, followed by:
    - Facial diplegia
    - Dysarthria and dysphagia
    - Neck weakness → limb weakness → respiratory weakness
    - Autonomic involvement: mydriasis, constipation or diarrhea, nausea, and bowel ileus
- Investigations
  - Botulinum toxin in serum or stool
  - Nerve conduction study typically shows normal sensory nerve action potentials (SNAPs), and absent or low-amplitude compound muscle action potential (CMAP).
  - Needle electromyography (EMG) may be normal, or demonstrates motor unit action potentials (MUAPs) that are unstable and/or short in duration and low in amplitudes with polyphasia ("myopathic").
  - RNS
    - Slow (low-frequency) RNS: decremental response
    - Rapid (high-frequency) RNS: modest incremental response (usually 40%–100% increment)
  - Single-fiber EMG
    - Abnormal jitter and blocking
    - Cannot differentiate botulism from other neuromuscular junction disorders

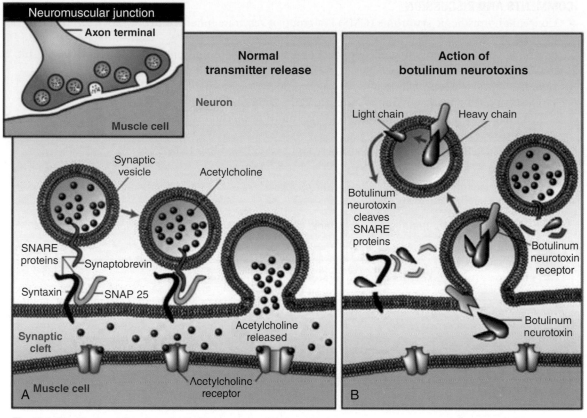

**Fig. 16.8 Mechanism of action of botulinum toxin.** (A) Normal fusion and exocytosis require SNARE proteins. (B) Botulinum toxins internalize into the presynpatic nerve terminal, and then cleaves specific SNARE proteins depending on the subtype, preventing the formation of the SNARE complex necessary for vesicle fusion and release. From Dureja G.P., *Handbook of Pain Medicine.* 2nd ed., Elsevier, 2013;34:409.

**TABLE 16.5** Botulinum toxin subtypes and affected SNARE protein.

| Subtype of botulinum toxin | SNARE protein affected by the toxin |
|---|---|
| A | SNAP-25 |
| B | Synaptobrevin |
| C | Syntaxin and SNAP-25 |
| D | Synaptobrevin |
| E | SNAP-25 |
| F | Synaptobrevin |
| G | Synaptobrevin |

*SNAP-25,* synaptosome-associated protein of 25 kDa; *SNARE,* soluble *N*-ethylmaleimide-sensitive factor attachment protein receptor

**QUESTION 29.** An 18-year-old man presents with long-standing, slowly progressive, generalized, weakness since he was a toddler. Examination showed slow pupillary light responses, scoliosis and reduced muscle bulk throughout. Neck flexors were graded 3+/5. Motor power was 4+/5 throughout. Reflexes were normal. He had a normal creatine kinase (CK) level, electromyography (EMG), and muscle biopsy. Motor conduction studies did not show repetitive compound muscle action potentials (CMAPs). You suspect a congenital myasthenic syndrome. This patient most likely has a mutation in which of the following genes?

A. *CHRNE*
B. *RAPSN*
C. *COLQ*
D. *DOK7*
E. *CHAT*

**ANSWER:** C. *COLQ*

## COMMENTS AND DISCUSSION

- Congenital myasthenic syndrome (CMS) is a group of very rare inherited neuromuscular junction diseases.
- Several mutations in genes that encode proteins around the neuromuscular junction (NMJ can result in CMS (Table 16.6 and Fig. 16.9).
- General clinical features of CMS
  - Onset at birth or early childhood, rarely in early adulthood
  - Generalized weakness that also affects ocular, bulbar, axial, and respiratory muscles
  - No cardiac involvement
- Some clinical clues may suggest certain subtypes of CMS (see Table 16.6).

**TABLE 16.6** Subtypes of congenital myasthenic syndromes (CMS) with their associated genes and clinical clues.

| CMS subtypes (with associated genes) | Percentage of all CMS | Clinical clues |
|---|---|---|
| **Presynaptic CMS** | | |
| Choline acetyltransferase (*CHAT*) | 5% | • Sudden and unexpected episodic apnea triggered by crying, excitement, and fever<br>• Sudden infant death syndrome<br>• Ptosis |
| **Synaptic CMS** | | |
| End plate acetylcholinesterase deficiency (*COLQ*) | 10%-15% | • Usually severe weakness, especially in the axial muscles<br>• Ophthalmoparesis<br>• *Slow pupillary light response* |
| **Postsynaptic CMS** | | |
| Acetylcholine receptor deficiency (*CHRNA1, CHRNB1, CHRND, CHRNE*) | | • Ptosis and ophthalmoplegia<br>• Bulbar weakness |
| Slow-channel CMS (*CHRNA1, CHRNB1, CHRND, CHRNE*) | 50% | • Wrist and finger extensor weakness |
| Fast-channel CMS (*CHRNA1, CHRND, CHRNE*) | | • No clinical clue, can be mild-to-severe weakness |
| Defects in AChR clustering pathway | | |
| • Rapsyn deficiency (*RAPSN*) | 15%–20% | • Arthrogryposis, contractures, episodic apnea<br>• Can mimic seronegative MG |
| • *DOK7* | 10%–15% | • Limb-girdle weakness, ptosis, stridor, vocal cord paralysis |
| • *LRP4* | <1% | • Respiratory failure at birth, ptosis, ophthalmoplegia, limb weakness |
| • *MUSK* | <1% | • Various phenotypes<br>  • Prenatal onset<br>  • Early onset with ophthalmoplegia and respiratory failure<br>  • Isolated vocal cord paralysis<br>  • Limb-girdle pattern |

*AChR*, acetylcholine receptor; *MG*, myasthenia gravis.
Adapted from Ciafaloni E. Myasthenia gravis and congenital myasthenic syndromes. *Continuum (Minneap Minn)*. 2019;25(6):1767–1784; and Abicht A, Müller JS, Lochmüller H. Congenital myasthenic syndromes overview. 2003[Updated 2021 Dec 23]. In: Adam MP, Ardinger HH, Pagon RA, et al., eds. GeneReviews® [Internet]. Seattle (WA): University of Washington, Seattle; 1993–2022.

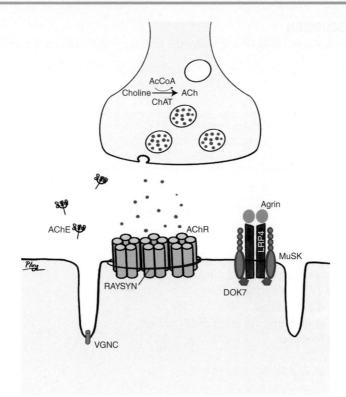

**Fig. 16.9** Location of protein products in the neuromuscular junction for genes commonly associated with congenital myasthenic syndrome.

**QUESTION 30.** An 18-year-old man is sent to the electromyography (EMG) lab for evaluation of possible seronegative myasthenia gravis (MG). He has bilateral ptosis and generalized weakness. On nerve conduction studies, you observe a small wave following the compound muscle action potential (CMAP) as in the following figure. What is the **MOST LIKELY** diagnosis?

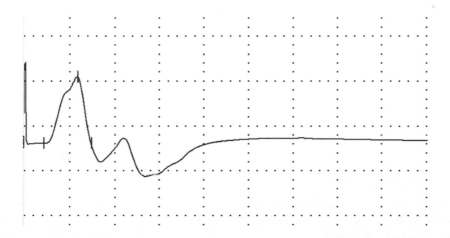

A. Agrin antibody–associated MG
B. Slow-channel congenital myasthenic syndrome
C. Mitochondrial myopathy
D. McArdle disease
E. Myofibrillar myopathy

**ANSWER:** B. Slow-channel congenital myasthenic syndrome

## COMMENTS AND DISCUSSION

- In the figure, there is a small CMAP following the initial CMAP called a "repetitive CMAP" or "double CMAP."

## 🔑 KEY POINT

> Double (aka repetitive) CMAP is a feature in
> - Slow-channel congenital myasthenic syndrome
> - *COLQ*--related endplate acetylcholinesterase deficiency

- In slow-channel congenital myasthenic syndrome, patients usually have ptosis, generalized weakness, and wrist and finger extensor weakness.

**QUESTION 31.** Which two congenital myasthenic syndromes (CMSs) worsen with pyridostigmine?
   A. Choline acetyltransferase (*CHAT*) and *RAPSN*-related
   B. Slow-channel and *DOK7*-related
   C. Fast-channel and slow-channel
   D. Acetylcholine receptor deficiency and *CHAT*-related
   E. *RAPSN* and *DOK7*-related

**ANSWER:** B. Slow-channel and *DOK7*-related

## COMMENTS AND DISCUSSION

- Congenital myasthenic syndromes may respond to some medications.
- Several CMS subtypes are responsive to pyridostigmine and 3,4-DAP, but some have no response or worsening with pyridostigmine and 3,4-DAP (Table 16.7).
- Response or failure to specific medications can provide important clues for the diagnosis of CMS subtypes.
- CMS subtypes that are responsive to pyridostigmine (mutations shown in parentheses)
  - Choline acetyltransferase deficiency (*CHAT*)
  - Acetylcholine receptor (AChR deficiency (*CHRNA1, CHRNB1, CHRND, CHRNE*)
  - Fast-channel CMS (*CHRNA1, CHRND, CHRNE*)
  - Rapsyn deficiency (*RAPSN*)
- CMS subtypes that are responsive to 3,4-DAP
  - AChR deficiency (*CHRNA1, CHRNB1, CHRND, CHRNE*)
  - Fast-channel CMS (*CHRNA, CHRND, CHRNE*)
  - Rapsyn deficiency (*RAPSN*)
- CMS subtypes that worsen with pyridostigmine and 3,4-DAP
  - Slow-channel CMS (*CHRNA1, CHRNB1, CHRND, CHRNE*)
- CMS subtypes with no response or worsening with pyridostigmine and 3,4-DAP
  - End plate acetylcholinesterase deficiency (*COLQ*)
  - *DOK7*-related CMS
- CMS subtypes that respond to albuterol
  - AChR deficiency (*CHRNA, CHRNB, CHRND, CHRNE*)
  - Rapsyn deficiency (*RAPSN*)
  - *DOK7*-related CMS
- CMS subtypes that respond to fluoxetine
  - Slow-channel CMS (*CHRNA1, CHRNB1, CHRND, CHRNE*)

**TABLE 16.7** Responses to therapy in common congenital myasthenic syndromes.

| CMS subtypes (with associated genes) | Response to therapy |
| --- | --- |
| **Presynaptic CMS** | |
| Choline acetyltransferase (*CHAT*) | • Improvement with pyridostigmine<br>• Intramuscular neostigmine can improve sudden apnea |
| **Synaptic CMS** | |
| End plate acetylcholinesterase deficiency (*COLQ*) | • No improvement or worsening with pyridostigmine and 3,4-DAP |
| **Postsynaptic CMS** | |
| AChR deficiency (*CHRNA1, CHRNB1, CHRND, CHRNE*) | • Improvement with pyridostigmine, 3,4-DAP and albuterol |
| Slow-channel CMS (*CHRNA1, CHRNB1, CHRND, CHRNE*) | • Worsening with pyridostigmine and 3,4-DAP<br>• Improvement with fluoxetine, quinine, quinidine |
| Fast-channel CMS (*CHRNA1, CHRND, CHRNE*) | • Improvement with pyridostigmine and 3,4-DAP |
| Defects in AChR clustering pathway | |
| • Rapsyn deficiency (*RAPSN*) | • Improvement with pyridostigmine, 3,4-DAP and albuterol |
| • *DOK7* | • No improvement or worsening with pyridostigmine<br>• Improvement with ephedrine and albuterol |
| • *LRP4* | • No data |
| • *MUSK* | • No improvement or worsening with pyridostigmine |

*3,4-DAP,* 3,4-diaminopyridine; *AChR,* acetylcholine receptor.
Adapted from Ciafaloni E. Myasthenia gravis and congenital myasthenic syndromes. *Continuum (Minneap Minn).* 2019;25(6):1767–1784.

**QUESTION 32.** A 42-year-old man had hypotonia, delayed motor milestones, and weakness since birth but without arthrogryposis. He had several episodes of severe weakness with spontaneous improvement for unknown reasons. His older sister also has similar symptoms. On examination, he has a myopathic facies, ptosis, and facial weakness. Weakness is most severe in the shoulder girdle and trunk. Creatine kinase (CK) level was normal. There were mild "myopathic" changes on needle electromyography (EMG) and muscle biopsy. Slow repetitive nerve stimulation (RNS) showed a significant decremental response. Which type of the following congenital myasthenic syndrome (CMS) can mimic the presentation of limb-girdle congenital muscular dystrophy?

A. Choline acetyltransferase deficiency (*CHAT* mutation)
B. Slow-channel syndrome
C. Rapsyn deficiency (*RAPSN* mutation)
D. Acetylcholine receptor (AChR) deficiency
E. *DOK7*-related CMS

**ANSWER:** E. *DOK7*-related CMS

**COMMENTS AND DISCUSSION**

• Several subtypes of congenital myasthenic syndromes, mostly *COLQ*- and *DOK7*-related, present with a limb-girdle pattern of weakness, mimicking limb-girdle muscular dystrophy (Table 16.8).
• Clinical presentation of "limb-girdle" CMS includes:
  ◦ Limb-girdle pattern of weakness
  ◦ Ptosis
  ◦ Waddling gait

**🔑 KEY POINT**

In patients with a limb-girdle pattern of weakness since early childhood, who have a negative workup for limb-girdle muscular dystrophy, congenital myasthenic syndrome should be considered.

**TABLE 16.8** Limb-girdle congenital myasthenic syndromes and their associated clincial features. Common subtypes are shown in bold. Abbreviations: Y, yes (present); N, no (absent).

| | Ptosis | Ophthalmoparesis | Respiratory weakness | Bulbar weakness | Tongue weakness |
|---|---|---|---|---|---|
| *DOK7* | Y | N | Y | Y | Y |
| *COLQ* | Y | Y (also slow pupillary light response) | Y | Y | N |
| *DPAGT1** | N | N | N | N | N |
| *GFPT1** | N | N | N | N | N |
| *GMPPB** | N | N | N | N | N |

*These are mutations involved in glycosylation pathways, resulting in both pre- and postsynaptic defects. Modified from Evangelista T, Hanna M, Lochmüller H. Congenital myasthenic syndromes with predominant limb girdle weakness. *J Neuromuscul Dis*. 2015;2(Suppl 2):S21–S29.

## SUGGESTED READINGS

Alshekhlee A, Miles DJ, Katirji B, Preston DC, Kaminski HJ. Incidence and mortality rates of myasthenia gravis and myasthenic crisis in U.S. hospitals. *Neurology*. 2009;72:1548-1554.

Bansal R, Goyal MK, Modi M. Management of myasthenia gravis during pregnancy. *Indian J Pharmacol*. 2018;50(6):302-308.

Carr AS, Cardwell CR, McCarron PO, et al. A systematic review of population based epidemiological studies in myasthenia gravis. *BMC Neurol*. 2010;10:46.

Cavalcante P, Le Panse R, Berrih-Aknin S, et al. The thymus in myasthenia gravis: Site of "innate autoimmunity"? *Muscle Nerve*. 2011;44:467-484.

Ciafaloni E. Myasthenia gravis and congenital myasthenic syndromes. *Continuum (Minneap Minn)*. 2019;25(6):1767-1784.

Conti-Fine BM, Diethelm-Okita B, Ostlie N, Wang W, Milani M. Immunopathogenesis of myasthenia gravis. In: Kaminski HJ, ed. *Myasthenia Gravis and Related Disorders*. Current Clinical Neurology. Totowa, NJ: Humana Press; 2003:53-91.

Elsheikh B, Arnold WD, Gharibshahi S, Reynolds J, Freimer M, Kissel JT. Correlation of single-breath count test and neck flexor muscle strength with spirometry in myasthenia gravis. *Muscle Nerve*. 2016;53(1):134-136.

Engel A. The anatomy and molecular architecture of the neuromuscular junction. In: Engel A, ed. *Myasthenia Gravis and Myasthenic Disorders*. 2nd ed. New York: Oxford University Press; 2012:1-36.

Engel A, Shen X, Ohno K, et al. Congenital myasthenic syndrome. In: Engel A, ed. *Myasthenia Gravis and Myasthenic Disorders*. 2nd ed. New York: Oxford University Press; 2012:173-230.

Evangelista T, Hanna M, Lochmüller H. Congenital myasthenic syndromes with predominant limb girdle weakness. *J Neuromuscul Dis*. 2015;2(suppl 2):S21-S29.

Gorelick PB, Rosenberg M, Pagano RJ. Enhanced ptosis in myasthenia gravis. *Arch Neurol*. 1981;38:531.

Graus F, Lang B, Pozo-Rosich P, Saiz A, Casamitjana R, Vincent A. P/Q type calcium-channel antibodies in paraneoplastic cerebellar degeneration with lung cancer. *Neurology*. 2002;59:764-766.

Grob D, Brunner N, Namba T, Pagala M. Lifetime course of myasthenia gravis. *Muscle Nerve*. 2008;37(2):141-149.

Guidon AC. Lambert-Eaton myasthenic syndrome, botulism, and immune checkpoint inhibitor-related myasthenia gravis. *Continuum (Minneap Minn)*. 2019;25(6):1785-1806.

Guptill JT, Sanders DB. Disorders of neuromuscular transmission. In: Jankovic J, Mazziotta JC, Pomeroy SL, Newman NJ, eds. *Bradley and Daroff's Neurology in Clinical Practice*. 8th ed. USA: Elsevier Inc; 2021:1958-1977.

Harper CM, Lennon VA. Lambert-Eaton syndrome. In: Kaminski HJ, ed. *Myasthenia Gravis and Related Disorders*. Current Clinical Neurology. Totowa, NJ: Humana Press; 2003:269-291.

Juel VC, Sanders DB. The Lambert-Eaton myasthenic syndrome. In: Engel A, ed. *Myasthenia Gravis and Myasthenic Disorders*. 2nd ed. New York: Oxford University Press; 2012:156-172.

Kuks JBM, Oosterhuis HJGH. Clinical presentation and epidemiology of myasthenia gravis. Current Clinical Neurology. In: Kaminski HJ, ed. *Myasthenia Gravis and Related Disorders*. Totowa, NJ: Humana Press; 2003:93-113.

Meriggioli MN, Sanders DB. Myasthenia gravis: diagnosis. *Semin Neurol*. 2004;24:31-39.

Moczydlowski EG. Synaptic transmission and the neuromuscular junction. In: Boron WF, Boulpaep EL, eds. *Medical Physiology*. 3rd ed. Philadelphia, PA: Elsevier; 2017:204-227.

Muley SA, Gomez CM. Congenital myasthenic syndromes. In: Kaminski HJ, ed. *Myasthenia Gravis and Related Disorders*. Current Clinical Neurology. Totowa, NJ: Humana Press; 2003:309-326.

Narayanaswami P, Sanders DB, Wolfe G, et al. International Consensus Guidance for management of myasthenia gravis: 2020 update. *Neurology*. 2021;96(3):114-122.

Nishimune H, Shigemoto K. Practical anatomy of the neuromuscular junction in health and disease. *Neurol Clin*. 2018;36(2):231-240.

Phillips WD, Vincent A. Pathogenesis of myasthenia gravis: update on disease types, models, and mechanisms. *F1000Res*. 2016;5:F1000 Faculty Rev-1513. Published Jun 27, 2016.

Rivner MH, Quarles BM, Pan JX, et al. Clinical features of LRP4/agrin-antibody-positive myasthenia gravis: a multicenter study. *Muscle Nerve*. 2020;62(3):333-343.

Romi F. Thymoma in myasthenia gravis: from diagnosis to treatment. *Autoimmune Dis*. 2011;2011:474512.

Ruff RL. Neuromuscular junction physiology and pathophysiology. In: Kaminski HJ, ed. *Myasthenia Gravis and Related Disorders*. Current Clinical Neurology. Totowa, NJ: Humana Press; 2003:1-13.

Singman EL, Matta NS, Silbert DI. Use of the Cogan lid twitch to identify myasthenia gravis. *J Neurophthalmol*. 2011;31:239-240.

Sussman J, Farrugia ME, Maddison P, et al. Myasthenia gravis: Association of British Neurologists' management guidelines. *Pract Neurol*. 2015;15:199-206.

Witzemann V, Chevessier F, Pacifici PG, Yampolsky P. The neuromuscular junction: selective remodeling of synaptic regulators at the nerve/muscle interface. *Mech Dev*. 2013;130(6–8):402-411.

Witzemann V, Chevessier F, Pacifici PG, et al. Myasthenia gravis seronegative for acetylcholine receptor antibodies. *Ann N Y Acad Sci*. 2008;1132:84-92.

Waterman SA. Autonomic dysfunction in Lambert-Eaton myasthenic syndrome. *Clin Auton Res*. 2001;11(3):145-154.

Wendell LC, Levine JM. Myasthenic crisis. *Neurohospitalist*. 2011;1(1):16-22.

Wolfe GI, Kaminski HJ, Aban IB, et al. Randomized trial of thymectomy in myasthenia gravis. *N Engl J Med*. 2016;375:511-522.

Wolfe GI, Kaminski HJ, Aban IB, et al. Long-term effect of thymectomy in patients with non-thymomatous myasthenia gravis treated with prednisone: 2-year extension of the MGTX randomised trial. *Lancet Neurol*. 2019;18(3):259-268.

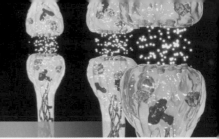

# CHAPTER 17

# Acquired Myopathies

## PART 1 | PRACTICE TEST

**Q1.** A 58-year-old man presents with a 2-year history of progressive muscle weakness. He reports difficulty getting up from a chair, climbing upstairs, and opening jars. Examination reveals asymmetrical atrophy of forearms and anterior thighs. Muscle strength of long finger flexors is grade 4 on the left, and 4+ on the right. Quadriceps strength is grade 4 on the right, and 4+ on the left. Bilateral ankle dorsiflexors are grade 4. Needle electromyography shows fibrillation potentials, small, short-duration polyphasic motor unit action potentials (MUAPs) in most muscles except in the rectus femoris, which shows both large, long-duration and small, short-duration polyphasic MUAPs with reduced recruitment. Which of the following antibodies is **MOST LIKELY** associated with this disorder?
A. Anti-Jo-1
B. Anti-Mi-2
C. Anti-signal recognition particle
D. Anti-cytosolic 5′-nucleotidase 1A
E. Anti-3-hydroxy-3-methyglutaryl-coenzyme A reductase

**Q2.** Which two groups of muscles are predominantly involved early in inclusion body myositis?
A. Deltoid and iliopsoas
B. Deltoid and quadriceps
C. Long finger flexors and quadriceps
D. Long finger extensors and quadriceps
E. Long finger extensors and hamstrings

**Q3.** Inclusion body myositis (IBM) is associated with abnormal accumulation of which of the following proteins?
1. Amyloid
2. Tau
3. TAR DNA-binding protein 43 (TDP-43)
4. Alpha-synuclein
   A. 1
   B. 1, 2
   C. 1, 3
   D. 1, 2, 3
   E. 1, 2, 3, 4

**Q4.** Which of the following statements is **CORRECT** regarding antibody to cytosolic 5′-nucleotidase 1A (NT5c1A) in inclusion body myositis (IBM)?
A. It is very sensitive and can be seen in almost all patients with IBM.
B. It is specific to IBM.
C. It is associated with earlier onset of the disease.
D. It is associated with bulbar dysfunction and respiratory compromise.
E. It can predict response to immunotherapies.

**Q5.** A 24-year-old woman presents with worsening symmetrical proximal muscle weakness in the past 3 months. On examination, she has erythema of both upper eyelids, anterior upper chest, and posterior upper back regions. In addition, there are plaques over the extensor surfaces of the metacarpophalangeal and proximal internal phalangeal joints of both hands. Motor strength is grade 3–4 proximally and grade 5 distally. Sensory examination is normal. Which of the following findings is expected to be seen on muscle biopsy in this patient?
A. Atrophy of muscle fibers at the center of each fascicle
B. Presence of predominant CD8+ T cells with increased MHC class I expression
C. Expression of myxovirus resistance protein A (MxA)
D. Vasculitis of epimysial blood vessels
E. 15–18-nm filamentous inclusions in muscles on electron microscopy

**Q6.** Which of the following shows the correct matching between the myositis-specific antibody and its associated feature?
A. Anti-Jo-1 – calcinosis cutis
B. Anti-MDA5 – classic dermatomyositis
C. Anti-Mi-2 – mechanic's hands
D. Anti-NXP2 – rapidly progressive interstitial lung disease
E. Anti-TIF1γ – strong association with cancer

**Q7.** A 46-year-old man presents with symmetrical proximal muscle weakness for 4 months. In addition, he has a worsening dry cough, difficulty breathing, and dyspnea on exertion. On examination, in addition to proximal muscle weakness, examination of his hands shows the findings in the following figure. Which of the following antibodies is **MOST LIKELY** to be positive in this patient?

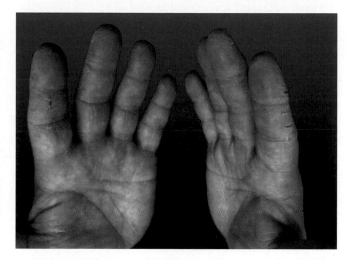

From Marco JL, Collins BF. Aug;34(4):101503. Photo courtesy of Greg Gardner.

A. Anti-cN1A
B. Anti-Jo-1
C. Anti-Mi-2
D. Anti-NXP2
E. Anti-3-hydroxy-3-methyglutaryl-coenzyme A reductase

**Q8.** A 57-year-old man with coronary artery disease, hypertension, diabetes, and dyslipidemia presents with progressive symmetrical proximal muscle weakness for 3 months. His medications include aspirin 81 mg/day, amlodipine 5 mg/day, glipizide 5 mg/day, and simvastatin 40 mg/day. On examination, muscle strength is grade 3 proximally and grade 4–5 distally. There is no sensory impairment. Muscle stretch reflexes are 1+ throughout. Serum creatine kinase is 5200 U/L. Serum anti-3-hydroxy-3-methyglutaryl-coenzyme A (anti-HMGCR) antibody is positive. Which of the following statements is most likely **CORRECT**?
A. All patients with this entity have a history of statin exposure.
B. Interstitial lung disease is commonly associated with this entity.
C. There is markedly increased risk of malignancy.
D. Muscle biopsy shows muscle necrosis and prominent lymphocytic endomysial infiltration.
E. This patient should have a good response to intravenous immunoglobulin.

**Q9.** Regarding immune-mediated necrotizing myopathy, which of the following features distinguishes anti-signal recognition particle (anti-SRP) antibody syndrome from anti-HMG-CoA reductase (anti-HMGCR) antibody syndrome?
A. More aggressive course of the disease
B. Higher association with malignancy
C. Fibrillation potentials on electromyography
D. More endomysial lymphocytic infiltration on muscle biopsy
E. Better response to intravenous immunoglobulin

**Q10.** A 36-year-old man has had progressive proximal muscle weakness in both arms and legs for 3 years. Serum creatine kinase was 12,543 U/L. Muscle biopsy of the biceps showed moderate variation of muscle fiber size and endomysial lymphocytic infiltration. He was diagnosed with polymyositis, and treated with oral prednisolone, intravenous immunoglobulin, mycophenolate mofetil, and, recently, rituximab, but there was no improvement. On examination, there is atrophy of proximal muscles and both calves. Muscle strength of bilateral upper and lower extremities is grade 4 proximally and grade 5 distally. Which of the following is the next best step in the management of this patient?
A. Repeat muscle biopsy
B. Antibody testing for anti-HMG-CoA reductase
C. Genetic testing of the dysferlin gene
D. Consider cyclophosphamide
E. Check CD19+ cells to monitor B-cell-depletion effects of rituximab

**Q11.** Which of the following enzymes is the **MOST** useful to differentiate between liver and muscle injury?
A. Aspartate aminotransferase (AST)
B. Alanine aminotransferase (ALT)
C. Alkaline phosphatase (ALP)
D. Gamma-glutamyl transferase (GGT)
E. Both A and B

**Q12.** Which of the following statements is **CORRECT** regarding myopathy related to thyroid disorders?
A. Fixed proximal muscle weakness is associated with hypothyroidism, but not hyperthyroidism.
B. Hyperthyroidism can be associated with periodic paralysis.
C. Muscle pain is usually absent in myopathy-related to hyperthyroidism but not hypothyroidism.
D. Delayed relaxation phase of muscle stretch reflexes is a feature of thyrotoxic myopathy.
E. Serum creatine kinase is usually normal in hypothyroid myopathy.

**Q13.** A 23-year-old man with HIV infection under a good control presents with progressive proximal muscle weakness and muscle pain for 3 months. He has been on zidovudine (AZT) and didanosine for over 2 years. His most recent CD4+ count is 720 /mm³ and viral load is 0. Zidovudine myopathy is suspected, and muscle biopsy is performed. Which of the following findings on muscle biopsy would confirm this diagnosis?
A. Autophagic vacuoles within muscle fibers
B. Fiber type grouping
C. Necrotic muscle fibers without lymphocytic infiltration
D. Ragged-red fibers
E. Type 2 muscle fiber atrophy

**Q14.** Which of the following is **NOT** a common feature between chloroquine-, hydroxychloroquine-, amiodarone-, and colchicine-induced myopathies?
A. Increased risk of myopathy in the setting of renal insufficiency
B. Coexisting neuropathy
C. Markedly elevated serum creatine kinase
D. Fibrillation potentials on needle electromyography
E. Autophagic vacuoles within muscle fibers on muscle biopsy

**Q15.** Which of the following statements is **FALSE** regarding statin-associated myopathy?
A. The risk increases with higher doses.
B. The risk increases when there is renal impairment.
C. The risk increases when using statin in combination with gemfibrozil or niacin.
D. Asymptomatic hyperCKemia can occur.
E. Intravenous immunoglobulin is the first-line treatment when there is persistently elevated serum creatine kinase.

**Q16.** In steroid myopathy, needle electromyography (EMG) and muscle biopsy most likely show which of the following findings?
A. Normal needle EMG and muscle biopsy
B. Myopathic findings on needle EMG and type 1 fiber atrophy on muscle biopsy
C. Myopathic findings on needle EMG and type 2 fiber atrophy on muscle biopsy
D. Normal needle EMG and type 1 fiber atrophy on muscle biopsy
E. Normal needle EMG and type 2 fiber atrophy on muscle biopsy

**Q17.** A 74-year-old woman was admitted to the intensive care unit (ICU) due to severe pneumonia, septic shock, renal failure, and respiratory failure requiring endotracheal intubation and ultimately tracheostomy. She was treated with intravenous fluids, intravenous norepinephrine, piperacillin and tazobactam, and intravenous corticosteroids. It was difficult to wean her from the ventilator and she developed weakness of all extremities. Examination on week 4 revealed severe weakness of all extremities, with proximal involvement being more pronounced. Muscle stretch reflexes were 1+ throughout. There was no sensory impairment. Nerve conduction studies showed low compound muscle action potential (CMAP) amplitudes but normal sensory nerve action potentials (SNAPs). Needle examination showed small, short-duration polyphasic motor unit action potentials with early recruitment. What is the **MOST LIKELY** finding on muscle biopsy in this patient?
A. Autophagic vacuoles within muscle fibers
B. Group atrophy and fiber type grouping
C. Muscle fiber necrosis and rimmed vacuoles within muscle fibers
D. Ragged-red fibers with cytochrome oxidase (COX)–deficient fibers
E. Loss of thick filaments on electron microscopic examination

**Q18.** Which of the following statements is **CORRECT** regarding myositis due to immune checkpoint inhibitors?
A. Examples of the offending agents include pembrolizumab, ipilimumab, and bortezomib.
B. The onset typically occurs after at least one year of immune checkpoint inhibitor use.
C. Myasthenia gravis and myocarditis may co-occur with myositis.
D. All patients require treatment with immunotherapies such as steroids and intravenous immunoglobulin.
E. Decrement on slow repetitive nerve stimulation is common in myositis.

**Q19.** A 79-year-old woman with hypertension, type 2 diabetes mellitus, and dyslipidemia presents with severe pain in the right thigh for 2 days. The pain develops acutely, and today she also notes swelling of the right thigh. Examination reveals swelling and marked tenderness at the right anterior thigh. Examination of the muscle strength of the right leg is markedly limited by pain. Examination of the other extremities is normal. Peripheral white blood cell count is 14,000 /μL with 75% neutrophils. Hemoglobin A1c is 9.3%. Erythrocyte sedimentation rate is 90 mm/h, and C-reactive protein is 71 mg/L. Serum creatine kinase is 396 U/L. What is the next best step of investigation to confirm the diagnosis in this patient?
A. Doppler ultrasound of the lower extremity
B. Serum myositis-specific antibodies
C. Electromyography
D. Muscle MRI
E. Muscle biopsy

**Q20.** A 24-year-old woman who is an immigrant from Thailand presents with swelling of the left thigh for 3 weeks. Four weeks ago, she had fever, abdominal pain, and diarrhea. These symptoms resolved after 1 week. In the past 3 weeks, she has also had muscle pain, fatigue, headache, and swelling around both eyes. Examination reveals periorbital edema, as well as grade 4 weakness and tenderness of the left quadriceps muscle. Complete blood count reveals white blood cell count of 11,250 /μL, with a differential count of 55% neutrophils, 26% lymphocytes, and 19% eosinophils. Muscle biopsy is performed and shows the finding in the following figure (hematoxylin and eosin staining, 400x). What is the **MOST LIKELY** causative organism in this patient?

A. *Naegleria fowleri*
B. *Taenia solium*
C. *Toxocara* spp.
D. *Toxoplasma gondii*
E. *Trichinella spiralis*

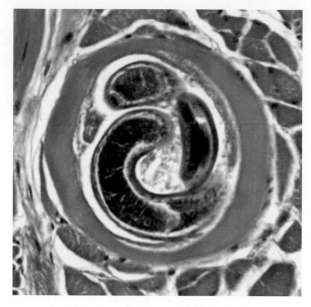

From Centers for Disease Control and Prevention.

## PART 2 | QUESTIONS WITH ANSWERS AND DISCUSSION

**QUESTION 1.** A 58-year-old man presents with a 2-year history of progressive muscle weakness. He reports difficulty getting up from a chair, climbing upstairs, and opening jars. Examination reveals asymmetrical atrophy of forearms and anterior thighs. Muscle strength of long finger flexors is grade 4 on the left, and 4+ on the right. Quadriceps strength is grade 4 on the right, and 4+ on the left. Bilateral ankle dorsiflexors are grade 4. Needle electromyography shows fibrillation potentials, small, short-duration polyphasic motor unit action potentials (MUAPs) in most muscles except in the rectus femoris, which shows both large, long-duration and small, short-duration polyphasic MUAPs with reduced recruitment. Which of the following antibodies is **MOST LIKELY** associated with this disorder?

A. Anti-Jo-1
B. Anti-Mi-2
C. Anti-signal recognition particle
D. Anti-cytosolic 5′-nucleotidase 1A
E. Anti-3-hydroxy-3-methyglutaryl-coenzyme A reductase

**ANSWER:** D. Anti-cytosolic 5′-nucleotidase 1A

### COMMENTS AND DISCUSSION

- The diagnosis in this patient is inclusion body myositis (IBM), one of the inflammatory myopathies.
- *Inflammatory myopathies*
  - Can be conventionally classified into four main categories:
    - Polymyositis
    - Dermatomyositis
    - Inclusion body myositis
    - Immune-mediated necrotizing myopathy
  - However, studies have shown that polymyositis is less common than previously thought. Many cases diagnosed as polymyositis have IBM or limb-girdle muscle dystrophies (LGMDs), such as LGMD2B (dysferlinopathy)

**HIGH-YIELD FACT**

In cases of "refractory polymyositis," it is crucial to reassess the diagnosis. These patients may have other disorders with evidence of inflammation on muscle biopsy such as:
- Inclusion body myositis (IBM)
- Limb-girdle muscular dystrophy type 2B (LGMD2B)
- Facioscapulohumeral dystrophy (FSHD)

   ◦ There have been attempts to incorporate myositis-specific antibodies into muscle histopathology for the classification of inflammatory myopathies (Fig. 17.1). The well-known categories include:
- Anti-synthetase syndrome
  - Associated with anti-synthetase antibodies
  - Anti-Jo-1 is associated with anti-synthetase syndrome
  - Anti-synthetase syndrome is mostly associated with dermatomyositis pathology.
- Dermatomyositis and immune-mediated necrotizing myopathies can be linked with various antibodies. These antibodies have different clinical presentations. For example, anti-Mi-2 is typically associated with classic dermatomyositis.
  - Anti-3-hydroxy-3-methylglutaryl-coenzyme A reductase (anti-HMG-CoA reductase or anti-HMGCR) and anti-signal recognition particle (anti-SRP) are associated with immune-mediated necrotizing myopathy.
- Overlap syndromes (aka, overlap myositis) refers to cases where inflammatory myopathies are accompanied by other connective tissue diseases such as systemic lupus erythematosus, systemic sclerosis, among others.

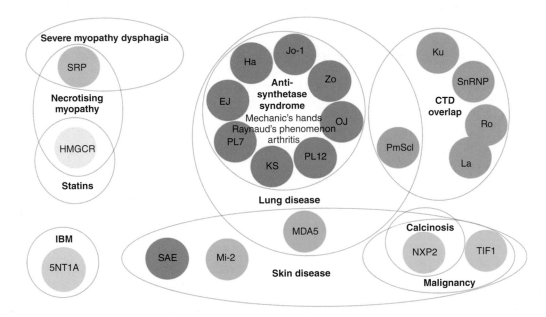

**Fig. 17.1 Association between myositis-specific antibodies and clinical phenotypes.** *5NT1A,* cytosolic 5′ nucleotidase 1A; *CTD,* connective tissue disease; *EJ,* glycyl tRNA synthetase; *Ha,* tyrosyl tRNA synthetase; *HMGCR,* 3-hydroxy-3-methylglutaryl-coenzyme A reductase; *IBM,* inclusion body myositis; *Jo-1,* histidyl tRNA synthetase; *KS,* asparaginyl tRNA synthetase; *MDA5,* melanoma differentiation-associated gene 5; *Mi-2,* nucleosome-remodeling deacetyalse complex; *NXP2,* nuclear matrix protein 2; *OJ,* isoleucyl tRNA synthetases; *PL7,* threonyl tRNA synthetase; *PL12,* alanyl tRNA synthetase; *SAE,* small ubiquitin-like modifier activating enzyme; *snRNP,* small nuclear ribonucleic protein; *SRP,* signal recognition particle; *TIF1,* transcription intermediary factor 1; *Zo,* phenylalanyl tRNA synthetase. From Betteridge Z, McHugh N. Myositis-specific autoantibodies: an important tool to support diagnosis of myositis. *J Intern Med.* 2016;280(1):8–23.

- *Inclusion body myositis (IBM)*
  - The most common inflammatory myopathy in individuals older than age 50 and also the most common new-onset myopathy in this age group.
  - Clinical features
    - Typical onset after the age of 45
    - Very slowly progressive, with a typical time course between initial symptoms and diagnosis of several years
    - Muscle atrophy and weakness (Fig. 17.2)
      - Asymmetric involvement is common.
      - Pattern of weakness: predilection of the long finger flexors (i.e., flexor digitorum superficialis, flexor digitorum profundus) and quadriceps. Involvement of the tibialis anterior and biceps can also be seen.
      - Atrophy of the ventral forearm and/or anterior thigh due to involvement of these muscles is common. There is sometimes obvious sparing of the rectus femoris, which gives the anterior thigh a characteristic diamond shape.
      - Patients frequently have dysphagia, which may be the initial symptom.

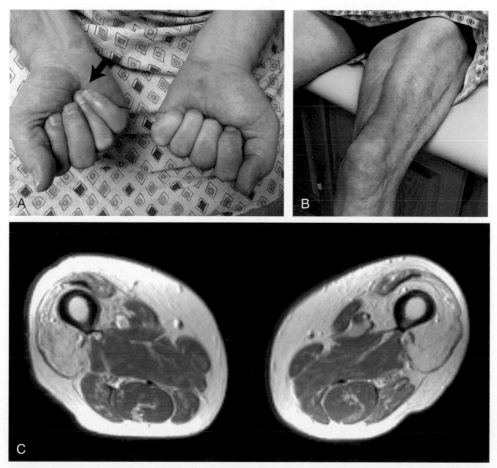

**Fig. 17.2** Clinical and imaging features in inclusion body myositis. (A) Asymmetric weakness of the long finger flexor muscles, more prominent on the right. There is incomplete flexion of the right fingers (arrow). (B) Severe atrophy of the quadriceps muscle. (C) Fat infiltration of the quadriceps, especially vastus medialis and vastus lateralis, demonstrated as hyperintensities on a proton density–weighted image of the muscle MRI. (C) from Needham M, Mastaglia FL. Inclusion body myositis: Current pathogenetic concepts and diagnostic and therapeutic approaches. *Lancet Neurol.* 2007;6(7):620–631.

**HIGH-YIELD FACT**

Classic muscle involvement in IBM = Long finger flexors + quadriceps.
Asymmetry is common.

- ∘ Laboratory features
  - Serum creatine kinase (CK): normal or mildly elevated; typically less than 10 times of upper normal limit
  - Antibody to cytosolic 5′-nucleotidase 1A (anti-cN1A, aka. NT5c1A)
    - Sensitivity: found in 40%–60% of patients with IBM
    - Specificity: can also be found in other disorders such as other inflammatory myopathies (e.g., anti-synthetase syndrome, dermatomyositis, and immune-mediated necrotizing myopathy), systemic autoimmune diseases (e.g., Sjögren syndrome, systemic lupus erythematosus) and motor neuron diseases
    - Seropositivity of NT5c1A is associated with more severe phenotypes and higher morbidity, including bulbar dysfunction (e.g., dysphagia), facial weakness, and respiratory compromise (e.g., reduced forced vital capacity).

 **HIGH-YIELD FACT**

NT5c1A in IBM is associated with more severe clinical phenotypes and higher mortality, including bulbar dysfunction (e.g., dysphagia), respiratory compromise, and facial weakness.

- Needle EMG: fibrillation potentials can be seen. There can be mixed myopathic features (small, short-duration polyphasic motor unit action potentials [MUAPs] with early recruitment) and neurogenic features (large, long-duration MUAPs with reduced recruitment) in inclusion body myositis.

 **HIGH-YIELD FACT**

- Fibrillation potentials or positive sharp waves are often seen in inflammatory myopathies.
- In inclusion body myositis, there can be mixed features of myopathic and neurogenic motor unit action potentials and recruitment on needle EMG.

- Muscle MRI: early fat infiltration (hyperintensity of T1-weighted images of the quadriceps) with relative sparing of muscles in the posterior thigh compartment (Fig. 17.2)
- Muscle biopsy (see also comments and discussion from Questions 6, and 11–13 in Chapter 10)
  - Myopathic features: variation of muscle fiber size
  - Rimmed vacuoles can be seen on hematoxylin and eosin (H&E) and modified Gomori trichrome (mGT) stains (Fig. 10.15C)
    - These vacuoles contain amyloid. On Congo red stain, amyloid has apple-green birefringence under polarized light. Hence, IBM is sometimes referred to as the "Alzheimer disease of the muscle."
  - Accumulation of other proteins within muscle fibers can be demonstrated on special immunostaining. These proteins include:
    - TAR DNA-binding protein 43 (TDP-43)
    - Paired helical filament (PHF)-tau (demonstrated on SMI-31 stain)
    - p62 (sequestosome-1, an autophagosome cargo protein involving in autophagy), which indicates abnormal autophagy
  - Inflammation: endomysial infiltration of T cells, specifically. CD8+ T cells or cytotoxic T cells. There is invasion of non-necrotic fibers, similar to polymyositis.
  - Evidence of mitochondrial dysfunction
    - Presence of abundant cytochrome oxidase (COX)–negative fibers
  - Electron microscopy: accumulation of 15–18-nm filamentous inclusions in muscle fibers

**HIGH-YIELD FACT**

In IBM, there is an abnormal accumulation of proteins including amyloid, TDP-43, tau (demonstrated on SMI-31 immunostaining), and p62 (involved in autophagy).

- o Pathogenesis
  - There are both neurodegenerative and inflammatory processes involved in IBM. The links between these two processes have been an active area of research.
- o Treatment
  - Response to immunotherapies is generally poor, and most clinicians discontinue or do not offer them in established IBM.
  - Multiple drugs have been studied in clinical trials.

**QUESTION 2.** Which two groups of muscles are predominantly involved early in inclusion body myositis?
  A. Deltoid and iliopsoas
  B. Deltoid and quadriceps
  C. Long finger flexors and quadriceps
  D. Long finger extensors and quadriceps
  E. Long finger extensors and hamstrings

**ANSWER:** C. Long finger flexors and quadriceps

**COMMENTS AND DISCUSSION (see also comments and discussion from Question 1)**
- In IBM, muscles that are involved early in the course of the disease include the long finger flexors (flexor digitorum superficialis, flexor digitorum profundus), quadriceps and, to a lesser extent, tibialis anterior and biceps.
  - o The involvement is commonly asymmetric. Due to preferential involvement of these muscles, there are the following clinical features:
    - Atrophy of the ventral forearm and anterior thigh
    - Weakness of finger flexion and knee extension and sometimes additional weakness of ankle dorsiflexion and elbow flexion.
  - o Deltoid is relatively spared.
- Unlike IBM, other types of inflammatory myopathies such as dermatomyositis, polymyositis, anti-synthetase syndrome, immune-mediated necrotizing myopathy tend to involve proximal muscles, including the deltoid, trapezius, biceps, triceps, iliopsoas, and gluteal muscles.

**QUESTION 3.** Inclusion body myositis (IBM) is associated with abnormal accumulation of which of the following proteins?
  1. Amyloid
  2. Tau
  3. TAR DNA-binding protein 43 (TDP-43)
  4. Alpha-synuclein
     A. 1
     B. 1, 2
     C. 1, 3
     D. 1, 2, 3
     E. 1, 2, 3, 4

**ANSWER:** D. 1, 2, 3

**COMMENTS AND DISCUSSION (see also comments and discussion from Question 1)**
- Histopathology of inclusion body myositis (IBM) demonstrates rimmed vacuoles within muscle fibers. These rimmed vacuoles contain amyloid, which shows apple-green birefringence on Congo red staining under polarized light. Some consider IBM as "Alzheimer disease of the muscle."
- In addition to amyloid, there is also accumulation of other proteins including:
  - o Tau (demonstrated on SMI-31 immunostain)
  - o TDP-43
  - o p62, which indicates abnormal autophagy

- Cytochrome oxidase (COX)–negative fibers are also seen in IBM, indicating mitochondrial dysfunction.
- There is no abnormal accumulation of alpha-synuclein in IBM.

**QUESTION 4.** Which of the following statements is **CORRECT** regarding antibody to cytosolic 5′-nucleotidase 1A (NT5c1A) in inclusion body myositis (IBM)?
   A. It is very sensitive and can be seen in almost all patients with IBM.
   B. It is specific to IBM.
   C. It is associated with earlier onset of the disease.
   D. It is associated with bulbar dysfunction and respiratory compromise.
   E. It can predict response to immunotherapies.

**ANSWER:** D. It is associated with bulbar dysfunction and respiratory compromise.

**COMMENTS AND DISCUSSION (see also comments and discussion from Question 1)**
- NT5c1A (aka. anti-cytosolic 5′-nucleotidase 1A, anti-cN1A) is an antibody associated with inclusion body myositis (IBM).
   - Sensitivity: 40%–60%
   - Specificity: 80%–100% from various studies. It can be seen in other disorders such as dermatomyositis, immune-mediated necrotizing myopathy, systemic lupus erythematosus, and Sjögren syndrome, among others.
   - This antibody is associated with more severe phenotypes.
      - Bulbar dysfunction including dysphagia, respiratory involvement including reduced forced vital capacity and respiratory compromise
      - Higher morbidity
- NT5c1A is *not* associated with the age at onset or duration of the disease.
- NT5c1A has *no* utility in predicting response to immunotherapies in IBM.

**QUESTION 5.** A 24-year-old woman presents with worsening symmetrical proximal muscle weakness in the past 3 months. On examination, she has erythema of both upper eyelids, anterior upper chest, and posterior upper back regions. In addition, there are plaques over the extensor surfaces of metacarpo-phalangeal and proximal internal phalangeal joints of both hands. Motor strength is grade 3–4 proximally and grade 5 distally. Sensory examination is normal. Which of the following findings is expected to be seen on muscle biopsy in this patient?
   A. Atrophy of muscle fibers at the center of each fascicle
   B. Presence of predominant CD8+ T cells with increased MHC class I expression
   C. Expression of myxovirus resistance protein A (MxA)
   D. Vasculitis of epimysial blood vessels
   E. 15–18-nm filamentous inclusions in muscles on electron microscopy

**ANSWER:** C. Expression of myxovirus resistance protein A (MxA)

**COMMENTS AND DISCUSSION**
- The diagnosis in this patient is *dermatomyositis*. There is symmetric progressive proximal muscle weakness and cutaneous manifestations including heliotrope rash, V sign, shawl sign, and Gottron papules.
- Clinical features of dermatomyositis
   - Onset in children (juvenile dermatomyositis) and adults
   - Proximal muscle weakness: often symmetric
      - Muscle pain can be present.
   - Cutaneous manifestations (Fig. 17.3)
      - Heliotrope rash: violaceous erythema of the upper eyelids
      - Malar rash: erythema of the bilateral cheeks, which also involves the nasolabial fold. This is in contrast to the malar rash in systemic lupus erythematosus, which spares the nasolabial fold.
      - V sign and shawl sign: erythema of the anterior upper chest and posterior upper back
      - Gottron papules: erythematous papules or plaques on the extensor surface of the metacarpopha-langeal, proximal interphalangeal joints of the hand, as well as the extensor surfaces of the elbow and knee

- Periungual telangiectasia
- Mechanic's hands: thickening of the skin of the hands with cracking and fissuring, especially at the palm, fingertips, and lateral aspects of the fingers
  - Usually associated with anti-Jo-1 antibody, one of the anti-synthetase antibodies
- Calcinosis cutis: usually associated with anti-NXP2

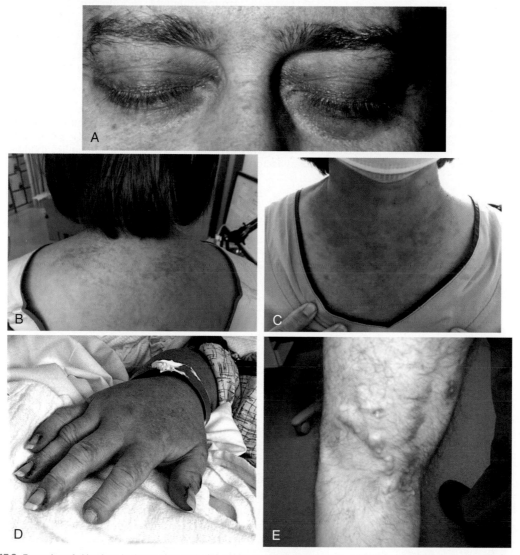

**Fig. 17.3** Examples of skin signs in dermatomyositis. (A) Heliotrope rash. (B) Shawl sign. (C) V sign. (D) Gottron papules with periungual telangiectasia. (E) Calcinosis cutis. (A) from Dugan EM, Huber AM, Miller FW, Rider LG. International Myositis Assessment and Clinical Studies Group. Photoessay of the cutaneous manifestations of the idiopathic inflammatory myopathies. *Dermatol Online J.* 2009;15(2):1.

- o Other systemic involvement
  - Interstitial lung disease: usually associated with anti-MDA5 and all anti-synthetase antibodies
  - Patients with anti-MDA5 typically have an amyopathic form with minimal or no muscle weakness.
  - Malignancy: usually associated with anti-TIF1γ and anti-NXP2
- Laboratory features of dermatomyositis
  - o Serum creatine kinase: usually elevated, up to 50 times of the upper normal limit
  - o Myositis-specific antibodies
    - Key features associated with each antibody are summarized in Table 17.1.

**TABLE 17.1** Myositis-specific antibodies and associated key features.

| Myositis-specific antibodies | Key features |
|---|---|
| Anti-Mi-2 | Classic DM |
| Anti-TIF1γ | High association with malignancy |
| Anti-NXP2 | Calcinosis cutis, association with malignancy |
| Anti-MDA5 | Amyopathic DM, rapidly progressive ILD |
| Anti-SAE | May begin with amyopathic DM, dysphagia |
| Anti-synthetase (anti-Jo-1, anti-PL-7, anti-PL-12, anti-EJ, anti-OJ, anti-KS, anti-Zo, anti-Ha) | Severe ILD; mechanic's hands (only anti-Jo-1) |

Of note, all in the table except anti-synthetase antibodies (i.e., antibodies to aminoacyl-transfer RNA synthetases) are dermatomyositis-specific antibodies. Amyopathic dermatomyositis (DM) is DM with no or minimal muscle involvement.
*DM*, dermatomyositis; *EJ*, glycyl tRNA synthetase; *Ha*, tyrosyl tRNA synthetase; *ILD*, interstitial lung disease; *Jo-1*, histidyl tRNA synthetase; *KS*, asparaginyl tRNA synthetase; *MDA5*, melanoma differentiation-associated gene 5; *Mi-2*, nucleosome-remodeling deacetylase complex; *NXP2*, nuclear matrix protein 2; *OJ*, isoleucyl tRNA synthetases; *PL7*, threonyl tRNA synthetase; *PL12*, alanyl tRNA synthetase; *SAE*, small ubiquitin-like modifier activating enzyme; *TIF1γ*, transcription intermediary factor 1 gamma; *Zo*, phenylalanyl tRNA synthetase.

## MNEMONICS

Myositis-specific antibodies
- High association with malignancy: anti-**T**IF1γ, anti-**N**XP2. **T**umors and **N**odes
- **A**myopathic DM: anti-MD**A**5, anti-S**A**E. These have letter "**A**" in their names.
- High association with interstitial lung disease: anti-MDA**5**, anti-synthetase. Lungs have totally **5 lobes** (3 on the right, and 2 on the left).

- Needle EMG: myopathic motor unit action potentials with fibrillation potentials and positive sharp waves
- Muscle MRI: edema in subcutaneous tissue and fascia demonstrated as hyperintensities on short tau inversion recovery (STIR) sequences. Calcinosis cutis (e.g., in anti-NXP2-associated dermatomyositis) can also be demonstrated.
- Muscle biopsy (see also comments and discussion from Questions 6, 21, and 29 in Chapter 10)
  - Perifascicular atrophy: the key feature of dermatomyositis, seen as atrophy of muscle fibers at the periphery of the muscle fascicle
  - Microvasculitis of perimysial (not epimysial) blood vessels
    - Microvasculitis is thought to result in microinfarcts and perifascicular atrophy.
    - Deposition of C5b-9 membrane attack complex in blood vessel walls
  - Infiltration of CD4+ cells including T cells and plasmacytoid dendritic cells in perimysium and blood vessel walls
  - Expression of myxovirus resistance protein A (MxA)
  - Upregulation of major histocompatibility complex (MHC) class I can also be seen in polymyositis, dermatomyositis, and also immune-mediated necrotizing myopathy.
  - Electron microscopy: tubuloreticular inclusions in the capillary endothelium

## ◎ HIGH-YIELD FACT

Patients with dermatomyositis require screening of malignancy (e.g., CT chest, abdomen and pelvis; age-appropriate screening) and interstitial lung disease (e.g., CT chest).

- In dermatomyositis, perifascicular atrophy characterized by atrophy of muscle fibers at the periphery (not the center) of muscle fascicles is a key feature.
- CD8+ T cells are the predominant inflammatory cells in polymyositis. In dermatomyositis, CD4+ cells including CD4+ T cells and plasmacytoid dendritic cells are the main inflammatory cells. Increased MHC class I expression can be seen in both polymyositis and dermatomyositis.
- 15–18-nm filamentous inclusions in muscles are seen in IBM.

**QUESTION 6.** Which of the following shows the correct matching between the myositis-specific antibody and its associated feature?
A. Anti-Jo-1 – calcinosis cutis
B. Anti-MDA5 – classic dermatomyositis
C. Anti-Mi-2 – mechanic's hands
D. Anti-NXP2 – rapidly progressive interstitial lung disease
E. Anti-TIF1γ – strong association with cancer

**ANSWER:** E. Anti-TIF1γ – strong association with cancer

**COMMENTS AND DISCUSSION (see also comments and discussion from Question 5)**
- All of the options are dermatomyositis-specific antibodies except anti-Jo-1, which is associated with anti-synthetase syndrome.
- Anti-Jo-1 is one of the anti-synthetase antibodies. Anti-Jo-1 is associated with myopathy, mechanic's hands, and severe interstitial lung disease. Patients with anti-Jo-1 may have mild skin rash.
- Anti-MDA5 is associated with amyopathic dermatomyositis and rapidly progressive interstitial lung disease.
- Anti-Mi-2 is associated with classic dermatomyositis in which patients have proximal muscle weakness, typical cutaneous manifestations, and a good response to immunotherapies.
- Anti-NXP2 is associated with calcinosis cutis and risk of malignancy.
- Anti-TIF1γ is associated with high risk of malignancy.

**QUESTION 7.** A 46-year-old man presents with symmetrical proximal muscle weakness for 4 months. In addition, he has a worsening dry cough, difficulty breathing, and dyspnea on exertion. On examination, in addition to proximal muscle weakness, examination of his hands shows findings in the following figure. Which of the following antibodies is **MOST LIKELY** to be positive in this patient?

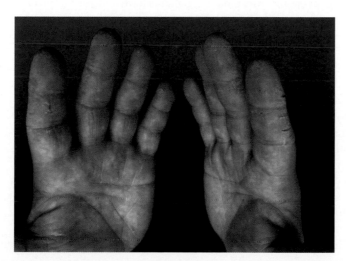

From Marco JL, Collins BF. Clinical manifestations and treatment of anti-synthetase syndrome. *Best Pract Res Clin Rheumatol.* 2020 Aug;34(4):101503. Photo courtesy Greg Gardner.

A. Anti-cN1A
B. Anti-Jo-1
C. Anti-Mi-2
D. Anti-NXP2
E. Anti-3-hydroxy-3-methyglutaryl-coenzyme A reductase

**ANSWER:** B. Anti-Jo-1

**COMMENTS AND DISCUSSION**
- The diagnosis in this patient is anti-synthetase syndrome. Among all anti-synthetase antibodies, anti-Jo-1 has been classically associated with mechanic's hands.

- The figure demonstrates classic mechanic's hands: thickened skin of the hands, and cracking and fissuring of the fingertips, lateral aspect of the fingers, and palms.
- *Anti-synthetase syndrome*
    - Associated with antibodies to aminoacyl-transfer RNA synthetases
    - Clinical features
        - Myopathy: symmetric proximal muscle weakness
        - Interstitial lung disease: can be severe or rapidly progressive
        - Mechanic's hands
        - Raynaud phenomenon
        - Arthritis
        - Fever
    - Laboratory features
        - Serum creatine kinase: usually elevated, up to 50 times the upper limit of normal
        - Anti-synthetase antibodies
            - Include anti-Jo-1, anti-PL-7, anti-PL-12, anti-EJ, anti-OJ, anti-KS, anti-Ha, anti-Zo
            - The most common is anti-Jo-1, which is classically associated with mechanic's hands.
        - Electromyography: myopathic findings with fibrillation potentials and positive sharp waves
        - Muscle biopsy
            - Most patients have features of dermatomyositis including perifascicular atrophy. However, there is no sarcoplasmic expression of myxovirus resistance protein A (MxA) or membrane attack complex in blood vessel walls.
            - Electron microscopy: nuclear actin aggregation, which is unique to anti-synthetase syndrome
- Anti-cN1A (aka, NT5c1A) is associated with IBM.
- Anti-Mi-2 is found in classic dermatomyositis with the typical skin rash.
- Anti-NXP2 is found in dermatomyositis. It is often associated with calcinosis cutis and increased risk of malignancy.
- Anti-3-hydroxy-3-methylglutaryl-coenzyme A reductase (anti-HMGCR) is associated with immune-mediated necrotizing myopathy. Most, not all, patients have a history of prior statin use.

**QUESTION 8.** A 57-year-old man with coronary artery disease, hypertension, diabetes, and dyslipidemia presents with progressive symmetrical proximal muscle weakness for 3 months. His medications include aspirin 81 mg/day, amlodipine 5 mg/day, glipizide 5 mg/day, and simvastatin 40 mg/day. On examination, muscle strength is grade 3 proximally and grade 4–5 distally. There is no sensory impairment. Muscle stretch reflexes are 1+ throughout. Serum creatine kinase is 5200 U/L. Serum anti-3-hydroxy-3-methylglutaryl-coenzyme A (anti-HMGCR) antibody is positive. Which of the following statements is most likely **CORRECT**?

A. All patients with this entity have history of statin exposure.
B. Interstitial lung disease is commonly associated with this entity.
C. There is markedly increased risk of malignancy.
D. Muscle biopsy shows muscle necrosis and prominent lymphocytic endomysial infiltration.
E. This patient should have a good response to intravenous immunoglobulin.

**ANSWER:** E. This patient should have a good response to intravenous immunoglobulin.

**COMMENTS AND DISCUSSION**
- This patient has *immune-mediated necrotizing myopathy* (IMNM, aka necrotizing autoimmune myopathy [NAM]) associated with anti-HMGCR antibody.
- IMNM is a group of inflammatory myopathies with a unique pathological feature of muscle necrosis without evidence of inflammation.
- IMNM patients present with symmetrical proximal muscle weakness, similar to dermatomyositis and polymyositis.
- All IMNMs do *not* have skin lesions, in contrast to dermatomyositis.
- Almost all IMNMs are not associated with interstitial lung disease, except a minority of patients with anti-SRP antibody.
- IMNM is associated with two main antibodies and can be classified into three subtypes (Table 17.2).
    - Anti-3-hydroxy-3-methylglutaryl-coenzyme A reductase (anti-HMGCR)
        - Associated with statin use or prior statin exposure. Of note, statins are HMG-CoA reductase inhibitors.

**TABLE 17.2** Comparison between subtypes of immune-mediated necrotizing myopathy.

|  | Anti-HMGCR | Anti-SRP | Seronegative |
|---|---|---|---|
| Severity and progression of the disease | + | +++ | + |
| Dermatologic involvement | - | - | - |
| Interstitial lung disease | - | + | - |
| Increased risk of malignancy | + | - | +++ |
| Response to conventional immunotherapies | +++ Good response to IVIG | - Good response to rituximab | + |

*Anti-HMGCR*, anti-3-hydroxy-3-methyglutaryl-coenzyme A reductase; *anti-SRP*, anti-signal recognition particle; IVIG, intravenous immunoglobulin
- indicates no association; + indicates presence of association; +++ indicates strong association

- Thirty percent of IMNM with positive anti-HMGCR antibody do not have a history of prior statin exposure.
- Symptoms continue to progress even after the discontinuation of statin.
- Increased risk of malignancy, but the association is not as strong as seronegative IMNM
- Good response to immunotherapies, especially intravenous immunoglobulin, in addition to discontinuation of statin.
  - Anti-signal recognition particle (anti-SRP)
    - Associated with a more severe disease course, compared to IMNM patients with anti-HMGCR. Patients can have rapid progression, severe muscle weakness, and dysphagia.
    - Ten to twenty percent of patients with anti-SRP have interstitial lung disease.
    - Not associated with increased risk of cancer
    - Poor response to corticosteroids and even intravenous immunoglobulin
    - Good response to rituximab has been shown in several reports.
  - Seronegative IMNM
    - IMNM with negative anti-HMGCR and anti-SRP antibodies
    - Increased risk of malignancy

## ◎ HIGH-YIELD FACT

Key features of each subtype of IMNM
- Anti-HMGCR: association with statin in 70%; favorable response to IVIG
- Anti-SRP: aggressive course of the disease, poor response to conventional immunotherapies, but good response to rituximab
- Seronegative: strong association with malignancy

- Laboratory features of IMNM
  - Serum creatine kinase (CK): markedly elevated, typically in the several thousand range, up to 50 times of upper normal limit
  - Electromyography: fibrillation potentials and/or positive sharp waves, which can be prominent, as well as myopathic features
  - Muscle MRI
    - Hyperintensities on short tau inversion recovery (STIR), which represents muscle edema and inflammation, and on T1, which represents fat infiltration within muscle fibers. However, unlike dermatomyositis, there are no hyperintensities in the fascia.

## MNEMONICS

Anti-HMG**C**R is associated with increased risk of **C**ancer (stronger association in seronegative IMNM).
Anti-SR**P** is associated with **P**ulmonary involvement in some patients.

○ Muscle biopsy (see also comments and discussion from Question 6 and Fig. 10.6D in Chapter 10)
  - Variation of muscle fiber size
  - Muscle fiber necrosis and regeneration (seen as small bluish fibers on hematoxylin and eosin [H&E] staining)
  - Absent or minimal inflammation including endomysial lymphocytic infiltration
  - Macrophages at or around necrotic muscle fibers can be seen. These macrophages have a role in phagocytosis and removal of cellular debris.
  - Expression of membrane attack complex and upregulation of major histocompatibility complex (MHC) class I expression

 **HIGH-YIELD FACT**

The key histopathologic feature of immune-mediated necrotizing myopathy is muscle fiber necrosis with **NO** or **MINIMAL** lymphocytic infiltration.
Of note, macrophages at or around necrotic fibers can be seen.

**QUESTION 9.**  Regarding immune-mediated necrotizing myopathy, which of the following features distinguishes anti-signal recognition particle (anti-SRP) antibody syndrome from anti-HMG-CoA reductase (anti-HMGCR) antibody syndrome?
A. More aggressive course of the disease
B. Higher association with malignancy
C. Fibrillation potentials on electromyography
D. More endomysial lymphocytic infiltration on muscle biopsy
E. Better response to intravenous immunoglobulin

**ANSWER:** A. More aggressive course of the disease

**COMMENTS AND DISCUSSION (see also comments and discussion from Question 8)**
- In immune-mediated necrotizing myopathy (IMNM), anti-signal recognition particle (anti-SRP) is associated with a more aggressive course of the disease. Patients typically have more severe muscle weakness with rapid progression, compared to patients with anti-3-hydroxy-3-methyglutaryl-coenzyme A reductase (anti-HMG-CoA reductase or anti-HMGCR). Dysphagia can be present.
- IMNM patients with anti-SRP generally have poor response to conventional immunotherapies including corticosteroids or intravenous immunoglobulin (IVIG). This is in contrast to IMNM patients with anti-HMGCR that generally have favorable response to IVIG. Patients with anti-SRP have been reported to have good response to rituximab.
- There is no increased risk of malignancy in IMNM patients with anti-SRP. Increased risk of malignancy is associated with seronegative IMNM patients, and to a lesser degree, IMNM patients with anti-HMGCR.
- Fibrillation potentials and positive sharp waves on electromyography can be seen in all subtypes of immune-mediated necrotizing myopathy, regardless of the antibody status. These may be more prominent in IMNM, compared to other inflammatory myopathies such as dermatomyositis.
- Endomysial lymphocytic infiltration is not seen in any subtypes of IMNM. The key histopathologic feature of IMNM is muscle fiber necrosis (and regeneration) without evidence of lymphocytic infiltration. However, macrophage infiltration at or around necrotic fibers is common. These macrophages scavenge cellular debris of necrotic fibers.

**QUESTION 10.** A 36-year-old man has had progressive proximal muscle weakness in both arms and legs for 3 years. Serum creatine kinase was 12,543 U/L. Muscle biopsy of the biceps showed moderate variation of muscle fiber size and endomysial lymphocytic infiltration. He was diagnosed with polymyositis, and treated with oral prednisolone, intravenous immunoglobulin, mycophenolate mofetil and recently rituximab, but there was no improvement. On examination, there is atrophy of proximal muscles and both calves. Muscle strength of bilateral upper and lower extremities is grade 4 proximally, and grade 5 distally. Which of the following is the next best step in the management of this patient?

A. Repeat muscle biopsy
B. Antibody testing for anti-HMG-CoA reductase
C. Genetic testing of the dysferlin gene
D. Consider cyclophosphamide
E. Check CD19+ cells to monitor B-cell depletion effects of rituximab

**ANSWER:** C. Genetic testing of the dysferlin gene

**COMMENTS AND DISCUSSION**

- This patient carries to diagnosis of polymyositis, but refractory to multiple immunotherapies. This raises an important red flag for this diagnosis.
- In this patient, markedly elevated serum creatine kinase (CK) and atrophy of the posterior leg compartment are clues for the diagnosis of dysferlinopathy (aka limb-girdle muscular dystrophy type 2A [LGMD2A]). Genetic testing of the *DYSF* gene encoding for dysferlin is the appropriate next step in the management.
- In any patients with "refractory polymyositis", the diagnosis should be reconsidered. Endomysial lymphocytic infiltration on muscle biopsy can be misleading, since this can also be seen in other disorders such as:
  ○ Inclusion body myositis (IBM)
    - Rimmed vacuoles may be present in less than 10% of muscle fibers, and can be missed.
    - Demonstration of abnormal protein accumulation (such as TDP-43, tau, p62) by special immunostaining and cytochrome oxidase (COX)-negative fibers has an important role in the diagnosis.
  ○ LGMD2A (aka dysferlinopathy)
    - Patients with LGMD2A can have proximal muscle weakness and markedly elevated serum CK, mimicking inflammatory myopathies.
    - It is important to keep a high index of suspicion and search for other important clues such as involvement of the posterior leg compartment.
  ○ Facioscapulohumeral dystrophy (FSHD)
    - Endomysial lymphocytic infiltration without invasion of non-necrotic muscle fibers is present in up to one-third of FSHD patients.
- Polymyositis is now thought to be a relatively rare diagnosis. Many patients previously diagnosed with polymyositis are subsequently found to have other diagnoses including the ones mentioned above such as IBM, as well as anti-synthetase syndrome and immune-mediated necrotizing myopathy (IMNM).
- The appropriate next step in the management is reconsideration of the diagnosis, instead of escalating the treatment. Use of cyclophosphamide or evaluation of B-cell depletion by rituximab is unlikely to be useful in this patient.
- Repeated muscle biopsy is unlikely to be useful, since the previous muscle biopsy already demonstrated endomysial lymphocytic infiltration which is a known finding in dysferlinopathy.
- Antibody testing for IMNM is unlikely to be useful. Endomysial lymphocytic infiltration is not a finding in this disorder. In addition, no response to multiple immunotherapies including intravenous immunoglobulin (IVIG) and rituximab is unusual for IMNM, especially anti-HMGCR-associated IMNM which typically has a favorable response to IVIG.

**QUESTION 11.** Which of the following enzymes is the most useful to differentiate between liver and muscle injury?

A. Aspartate aminotransferase (AST)
B. Alanine aminotransferase (ALT)
C. Alkaline phosphatase (ALP)
D. Gamma-glutamyltransferase (GGT)
E. Both A and B

**ANSWER:** D. Gamma-glutamyltransferase (GGT)

**COMMENTS AND DISCUSSION**

- The transaminase enzymes including aspartate aminotransferase (AST, aka SGOT), and alanine aminotransferase (ALT, aka SGPT) can be elevated when there is liver or muscle injury. In other words, elevation of AST and ALT can also be due to muscle injury, in addition to the well-known hepatocellular injury.
- Gamma-glutamyltransferase (GGT) is useful to differentiate between liver injury and muscle injury, when AST and ALT are elevated. GGT is specific to the liver, and is not elevated in cases of muscle injury.
- AST/ALT ratio can also be useful to differentiate between the liver and muscle injury.
  - In liver injury, AST/ALT ratio is less than 1.
  - In cases of skeletal or cardiac muscle injury such as myocardial infarction, AST/ALT ratio is greater than 1. During the acute phase of muscle damage (the first few days), AST/ALT ratio is usually greater than 3.
- Elevation of alkaline phosphatase (ALP) is can be due to:
  - Hepatic causes, especially cholestasis and space occupying lesions within the liver. In cholestasis, there is an elevation of ALP out of proportion to the aminotransferases. In cases of a space occupying lesion, there may be an isolated elevation of ALP.
  - Non-hepatic causes, especially bony diseases. Other less common causes include cardiac and renal failure, and hyperthyroidism, among others.
- Lactate dehydrogenase (LDH) is also not specific to the liver. It is found in almost every cell type in the body. The common causes of elevated LDH include hemolysis, muscle injury, hematologic malignancies (e.g., lymphoma), and liver diseases, among others.

**QUESTION 12.** Which of the following statements is **CORRECT** regarding myopathy related to thyroid disorders?
A. Fixed proximal muscle weakness is associated with hypothyroidism, but not hyperthyroidism.
B. Hyperthyroidism can be associated with periodic paralysis.
C. Muscle pain is usually absent in myopathy-related to hyperthyroidism but not hypothyroidism.
D. Delayed relaxation phase of muscle stretch reflexes is a feature of thyrotoxic myopathy.
E. Serum creatine kinase is usually normal in hypothyroid myopathy.

**ANSWER:** B. Hyperthyroidism can be associated with periodic paralysis.

**COMMENTS AND DISCUSSION**

- Both hypothyroidism and hyperthyroidism can cause myopathy with predominantly proximal muscle weakness. Myalgia and fatigue are common symptoms in both hypothyroid myopathy and thyrotoxic myopathy.
  - *Hypothyroid myopathy*
    - Examination may show delayed relaxation phase of muscle stretch reflexes.
    - Rhabdomyolysis may rarely occur.
    - Serum creatine kinase (CK) is usually markedly elevated.
  - *Thyrotoxic myopathy*
    - Associated with other signs of hyperthyroidism such as thyroid eye disease (exophthalmos or ophthalmoparesis in Graves' disease).
    - Serum CK is usually normal.
- In addition to fixed weakness, thyrotoxic myopathy can be associated with periodic paralysis, called thyrotoxic periodic paralysis (TPP).
  - In TPP, there is a male predominance. This is in contrast to hyperthyroidism which predominantly affects females.
  - One-third of patients with TPP have mutations in the *KCNJ18* gene encoding Kir2.6, an inward rectifier potassium channel 18.
- Of note, hyperparathyroidism and osteomalacia can also be associated with myopathy. Serum CK is usually normal. Hypoparathyroidism is usually not associated with myopathy.

**QUESTION 13.** A 23-year-old man with HIV infection under a good control presents with progressive proximal muscle weakness and muscle pain for 3 months. He has been on zidovudine (AZT) and didanosine for over 2 years. His most recent CD4+ count is 720 /mm³, and viral load is 0. Zidovudine myopathy is suspected, and muscle biopsy is performed. Which of the following findings on muscle biopsy would confirm this diagnosis?

A. Autophagic vacuoles within muscle fibers
B. Fiber type grouping
C. Necrotic muscle fibers without lymphocytic infiltration
D. Ragged-red fibers
E. Type 2 muscle fiber atrophy

**ANSWER:** D. Ragged-red fibers

**COMMENTS AND DISCUSSION (see also comments and discussion from Question 8 in Chapter 10)**

- Zidovudine (AZT) is an antiretroviral drug in the class of nucleoside reverse transcriptase inhibitors. It is now much less commonly used, due to the availability of newer antiretroviral agents.
- *Zidovudine myopathy*
  - Symmetrical proximal muscle weakness
  - Serum creatine kinase: mildly elevated
  - Electromyography: myopathic features with fibrillation potentials, as seen in most drug-induced or toxic myopathies
  - Muscle biopsy
    - Zidovudine also inhibits DNA polymerase γ resulting in mitochondrial dysfunction. Hence, the key histopathologic findings in zidovudine myopathy demonstrate evidence of mitochondrial dysfunction, similar to that seen in mitochondrial myopathy.
    - Key histopathologic findings
      - Ragged-red fibers on modified Gomori trichrome (mGT) stain
      - Cytochrome oxidase (COX)-negative fibers on COX stain
      - Paracrystalline inclusions arranged in a "parking lot" pattern on electron microscopy. These represent abnormal mitochondria.
      - There should be no inflammation in zidovudine myopathy.
        - This contrasts with HIV-associated inflammatory myopathy where there is endomysial lymphocytic endomysial infiltration, similar to what is seen in polymyositis. Of note, HIV-associated inflammatory myopathy is not caused by direct infection, but rather inflammation induced by HIV.

### ◎ HIGH-YIELD FACT

> Defects in DNA polymerase γ results in mitochondrial dysfunction, and can be due to:
> - Genetic cause: as seen in *POLG*-related disorders (e.g., chronic progressive external ophthalmoplegia). These disorders can result in mitochondrial myopathy.
> - Acquired cause: zidovudine resulting in histopathologic findings, similar to those seen in mitochondrial myopathy

- Other antiviral agents that can cause myopathy with mitochondrial dysfunction, and histopathologic findings similar to zidovudine myopathy include:
  - Lamivudine: for treatment of HIV and hepatitis B virus infections
  - Clevudine: for treatment of hepatitis B virus infection
  - Entecavir: for treatment of hepatitis B virus infection
  - Telbivudine: for treatment of hepatitis B virus infection
    - Telbivudine can also cause neuropathy, in addition to myopathy, termed "neuromyopathy."

**QUESTION 14.** Which of the following is **NOT** a common feature between chloroquine-, hydroxychloroquine-, amiodarone-, and colchicine-induced myopathies?

A. Increased risk of myopathy in the setting of renal insufficiency
B. Coexisting neuropathy
C. Markedly elevated serum creatine kinase
D. Fibrillation potentials on needle electromyography
E. Autophagic vacuoles within muscle fibers on muscle biopsy

**ANSWER:** C. Markedly elevated serum creatine kinase

**COMMENTS AND DISCUSSION (see also comments and discussion from Questions 6 and 30 in Chapter 10)**

- These medications cause amphiphilic drug myopathy and anti-microtubular myopathy.
- Markedly elevated serum creatine kinase (CK) is generally found in colchicine myopathy, but not in the others.
- Chloroquine, hydroxychloroquine and amiodarone are amphiphilic drugs.
    - Amphi- means "both."
    - Amphiphilic molecules have both hydrophilic (water-soluble, polar) and hydrophobic (lipophilic, apolar) regions.
    - These molecules can have interaction with cell membranes and organelles.
- Colchicine is an anti-microtubular agent.
    - It binds to tubulin, and forms tubulin-colchicine complex preventing microtubule assembly.
    - It is also weakly amphiphilic.
- Both amphiphilic drug myopathy and anti-microtubular myopathy have several common features:
    - Myopathy: symmetrical proximal muscle weakness
    - Amphiphilic drugs (chloroquine, hydroxychloroquine, and amiodarone) and colchicine can cause polyneuropathy, in addition to myopathy, called *neuromyopathy*.
    - The risk of neuromyopathy is increased with renal failure and prolonged exposure to the medications (generally greater than 1 year).
    - Needle EMG
        - In cases of myopathy: fibrillation potentials or positive sharp waves, and myopathic features
        - In cases of neuromyopathy: mixed myopathic features (especially in proximal muscles) and neuropathic features (especially in distal muscles)
    - Muscle biopsy (Figure 17.4)
        - Autophagic vacuoles within muscle fibers. Vacuoles can also be seen in nerves on nerve biopsy, in cases of neuromyopathy.
        - These autophagic vacuoles are due to accumulation of abnormal lysosomes, and thus show positive acid phosphatase staining within muscle fibers.
        - On electron microscopy, autophagic vacuoles contain lamellar myeloid bodies or curvilinear bodies. These are lipid-containing inclusions.

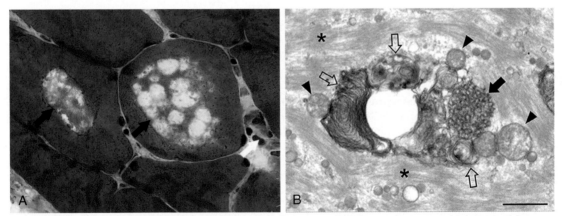

**Fig. 17.4  Drug-induced vacuolar myopathy.** (A) Colchicine myopathy. This muscle biopsy demonstrates multiple vacuoles (*arrows*) within muscle fibers on hematoxylin and eosin staining. (B) Electron microscopy shows a vacuole with adjacent typical curvilinear bodies (*filled arrow*) and myelinoid bodies (*open arrows*). Also present are mitochondria (*arrowheads*) and myofilaments (*asterisks*) (A) From Sista SR, Nyce MQ, Bach SE, Blume GM. Teaching Neurolmages: Colchicine-induced vacuolar myopathy. *Neurology.* 2019;93(24):e2306–e2307. (B) From Pamphlett R, Wang MX, Chan RC. Challenges in diagnosing hydroxychloroquine myopathy during the COVID-19 pandemic. *Intern Med J.* 2020 Dec;50(12):1559-1562. doi: 10.1111/imj.15092. PMID: 33354884.

- Serum CK levels differ between amphiphilic drug myopathy and anti-microtubular myopathy.
    - Amphiphilic drug myopathy: CK is usually normal or mildly elevated.
    - Colchicine myopathy: CK is markedly elevated.

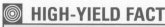 **HIGH-YIELD FACT**

**Medications that can cause "neuromyopathy" include**
- Amphiphilic drugs: chloroquine, hydroxychloroquine, amiodarone
- Anti-microtubular drug: colchicine (also weakly amphiphilic)
- Antiviral drug: telbivudine

**Muscle biopsy**
- Amphiphilic drugs and colchicine myopathies show autophagic vacuoles.
- Telbivudine myopathy shows mitochondrial pathology (i.e., ragged-red fibers and COX-negative fibers), but does not have vacuoles.

**QUESTION 15.** Which of the following statements is **FALSE** regarding statin-associated myopathy?
A. The risk increases with higher doses.
B. The risk increases when there is renal impairment.
C. The risk increases when using statin in combination with gemfibrozil or niacin.
D. Asymptomatic hyperCKemia can occur.
E. Intravenous immunoglobulin is the first-line treatment when there is persistently elevated serum creatine kinase.

**ANSWER:** E. Intravenous immunoglobulin is the first-line treatment when there is persistently elevated serum creatine kinase

**COMMENTS AND DISCUSSION (see also comments and discussion from Question 8)**
- When statin-associated myopathy is suspected, the first step in management is to discontinue the statin and monitor serum creatine kinase (CK) levels.
  - It is important to differentiate between toxic necrotizing myopathy and statin-associated immune-mediated necrotizing myopathy (IMNM, aka necrotizing immune myopathy, NAM).
  - If serum CK does not return to normal within 1-2 months after discontinuation of statin, IMNM should be suspected and confirmed with anti-HMG-CoA reductase (anti-HMGCR) testing and muscle biopsy
  - Once the diagnosis of IMNM is confirmed (or highly suspected when confirmatory tests are still pending), treatment with intravenous immunoglobulin (IVIG) can be considered
- Statins can cause a spectrum of adverse effects on the muscle with varying degrees of severity, including:
  - Asymptomatic hyperCKemia
  - Myalgia and cramps
  - Toxic myopathy: due to direct toxic effects of statins on muscle
    - Toxic necrotizing myopathy
    - Rhabdomyolysis in the severe form
  - Immune-mediated necrotizing myopathy (IMNM): due to an immune response
    - Associated with anti-HMGCR antibody
    - How to differentiate statin-associated IMNM from toxic necrotizing myopathy?
      - In toxic necrotizing myopathy, after discontinuation of statin, serum CK should return to normal within 1-2 months.
      - Positive anti-HMGCR supports the diagnosis of IMNM, but a negative result does not exclude the possibility of IMNM.
      - If serum CK remains elevated after discontinuation of statin and anti-HMGCR is negative, muscle biopsy should be performed. The upregulation of major histocompatibility complex (MHC) class I and membrane attack complex (MAC) expression in the non-necrotic fibers supports the diagnosis of IMNM.
      - IMNM requires different treatment strategies from toxic necrotizing myopathy. IMNM is treated with immunotherapies such as IVIG and/or corticosteroids.
- Risk factors of toxic necrotizing myopathy from statins
  - Combined use with other medications such as
    - Other lipid lowering agents including fibrates (e.g., gemfibrozil), niacin, ezetimibe
      - It is important to note that these medications can also cause myopathy when used alone without a statin.
    - Medications that inhibit cytochrome P450 3A4 (CYP3A4):
      - Amiodarone
      - Colchicine
      - Cyclosporine

- Protease inhibitors such as ritonavir
- Antifungal agents such as ketoconazole and itraconazole
- Macrolide antibiotics
- Calcium channel blockers such as verapamil
- Grapefruit juice
  - Use of high-dose statin
  - Increased age
  - Renal insufficiency or liver failure
  - Hypothyroidism
  - Presence of a single nucleotide polymorphism in the *SLCO1B1* gene

 **HIGH-YIELD FACT**

Statin use in combination with other lipid-lowering agents (e.g., gemfibrozil, niacin, ezetimibe), or cytochrome P450 3A4 inhibitors (e.g., amiodarone, colchicine) increases the risk of myopathy.

**QUESTION 16.** In steroid myopathy, needle electromyography (EMG) and muscle biopsy most likely show which of the following findings?
A. Normal needle EMG and muscle biopsy
B. Myopathic findings on needle EMG and type 1 fiber atrophy on muscle biopsy
C. Myopathic findings on needle EMG and type 2 fiber atrophy on muscle biopsy
D. Normal needle EMG and type 1 fiber atrophy on muscle biopsy
E. Normal needle EMG and type 2 fiber atrophy on muscle biopsy

**ANSWER:** E. Normal needle EMG and type 2 fiber atrophy on muscle biopsy

**COMMENTS AND DISCUSSION**
- *Steroid myopathy*
  - Risk factors: high doses, prolonged use or both
  - Clinical features: symmetrical proximal muscle weakness; only extremities are involved
  - Serum creatine kinase: normal
  - Needle electromyography: normal
    - No fibrillation potentials or positive sharp waves
    - During normal voluntary activation, type 1 muscle fibers are predominantly recruited.
    - Since steroid mainly affects type 2 muscle fibers, voluntary activation on needle EMG is typically normal.
  - Muscle biopsy
    - Type 2 muscle fiber atrophy. This finding can also be seen in disuse atrophy.
    - No inflammatory features
- Since patients with muscle weakness and inflammatory myopathies often receive treatment with steroids, a common clinical question is whether worsening weakness is due to steroid myopathy or worsening disease itself. Table 17.3 demonstrates some clues to help distinguish between these two, by using polymyositis as an example.

**TABLE 17.3** Differentiating between steroid myopathy and worsening of an underlying inflammatory myopathy using polymyositis as an example.

|  | Steroid myopathy | Worsening polymyositis |
|---|---|---|
| Serum CK | Stable or normalized from previous values (steroid myopathy has normal CK) | Rising from previous values |
| Needle EMG | No fibrillation potentials or positive sharp waves | More fibrillation potentials or positive sharp waves |
|  | Normal voluntary activity | Small short-duration polyphasic MUAPs with early recruitment |
| Muscle biopsy* | Type 2 fiber atrophy | Endomysial lymphocytic infiltration |
| Trial of reduction or discontinuation of steroids | Clinically improved | Clinically worse |

*Often not necessary to perform
*CK*, creatine kinase; *EMG*, electromyography; *MUAP*, motor unit action potential

**QUESTION 17.** A 74-year-old woman was admitted to the intensive care unit (ICU) due to severe pneumonia, septic shock, renal failure and respiratory failure requiring endotracheal intubation and ultimately tracheostomy. She was treated with intravenous fluids, intravenous norepinephrine, piperacillin and tazobactam and intravenous corticosteroids. It was difficult to wean her off the ventilator and she developed weakness of all extremities. Examination on week 4 revealed severe weakness of all extremities, worse proximally. Muscle stretch reflexes were 1+ throughout. There was no sensory impairment. Nerve conduction studies showed low compound muscle action potential (CMAP) amplitudes, but normal sensory nerve action potentials (SNAPs). Needle examination showed small, short-duration polyphasic motor unit action potentials with early recruitment. What is the **MOST LIKELY** finding on muscle biopsy in this patient?

A. Autophagic vacuoles within muscle fibers
B. Group atrophy and fiber type grouping
C. Muscle fiber necrosis and rimmed vacuoles within muscle fibers
D. Ragged-red fibers with cytochrome oxidase (COX)-deficient fibers
E. Loss of thick filaments on electron microscopic examination

**ANSWER:** E. Loss of thick filaments on electron microscopic examination

**COMMENTS AND DISCUSSION**

- The diagnosis in this patient is *critical illness myopathy (CIM)*.
  - She had a prolonged stay in intensive care unit, sepsis, multiorgan failure including respiratory and renal failure, as well as corticosteroid use.
  - She had difficult weaning and predominantly proximal muscle weakness in all extremities.
  - Low CMAP amplitudes with preserved SNAPs and normal conduction velocities, along with myopathic findings on needle EMG are compatible with severe myopathy.
  - There was no evidence of coexisting neuropathy on clinical examination and electrodiagnostic studies (normal sensation and normal SNAPs).
  - Loss of myosin (thick filaments) can be seen on muscle biopsy in some patients with CIM, but not in all cases.
- Critical illness-associated persistent neuromuscular weakness includes:
  - Critical illness myopathy (CIM), previously called "acute quadriplegic myopathy."
  - Critical illness polyneuropathy (CIP)
  - Critical illness myopathy and polyneuropathy (CIM/CIP)
- Risk factors of CIM, CIP, and CIM/CIP
  - Sepsis
  - Multiorgan system failure
  - Long duration of mechanical ventilation
  - Immobility
  - Hyperglycemia
  - Use of glucocorticoids or neuromuscular blocking agents or both. However, some studies showed that these agents did not increase risks of CIM and CIP.
- Several features can be used to differentiate between CIM and CIP, as outlined in Table 17.4.
- Autophagic vacuoles within muscle fibers are associated with amphiphilic drug (chloroquine, hydroxychloroquine, amiodarone) myopathy and anti-microtubular (colchicine) myopathy. These vacuoles contain the accumulation of abnormal lysosomes and are positive for acid phosphatase staining. In addition, autophagic vacuoles can also be seen in Pompe disease, but the vacuoles in this disorder also contain glycogen which is positive for periodic acid-Schiff (PAS) staining.
- Group atrophy and fiber type grouping are neurogenic changes. These can be seen in CIP, but not in CIM.
- Muscle fiber necrosis and rimmed vacuoles within muscle fibers are features seen in IBM.
- Ragged-red fibers and cytochrome oxidase (COX)-deficient fibers are indicative of mitochondrial dysfunction. These findings can be seen in mitochondrial myopathies, as well as in myopathies induced by drugs that are toxic to mitochondria such as zidovudine.

**TABLE 17.4** Comparison between critical illness myopathy (CIM) and critical illness polyneuropathy (CIP). CIM/CIP has mixed features of both CIM and CIP.

|  | CIM | CIP |
|---|---|---|
| Pattern of weakness | Predominantly proximal | Predominantly distal |
| Sensory impairment | No | Yes |
| Reflexes | Usually reduced or absent | Reduced or absent |
| Serum CK | Normal or mildly-to-moderately elevated (more elevation in acute period) | Normal |
| Nerve conduction study | Reduced CMAP amplitudes | Reduced CMAP amplitudes |
|  | Normal SNAPs | Reduced SNAP amplitudes |
|  | Normal or minimally reduced CVs | Normal or minimally reduced CVs |
| Needle EMG | Fibrillation potentials and/or positive sharp waves can be seen | Fibrillation potentials and/or positive sharp waves |
|  | Small short-duration polyphasic MUAPs with early recruitment | Large long-duration polyphasic MUAPs with reduced recruitment |
| Direct muscle stimulation | Reduced muscle excitability | Normal muscle excitability |
|  | Nerve: muscle ratio ~ 1 | Nerve: muscle ratio < 0.5 |
| Muscle biopsy | Type 2 muscle fiber atrophy | Denervation atrophy |
|  | Loss of myosin (thick filaments) in some patients (not in all cases) | Fiber type grouping |
| Prognosis | Better with more rapid and complete recovery | Poorer with slower and incomplete recovery |

CMAP, compound muscle action potential; CK, creatine kinase; CV, conduction velocity; EMG, electromyography; SNAP, sensory nerve action potential; MUAP, motor unit action potential.

**QUESTION 18.** Which of the following statements is **CORRECT** regarding myositis due to immune checkpoint inhibitors?
  A. Examples of the offending agents include pembrolizumab, ipilimumab, and bortezomib.
  B. The onset typically occurs after at least one year of immune checkpoint inhibitor use.
  C. Myasthenia gravis and myocarditis may co-occur with myositis.
  D. All patients require treatment with immunotherapies such as steroids and intravenous immunoglobulin.
  E. Decrement on slow repetitive nerve stimulation is common in myositis.

**ANSWER:** C. Myasthenia gravis and myocarditis may co-occur with myositis.

## COMMENTS AND DISCUSSION
- *Immune checkpoint inhibitors* are a relatively new group of cancer immunotherapies.
  - Ipilimumab is the first immune checkpoint inhibitor approved by the US FDA for the treatment of melanoma in 2011.
  - Since then, medications in this group and their indications have been expanding.
  - Immune checkpoints affect the interaction between immune cells (i.e., cytotoxic T cells) and other cells (i.e., tumor cells and antigen-presenting cells) (Table 17.5). Immune checkpoints have a role in preventing overactivation of the immune system.
  - When immune checkpoints are inhibited (Fig. 17.5):
    - Immune cells become more active, and kill tumor cells.
    - Immune cells that are overactivated can have off-target effects to cells other than tumor cells resulting in complications, including:
      - Neurologic complications: encephalitis, hypophysitis, myopathy, myasthenia gravis (MG), neuropathies (e.g., Guillain-Barré syndrome)
      - Non-neurologic complications: colitis, hepatitis, pneumonitis, myocarditis, retinopathy, pancreatitis

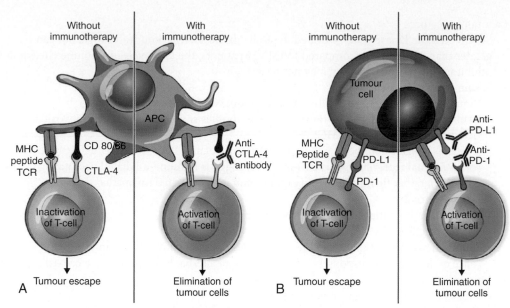

**Fig. 17.5** Immune checkpoints and the mechanisms of action of immune checkpoint inhibitors. (A) The interaction between CTLA-4 on T cell and CD80 ligand on antigen-presenting cells inhibits activation of T cells *(left)*. With anti-CTLA-4 antibodies, T cells become active, and can kill tumor cells. (B) The interaction between PD-1 on T cells and PD-L1 ligands on tumor cells results in T cell anergy (self-tolerance) and tumor escape. With anti-PD-1 or anti-PD-L1 antibodies, T cells can kill tumor cells. From Lewis AL, Chaft J, Girotra M, Fischer GW. Immune checkpoint inhibitors: A narrative review of considerations for the anaesthesiologist. *Br J Anaesth.* 2020;124(3):251–260.

**TABLE 17.5** Immune checkpoints and immune checkpoint inhibitors.

| T cell receptor | Ligand | Relevant immune checkpoint inhibitors |
|---|---|---|
| PD-1 | PD-L1 on tumor cell | PD-1 inhibitors: pembrolizumab, nivolumab |
| | | PD-L1 inhibitors: atezolizumab, avelumab, durvalumab |
| CTLA-4 | B7 (CD80 ligand) on antigen presenting-cell | CTLA-4 inhibitors: ipilimumab |

*CTLA-4*, cytotoxic T-lymphocyte-associated antigen 4; *PD-1*, programmed cell death-1; *PD-L1*, programmed death-ligand 1

**MNEMONICS**

**P**D-1 inhibitors: **P**embrolizumab, **N**ivolumab. The names begin with **P** and **N** (which is close to P).
**P**D-**L**1 inhibitors: **A**tezolizumab, **A**velumab, **D**urvalumab. The names begin with alphabets with **L**onger distance from P, specifically the **very first alphabets**.

- *Immune checkpoint inhibitor-associated myopathy*
  - Clinical features
    - Onset is typically within the first 2 months or after 1-2 cycles of treatment.
    - Muscle weakness
      - Limb-girdle pattern of weakness: proximal upper and lower extremities
      - Axial weakness: weakness of neck flexors (can present with dropped head syndrome), neck extensors
      - Oculobulbar weakness: ptosis, ophthalmoparesis (due to weakness of extraocular muscles), dysphagia, respiratory muscle weakness.
        - Oculobulbar weakness may occur with limb-girdle weakness or in isolation.
        - This can mimic MG. However, in some cases, patients may have coexisting MG and myopathy.
    - Myalgia is common.
    - Patients can also have MG and/or myocarditis.

- Laboratory features
  - Serum creatine kinase (CK): elevated, typically in the several thousand range, but can be greater than 10,000 U/L. Compared to IMNM patients, the CK levels in immune checkpoint inhibitor-associated myopathy may not be as high.
  - Serum autoantibodies
    - Some patients may have positive anti-striational antibodies.
    - Anti-acetylcholine receptor (anti-AChR) antibodies should be negative in myositis. Positive results suggest associated MG.
    - Myositis-specific antibodies are negative. Presence of anti-HMG-CoA reductase (anti-HMGCR) or anti-signal recognition particle (anti-SRP) suggests immune-mediated necrotizing myopathy (IMNM), rather than immune checkpoint inhibitor-associated myopathy.
  - Electromyography
    - Fibrillation potentials and/or positive sharp waves
    - Myopathic features
    - Repetitive nerve stimulation at low frequencies does not show decremental responses. Presence of decremental responses suggests MG as an alternative diagnosis or a coexisting disease.
  - Muscle biopsy
    - Muscle fiber necrosis and regeneration
    - Endomysial lymphocytic infiltration, predominantly by CD8+ T cells, has been demonstrated in some reports. The inflammation might be focal.
    - However, some reports have described no or minimal lymphocytic infiltration, similar to IMNM.
- Differential diagnosis
  - Myasthenia gravis (MG)
    - Positive anti-AChR antibodies
    - Decremental responses on low-frequency repetitive nerve stimulation
  - Immune-mediated necrotizing myopathy (IMNM)
    - Positive anti-HMGCR or anti-SRP
    - Presence of endomysial lymphocytic infiltration argues against the diagnosis of IMNM.
- Treatment
  - Discontinuing the immune checkpoint inhibitor
  - The need for immunotherapies depends on the severity of the disease.
    - In mild cases, only discontinuing the immune checkpoint inhibitor may be sufficient. Corticosteroids may be used.
    - In more severe cases, intravenous immunoglobulin (IVIG) and/or plasma exchange (PLEX) can be considered.
  - In mild cases, immune checkpoint inhibitor may be rechallenged. However, this was not attempted in most cases reported in the literature.
- Prognosis
  - Prognosis of myopathy
    - Patients typically improve within several weeks, and corticosteroids can be tapered. Serum CK levels usually return to normal within several weeks to up to 3 months.
  - Prognosis of cancer
    - Patients who develop and can tolerate the severe adverse effects associated with immune checkpoint inhibitors generally have good cancer prognoses and survivals.
- While pembrolizumab and ipilimumab are immune checkpoint inhibitors, bortezomib is not. Bortezomib is a selective 26S proteasome inhibitor used for treatment of multiple myeloma and mantle cell lymphoma.
- The onset of immune checkpoint inhibitor-associated myopathy is usually within 1-2 months after initiation of the immune checkpoint inhibitor, typically within the first two cycles.
- Not all patients with immune checkpoint inhibitor-associated neurologic complications require immunotherapies. Patients with mild symptoms may improve after discontinuation of the immune checkpoint inhibitor. In patients with insufficient improvement or more severe symptoms, corticosteroids, IVIG, and/or PLEX can be considered.
- Decrement on slow repetitive nerve stimulation is not seen in myositis and suggests coexisting MG.

**QUESTION 19.** A 79-year-old woman with hypertension, type 2 diabetes mellitus and dyslipidemia presents with severe pain in the right thigh for 2 days. The pain develops acutely, and today she also notes swelling of the right thigh. Examination reveals swelling and marked tenderness at the right anterior thigh. Examination of the muscle strength of the right leg is markedly limited by pain. Examination of the other extremities is normal. Peripheral white blood cell count is 14,000 /μL with 75% neutrophils. Hemoglobin A1c is 9.3%. Erythrocyte sedimentation rate is 90 mm/h, and C-reactive protein is 71 mg/L. Serum creatine kinase is 396 U/L. What is the next best step of investigation to confirm the diagnosis in this patient?

A.  Doppler ultrasound of the lower extremity
B.  Serum myositis-specific antibodies
C.  Electromyography
D.  Muscle MRI
E.  Muscle biopsy

**ANSWER:** D. Muscle MRI

**COMMENTS AND DISCUSSION**

- The diagnosis in this patient is diabetic muscle infarction (aka., diabetic myonecrosis), a rare complication of diabetes mellitus.
- Clinical features of diabetic muscle infarction
  - This typically involves the lower extremity including thigh or calf. Upper extremity involvement is much less common but can occur. There can be bilateral involvement.
  - Acute painful swelling of the involved extremity
  - Associated with poor glycemic control. Patients often have other diabetic complications such as retinopathy, nephropathy, and neuropathy.
- Pathophysiology
  - Microvascular infarct. Diabetic muscle infarct is considered one of the microvascular complications of diabetes mellitus.
- Laboratory investigations
  - Serum creatine kinase (CK): normal or elevated (in about one-third of patients)
  - The investigation of choice is muscle MRI.
    - On short tau inversion recovery (STIR) or T2-weighted images, there are hyperintensities within the involved muscle(s) representing muscle edema (Fig. 17.6).
  - Muscle ultrasound: loss of normal muscle striations, subcutaneous edema
  - Muscle biopsy should be avoided, since it is associated with the risk of procedural-related complications and longer time to symptom improvement.

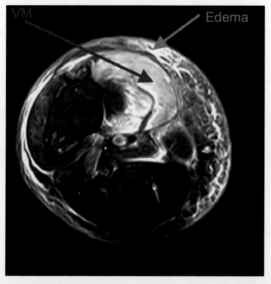

**Fig. 17.6** Muscle magnetic resonance imaging (MRI) in diabetic muscle infarct. This short tau inversion recovery (STIR) image demonstrates hyperintensities in the vastus medialis (*red arrow*), adjacent muscles (especially vastus intermedius), and subcutaneous tissue (*blue arrow*). These represent edema within the muscles and subcutaneous tissue. From Verjee MA, Abdelsamad NA, Qureshi S, Malik RA. Diabetic muscle infarction: Often misdiagnosed and mismanaged. *Diabetes Metab Syndr Obes.* 2019;12:285–290.

- Treatment
  - Main treatment includes bed rest and pain control with non-steroidal anti-inflammatory agents.
  - Surgery and rehabilitation should be avoided, since they are associated with longer time to improvement of symptoms. Surgery is associated with high risk of recurrence.

## ◎ HIGH-YIELD FACT

Muscle MRI is the investigation of choice for diabetic muscle infarction.
Muscle biopsy, surgery, and rehabilitation should be **avoided** in this disorder.

- While muscle ultrasound can be useful in diabetic muscle infarct, Doppler ultrasound of the lower extremity is used to search for deep vein thrombosis which is not suspected in this patient.
- Serum myositis-specific antibodies are not useful in this case, since inflammatory myopathies are not suspected.
- Electromyography is unlikely to provide additional information for the diagnosis.
- While muscle biopsy will show mostly necrosis and ischemia of muscle and can provide definitive findings and diagnosis, it is not recommended.

**QUESTION 20.** A 24-year-old woman who is an immigrant from Thailand presents with swelling of the left thigh for 3 weeks. Four weeks ago, she had fever, abdominal pain, and diarrhea. These symptoms resolved after 1 week. In the past 3 weeks, she has also had muscle pain, fatigue, headache, and swelling around both eyes. Examination reveals periorbital edema, as well as grade 4 weakness and tenderness of the left quadriceps muscle. Complete blood count reveals white blood cell count of 11,250 /μL, with a differential count of 55% neutrophils, 26% lymphocytes, and 19% eosinophils. Muscle biopsy is performed and shows the finding in the figure below (hematoxylin and eosin staining, 400x). What is the **MOST LIKELY** causative organism in this patient?

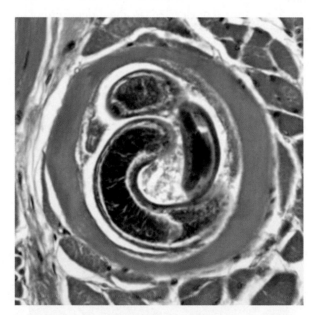

From www.cdc.gov/dpdx/trichinellosis/index.html. Centers for Disease Control and Prevention

A. *Naegleria fowleri*
B. *Taenia solium*
C. *Toxocara* spp.
D. *Toxoplasma gondii*
E. *Trichinella spiralis*

**ANSWER:** E. *Trichinella spiralis*

## COMMENTS AND DISCUSSION

- This patient has *trichinosis* (aka., trichinellosis). The muscle biopsy shows an encysted larva within the muscle.
- Trichinosis is due to infection by nematodes *Trichinella* spp. One of the most common species is *Trichinella spiralis*. There are also others that can cause trichinosis.
- Pathogenesis of trichinosis
  - Ingestion of meat containing pseudocysts → Release of larvae in small intestine → Fertilization in small intestine → Migration of young larvae via intestinal mucosa into bloodstream and muscle → Formation of encysted larvae within the muscle
- Clinical features of trichinosis
  - Incubation period after consuming meat containing pseudocysts is usually 2-12 days.
  - Prodromal symptoms: abdominal pain, diarrhea
  - In the second week: fever, subconjunctival hemorrhage, periorbital edema, myalgia
  - Myositis
    - Pain, swelling, weakness
    - Involved muscles: extraocular muscles, any striated muscles including muscles in the extremities, intercostal muscles, and diaphragm
    - Symptoms decrease after thickening of the capsule around the larva and calcification.
- Laboratory features of trichinosis
  - Complete blood count: eosinophilia
  - Serum creatine kinase (CK): elevated in the acute period
  - Electromyography: fibrillation potentials or positive sharp waves, myopathic features
  - Antibodies against *Trichinella*: usually takes 3-5 weeks to be positive
  - Muscle biopsy: encysted larva within muscle tissue
- Treatment: albendazole, mebendazole
- *Taenia solium* can cause cysticercosis and taeniasis in humans.
  - Cysticercosis occurs when humans become an intermediate host after ingesting ova in the feces that are contaminated in food or water. Cysticerci develop within muscle tissue.
  - In taeniasis, humans are a definitive host. Taeniasis occurs when humans ingest poorly cooked pork that contain the adult form of the pork tapeworm (*Taenia solium*).
- *Nuegleria fowleri* is an amoeba that can cause encephalitis when freshwater contaminated with the organism enters the brain through the nose.
- *Toxocara* spp. are nematodes (roundworm).
- *Toxoplasma gondii* is a protozoon. *Toxocara* spp. and *Toxoplasma gondii* can also cause infectious myopathy.

## SUGGESTED READINGS

Allenbach Y, Keraen J, Bouvier AM, et al. High risk of cancer in autoimmune necrotizing myopathies: usefulness of myositis specific antibody. *Brain.* 2016;139:2131-2135.

Allenbach Y, Mammen AL, Benveniste O, Stenzel W, Immune-Mediated Necrotizing Myopathies Working Group. 224th ENMC International Workshop: clinico-sero-pathological classification of immune-mediated necrotizing myopathies. Zandvoort, The Netherlands, 14-16 October 2016. *Neuromuscul Disord.* 2018;28:87-99.

Anquetil C, Boyer O, Wesner N, Benveniste O, Allenbach Y. Myositis-specific autoantibodies: a cornerstone in immune-mediated necrotizing myopathy. *Autoimmun Rev.* 2019;18:223-230.

Ansari R, Katirji B. Serum muscle enzymes in neuromuscular disease. In: Katirji B, Kaminski HJ, Ruff RL, eds. *Neuromuscular Disorders in Clinical Practice.* New York: Springer; 2014:39-50.

Bolton CF. Neuromuscular manifestations of critical illness. *Muscle Nerve.* 2005;32:140-163.

Boonyapisit K. Infectious and granulomatous myopathies. In: Katirji B, Kaminski HJ, Ruff RL, eds. *Neuromuscular Disorders in Clinical Practice.* New York: Springer; 2014:1389-1408.

Dalakas MC. Toxic and drug-induced myopathies. *J Neurol Neurosurg Psychiatry.* 2009;80:832-838.

Dalakas MC. Neurological complications of immune checkpoint inhibitors: what happens when you 'take the brakes off' the immune system. *Ther Adv Neurol Disord.* 2018;11.

Dalakas MC, Illa I, Pezeshkpour GH, et al. Mitochondrial myopathy caused by long-term zidovudine therapy. *N Engl J Med.* 1990;322;1098-1105.

Doughty CT, Amato AA. Toxic myopathies. *Continuum (Minneap Minn).* 2019;25:1712-1731.

El-Beshbishi SN, Ahmed NN, Mostafa SH, El-Ganainy GA. Parasitic infections and myositis. *Parasitol Res.* 2012;110:1-18.

Goyal NA. Immune-mediated myopathies. *Continuum (Minneap Minn).* 2019;25:1564-1585.

Goyal NA, Cash TM, Alam U, et al. Seropositivity for NT5c1A antibody in sporadic inclusion body myositis predicts more severe motor, bulbar and respiratory involvement. *J Neurol Neurosurg Psychiatry.* 2016;87:373-378.

Greenberg SA. Inclusion body myositis: clinical features and pathogenesis. *Nat Rev Rheumatol.* 2019;15:257-272.

Group SC, Link E, Parish S, et al. SLCO1B1 variants and statin-induced myopathy—a genomewide study. *N Engl J Med.* 2018;359:789-799.

Horton WB, Taylor JS, Ragland TJ, Subauste AR. Diabetic muscle infarction: a systematic review. *BMJ Open Diabetes Res Care.* 2015;3:e000082.

Janssen L, Allard NAE, Saris CGJ, et al. Muscle toxicity of drugs: When Drugs turn physiology into pathophysiology. *Physiol Rev.* 2020;100:633-672.

Kress JP, Hall JB. ICU-acquired weakness and recovery from critical illness. *N Engl J Med.* 2014;370:1626-1635.

Lundberg IE, Fujimoto M, Vencovsky J, et al. Idiopathic inflammatory myopathies. *Nat Rev Dis Primers.* 2021;7:86.

Rodolico C, Bonanno C, Pugliese A, et al. Endocrine myopathies: clinical and histopathological features of the major forms. *Acta Myol.* 2020;39:130-135.

Shelly S, Triplett JD, Pinto MV, et al. Immune checkpoint inhibitor-associated myopathy: a clinicoseropathologically distinct myopathy. *Brain Commun.* 2020;2:fcaa181.

Supakornnumporn S, Katirji B. Guillain-Barre syndrome triggered by immune checkpoint inhibitors: a case report and literature review. *J Clin Neuromuscul Dis.* 2017;19:80-83.

Touat M, Maisonobe T, Knauss S, et al. Immune checkpoint inhibitor-related myositis and myocarditis in patients with cancer. *Neurology.* 2018;91:e985-e994.

Uruha A, Nishikawa A, Tsuburaya RS, et al. Sarcoplasmic MxA expression: a valuable marker of dermatomyositis. *Neurology.* 2017;88:493-500.

Valiyil R, Christopher-Stine L. Drug-related myopathies of which the clinician should be aware. *Curr Rheumatol Rep.* 2010;12:213-220.

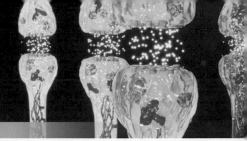

# CHAPTER 18

# Hereditary Myopathies

## PART 1: PRACTICE TEST

**Q1.** A 4-year-old boy presents with toe walking, difficulty running, and proximal muscle weakness. Calf hypertrophy is noted on examination. Serum creatine kinase level is 12,000 U/L. Muscle biopsy reveals absent dystrophin staining. Which of the following statements is **CORRECT** regarding this disorder?
A. Neck flexors are typically spared.
B. Gowers sign is specific to this condition.
C. This disorder is associated with restrictive cardiomyopathy.
D. Cognition is spared in this condition.
E. Patients typically become wheelchair dependent around the age of 12 years.

**Q2.** Which of the following laboratory tests is the most useful in differentiating Duchenne muscular dystrophy from Becker muscular dystrophy?
A. Serum creatine kinase
B. Hematoxylin and eosin staining on muscle biopsy
C. Western blot analysis of muscle tissue
D. Needle electromyography
E. Muscle ultrasonography

**Q3.** Which of the following mutations is the most common among patients with dystrophinopathies?
A. Large deletions
B. Large duplications
C. Point mutations
D. Trinucleotide repeat expansions
E. Chromosomal translocations

**Q4.** Which of the following statements is **CORRECT** regarding corticosteroid treatment in Duchenne muscular dystrophy?
A. Corticosteroids provide symptomatic benefit without slowing the progression of the disease.
B. Corticosteroids increase the risk of scoliosis.
C. An intermittent dosing regimen of prednisone has higher efficacy than a daily dosing regimen.
D. Deflazacort is preferred due to its higher efficacy than prednisone.
E. Weight gain is less with deflazacort, compared to prednisone.

**Q5.** Eteplirsen is a gene therapy that was approved by the US Food and Drug Administration (FDA) in 2016 for the treatment of Duchenne muscular dystrophy. What is the mechanism of this treatment?
A. Skipping of exon 51 of the dystrophin gene
B. Integration of exon 51
C. Readthrough of premature stop codons
D. Transferring of dystrophin gene by a viral vector
E. Antibody to myostatin

**The following answer options are for QUESTIONS 6 through 10.**

> **Match each dystrophy-related protein with its location in muscle.**
> A. Sarcolemma
> B. Sarcomere
> C. Nuclear membrane
> D. Extracellular matrix

**Q6.** Dystrophin
**Q7.** Dystroglycan
**Q8.** Emerin
**Q9.** Dysferlin
**Q10.** Collagen VI

**Q11.** A 35-year-old woman developed toe walking around the age of 7 years. Around the early teenage years she had difficulty combing her hair and walking upstairs. She became wheelchair dependent in her early 30s. Examination reveals bilateral scapular winging, prominent (grade 1–2) weakness of proximal muscles and mild weakness of distal muscles. Serum creatine kinase is 3853 U/L. Muscle biopsy demonstrates eosinophilic infiltration on hematoxylin and eosin (H&E) staining and lobulated fibers on nicotinamide adenine dinucleotide (NADH) stain. What is the most likely diagnosis?
A. Becker muscular dystrophy
B. Duchenne muscular dystrophy
C. Facioscapulohumeral dystrophy
D. Limb-girdle muscular dystrophy type 2A (calpainopathy)
E. Limb-girdle muscular dystrophy type 2B (dysferlinopathy)

**Q12.** Which of the following findings is **LEAST** likely to be seen in calpainopathy (LGMD2A)?
  A. Ankle contracture
  B. Scapular winging
  C. Cardiac abnormalities
  D. Respiratory involvement
  E. Medial gastrocnemius weakness

**Q13.** A 25-year-old man had difficulty standing on his toes and playing sports 3–4 years earlier. Subsequently he developed difficulty climbing stairs and flexing his elbows. Examination revealed prominent atrophy of both calves, more prominent on the right. There were no winged scapulae. Motor strength showed grade 4 weakness throughout. Reflexes were 1+ in the biceps and quadriceps, and 0 at both ankles. Serum creatine kinase was 19,000 U/L. Muscle biopsy revealed variation of muscle fiber size and endomysial lymphocytic infiltration. What is the most likely diagnosis?
  A. Becker muscular dystrophy
  B. Dysferlinopathy
  C. Inclusion body myositis
  D. Polymyositis
  E. Sarcoglycanopathy

**Q14.** Which of the following distal myopathies is characterized by weakness of the posterior leg compartment muscles?
  A. Miyoshi myopathy
  B. Nonaka myopathy
  C. Laing myopathy
  D. Udd myopathy
  E. Welander myopathy

**Q15.** Which of the following features is **LEAST** likely to be seen in dysferlinopathy (LGMD2B)?
  A. Asymmetric involvement
  B. Inability to walk on toes
  C. Cardiac involvement
  D. Serum creatine kinase of 30,000 U/L
  E. Endomysial infiltration on muscle biopsy

**Q16.** A 6-year-old Amish boy did not walk until the age of 24 months. He had tongue and calf hypertrophy, scapular winging, lumbar lordosis, and proximal muscle weakness. Serum creatine kinase was persistently elevated in the range of 10,000–20,000 U/L. Muscle biopsy showed dystrophic features but normal immunoreactivity to dystrophin antibodies. Transthoracic echocardiography revealed mild left ventricular systolic dysfunction. What is the most likely diagnosis?
  A. Becker muscular dystrophy
  B. Calpainopathy
  C. Dysferlinopathy
  D. Emery-Dreifuss muscular dystrophy
  E. Sarcoglycanopathy

**Q17.** The disorder associated with a deficiency of which of the following proteins has clinical features most comparable to those of Duchenne muscular dystrophy?
  A. Anoctamin 5
  B. Calpain
  C. Dysferlin
  D. Fukutin-related protein
  E. Merosin

**Q18.** Which of the following features distinguish anoctaminopathy (LGMD2L) from dysferlinopathy (LGMD2B/Miyoshi myopathy)?
  A. Inability to walk on toes
  B. Asymmetric muscle atrophy and weakness
  C. Cardiac involvement
  D. Respiratory involvement
  E. Creatine kinase level of 10,000 U/L

**Q19.** A 29-year-old man presented with an acute embolic stroke in the right middle cerebral artery territory and newly-diagnosed atrial fibrillation. The patient's left hemiparesis gradually improved to almost normal strength of the left arm and leg. Rivaroxaban was started. On examination, there was contracture of the elbows and ankles and grade 4 weakness of bilateral biceps, triceps, and gastrocnemius. The patient reported that his elbow and ankle contractures had been gradually worsening since his early teens and muscle weakness started in his early 20s. Additionally, his maternal grandfather developed similar symptoms in his 40s and had a cardiac problem requiring pacemaker placement. What is the most likely diagnosis in this patient?
  A. Bethlem myopathy
  B. Calpainopathy
  C. Dystrophinopathy
  D. Emery-Dreifuss muscular dystrophy
  E. Sarcoglycanopathy

**Q20.** Which of the following proteins is **NOT** associated with Emery-Dreifuss muscular dystrophy?
  A. Emerin
  B. Four and a half LIM domains
  C. Lamin A/C
  D. Laminin α2
  E. Nesprin

**Q21.** A 4-year-old girl has had frequent falls and progressive generalized muscle weakness since the age of 3 years. Examination reveals generalized hypotonia and reduced muscle mass. Motor strength of the upper and lower extremities is grade 3 proximally and grade 4 distally. There are contractures of both elbows, hyperlaxity of both wrists and ankles, and prominent soft tissue over the calcaneal region of both feet. This disorder is due to abnormality in which of the following proteins?
  A. α-Dystroglycan
  B. Collagen VI
  C. Emerin
  D. Merosin
  E. Selenoprotein N

**Q22.** A 32-year-old man presents with chronic slowly progressive proximal muscle weakness for over 10 years. On examination, finger flexion contracture is noted as in the following figure. What is the most likely diagnosis?

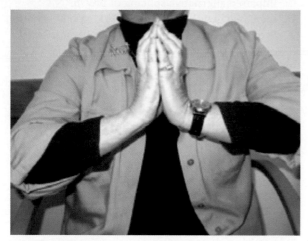

From Bönnemann CG. *Nat Rev Neurol.* 2011 Jun 21;7(7):379–390.

    A. Bethlem myopathy
    B. Emery-Dreifuss muscular dystrophy
    C. Kearns-Sayre syndrome
    D. Rigid spine muscular dystrophy
    E. Welander distal myopathy

**Q23.** Which of the following distal myopathies has preferential muscle involvement in the leg compartment that is different from the others?
    A. Nonaka myopathy (distal myopathy with rimmed vacuoles)
    B. Miyoshi myopathy
    C. Laing myopathy
    D. Markesbery-Griggs myopathy
    E. Udd myopathy

**Q24.** A 45-year-old man developed slowly progressive generalized muscle weakness around the age of 32. In the past year, he has also experienced behavioral changes including disinhibition. Multiple family members in every generation have similar symptoms. Frontotemporal dementia is suspected, and magnetic resonance imaging (MRI) of the brain reveals bilateral frontotemporal atrophy. However, proximal and distal muscle weakness is also noted in the bilateral upper and lower extremities. Muscle biopsy is performed and is compatible with inclusion body myositis (IBM). This disorder is most likely due to mutations in which of the following genes?
    A. *C9orf72*
    B. *FUS*
    C. *GNE*
    D. *VCP*
    E. *SOD1*

**Q25.** Which of the following genes is **NOT** associated with myofibrillar myopathy?
    A. *FHL1*
    B. *FLNC* (encoding filamin C)
    C. *LMNA* (encoding lamin A/C)
    D. *MYOT* (encoding myotilin)
    E. *ZASP*

**Q26.** Five years prior, a 29-year-old man developed difficulty puffing his cheeks, drinking water from a straw, and whistling. In addition, he noted increasing difficulty raising his arms above his head. Examination reveals facial diplegia, especially in the lower facial region, weakness of the bilateral shoulder girdle muscles, and mild scapular winging. There is no limitation of extraocular movements. Muscle biopsy shows endomysial lymphocytic infiltration. What is the most likely underlying pathomechanism of the disease in this patient?
    A. Autoimmune process resulting in inflammatory myopathy
    B. Contraction of D4Z4 repeats in the *FSHD* gene
    C. Mutation in the mitochondrial DNA
    D. Mutation in the dysferlin (*DYSF*) gene
    E. Trinucleotide repeat expansion in the *PABPN1* gene

**Q27.** Which of the following genetic mechanisms is common among all types of facioscapulohumeral muscular dystrophy?
    A. D4Z4 repeat contraction
    B. *SMCHD1* mutation
    C. Hypermethylation of the D4Z4 region
    D. 4qB haplotype
    E. Presence of *DUX4* transcript

**Q28.** All of the following signs can be seen in facioscapulohumeral muscular dystrophy **EXCEPT:**
    A. Beevor sign.
    B. diamond on quadriceps sign.
    C. poly-hill (triple hump) sign.
    D. Popeye sign.
    E. reversed axillary fold.

**Q29.** Which of the following statements is **CORRECT** regarding the extramuscular manifestations of facioscapulohumeral muscular dystrophy (FSHD)?
    A. These include cardiomyopathy, retinal vasculopathy, and hearing loss.
    B. Hearing loss is typically associated with late-onset FSHD.
    C. Retinal vasculopathy is typically associated with late-onset FSHD.
    D. Coats disease is associated with early-onset FSHD.
    E. Hearing loss and retinal vasculopathy are associated with high numbers of D4Z4 repeats.

**Q30.** Scapular winging is a common clinical feature in the following disorders **EXCEPT:**
A. calpainopathy.
B. dysferlinopathy.
C. facioscapulohumeral muscular dystrophy.
D. sarcoglycanopathy.
E. valosin-containing protein (VCP)–related myopathy.

**Q31.** A 45-year-old man reports difficulty using his hands including opening jars and buttoning in the past 2 years. His younger sister has early cataracts. His father died of sudden cardiac death in his 50s. When you shake the patient's hand, he has difficulty releasing his hand from yours. Motor strength is grade 4 for finger flexion bilaterally, while the other muscles are grade 5. What is the most likely genetic abnormality in this patient?
A. CTG repeat expansion in the *DMPK* gene
B. CCTG repeat expansion in the *CNBP* gene
C. Mutation in the *CLCN1* gene encoding for a chloride channel
D. Mutation in the *SCN4A* gene encoding for a sodium channel
E. Mutation in the *MYH7* gene encoding for myosin heavy chain

**Q32.** Which of the following features is more prominent in myotonic dystrophy type 2, compared to type 1?
A. Distal weakness
B. Myotonia
C. Pain
D. Cataracts
E. Cardiac conduction defect

**Q33.** Which of the following is the leading cause of death in patients with myotonic dystrophy?
A. Aspiration from dysphagia
B. Cardiac conduction abnormalities
C. Diabetic ketoacidosis
D. Neuromuscular respiratory failure
E. Sleep apnea

**Q34.** A newborn baby born from a mother with myotonic dystrophy type 1 has respiratory and feeding difficulties requiring admission to the neonatal intensive care unit. Examination reveals generalized hypotonia and bilateral talipes equinovarus. Which of the following statements is **CORRECT**?
A. Oligohydramnios can be a finding during the prenatal period.
B. This is due to placental transmission of autoantibodies from a mother to a baby.
C. The baby most likely has a number of CTG repeats in the *DMPK* gene greater than 1000.
D. The baby is more likely to have an affected father than an affected mother.
E. This disorder does not affect intellectual skills.

**Q35.** Which of the following **BEST** describes the pathophysiology of myotonic dystrophy type 1?
A. Impaired glycosylation
B. Defects in muscle membrane repair
C. Impaired alternative splicing of pre-mRNA
D. Increased gene expression due to hypomethylation
E. Premature stop codon resulting in truncation of protein

**Q36.** Which of the following statements is **CORRECT** regarding mexiletine?
A. It reduces myotonia by blocking chloride channels.
B. It can improve muscle strength.
C. It is used in dystrophic myotonias but not nondystrophic myotonias.
D. It can be used in patients with coexisting cardiac conduction defects.
E. Gastrointestinal discomfort is a common side effect.

**Q37.** In addition to limb-girdle muscular dystrophy type 1C, mutations in the caveolin-3 (*CAV3*) gene are associated with which of the following disorders?
A. Miyoshi myopathy
B. Emery-Dreifuss muscular dystrophy
C. Hypokalemic periodic paralysis
D. Myotonia congenita
E. Rippling muscle disease

**Q38.** Which of the following features is the most useful to differentiate between congenital muscular dystrophy and congenital myopathy?
A. Cardiac involvement
B. Central nervous system involvement
C. Contracture
D. Facial muscle weakness
E. Respiratory involvement

**Q39.** A 1-week-old baby boy is referred for evaluation of generalized hypotonia and muscle weakness. He also has respiratory failure requiring endotracheal intubation and feeding difficulty requiring nasogastric tube placement. On examination, marked limitation of eye movements in multiple directions is noted. Serum creatine kinase is 40 U/L. Brain magnetic resonance imaging (MRI) is normal. Muscle biopsy shows internalized nuclei in most muscle fibers. This patient most likely has a mutation in which of the following genes?
A. *ACTA1* encoding α-actin 1
B. *DNM2* encoding dynamin 2
C. *MTM1* encoding myotubularin
D. *RYR1* encoding ryanodine receptor 1
E. *SEPN1* encoding selenoprotein N

**Q40.** Mutations in which of the central core disease genes are associated with an increased risk of malignant hyperthermia?
A. *ACTA1* encoding α-actin 1
B. *MYH7* encoding myosin heavy chain 7
C. *RYR1* encoding ryanodine receptor
D. *SELENON (SEPN1)* encoding selenoprotein N
E. *TTN* encoding titin

**Q41.** Which of the following disorders is **NOT** associated with mutations in the *RYR1* gene?
A. Centronuclear myopathy
B. Central core myopathy
C. Malignant hyperthermia
D. Multiminicore myopathy
E. Reducing body myopathy

**Q42.** Which of the following statements is **CORRECT** regarding nemaline myopathy?
A. The onset can vary from the neonatal period to late adulthood.
B. Ophthalmoparesis is a frequent clinical feature.
C. Cardiac involvement is absent.
D. Mutations in the *ACTA1* gene are the most common.
E. Nemaline rods are best demonstrated on NADH stain.

**Q43.** Which of the following is a muscle biopsy feature typically seen in congenital fiber-type disproportion?
A. Type 1 muscle fiber atrophy and predominance
B. Type 2 muscle fiber atrophy and predominance
C. Type 1 muscle fiber atrophy and type 2 muscle fiber predominance
D. Type 2 muscle fiber atrophy and type 1 muscle fiber predominance
E. Type 2 muscle fiber predominance without atrophy

**Q44.** Which of the following phenotypes is **NOT** associated with α-dystroglycanopathies?
A. Limb-girdle muscular dystrophy
B. Fukuyama congenital muscular dystrophy
C. Merosin-deficient congenital muscular dystrophy
D. Muscle-eye-brain disease
E. Walker-Warburg syndrome

**Q45.** A newborn has severe hypotonia, contractures of multiple joints, and generalized muscle weakness at birth. A few days later, he develops feeding difficulty and respiratory failure. Brain magnetic resonance imaging (MRI) reveals hyperintense signals in the bilateral subcortical white matter on T2-weighted images. Serum creatine kinase is 1546 U/L. Muscle biopsy revealed absent merosin staining. This disorder is due to abnormalities in which of the following proteins?
A. α-Dystroglycan
B. Collagen VI
C. Dystrophin
D. Laminin α2
E. Selenoprotein N

**Q46.** Which of the following statements is **CORRECT** regarding mitochondrial myopathies?
A. The ratio of mutated mitochondrial DNA is identical among all tissues in mitochondrial encephalomyopathy, lactic acidosis, and stroke-like episodes (MELAS).
B. Mitochondrial myopathies may be due to mutations in the nuclear DNA.
C. Mitochondrial DNA depletion syndrome is due to a primary defect in the mitochondrial DNA.
D. All patients with Leigh syndrome inherit the disease from their mothers.
E. Ragged-red fibers on muscle biopsy are best demonstrated with cytochrome oxidase (COX) staining.

**Q47.** Which of the following phenotypes is **NOT** associated with *POLG* mutations?
A. Myocerebrohepatopathy in a toddler
B. Myoclonic epilepsy, myopathy, and sensory ataxia
C. Progressive external ophthalmoplegia
D. Sideroblastic anemia with pancreatic dysfunction
E. Sensory ataxia, neuropathy, dysarthria, and ophthalmoplegia

**Q48.** A 30-year-old man presents for further evaluation of weakness. He has had difficulty swallowing, chronic nausea, frequent vomiting after meals, abdominal pain, and diarrhea for more than 5 years. On examination, his weight is 70 lb (32 kg) and height is 168 cm (5 ft 6 in). He has bilateral ptosis, limitations of extraocular movements, and generalized and symmetrical muscle weakness, grade 3 proximally and grade 4 distally. Reflexes are diffusely reduced. This disorder is due to an abnormality in which of the following proteins?
A. Acid maltase
B. Docking protein 7 (DOK7)
C. Myophosphorylase
D. DNA polymerase-gamma
E. Thymidine phosphorylase

**Q49.** A 52-year-old woman has long-standing ptosis, limited eye movements, and proximal muscle weakness for more than two decades. She has been diagnosed with myasthenia gravis and treated with pyridostigmine and immunosuppressive agents with no response. She denies diplopia. She has a medical history of second-degree atrioventricular block requiring pacemaker placement. On examination, there is prominent bilateral non-fatigable ptosis, and moderately limited eye movements in both the horizontal and vertical directions. Muscle strength is grade 4 proximally and grade 5 distally in all extremities. What is the most likely genetic abnormality in this patient?
A. Mutation in the *DOK7* gene in the nuclear DNA
B. Mutation in the *POLG* gene in the nuclear DNA
C. Mutation in the mitochondrial tRNA^Leu gene
D. Large deletion in the mitochondrial DNA
E. Mitochondria DNA depletion

**Q50.** Which of the following is **CORRECT** regarding forearm exercise testing?
A. The test is indicated in a patient with nocturnal muscle cramps.
B. Blood pressure cuff insufflation above systolic blood pressure is the generally preferred method.
C. The venous blood is drawn at baseline and 10 minutes after exercise.
D. Each blood sample is tested for ammonia, lactate, and triglyceride.
E. If a patient develops muscle contracture, the test should be terminated.

**Q51.** A 22-year-old man comes for an evaluation of exercise-induced muscle cramps. Forearm exercise test shows no rise in venous lactate levels, but a six-fold rise in venous ammonia levels from baseline. Which of the following disorders is most compatible with this finding?
A. Acid maltase deficiency
B. Carnitine palmitoyltransferase II (CPT II) deficiency
C. Myoadenylate deaminase deficiency
D. Myophosphorylase deficiency
E. This result cannot be interpreted due to poor patient effort.

**Q52.** A 22-year-old man presents with recurrent episodes of muscle pain and cramps after intense running for about 5–10 minutes. He gets some relief of muscle pain and cramps after a few minutes of rest and then can continue his exercise. During some episodes his urine turns rusty in color. He feels normal at rest and denies weakness between these episodes. Serum creatine kinase level was 4552 U/L after one episode. What is the most likely diagnosis in this patient?
A. Acid maltase deficiency
B. Carnitine palmitoyltransferase II deficiency
C. Glycogen debranching enzyme deficiency
D. Myophosphorylase deficiency
E. Phosphofructokinase deficiency

**Q53.** Which of the following features is **LEAST** likely to be seen in phosphofructokinase deficiency?
A. Exercise intolerance
B. Hemolytic anemia
C. Myoglobinuria
D. Second wind phenomenon
E. Worsening of symptoms after glucose administration

**Q54.** Which of the following statements is **CORRECT** regarding lipid storage myopathies?
A. Absence of lipid vacuoles on muscle biopsy excludes lipid storage myopathies.
B. Carnitine palmitoyltransferase II (CPT II) deficiency typically presents with fixed weakness.
C. Primary carnitine deficiency rarely presents with encephalopathy.
D. Multiple acyl-CoA dehydrogenase deficiency (MADD) has second wind phenomenon.
E. MADD is a riboflavin-responsive disorder.

**Q55.** A 4-month-old infant presents with generalized hypotonia and weakness. He also has feeding difficulty, respiratory failure, and hypertrophic cardiomyopathy. An enlarged tongue is noted on physical examination. Serum creatine kinase is 1210 U/L. Muscle biopsy shows extensive large vacuoles within muscle fibers, which demonstrate positive periodic acid–Schiff staining with sensitivity to diastase and positive acid phosphatase staining. What is the most likely deficient enzyme in this patient?
A. Alpha-glucosidase
B. Alpha-galactosidase
C. Glycogen debranching enzyme
D. Myophosphorylase
E. Phosphofructokinase

**Q56.** A 51-year-old man has mild proximal muscle weakness for 3 years with shortness of breath, especially on exertion. He is admitted because of acute respiratory failure requiring endotracheal intubation. Electromyography shows small polyphasic motor unit action potentials with early recruitment in the proximal muscles. Myotonic discharges are detected in paraspinal muscles. Which of the following is most likely to be encountered in this patient?
A. CTG repeat expansion in the *DMPK* gene
B. Degeneration of anterior horn cells and corticospinal tracts
C. Deficiency of acid maltase enzyme
D. Mutation in the *DYSF* gene
E. Mutation in the *DOK7* gene

**Q57.** Which of the following statements is **CORRECT** regarding alglucosidase alfa, an enzyme replacement therapy (ERT) in Pompe disease?
A. It has no benefit in the late-onset form.
B. It does not improve cardiac muscle function.
C. It provides symptomatic benefit without altering the natural history of the disease.
D. It has no impact on survival outcome.
E. It should be initiated as early as possible.

**Q58.** A 17-year-old woman presents with proximal muscle weakness. He has a hypertrophic cardiomyopathy and Wolff-Parkinson-White syndrome. Examination shows mild (grade 4) symmetrical weakness of the proximal muscles in the upper and lower extremities. Muscle biopsy demonstrates periodic acid–Schiff (PAS)-positive and acid phosphatase–positive vacuoles within muscle fibers. Biochemical testing shows normal alpha-glucosidase activity, and genetic testing shows no mutation in the *GAA* gene. Deficiency of which of the following proteins is most likely responsible for the disorder in this patient?
A. Alpha-galactosidase
B. Glycogen debranching enzyme
C. Lysosome-associated membrane protein 2
D. Myophosphorylase
E. Titin

**Q59.** A 24-year-old man presents with slowly progressive weakness, affecting mainly his hands and feet, for over a decade. He also has a history of cardiomyopathy. Examination reveals hepatomegaly, as well as prominent atrophy and grade 3–4 weakness of muscles in the distal upper and lower extremities. The clinician suspects motor neuron disease. Needle electromyography (EMG) reveals small polyphasic short-duration motor unit action potentials with early recruitment. Muscle biopsy reveals periodic acid–Schiff (PAS)–positive, acid phosphatase–negative vacuoles within muscle fibers, which are sensitive to diastase. This patient most likely has a deficiency in which of the following enzymes?
A. Acid maltase
B. Carnitine palmitoyltransferase II
C. Glycogen debranching enzyme
D. Myophosphorylase
E. Phosphofructokinase

**Q60.** A 9-year-old boy presents with stiffness of his legs when walking for 2 years. After walking or running for a while, he feels better. Stiffness is worse with cold temperature. Examination reveals no muscle weakness. There is grip myotonia of both hands, which improves after repetitive hand opening and closing. Needle electromyography (EMG) shows myotonia in several proximal and distal muscles. The disorder in this patient is most likely caused by an abnormality in which of the following channels?
A. Sodium channel
B. Potassium channel
C. Calcium channel
D. Chloride channel
E. Either sodium or chloride channel

**Q61.** Which of the following features is seen in paramyotonia congenita, but **NOT** in myotonia congenita?
A. Episodic weakness
B. Eyelid myotonia
C. Myotonia provoked by cold
D. Myotonia provoked by exercise
E. Warm-up phenomenon

**Q62.** Which of the following disorders is **NOT** associated with sodium channelopathies?
A. Episodic ataxia type 1
B. Familial erythromelalgia
C. Hypokalemic periodic paralysis
D. Hyperkalemic periodic paralysis
E. Potassium-aggravated myotonia

**Q63.** A 12-year-old girl presents with multiple attacks of generalized muscle weakness, sometimes associated with pain. These attacks usually occur after prolonged rest. On examination, you note dysmorphic features including low-set ears, broad nose, hypertelorism, and clinodactyly, in addition to short stature. Electrocardiography demonstrates a prolonged QT interval. This disorder is due to an abnormality in which of the following channels?
A. Sodium
B. Potassium
C. Chloride
D. Calcium
E. None of the above

**Q64.** Which of the following conditions is **NOT** electrically silent on needle electromyography?
A. Contracture in McArdle disease
B. Contracture after muscle cooling in paramyotonia congenita
C. Cramps
D. Severe paralytic attack of hypokalemic periodic paralysis
E. Rippling muscle disease

**Q65.** A 55-year-old man presents with slowly progressive proximal muscle weakness over 5 years. In addition, he reports difficulty swallowing for over a decade and has mild aspiration, especially when drinking water. He also complains of mild diplopia. His younger sister and mother have similar symptoms beginning in their late 40s. On examination, he has bilateral ptosis, which has remained unchanged since his early 40s according to his report. Extraocular movement examination shows mild limitation of upward gaze. There is grade 4 weakness of the proximal muscles in both arms and legs. Distal muscles are grade 5. What is the most likely underlying etiology of the disorder in this patient?
A. Autoimmunity to the postsynaptic acetylcholine receptor
B. CTG repeat expansion in the *DMPK* gene
C. GCN repeat expansion in the *PABPN1* gene
D. Large deletion in the mitochondrial DNA
E. Mutation in the *POLG* gene encoding DNA polymerase-gamma

## PART 2: QUESTIONS WITH ANSWERS AND DISCUSSION

**QUESTION 1.** A 4-year-old boy presents with toe walking, difficulty running, and proximal muscle weakness. Calf hypertrophy is noted on examination. Serum creatine kinase level is 12,000 U/L. Muscle biopsy reveals absent dystrophin staining. Which of the following statements is **CORRECT** regarding this disorder?
A. Neck flexors are typically spared.
B. Gowers sign is specific to this condition.
C. This disorder is associated with restrictive cardiomyopathy.
D. Cognition is spared in this condition.
E. Patients typically become wheelchair dependent around the age of 12 years.

**ANSWER:** E. Patients typically become wheelchair dependent around the age of 12 years.

### COMMENTS AND DISCUSSION

- The diagnosis in this boy is *Duchenne muscular dystrophy (DMD)*.
- Clinical spectrum of dystrophinopathies
  - Muscular dystrophy
    - Duchenne muscular dystrophy: loss of ambulation by the age of 12 years
    - Intermediate phenotype: loss of ambulation between the ages of 12 and 16 years
    - Becker muscular dystrophy (BMD): loss of ambulation after the age of 16 years
    - However, if a patient receives steroid treatment, loss-of-ambulation may be delayed. Patients with DMD who are treated with steroids may still be able to ambulate after the age of 12 years.
  - Other phenotypes
    - X-linked cardiomyopathy
    - Asymptomatic hyperCKemia
- Clinical features of Duchenne muscular dystrophy
  - Progressive proximal muscle weakness
  - Symptom onset is usually in the first 1–2 years of life.
  - Diagnosis is frequently delayed by several years.
  - Delay in developmental motor milestone.
  - Toe walking due to Achilles tendon shortening.
  - Neck flexor weakness can be an early finding.
  - Tongue hypertrophy is a frequent sign.
  - Lumbar lordosis due to weakness of hip extensors and knee extensors.
  - Waddling gait due to weakness of pelvic girdle muscles; gait can also be wide-based.
  - Gowers sign
    - A child uses his hands to climb onto his knees when arising from the floor.
    - Due to weakness of pelvic girdle and knee extensors
    - This sign is not specific to dystrophinopathies and can also be seen in other disorders with pelvic girdle weakness.
  - Calf pseudohypertrophy
    - This is due to fatty infiltration of calf muscles, but the calf muscles themselves are indeed atrophic and replaced by excessive fibrotic tissue. Thus this is referred to as "pseudohypertrophy."
  - Patients with DMD can also have intellectual impairment and learning disabilities.
  - Systemic features
    - Cardiac involvement: dilated (not restrictive) cardiomyopathy with electrocardiography showing sinus tachycardia in most patients.
    - Respiratory involvement
      - Weakness of respiratory muscles including the diaphragm results in impaired ventilatory function. Progressive kyphoscoliosis can also lead to restrictive lung disease.
      - Patients have nocturnal hypoventilation as an early sign.
      - Non-invasive ventilation (NIV) and tracheostomy with assisted ventilation may be needed by the age of 18–20 years.
- The clinical features of BMD are similar to DMD, but BMD has a later and more variable onset of symptoms (late childhood to early adulthood) and is milder, with a slower rate of progression. In fact, most patients are able to maintain ambulation well beyond the age of 16 years.

**HIGH-YIELD FACT**

Weakness of neck flexors is one of the early signs in Duchenne muscular dystrophy.

**QUESTION 2.** Which of the following laboratory tests is the most useful in differentiating Duchenne muscular dystrophy from Becker muscular dystrophy?
A. Serum creatine kinase
B. Hematoxylin and eosin staining on muscle biopsy
C. Western blot analysis of muscle tissue
D. Needle electromyography
E. Muscle ultrasonography

**ANSWER:** C. Western blot analysis of muscle tissue

### COMMENTS AND DISCUSSION

- Laboratory testing in dystrophinopathies
  - Serum creatine kinase
    - 50–200 times of the upper normal limit (UNL) in Duchenne muscular dystrophy (DMD). Creatine kinase (CK) levels decline with age and the use of corticosteroids.
    - 20–200 times of UNL in Becker muscular dystrophy (BMD)
    - There is significant overlap of CK levels between DMD and BMD.
  - Electrodiagnostic studies show myopathic changes, which are low-amplitude, short-duration and polyphasic motor unit action potentials (MUAPs), with early recruitment on needle electromyography (EMG). These findings are not specific to DMD or BMD. While fibrillation potentials are common in DMD, they are not specific to the disease. Nerve conduction studies are normal but low compound muscle action potential (CMAP) amplitudes may be encountered in advanced cases.
  - Muscle biopsy
    - Hematoxylin and eosin (H&E) staining (see Fig. 10.3)
      - Variation of muscle fiber size
      - Dystrophic changes: myofiber degeneration and regeneration. Degenerating fibers are usually pink on H&E, whereas regenerating fibers are small and bluish in color.
      - H&E staining alone cannot precisely differentiate DMD from BMD, although DMD tends to have more severe pathological changes.
    - Immunohistochemistry (Table 18.1)
      - By using dystrophin antibodies, which include antibodies to the N-terminal domain, rod domain, and C-terminal domain (see Fig. 10.4)
      - Dystrophin is a sarcolemmal protein, more precisely, located in the subsarcolemmal region, and links actin to dystroglycan. Immunohistochemistry of the normal muscle fibers by using dystrophin antibodies exhibits sarcolemmal staining.

**TABLE 18.1** Comparison between Duchenne and Becker muscular dystrophies.

| | Duchenne muscular dystrophy | Becker muscular dystrophy |
|---|---|---|
| Onset of symptoms | 1–2 years of age | Variable (late childhood to early adulthood) |
| Severity of symptoms | More severe | Less severe |
| Ambulatory function (when not treated with steroids) | Loss of ambulation by the age of 12 years | Remains ambulatory after the age of 16 years |
| Immunohistochemistry to dystrophin | Absent or markedly reduced | Reduced, but not absent |
| Western blot analysis of dystrophin | Absent or markedly reduced (0%–5% of normal) | Reduced in amount and/or size of dystrophin |
| Genetic abnormalities, in case of deletions | Out-of-frame deletions resulting in no dystrophin production | In-frame deletions resulting in shorter dystrophin protein |

- Antibodies to the C-terminal domain are the most sensitive immunohistochemical study to detect the pathology (most likely to be reduced or absent), since the C-terminal domain is translated after the N-terminal and rod domains. Therefore, it is more likely to be affected when there is a premature stop codon (see also comments and discussion from Question 3).
    - DMD: *absent or markedly reduced* dystrophin staining
    - BMD: *reduced* dystrophin staining
    - Revertant fibers can be found in DMD in less than 1% of all muscle fibers. These are fibers with preserved dystrophin staining. The exact pathomechanism remains unclear.
  - Western blot analysis of muscle tissue
    - Detects the amount and size of dystrophin protein
    - DMD: absent or markedly reduced dystrophin, 0%–5% of normal
    - BMD: reduced the amount and/or size of dystrophin
  - Muscle ultrasound
    - Non-invasive method; useful to follow changes over time
    - Muscle echogenicity can reflect the degree of fat infiltration and muscle fibrosis. Muscle atrophy can also be demonstrated.
    - However, muscle ultrasound cannot be used to differentiate DMD from BMD.
  - Genetic testing will be discussed in Question 3.

**QUESTION 3.**   Which of the following mutations is the most common among patients with dystrophinopathies?
A. Large deletions
B. Large duplications
C. Point mutations
D. Trinucleotide repeat expansions
E. Chromosomal translocations

**ANSWER:** A. Large deletions

**COMMENTS AND DISCUSSION**
- Dystrophinopathies are X-linked recessive disorders.
  - There is no male-to-male transmission.
  - Males are predominantly affected. Daughters of affected males are obligatory carriers.
  - Females can also be affected, termed manifesting carrier. This is due to skewed inactivation of the X chromosome. Affected females typically have milder and much later onset of symptoms than males.
- Dystrophin is a large gene located on chromosome Xp21.
- Mutations in dystrophinopathies
  - Deletions of one or more exons (large deletions): most common, ~60%–70% of all patients
    - DMD: out-of-frame deletions disrupt the reading frame. This results in a premature stop codon and subsequently no dystrophin protein production.
    - BMD: in-frame deletions still preserve the reading frame. Transcription and translation can still occur but the protein product is shorter than normal.
  - Duplications of one or more exons (large duplications): in about 5%–10%
  - Point mutations: in about 20%–30%
  - Thus the diagnostic approach when dystrophinopathies are suspected is as follows:
    - Detecting large deletions first by multiplex ligation–dependent probe amplification (MLPA) or array comparative genomic hybridization (aCGH). MLPA and aCGH can also detect large duplications.
    - Gene sequencing to detect point mutations is usually performed after the first two methods, given the large size of the gene.
    - Muscle biopsy can also be done to detect absent or reduced dystrophin, but this is more invasive.
- X-autosome translocations with breakpoints at the dystrophin gene locus are one of the causes of manifesting (female) carriers which are rare in DMD.
- Trinucleotide repeat expansion is not responsible for dystrophinopathies. CAG repeat expansion on the X chromosome is associated with Kennedy disease (i.e., X-linked spinobulbar muscular atrophy). Myotonic dystrophy types 1 and 2 are associated with CTG and CCTG repeat expansions, respectively.

**MNEMONICS**

Frequency of mutations in dystrophinopathies (in the order from the most common):
**De**letions > **Du**plications > **P**oint mutations
These are in an alphabetical order.

**QUESTION 4.** Which of the following statements is **CORRECT** regarding corticosteroid treatment in Duchenne muscular dystrophy?
A. Corticosteroids provide symptomatic benefit without slowing the progression of the disease.
B. Corticosteroids increase the risk of scoliosis.
C. An intermittent dosing regimen of prednisone has higher efficacy than a daily dosing regimen.
D. Deflazacort is preferred due to its higher efficacy than prednisone.
E. Weight gain is less with deflazacort, compared to prednisone.

**ANSWER:** E. Weight gain is less with deflazacort, compared to prednisone.

**COMMENTS AND DISCUSSION**
- Corticosteroids are considered a disease-modifying therapy in dystrophinopathies, since they:
  - Slow the disease progression and prolong the ambulatory period
  - Reduce the risk of scoliosis
  - Help stabilize cardiopulmonary function
- The mechanisms may not be due simply to their anti-inflammatory effect, but to their effects on muscle growth and repair function.
- Types and regimens of corticosteroids
  - Prednisone
    - Daily regimen: 0.75 mg/kg/day; lower dose is not as effective
    - Intermittent regimens: At least two regimens are generally accepted.
      - 10 days on and 10 days off
      - High doses only during the weekends
    - The main purpose of intermittent regimens is to reduce side effects, but the efficacy is not superior to the daily dosing regimen.
  - Deflazacort
    - Approved by the US Food and Drug Administration (FDA) in 2017
    - 0.9–1.2 mg/kg/day
    - Equally effective as prednisone, but with fewer side effects.
    - Compared to prednisone, deflazacort is associated with less weight gain but higher risk of cataracts.

◎ **HIGH-YIELD FACT**

Compared to prednisone, deflazacort is associated with LESS weight gain, but MORE cataracts.

**QUESTION 5.** Eteplirsen is a gene therapy that was approved by the US Food and Drug Administration (FDA) in 2016 for the treatment of Duchenne muscular dystrophy. What is the mechanism of this treatment?
A. Skipping of exon 51 of the dystrophin gene
B. Integration of exon 51
C. Readthrough of premature stop codons
D. Transferring of dystrophin gene by a viral vector
E. Antibody to myostatin

**ANSWER:** A. Skipping of exon 51 of the dystrophin gene

**COMMENTS AND DISCUSSION**
- The field of gene therapy has shown promising results in several neuromuscular disorders including Duchenne muscular dystrophy (DMD) and spinal muscular atrophy.

- Eteplirsen is an antisense oligonucleotide (ASO) that binds to complementary pre-mRNA. It is mutation specific and can be used in about 14% of all DMD patients.
- Some mutations in DMD result in shifting of reading frames and premature stop codons in exon 51.
- Binding of eteplirsen to exon 51 results in skipping of exon 51 (and the premature stop codon). Thus the reading frame is restored. Translation can continue, but the dystrophin protein is shorter than normal. In other words, skipping exon 51 by eteplirsen is an attempt to convert DMD to the milder Becker muscular dystrophy (BMD) phenotype (Fig. 18.1).
- In the landmark study by Mendell and colleagues, 12 boys treated with eteplirsen showed statistically significant longer distance on the 6-minute walk test and less loss of ambulation, compared to 13 healthy controls.
- Since this study, the number of ASO skipping therapies for the treatment of DMD have increased to the following four (Table 18.2):
  - Eteplirsen, approved in 2016 for patients who have a confirmed mutation of the *DMD* gene that is amenable to exon 51 skipping.
  - Golodirsen, approved in 2019 for patients who have a confirmed mutation of the *DMD* gene that is amenable to exon 53 skipping.
  - Viltolarsen, approved in 2020 for patients who have a confirmed mutation of the *DMD* gene that is amenable to exon 53 skipping (second agent for this mechanism).
  - Casimersen, approved in 2021 for patients who have a confirmed mutation of the *DMD* gene that is amenable to exon 45 skipping.
- Other gene therapies that have been studied in DMD:
  - Dystrophin gene transfer by adeno-associated virus (AAV) vectors
  - Ataluren
    - Acts at the translation process
    - It promotes stop-codon readthrough by facilitating ribosomes and translation of a premature stop codon; near cognate-tRNA is recruited to the site of premature stop codon.
- Anti-myostatin antibody is not a gene therapy. Myostatin inhibits growth of muscle cells. Thus anti-myostatin antibodies have been studied in DMD in order to promote muscle growth and regeneration.

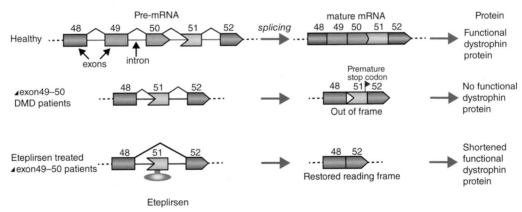

**Fig. 18.1** Mechanism of action of eteplirsen. Eteplirsen is an antisense oligonucleotide that binds to exon 51, resulting in skipping of this exon during splicing of pre-mRNA to mature mRNA. Skipping of this exon, which contains the premature stop codon, leads to restoration of the reading frame. Translation and production of the dystrophin protein can occur. However, the dystrophin protein is shorter than normal but can still be functional, as seen in Becker muscular dystrophy. From Tang Z, Zhao J, Pearson ZJ, Boskovic ZV, Wang J. RNA-Targeting splicing modifiers: drug development and screening assays. *Molecules.* 2021;26(8):2263.

**TABLE 18.2** Currently available antisense oligonucleotide (ASO) therapies for Duchenne muscular dystrophy and their genetic mechanisms.

| Genetic mechanism | ASO therapies |
| --- | --- |
| Exon 45 skipping | Casimersen |
| Exon 51 skipping | Eteplirsen |
| Exon 53 skipping | Golodirsen, viltolarsen |

- Exon integration is a mechanism of gene therapy in some disorders, but *not* in DMD. The important neuromuscular disorder treated with exon integration strategy is spinal muscular atrophy (SMA). Nusinersen is an ASO integrating exon 7 into the *SMN2* gene, thus converting the severe form of SMA to the milder forms. (see also Question 23 and Table 12.5 in Chapter 12.)

*The following answer options are for QUESTIONS 6 through 10.*

*Match each dystrophy-related protein with its location in muscle.*
  A. Sarcolemma
  B. Sarcomere
  C. Nuclear membrane
  D. Extracellular matrix

**QUESTION 6.** Dystrophin
**ANSWER:** A. Sarcolemma

**QUESTION 7.** Dystroglycan
**ANSWER:** A. Sarcolemma

**QUESTION 8.** Emerin
**ANSWER:** C. Nuclear membrane

**QUESTION 9.** Dysferlin
**ANSWER:** A. Sarcolemma

**QUESTION 10.** Collagen VI
**ANSWER:** D. Extracellular matrix

## COMMENTS AND DISCUSSION

- Muscular dystrophies are due to abnormalities of various proteins located within or linked to the muscle fiber. These proteins can be located at the sarcomeric unit, sarcolemma (muscle membrane), nuclear membrane, or extracellular matrix (Fig. 18.2).
  ○ Proteins located at the sarcolemma include dystroglycans, sarcoglycans, dysferlin, caveolin-3, and anoctamin-5.
  ○ Dystrophin is considered to be located at the sarcolemma as well. However, it is actually located at the subsarcolemmal region and links actin at the sarcomeric unit to dystroglycan at the sarcolemma.
  ○ Proteins located at the sarcomere or sarcomeric unit include titin, telethonin, and myotilin, among others.
  ○ Proteins located at the nuclear membrane include emerin.
  ○ Lamin A/C is located at the nuclear lamina next to the inner nuclear membrane.
  ○ Proteins located at the extracellular matrix include laminin α2 (aka merosin) and collagen VI.

**QUESTION 11.** A 35-year-old woman developed toe walking around the age of 7 years. Around the early teenage years she had difficulty combing her hair and walking upstairs. She became wheelchair dependent in her early 30s. Examination reveals bilateral scapular winging, prominent (grade 1–2) weakness of proximal muscles and mild weakness of distal muscles. Serum creatine kinase is 3853 U/L. Muscle biopsy demonstrates eosinophilic infiltration on hematoxylin and eosin (H&E) staining and lobulated fibers on nicotinamide adenine dinucleotide (NADH) stain. What is the most likely diagnosis?
  A. Becker muscular dystrophy
  B. Duchenne muscular dystrophy
  C. Facioscapulohumeral dystrophy
  D. Limb-girdle muscular dystrophy type 2A (calpainopathy)
  E. Limb-girdle muscular dystrophy type 2B (dysferlinopathy)

**ANSWER:** D. LGMD2A (calpainopathy)

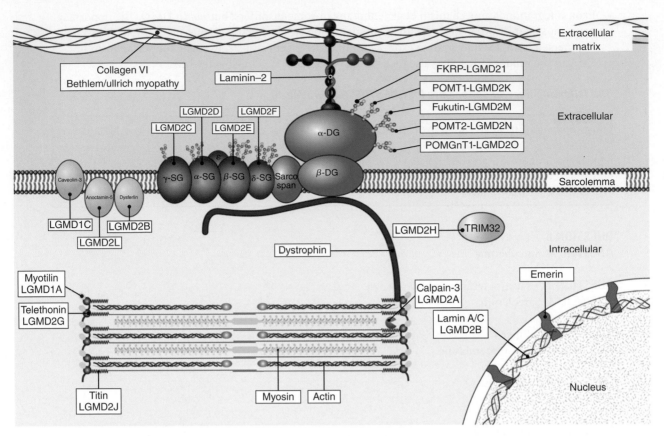

**Fig. 18.2** Proteins associated with various muscular dystrophies and their locations. From Wicklund MP. Limb-girdle muscular dystrophies. In: Aminoff MJ, Daroff RB, eds. *Encyclopedia of the Neurological Sciences.* 2nd edition. Oxford: Academic Press; 2014:890–896.

## COMMENTS AND DISCUSSION

- The most likely diagnosis in this patient is *calpainopathy* (limb-girdle muscular dystrophy type 2A or R1, according to the new nomenclature).
- Limb-girdle muscular dystrophies, as originally designated by Sir John Walton, encompass a group of hereditary myopathies characterized by progressive proximal muscle weakness and dystrophic changes on muscle biopsy. There are at least two sets of nomenclature
  - Originally accepted nomenclature
    - LGMD1 (alphabet) – autosomal dominant: LGMD1A, LGMD1B, LGMD1C, and so on.
    - LGMD2 (alphabet) – autosomal recessive: LGMD2A, LGMD2B, LGMD2C, and so on.
    - This nomenclature is limited in that the alphabets are not sufficient for the expanding number of the LGMD types.
  - Newly suggested nomenclature
    - LGMD D (number) – autosomal dominant: LGMD D1, LGMD D2, LGMD D3, and so on.
    - LGMD R (number) – autosomal recessive: LGMD R1, LGMD R2, LGMD R3, and so on.
  - In this book, the original nomenclature is used primarily.
- There are numerous types of LGMDs. The autosomal recessive forms are much more common. The most prevalent include LGMD2A (calpainopathy), LGMD2B (dysferlinopathy), and collagen VI– related disorders. Other worth knowing LGMDs include LGMD2C-F (sarcoglycanopathies), LGMD2I (related to fukutin-related protein), and LGMD2L (related to anoctamin-5). LGMD1B (due to lamin A/C deficiency) overlaps with Emery-Dreifuss muscular dystrophy (EDMD).
- LGMD2A (aka calpainopathy, LGMD R1) is the most common LGMD in the United States, caused by calpain-3 (*CAPN3*) gene mutations.
  - Clinical features
    - Typical onset between 5 and 20 years of age
    - Weakness of the hip extensors (especially gluteus maximus) and hip adductors; hamstrings can be involved resulting in knee flexor weakness
    - Scapular winging: seen in 20% of patients
    - Contracture of ankles, knees, or elbows

- Calf hypertrophy not as prominent as in dystrophinopathies
- Cardiac involvement is extremely rare; however, respiratory muscles may be involved with advanced disease.

◎ **HIGH-YIELD FACT**

Important LGMDs with **NO** cardiac involvement:
- Calpainopathy (LGMD2A)
- Dysferlinopathy (LGMD2B)

◎ **HIGH-YIELD FACT**

Hereditary myopathies with scapular winging:
- Facioscapulohumeral dystrophy (FSHD)
- Calpainopathy (LGMD2A) – seen in 20%
- Sarcoglycanopathies (LGMD2C–F)

- o Laboratory features
  - Serum creatine kinase (CK) typically 5–20 times of the upper normal limit.
  - Muscle magnetic resonance imaging (MRI): involvement (fat infiltration) of the medial gastrocnemius in the early stage
  - Muscle biopsy:
    - Variation of muscle fiber size, which is a nonspecific myopathic finding
    - Rarely eosinophilic infiltration can be seen on H&E stain (Fig. 18.3). These cases were often misdiagnosed as "idiopathic eosinophilic myositis." Lobulated fibers can be seen on NADH stain, although not specific to LGMD2A.

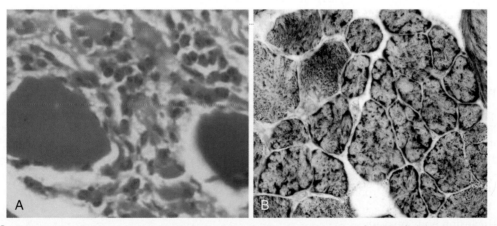

**Fig. 18.3** Histopathologic findings in calpainopathy (limb-girdle muscular dystrophy type 2A [LGMD2A]). (A) This hematoxylin and eosin (H&E) staining (400x) demonstrates eosinophilic infiltration. This finding was previously called "eosinophilic myositis", but later *CAPN3* mutations were found in these patients. (B) This nicotinamide adenine dinucleotide (NADH) staining demonstrates lobulated fibers. However, this finding is not specific to calpainopathy and has been observed in various myopathies. A from Oflazer PS, Gundesli H, Zorludemir S, Sabuncu T, Dincer P. Eosinophilic myositis in calpainopathy: Could immunosuppression of the eosinophilic myositis alter the early natural course of the dystrophic disease? *Neuromuscul Disord.* 2009;19(4):261–263. B from Dubowitz V, Sewry CA, Oldfors A. Muscular Dystrophies and Allied Disorders II: Limb-Girdle Muscular Dystrophies. In: Muscle biopsy. Philladelphia, PA: 5th ed. Elsevier; 2021:244.

◎ **HIGH-YIELD FACT**

Eosinophilic infiltration and lobulated fibers can be seen in calpainopathy.

- Western blot analysis to detect reduction in calpain-3. However, caution must be taken, since secondary calpain deficiency can also be seen in other LGMDs, especially in dysferlinopathy (LGMD2B) and titinopathy (LGMD2J).

- Genetic testing of the *CAPN3* gene
  - Calpain-3 is a calcium-dependent cysteine protease playing a role in sarcomere formation and remodeling.
- Becker muscular dystrophy and Duchenne muscular dystrophy are X-linked, with women often asymptomatic or mildly symptomatic as manifesting carriers. Dystrophinopathies are not associated with lobulated fibers on muscle biopsy. Lobulated fibers can be seen in facioscapulohumeral dystrophy, but eosinophilic infiltration should not be present in this disorder.
- Dysferlinopathy (LGMD2B) is not associated with scapular winging and often overlaps with Miyoshi distal myopathy, with prominent early gastrocnemius weakness and atrophy (see also comments and discussion from Questions 13-15).

**QUESTION 12.** Which of the following findings is **LEAST** likely to be seen in calpainopathy (LGMD2A)?
  A. Ankle contracture
  B. Scapular winging
  C. Cardiac abnormalities
  D. Respiratory involvement
  E. Medial gastrocnemius weakness

**ANSWER:** C. Cardiac abnormalities

**COMMENTS AND DISCUSSION (see also comments and discussion for Question 11)**
- Cardiac abnormalities are typically absent in some limb-girdle muscular dystrophies (LGMDs), most commonly in calpainopathy and dysferlinopathy. There have been only rare case reports of cardiac abnormalities in calpainopathy.
- Although cardiac involvement is typically absent in calpainopathy, respiratory involvement can be seen, especially in the late stage of the disease.
- Scapular winging can be a helpful clue, as it can be seen in some LGMDs, especially calpainopathy and sarcoglycanopathies, as well as in facioscapulohumeral muscular dystrophy (FSHD). In calpainopathy, scapular winging can be seen in ~20% of patients.
- Patients with calpainopathy can have contractures involving their ankles, knees, elbows, or hips. Elbow and ankle contracture may mimic Emery-Dreifuss muscular dystrophy (EDMD).
- Patients with calpainopathy can have atrophy of the medial gastrocnemius, and fat infiltration in this muscle can be demonstrated as an early finding on muscle magnetic resonance imaging (MRI).

**QUESTION 13.** A 25-year-old man had difficulty standing on his toes and playing sports 3–4 years earlier. Subsequently he developed difficulty climbing stairs and flexing his elbows. Examination revealed prominent atrophy of both calves, more prominent on the right. There were no winged scapulae. Motor strength showed grade 4 weakness throughout. Reflexes were 1+ in the biceps and quadriceps, and 0 at both ankles. Serum creatine kinase was 19,000 U/L. Muscle biopsy revealed variation of muscle fiber size and endomysial lymphocytic infiltration. What is the most likely diagnosis?
  A. Becker muscular dystrophy
  B. Dysferlinopathy
  C. Inclusion body myositis
  D. Polymyositis
  E. Sarcoglycanopathy

**ANSWER:** B. Dysferlinopathy

**COMMENTS AND DISCUSSION**
- The most likely diagnosis in this patient is *dysferlinopathy* (limb-girdle muscular dystrophy type 2B [LGMD2B] or LGMD R2).
- Dysferlinopathy (LGMD2B) is the second most common LGMD in the United States, after calpainopathy. It is more prevalent in the Asian population and may be the most common LGMD in several Asian countries.
- Dysferlinopathy (LGMD2B)
  - Clinical features
    - Age at onset typically between 10 and 30 years
    - Before the onset of the disease patients are quite active and often athletic. This feature is also seen in anoctaminopathy (LGMD2L), which is considered in the differential diagnosis.

- Weakness of the gastrocnemius (posterior compartment of the calf) resulting in an inability to walk on toes. This is an important early feature of the disease. The Achilles tendon reflex can be absent early.
  - Weakness of the gastrocnemius in LGMD2B demonstrates phenotypic overlap with Miyoshi myopathy, a form of distal myopathy that is allelic to LGMD2B.
  - Miyoshi myopathy is also due to mutations in the dysferlin (*DYSF*) gene, and has predominant involvement of the posterior compartment of the calf.
  - Patients with LGMD2B and Miyoshi myopathy can have overlapping features: those with LGMD2B can have some distal involvement, and those with Miyoshi myopathy can present with some proximal muscle weakness.

### ◎ HIGH-YIELD FACT

LGMD2B is allelic to Miyoshi myopathy. Both are dysferlinopathies.
There is a marked phenotypic overlap between these two disorders. LGMD2B can present with distal weakness, especially in the gastrocnemius. Miyoshi myopathy typically presents with predominant atrophy of the posterior leg compartment but may also have some degree of proximal weakness.

- Weakness can also involve the proximal legs and arms.
- Muscle involvement may be asymmetric between two sides.
- Relative sparing of the deltoid and periscapular muscles. Thus there is no scapular winging in LGMD2B.
- No significant cardiac and respiratory involvement
- Noteworthy signs in dysferlinopathies
  - "Diamond on quadriceps" sign: When a patient partially bends their knees, there is bulging of the mid-portion of the quadriceps muscle, due to atrophy of the proximal and distal parts of the muscle. This sign can be seen in both LGMD2B and Miyoshi myopathy (Fig. 18.4).
  - "Calf heads on a trophy" sign: This sign is seen when a patient with Miyoshi myopathy abducts and externally rotates his shoulder. It is due to selective weakness of some parts of the trapezius, supraspinatus and other shoulder girdle muscles, with sparing of the deltoid.
  ○ Laboratory features
  - Serum creatine kinase (CK) levels are typically markedly elevated, ranging from 50 to 150 times of the upper normal limit, often exceeding 10,000–20,000 U/L.

### ◎ HIGH-YIELD FACT

LGMDs with serum CK levels in the very high range, typically >100–150 times of the upper normal limit
- Dysferlinopathies (LGMD2B and Miyoshi myopathy)
- Sarcoglycanopathies (LGMD2C–F)

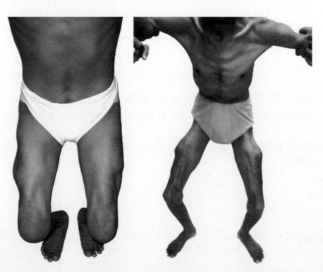

**Fig. 18.4** "Diamond on quadriceps" sign in dysferlinopathies. The left image shows a patient with limb-girdle muscular dystrophy type 2B (LGMD2B), and the right image shows a patient with Miyoshi myopathy. From Pradhan S. Diamond on quadriceps: A frequent sign in dysferlinopathy. *Neurology.* 2008;70(4):322.

- Muscle magnetic resonance imaging (MRI) demonstrates muscle involvement with a similar pattern of weakness (e.g., involvement of the gastrocnemius).
- Muscle biopsy
  - Variation of muscle fiber size (myopathic features), and muscle fiber necrosis and regeneration (dystrophic features)
  - Endomysial lymphocytic infiltration (Fig. 18.5). This finding, along with high serum CK levels, can mimic polymyositis. In clinical practice, this misdiagnosis can lead to unnecessary treatments for patients with dysferlinopathies.
  - Immunohistochemistry by using antibodies to dysferlin shows reduced or absent staining.

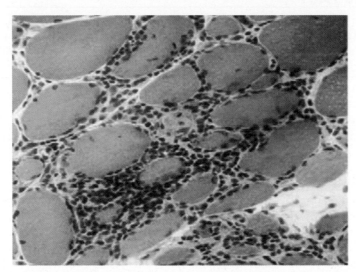

**Fig. 18.5** Muscle biopsy in dysferlinopathy. This figure demonstrates endomysial lymphocytic infiltration, which can mislead to the diagnosis of inflammatory myopathy. From Confalonieri P, Oliva L, Andreetta F, et al. Muscle inflammation and MHC class I up-regulation in muscular dystrophy with lack of dysferlin: An immunopathological study. *J Neuroimmunol.* 2003;142(1-2):130–136.

- Western blot: absent dysferlin protein. However, some patients still have relative normal dysferlin levels on western blot.

 **HIGH-YIELD FACT**

> Due to very high CK levels (>10,000–20,000 U/L) and endomysial lymphocytic infiltration seen on muscle biopsy, patients with dysferlinopathies may be misdiagnosed with polymyositis and received unnecessary treatments.

- Genetic testing
  - Mutations in the *DYSF* gene encoding for dysferlin
  - Dysferlin is located at the sarcolemma. It has a role in muscle membrane repair.

**QUESTION 14.** Which of the following distal myopathies is characterized by weakness of the posterior leg compartment muscles?
A. Miyoshi myopathy
B. Nonaka myopathy
C. Laing myopathy
D. Udd myopathy
E. Welander myopathy

**ANSWER:** A. Miyoshi myopathy

**COMMENTS AND DISCUSSION (see also comments and discussion from Question 13)**

- Limb-girdle muscular dystrophy type 2B (LGMD2B) and Miyoshi myopathy are allelic disorders. Both are due to mutations in the *DYSF* gene encoding dysferlin, and therefore classified as dysferlinopathies.
- Patients often have overlapping phenotypes between these two disorders.
  - Although patients with LGMD2B have predominant limb-girdle weakness, distal muscle weakness, especially in the gastrocnemius, is often seen and can be an early feature.
  - Although patients with Miyoshi myopathy have distal weakness with predominant involvement of the posterior compartment of the legs, proximal muscle weakness can also be seen.
- Patients with these two disorders often have very high serum CK levels, greater than 10,000–20,000 U/L, and endomysial lymphocytic infiltration on muscle biopsies.
- Preferential muscle involvement can be an important clue in distal myopathies.
  - Preferential involvement of the *posterior compartment* of the legs
    - Miyoshi myopathy (due to mutations in the *DYSF* gene)
    - Anoctaminopathy (LGMD2L) also called Miyoshi myopathy type 3.
  - Preferential involvement of the *anterior compartment* of the legs
    - Nonaka myopathy (due to mutations in the *GNE* gene), also called GNE myopathy, distal myopathy with rimmed vacuoles (since rimmed vacuoles are seen on muscle biopsy), hereditary inclusion body myopathy, or quadriceps sparing myopathy
    - Laing myopathy (due to mutations in the *MYH7* gene encoding for myosin heavy chain 7). In this disorder, weakness of neck flexors is often present, and weakness of the toe dorsiflexors can result in a "hanging big toe" sign
    - Markesbery-Griggs myopathy (due to mutations in the *ZASP* gene)
    - Udd myopathy (due to mutations in the *TTN* gene encoding for titin)
  - Preferential involvement of the wrist and finger extensors
    - Welander myopathy (due to mutations in the *TIA1* gene)

---

### MNEMONICS

Both Miyoshi and Nonaka are Japanese names. These two disorders involve different leg compartments.
Non**A**k**A** has **A** in the name, thus the **A**nterior leg compartment is predominantly involved.
Miyoshi involves the opposite: the posterior leg compartment.

---

**QUESTION 15.** Which of the following features is **LEAST** likely to be seen in dysferlinopathy (LGMD2B)?
  A. Asymmetric involvement
  B. Inability to walk on toes
  C. Cardiac involvement
  D. Serum creatine kinase of 30,000 U/L
  E. Endomysial infiltration on muscle biopsy

**ANSWER:** C. Cardiac involvement

**COMMENTS AND DISCUSSION (see comments and discussion for Question 13)**

- Asymmetry of muscle weakness/atrophy is common in dysferlinopathies.
- Inability to walk on toes due to weakness of the gastrocnemius can be seen in limb-girdle muscular dystrophy type 2B (LGMD2B; dysferlinopathy).
  - This can be an early feature.
  - In patients who cannot walk on toes within a few years after the onset of weakness, the differential diagnoses should include LGMD2B (dysferlinopathy) and LGMD2L (anoctaminopathy).
  - The calf or distal leg involvement demonstrates an overlapping feature between LGMD2B and its allelic disorder, Miyoshi myopathy.
- Dysferlinopathies typically have no cardiac and respiratory involvement. Cardiac involvement is rare and typically insignificant.
  - Calpainopathy also has no cardiac involvement.
- When encountering a very high serum creatine kinase level (in the range of 10,000 U/L or higher) along with endomysial lymphocytic infiltration on muscle biopsy, one should raise a clinical suspicion of dysferlinopathies. Many of these patients have been misdiagnosed with polymyositis.

**QUESTION 16.** A 6-year-old Amish boy did not walk until the age of 24 months. He had tongue and calf hypertrophy, scapular winging, lumbar lordosis, and proximal muscle weakness. Serum creatine kinase was persistently elevated in the range of 10,000–20,000 U/L. Muscle biopsy showed dystrophic features but normal immunoreactivity to dystrophin antibodies. Transthoracic echocardiography revealed mild left ventricular systolic dysfunction. What is the most likely diagnosis?

A. Becker muscular dystrophy
B. Calpainopathy
C. Dysferlinopathy
D. Emery-Dreifuss muscular dystrophy
E. Sarcoglycanopathy

**ANSWER:** E. Sarcoglycanopathy

**COMMENTS AND DISCUSSION**

- The most likely diagnosis in this patient is *sarcoglycanopathy* (LGMD2C–F or LGMD R3–6) with manifestations fairly similar to dystrophinopathies (Duchenne muscular dystrophy [DMD] and Becker muscular dystrophy [BMD]), but with an autosomal recessive inheritance rather than X-linked. Hence, the prior name of this condition was severe childhood autosomal recessive muscular dystrophy (SCARMD).
- All four sarcoglycanopathies (i.e., LGMD2C, LGMD2D, LGMD2E, and LGMD2F) have similar clinical features and cannot be distinguished from each other clinically.
- Sarcoglycanopathies have Duchenne- or Becker-like phenotypes.
  - Age at onset is typically early, around 2–15 years.
  - The severe form was previously called "severe childhood autosomal recessive muscular dystrophy (SCARMD)," mimicking DMD.
  - Later age at onset can mimic BMD.

◎ **HIGH-YIELD FACT**

LGMDs with dystrophinopathy (Duchenne or Becker)-like phenotypes:
- Sarcoglycanopathies (LGMD2C–F)
- Fukmembrane stabilizers utin-related protein (FKRP)-related LGMD (LGMD2I)
When a patient has clinical features similar to Duchenne or Becker muscular dystrophy, but muscle biopsy or genetic testing does not confirm the diagnosis similar to dystrophinopathy, one has to think about these LGMDs.

  - In addition to proximal muscle weakness, patients can have tongue and calf hypertrophy. Neck flexors can be involved, similar to dystrophinopathies.
  - Scapular winging is a frequent finding. This is a very important feature.
  - Patients can have muscle pain or cramps mimicking metabolic myopathies, called "pseudometabolic presentation."
  - Cardiac involvement: dilated cardiomyopathy is not a common feature.
  - Respiratory insufficiency
  - LGMD2C, LGMD2D, LGMD2E, and LGMD2F are caused by mutations in the γ-sarcoglycan, α-sarcoglycan, β-sarcoglycan, and δ-sarcoglycan, respectively.
  - Immunohistochemistry of the muscle biopsy specimen with antibodies to each subunit of sarcoglycan is useful to identify this group of disorders. However, identifying the specific type of sarcoglycanopathies from staining patterns can be challenging. The pattern is not straightforward, since reduction of one subunit of sarcoglycan can also affect other subunits within the sarcoglycan complex.
  - Genetic testing can be performed to confirm the diagnosis.
- Becker muscular dystrophy is unlikely in this patient, since dystrophin immunoreactivity is normal.
- Dysferlinopathies can present with very high serum CK levels, as seen in this patient. However, dysferlinopathies (and also calpainopathy) typically do not have cardiac involvement.

- Although patients with Emery-Dreifuss muscular dystrophy (EDMD) often have cardiac involvement, the common clinical features include early contracture and weakness in a humeroperoneal distribution. Serum CK levels can be normal or elevated up to 5 times of the upper normal limit, but not in the very high ranges as found in this patient.

**QUESTION 17.** The disorder associated with a deficiency of which of the following proteins has clinical features most comparable to those of Duchenne muscular dystrophy?
   A. Anoctamin 5
   B. Calpain
   C. Dysferlin
   D. Fukutin-related protein
   E. Merosin

**ANSWER:** D. Fukutin-related protein

**COMMENTS AND DISCUSSION**
- LGMDs that can have Duchenne- or Becker-like phenotypes include
   ○ Sarcoglycanopathies (limb-girdle muscular dystrophy types 2C–F [LGMD2C–F]); see also comments and discussion from Question 16.
   ○ Fukutin-related protein (FKRP)–related LGMD (LGMD2I)
- *FKRP-related LGMD (LGMD2I or LGMD R9)*
   ○ Higher prevalence in Northern Europe (Denmark and Norway)
   ○ Age at onset varies from 1–40 years with most patients having onset before the age of 5 years.
   ○ Patients with the c.826C>A homozygous mutations tend to have more severe phenotypes; if there is c.826C>A in only one allele, the phenotype is milder.
   ○ Duchenne-like phenotype: proximal muscle weakness, neck flexor weakness, lumbar lordosis
   ○ Hypertrophy the of calf, tongue, and brachioradialis
   ○ Patients can have episodes of weakness induced by febrile or acute illnesses prior to the onset of persistent weakness.
   ○ Cardiac involvement including dilated cardiomyopathy
   ○ Respiratory insufficiency
   ○ LGMD2I is due to mutations in the *FKRP* gene encoding fukutin-related protein (or FKRP).
   ○ FKRP is *not* identical to fukutin (which is encoded by the *FKTN* gene).
      - However, both FKRP and fukutin have similar function in *O*-mannosyl glycosylation of α-dystroglycan but involve different steps of the process.
      - In addition to the limb-girdle phenotype, mutations in the *FKRP* gene can result in congenital muscular dystrophy.
      - Both *FKRP* and *FKTN* gene mutations are associated with congenital muscular dystrophies.
- Calpainopathy (LGMD2A), dysferlinopathy (LGMD2B), and anoctaminopathy (LGMD2L) are associated with limb-girdle phenotypes. However, the phenotypes are not similar to Duchenne muscular dystrophy. In calpainopathy and dysferlinopathy, there is typically no cardiac involvement.
- Anoctaminopathy shares phenotypic similarities with dysferlinopathy, with the exception that it may also have cardiac abnormalities due to the expression of anoctamin 5 in cardiac muscle.

**QUESTION 18.** Which of the following features distinguish anoctaminopathy (LGMD2L) from dysferlinopathy (LGMD2B/Miyoshi myopathy)?
   A. Inability to walk on toes
   B. Asymmetric muscle atrophy and weakness
   C. Cardiac involvement
   D. Respiratory involvement
   E. Creatine kinase level of 10,000 U/L

**ANSWER:** C. Cardiac involvement

## COMMENTS AND DISCUSSION

- Anoctaminopathy (LGMD2L) has clinical features similar to those of dysferlinopathies (LGMD2B/Miyoshi myopathy).
- Anoctaminopathy is also called "Miyoshi myopathy type 3."
- Both patients with anoctaminopathy and dysferlinopathy can have an inability to walk on their toes in the early course of the disease as well as asymmetric weakness and muscle atrophy. The quadriceps and muscles biceps are commonly involved in anoctaminopathy.
- Both anoctaminopathy and dysferlinopathy have no significant respiratory involvement.
- Anoctamin 5 is also expressed in cardiac muscle. Cardiac abnormalities in anoctaminopathy include arrhythmias such as premature ventricular contractions (PVCs), cardiomyopathies, and impaired systolic function.
- Hence, the main distinguishing feature between anoctaminopathy and dysferlinopathy is cardiac abnormalities, which are present only in the former.
- Serum creatine kinase (CK) levels in anoctaminopathy are usually up to 50 times of the upper normal limit. Although this is not as high as in dysferlinopathies, there is significant overlap in CK levels between anoctaminopathy and dysferlinopathy.

## MNEMONIC

Dysferlinopathy + Cardiac abnormalities = Anoctaminopathy

**QUESTION 19.** A 29-year-old man presented with an acute embolic stroke in the right middle cerebral artery territory and newly-diagnosed atrial fibrillation. The patient's left hemiparesis gradually improved to almost normal strength of the left arm and leg. Rivaroxaban was started. On examination, there was contracture of the elbows and ankles, and grade 4 weakness of bilateral biceps, triceps, and gastrocnemius. The patient reported that his elbow and ankle contractures had been gradually worsening since his early teens and muscle weakness started in his early 20s. Additionally, his maternal grandfather developed similar symptoms in his 40s and had a cardiac problem requiring pacemaker placement. What is the most likely diagnosis in this patient?

A. Bethlem myopathy
B. Calpainopathy
C. Dystrophinopathy
D. Emery-Dreifuss muscular dystrophy
E. Sarcoglycanopathy

**ANSWER:** D. Emery-Dreifuss muscular dystrophy

## COMMENTS AND DISCUSSION

- The most likely diagnosis in this patient is *Emery-Dreifuss muscular dystrophy (EDMD)*, based on the classic clinical features of elbow and ankle contractures as an early presentation, weakness in the humeroperoneal distribution, cardiac abnormalities, as well as the and family history.
- EDMD can be due to mutations in various genes.
  - X-linked recessive forms:
    - *STA* gene (encoding emerin)
    - *FHL1* gene (encoding four and a half LIM domains protein)
  - Autosomal dominant forms:
    - *LMNA* gene (encoding lamin A/C)
    - *SYNE1* and *SYNE2* genes (encoding nesprin 1 and nesprin 2), which are rare
  - Autosomal recessive forms
    - *LMNA* gene is also associated with autosomal recessive EDMD
  - EDMD is a disorder of the muscle nuclear envelope (nuclear envelopathies) (Fig. 18.2).
    - Emerin and nesprin are at the nuclear membrane.
    - Lamin A/C is located at the nuclear lamina next to the inner nuclear membrane.
      - Mutations in the lamin A/C gene can also cause a variety of disorders that are allelic to EDMD. This represents phenotypic variability. Examples of laminopathies include:
        - Limb-girdle muscular dystrophy type 1B (LGMD1B). In the new classification, this was removed from the LGMD category.

- ○ *LMNA*-related congenital muscular dystrophy
- ○ Dilated cardiomyopathy
- ○ Familial partial lipodystrophy (Dunnigan type)
- ○ Hutchinson-Gilford progeria syndrome
- Clinical features of EDMD
  - ○ Age at onset: typically in childhood but can be variable (teenage or adulthood)
  - ○ Triad
    - Early contracture of the ankles, elbows, and posterior cervical muscles. Contracture often precedes the onset of weakness (Fig. 18.6).
    - Gradual weakness in the humeroperoneal distribution, especially involving the biceps, triceps, and gastrocnemius muscles.
    - Cardiac involvement:
      - Cardiac conduction defects including atrial conduction defects are common in EDMD.
      - Cardiomyopathy, including atrial standstill and dilated cardiomyopathy
      - Cardiac arrhythmias can result in syncopal episodes or stroke in the young.
      - Screening of cardiac abnormalities and cardiac surveillance are crucial in EDMD.
  - ○ EDMD due to various mutations has similar clinical features and cannot be distinguished clinically.

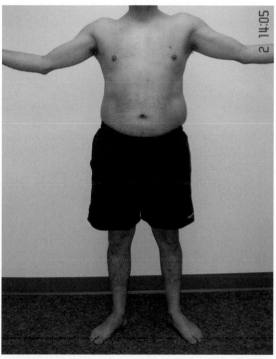

**Fig. 18.6** Flexion contracture of the elbows in a patient with Emery-Dreifuss muscular dystrophy. From Parmar MS, Parmar KS. Emery-Dreifuss humeroperoneal muscular dystrophy: Cardiac manifestations. *Can J Cardiol.* 2012;28(4):516.e1-3.

◎ **HIGH-YIELD FACT**

Clinical triad of Emery-Dreifuss muscular dystrophy
1. **Early** contracture of the ankles, elbows, posterior cervical muscles
2. Humeroperoneal weakness
3. Cardiac conduction defect with atrial and ventricular cardiomyopathy

◎ **HIGH-YIELD FACT**

Screening of cardiac abnormalities and cardiac surveillance are very important in Emery-Dreifuss muscular dystrophy.

- Laboratory features of EDMD
  - Serum creatine kinase (CK) levels can be normal or mildly elevated, 5 times of the upper normal limit
  - EMG and muscle biopsy typically show nonspecific myopathic features.
- Bethlem myopathy and Ullrich myopathy are collagen VI–related disorders. Bethlem myopathy typically presents in adulthood and is characterized by prominent finger contractures. When asked to place both palms togetherin a praying position, individuals with Bethlem myopathy are unable to fully extend their fingers due to contractures. This is referred to as the "prayer sign."
- Calpainopathy typically does not have cardiac abnormalities (see also comments and discussion from Question 11).
- Patients with dystrophinopathies can have cardiac abnormalities including dilated cardiomyopathy. However, early contracture before the development of prominent muscle weakness is not a feature of dystrophinopathies. In addition, cardiac arrhythmias or cardiac conduction defects are not common cardiac abnormalities in dystrophinopathies (see also Comments and discussion for Question 1).
- Sarcoglycanopathies may have cardiac involvement, especially dilated cardiomyopathy. However, early contracture is not a feature of these disorders (see also comments and discussion from Question 16).

**QUESTION 20.** Which of the following proteins is **NOT** associated with Emery-Dreifuss muscular dystrophy?
A. Emerin
B. Four and a half LIM domains
C. Lamin A/C
D. Laminin α2
E. Nesprin

**ANSWER:** D. Laminin α2

**COMMENTS AND DISCUSSION (see also comments and discussion from Question 19):**
- Several genes are associated with Emery-Dreifuss muscular dystrophy. These genes encode various proteins that are associated with the nuclear envelope (Table 18.3).
- Laminin α2, or merosin, is associated with congenital muscular dystrophy, not Emery-Dreifuss muscular dystrophy.

**TABLE 18.3** Genes associated with Emery-Dreifuss muscular dystrophy, their encoded proteins, and locations in the nuclear envelope.

| Gene | Protein | Location in the nuclear envelope | Mode of inheritance |
| --- | --- | --- | --- |
| STA | Emerin | Nuclear membrane | X-linked recessive |
| FHL1 | Four and a half LIM domains | Unclear (FHL1A located at sarcolemma, sarcomere, and nucleus) | X-linked recessive |
| LMNA | Lamin A/C | Nuclear lamina (next to inner nuclear membrane) | Autosomal dominant or Autosomal recessive |
| SYNE1, SYNE2 | Nesprin 1, Nesprin 2 | Nuclear membrane | Autosomal dominant |

**QUESTION 21.** A 4-year-old girl has had frequent falls and progressive generalized muscle weakness since the age of 3 years. Examination reveals generalized hypotonia and reduced muscle mass. Motor strength of the upper and lower extremities is grade 3 proximally and grade 4 distally. There are contractures of both elbows, hyperlaxity of both wrists and ankles, and prominent soft tissue over the calcaneal region of both feet. This disorder is due to abnormality in which of the following proteins?
A. α-Dystroglycan
B. Collagen VI
C. Emerin
D. Merosin
E. Selenoprotein N

**ANSWER:** B. Collagen VI

**COMMENTS AND DISCUSSION**

- The diagnosis in this patient is *Ullrich congenital muscular dystrophy*.
- Ullrich congenital muscular dystrophy is one of the two collagen VI–related disorders. The other disorder is Bethlem myopathy.
- Collagen VI is a component of the basal lamina (basement membrane), located in the extracellular matrix. It is important in stabilization of the sarcolemma.
- Ullrich congenital muscular dystrophy typically presents with more severe phenotypes and has an onset in infancy or early childhood. In contrast, Bethlem myopathy typically presents with less severe phenotypes and has a later onset. However, there significant phenotypic overlap between these two disorders.
- Both Ullrich congenital muscular dystrophy and Bethlem myopathy can be either autosomal recessive or autosomal dominant. These disorders cannot be differentiated by mode of inheritance, as originally thought. Both disorders are due to mutations in the *COL6A1*, *COL6A2*, and *COL6A3* genes encoding the collagen VI protein.

 **HIGH-YIELD FACT**

Collagen VI–related disorders
- Ullrich congenital muscular dystrophy: severe end of the spectrum
- Bethlem myopathy: mild end of the spectrum
- Both disorders can be either autosomal recessive or dominant.

- Ullrich congenital muscular dystrophy
  - Clinical features
    - Onset in infancy or early childhood
    - Generalized hypotonia. Patients can have congenital hip dysplasia.
    - Key features: contracture of proximal joints (e.g., elbows and knees) and hyperlaxity of distal joints (e.g., wrists and ankles); prominent calcaneal soft tissue; keratosis pilaris (gooseflesh-like bumping of skin); keloids (Fig. 18.7A, B)
    - Rigid spine, scoliosis, respiratory failure

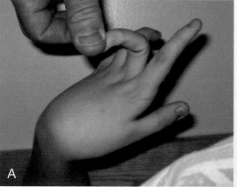 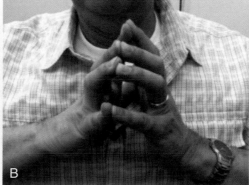 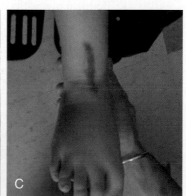

**Fig. 18.7** Clinical signs in collagen VI-related disorders. (A) Prominent distal laxity in a child with Ullrich myopathy. (B) Prayer sign in Bethlem myopathy. (C) Keloid in Ullrich congenital muscular dystrophy. A and B from Bönnemann CG, Voermans NC. Chapter 70 - ECM-Related Myopathies and Muscular Dystrophies. In: Hill JA, Olson EN, eds. Muscle. Boston/Waltham: Academic Press; 2012:984. C from Mercuri E, Muntoni F. Chapter 29 - Congenital Muscular Dystrophies. In: Darras BT, Jones HR, Ryan MM, De Vivo DC, eds. Neuromuscular Disorders of Infancy, Childhood, and Adolescence (Second Edition). San Diego: Academic Press; 2015:546.

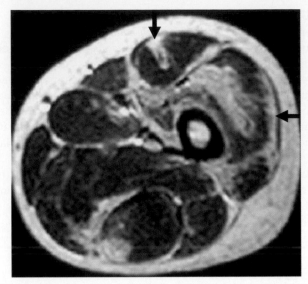

**Fig. 18.8** Muscle MRI in Ullrich congenital muscular dystrophy. T1-weighted sequence demonstrates increased signal in the central part of rectus femoris (called "central cloud"; *vertical arrow*) and increased signal in the periphery of vastus lateralis (*horizontal arrow*) From Mercuri E, Lampe A, Allsop J, et al. Muscle MRI in Ullrich congenital muscular dystrophy and Bethlem myopathy. *Neuromuscul Disord.* 2005;15(4):303–310.

- Laboratory features
  - Serum creatine kinase (CK) levels are normal or mildly elevated.
  - Muscle magnetic resonance imaging
    - T1-weighted image: Increased signal in the central part of rectus femoris (called "central cloud"), and in the periphery of the vastus lateralis (Fig. 18.8)
    - These features can also be seen in Bethlem myopathy.
  - Muscle biopsy
    - Increased endomysial connective tissue (therefore also called "scleroatonic" muscular dystrophy)
    - Absent or markedly reduced immunostaining of collagen VI
  - Genetic testing
    - Mutations in the *COL6A1*, *COL6A2*, or *COL6A3* genes
- Bethlem myopathy
  - Clinical features
    - Later age at onset compared to Ullrich congenital muscular dystrophy. The onset can range from 2 years of age to the seventh decade of life.
    - Phenotypes are similar to those of Ullrich congenital muscular dystrophy but typically milder.
    - More than half to two-thirds of patients with Bethlem myopathy lose ambulation by the age of 60.
    - Key feature: contracture of the interphalangeal joints, which gives rise to the characteristic "*prayer sign* (Fig. 18.7C)."
- Selenoprotein N is associated with *SEPN1*-related congenital muscular dystrophy. Patients with mutations in the *SEPN1* gene can have the phenotype of rigid spine syndrome. α-Dystroglycan and merosin (aka laminin α2) are also associated with congenital muscular dystrophies. However, contracture of the proximal joints and hyperlaxity of the distal joints are not features of these disorders.
- Emerin is associated with Emery-Dreifuss muscular dystrophy (EDMD). In EDMD, the onset is typically later. Patients can have prominent contracture of elbows. However, hyperlaxity of the distal joints and prominent calcaneal soft tissue are not features of EDMD.

**QUESTION 22.** A 32-year-old man presents with chronic slowly progressive proximal muscle weakness for over 10 years. On examination, finger flexion contracture is noted as in the following figure. What is the most likely diagnosis?

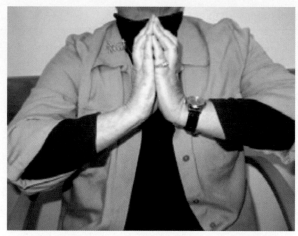

From Bönnemann CG. The collagen VI-related myopathies: muscle meets its matrix. *Nat Rev Neurol.* 2011 Jun 21;7(7):379–390.

A. Bethlem myopathy
B. Emery-Dreifuss muscular dystrophy
C. Kearns-Sayre syndrome
D. Rigid spine muscular dystrophy
E. Welander distal myopathy

**ANSWER:** A. Bethlem myopathy

**COMMENTS AND DISCUSSION (see also comments and discussion for Question 21)**
- The sign depicted in the figure above is the "*prayer sign*", which is caused by contractures of the long finger flexors in both hands. This sign is characteristic of Bethlem myopathy.
- Emery-Dreifuss muscular dystrophy typically has contracture of the elbows, ankles, and posterior cervical muscles, but not the long finger flexors.
- Kearns-Sayre syndrome is a mitochondrial myopathy with chronic progressive external ophthalmoplegia and cardiac conduction defects.
- Rigid spine muscular dystrophy is due to mutations in the *SEPN1* gene. Contracture is limited mainly to the spine, not in the peripheral joints.
- Welander distal myopathy is a distal myopathy, which has preferential involvement of the wrist extensor and long finger extensor muscles. Patients can have wrist and finger drop but contracture is not a typical feature.

**QUESTION 23.** Which of the following distal myopathies has preferential muscle involvement in the leg compartment that is different from the others?
A. Nonaka myopathy (distal myopathy with rimmed vacuoles)
B. Miyoshi myopathy
C. Laing myopathy
D. Markesbery-Griggs myopathy
E. Udd myopathy

**ANSWER:** B. Miyoshi myopathy

**COMMENTS AND DISCUSSION (see also comments and discussion from Question 14)**
- Distal myopathies represent a group of hereditary myopathies in which the distal muscles of the lower or upper extremities are predominantly affected. Preferential involvement of a specific muscle compartment (e.g., anterior versus posterior compartment of the leg) can be a useful phenotypic clue.
- Distal myopathies are summarized in Table 18.4.

**TABLE 18.4** Summary of distal myopathies.

| Disorder | Typical onset | Mode of inheritance | Gene | Preferential involvement | Other features |
|---|---|---|---|---|---|
| Miyoshi | Early adulthood | AR, sporadic | *DYSF* (encoding dysferlin) | Posterior leg compartment | Allelic to LGMD2B; levels in a very high range (50–150 time of UNL) |
| Nonaka[1] | Early adulthood | AR, sporadic | *GNE* | Anterior leg compartment | Quadriceps is spared |
| Udd | Late adulthood | AD | *TTN* (encoding titin) | Anterior leg compartment | |
| Markesbery-Griggs | Late adulthood | AD | *ZASP* | Anterior leg compartment | |
| Laing | Early adulthood | AD | *MYH7* (encoding myosin heavy chain 7) | Anterior leg compartment | Patients can have hanging big toe sign or dropped finger sign |
| Welander | Late adulthood | AD | *TIA1* | Long finger extensors, especially index | |

Abbreviations: *AD*, autosomal dominant; *AR*, autosomal recessive; *CK*, creatine kinase; *UNL*, upper normal limit.
[1]aka GNE myopathy, distal myopathy with rimmed vacuoles, hereditary inclusion body myopathy, and quadriceps-sparing myopathy.

 **HIGH-YIELD FACT**

Extensor digitorum brevis (EDB) is typically spared in distal myopathies. This can be a useful feature for differentiating between distal myopathy and neuropathy.

- Most distal myopathies have serum creatine kinase (CK) in the normal or mildly elevated levels except Miyoshi myopathy, which typically has serum CK levels in a very high range.
- Of all options listed, only Miyoshi myopathy has preferential involvement of the posterior leg compartment. The other disorders in this question have preferential involvement of the anterior leg compartment.

**QUESTION 24.** A 45-year-old man developed slowly progressive generalized muscle weakness around the age of 32. In the past year, he has also experienced behavioral changes including disinhibition. Multiple family members in every generation have similar symptoms. Frontotemporal dementia is suspected, and magnetic resonance imaging (MRI) of the brain reveals bilateral frontotemporal atrophy. However, proximal and distal muscle weakness is also noted in the bilateral upper and lower extremities. Muscle biopsy is performed and is compatible with inclusion body myositis (IBM). This disorder is most likely due to mutations in which of the following genes?
A. *C9orf72*
B. *FUS*
C. *GNE*
D. *VCP*
E. *SOD1*

**ANSWER:** D. *VCP*

**COMMENTS AND DISCUSSION**
- The most likely diagnosis in this patient is *inclusion body myopathy with Paget disease of bone and frontotemporal dementia (IBMPFD)*.
- IBMPFD
  - Autosomal dominant inheritance; due to mutations in the *VCP* gene that encodes valosin-containing protein
  - Clinical features: adult-onset proximal and distal muscle weakness, early-onset frontotemporal dementia, and Paget disease of bone resulting in high serum alkaline phosphatase (ALP)
- GGGGCC hexanucleotide repeat expansions in the *C9orf72* gene result in familial frontotemporal dementia associated with amyotrophic lateral sclerosis (FTD-ALS). However, this is not associated with IBM or Paget disease of bone.

- Mutations in the *FUS* and *SOD1* genes are associated with familial ALS but not the IBMPFB IBMPFD phenotype.
- Mutations in the *GNE* gene are associated with Nonaka myopathy, a form of distal myopathy. Muscle biopsy in this disorder shows rimmed vacuoles, which can sometimes be misdiagnosed as inclusion body myositis. Nonaka myopathy was previously called "hereditary inclusion body myopathy." However, after the discovery of the gene, it is now recognized as a distinct disorder that is not related to inclusion body myositis. Nonaka myopathy is not associated with FTD or Paget disease of bone.

**QUESTION 25.** Which of the following genes is **NOT** associated with myofibrillar myopathy?
   A. *FHL1*
   B. *FLNC* (encoding filamin C)
   C. *LMNA* (encoding lamin A/C)
   D. *MYOT* (encoding myotilin)
   E. *ZASP*

**ANSWER:** C. *LMNA* (encoding lamin A/C)

**COMMENTS AND DISCUSSION**
- *Myofibrillar myopathy (MFM)* is a heterogeneous group of disorders that share a common feature of myofibrillar dissolution and degradation on muscle pathology. Thus MFM is a pathological diagnosis rather than a clinical one.
- Genes associated with MFM include
   - Myotilin (*MYOT*): allelic to limb-girdle muscular dystrophy type 1A (LGMD1A)
   - Desmin (*DES*)
   - αβ-crystallin (*CRYAB*)
   - Filamin C (*FLNC*)
   - *ZASP*: allelic to Markesbery-Griggs distal myopathy
   - *BAG3*
   - Four and a half LIM domains 1 (*FHL1*): allelic to Emery-Dreifuss muscular dystrophy
   - Titin (*TTN*)
   - *DNAJB6*
- Among the options listed, all are associated with MFM except the *LMNA* gene (encoding lamin A/C). Mutations in this gene are associated with LGMD1B and Emery-Dreifuss muscular dystrophy, but not MFM.

**QUESTION 26.** Five years prior, a 29-year-old man developed difficulty puffing his cheek, drinking water from a straw, and whistling. In addition, he noted increasing difficulty raising his arms above his head. Examination reveals facial diplegia, especially in the lower facial region, weakness of the bilateral shoulder girdle muscles, and mild scapular winging. There is no limitation of extraocular movements. Muscle biopsy shows endomysial lymphocytic infiltration. What is the most likely underlying pathomechanism of the disease in this patient?
   A. Autoimmune process resulting in inflammatory myopathy
   B. Contraction of D4Z4 repeats in the *FSHD* gene
   C. Mutation in the mitochondrial DNA
   D. Mutation in the dysferlin (*DYSF*) gene
   E. Trinucleotide repeat expansion in the *PABPN1* gene

**ANSWER:** B. Contraction of D4Z4 repeats in the *FSHD* gene

**COMMENTS AND DISCUSSION**
- The diagnosis in this patient is *facioscapulohumeral muscular dystrophy (FSHD)*.
- FSHD
   - Autosomal dominant. FSHD can be classified into two types: FSHD type 1 (FSHD1) and FSHD type 2 (FSHD2).
   - FSHD1
     - 95% of FSHD patients
     - Due to contraction of D4Z4 repeats in the *FSHD* gene on chromosome 4
     - In normal individuals with normal D4Z4 repeats → tight chromatin (heterochromatin or closed chromatin) → no gene expression (Fig. 18.9)
     - Contraction of D4Z4 repeats → hypomethylation of the D4Z4 region → relaxed (open) chromatin → expression of the *DUX4* gene (transcription of the gene). The *DUX4* gene is located within a D4Z4 repeat array in the subtelomeric region of chromosome 4q.

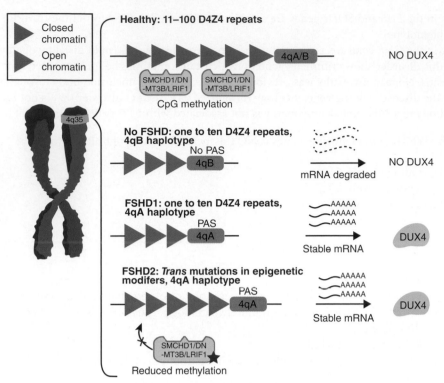

**Fig. 18.9** Genetic mechanisms of facioscapulohumeral muscular dystrophy (FSHD). In healthy individuals with a normal number of D4Z4 repeats, the D4Z4 region is characterized by closed (tight) chromatin (blue triangle), which results in no *DUX4* gene expression and absent *DUX4* transcript production. However, in FSHD1, contraction of the D4Z4 repeats leads to hypomethylation of the D4Z4 region (not shown), resulting in open (relaxed) chromatin (orange triangle), subsequent *DUX4* gene expression, and production of the *DUX4* transcript and DUX4 protein. It is important to note that the presence of the A allele rather than the B allele is required for polyadenylation and stabilization of the *DUX4* transcript. In the presence of D4Z4 contraction but without the A allele, there is no production of the DUX4 protein. FSHD2 is caused by mutations in genetic modifier genes such as the *SMCHD1* gene. These mutations can lead to reduced methylation of the D4Z4 region, resulting in open chromatin, subsequent gene expression, and production of the *DUX4* transcript and DUX4 protein. This also requires the presence of the A allele. From Cohen J, DeSimone A, Lek M, Lek A. Therapeutic approaches in facioscapulohumeral muscular dystrophy. *Trends Mol Med.* 2021;27(2):123–137.

- Expression of the *DUX4* gene + A allele (*not* B allele) → stabilized *DUX4* transcript
- DUX4 is a protein and transcription factor that is thought to be a key player in the pathophysiology of FSHD.
- The genetics of FSHD represent the role of epigenetic mechanism resulting in abnormalities of gene expression.
  ○ FSHD2
    - 5% of FSHD patients
    - Due to mutations in the genetic modifier genes (e.g., *SMCHD1* gene) → hypomethylation of the D4Z4 region → expression of the gene
    - Expression of the gene + A allele → DUX4 transcript
    - Thus hypomethylation of the D4Z4 region resulting in expression of the *DUX4* gene, along with the presence of the A allele is the shared genetic mechanism between FSHD1 and FSHD2.

◎ **HIGH-YIELD FACT**

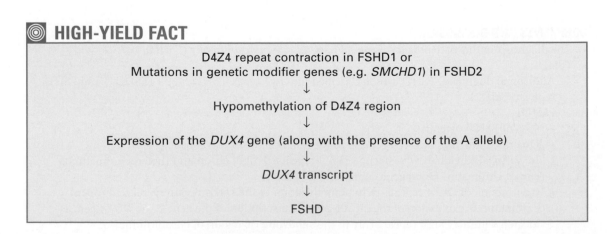

D4Z4 repeat contraction in FSHD1 or
Mutations in genetic modifier genes (e.g. *SMCHD1*) in FSHD2
↓
Hypomethylation of D4Z4 region
↓
Expression of the *DUX4* gene (along with the presence of the A allele)
↓
*DUX4* transcript
↓
FSHD

- Clinical features of FSHD
  - Onset of weakness varies from the infantile period to late adulthood, typically occurring in the teenage or early adulthood years.
  - Weakness, which may be asymmetric, involves:
    - Facial muscles: inability to whistle, pucker, or use a straw
    - Rhomboids and serratus anterior: These muscles stabilize the scapula to the rib cage, and weakness results in scapular winging. The medial border of the scapula separates from the rib cage.
    - Shoulder girdle muscles. Patients have difficulty lifting or abducting arms.
    - Biceps and triceps with relative sparing of the deltoid giving the classic "*Popeye arm*" sign.
    - Tibialis anterior resulting in foot drop
    - Abdominal muscles, especially lower abdominal muscles resulting in positive *Beevor sign*, which is characterized by upward movement of the umbilicus when the individual sits up
  - Noteworthy signs in FSHD
    - *Poly-hill sign* (aka triple hump sign): when a patient holds their arms in abduction, there are three humps, from medial to lateral, as follows (Fig. 18.10):
      - Upper border of the scapula
      - Displaced acromioclavicular joint
      - Relative sparing of the deltoid muscle
    - *Reversed axillary fold*: anterior axillary fold points upward medially instead of upward laterally to the shoulder
    - *Popeye sign*: due to atrophy of the biceps and triceps with relative sparing of the deltoid
    - *Beevor sign*: upward movement of the umbilicus when the patient is sitting up
  - Extramuscular manifestations
    - Retinal vasculopathy
      - Coats disease (representing a severe form of retinal vasculopathy): abnormal development of the retinal blood vessels (e.g., retinal telangiectasia)
    - High-frequency hearing loss
- Both retinal vasculopathy and hearing loss are often associated with early-onset FSHD, typically caused by a very low number of D4Z4 repeats or marked D4Z4 repeat contractions (1–3 repeats; normal 11–150).
- Laboratory features of FSHD
  - Muscle magnetic resonance imaging (MRI): selective involvement of the hamstrings, especially semimembranosus, and abdominal muscles
  - Needle electromyography (EMG): myopathic features
  - Muscle biopsy: dystrophic features. Endomysial lymphocytic infiltration, typically without invasion of non-necrotic muscle fibers, may be seen in up to one-third of patients with FSHD.

## ◎ HIGH-YIELD FACT

A very low number of D4Z4 repeats (1–3 repeats) is associated with
- Early (infantile)–onset FSHD
- Extramuscular manifestations include
  - Retinal vasculopathy such as Coats disease
  - High-frequency hearing loss

- Endomysial lymphocytic infiltration seen on muscle biopsy of individuals with FSHD may be misinterpreted as inflammatory myopathy. This may result in inappropriate treatment with steroids. It is important to recognize that this endomysial lymphocytic infiltration can be present in up to one-third of patients with FSHD.
  - In inflammatory myopathies, lymphocytes invade non-necrotic fibers. However, in FSHD, this feature is not seen: there is only lymphocytic infiltration of necrotic muscle fibers.

## ◎ HIGH-YIELD FACT

Endomysial lymphocytic infiltration on muscle biopsy may be seen in:
- Inflammatory myopathies, including polymyositis (with invasion of non-necrotic fibers)
- Dysferlinopathies
- Facioscapulohumeral muscular dystrophy (FSHD)

- Many mitochondrial myopathies may involve extraocular muscles manifesting as chronic progressive external ophthalmoplegia such as with Kearns-Sayre syndrome. However, extraocular muscles are spared in patients with FSHD.
- Dysferlinopathies may have endomysial lymphocytic infiltration on muscle biopsy, mimicking inflammatory myopathies. However, patients with dysferlinopathies present with a limb-girdle phenotype or distal myopathy (Miyoshi myopathy), not weakness of the facial muscles as seen in FSHD. Scapular winging is a common feature in FSHD, calpainopathy, and sarcoglycanopathies, but not in dysferlinopathies.
- GCN trinucleotide repeat expansion in the *PABPN1* gene is associated with oculopharyngeal muscular dystrophy (OPMD). In OPMD, patients often have ptosis, weakness of extraocular muscles, and dysphagia, which were not present in this patient.

**QUESTION 27.** Which of the following genetic mechanisms is common among all types of facioscapulo-humeral muscular dystrophy?
A. D4Z4 repeat contraction
B. *SMCHD1* mutation
C. Hypermethylation of the D4Z4 region
D. 4qB haplotype
E. Presence of *DUX4* transcript

**ANSWER:** E. Presence of *DUX4* transcript

**COMMENTS AND DISCUSSION (see also comments and discussion from Question 26):**
- Facioscapulohumeral muscular dystrophy type 1 (FSHD1) represents ~95% of all patients with FSHD, and is caused by a D4Z4 repeat contraction.
- FSHD2 represents ~5% of all patients with FSHD and is caused by mutations in the genetic modifier genes such as *SMCHD1*.
- Both FSHD1 and FSHD2 will result in hypomethylation (not hypermethylation) of the D4Z4 region → relaxed (open) chromatin → gene expression. The *DUX4* gene, which is located within the D4Z4 repeat array in the subtelomeric region of chromosome 4q, will be transcribed (Fig. 18.9).
- In the setting of the A allele or 4qA haplotype (not 4qB haplotype), *DUX4* transcript will be polyadenylated and stabilized, leading to subsequent translation of this transcript and production of the DUX4 protein
- Thus, the common genetic mechanisms among all types of FSHD include hypomethylation of the D4Z4 region, presence of the 4qA haplotype, and presence of the *DUX4* transcript (with subsequent translation to the DUX4 protein).
- The DUX4 protein is thought to be key in the pathophysiology of FSHD, and research is currently ongoing to develop gene therapies that target this protein.

**QUESTION 28.** All of the following signs can be seen in facioscapulohumeral muscular dystrophy **EXCEPT:**
A. Beevor sign.
B. diamond on quadriceps sign.
C. poly-hill (triple hump) sign.
D. Popeye sign.
E. reversed axillary fold.

**ANSWER:** B. diamond on quadriceps sign.

**COMMENTS AND DISCUSSION (see also comments and discussion from Question 26):**
- All of the signs listed can be seen in facioscapulohumeral muscular dystrophy (FSHD) except the diamond on quadriceps sign, which is typically seen in dysferlinopathies.
  - Beevor sign is upward displacement of the umbilicus when a patient is sitting up. This can be seen in FSHD and indicates weakness of the lower abdominal muscles.
  - Poly-hill (aka triple hump) sign is due to atrophy of the shoulder girdle muscles. Three humps are seen when a patient abducts his/her arms (Fig. 18.10).
    - The most medial hump is the upper border of the scapula due to atrophy of the trapezius muscle.
    - The middle hump is the acromioclavicular joint.
    - The lateral hump is due to relative sparing of the muscle bulk of the distal deltoid, which is more prominent when there is atrophy of the proximal deltoid muscle.
  - Popeye sign is due to atrophy of the biceps muscle.

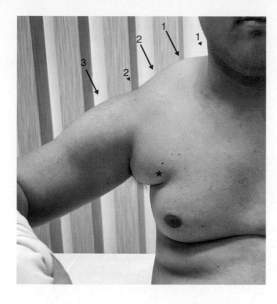

**Fig. 18.10** Signs in facioscapulohumeral muscular dystrophy (FSHD). Poly-hill sign or triple hump sign is characterized by three humps, including the upper border of the scapula (*arrow 1*), the acromioclavicular joint (*arrow 2*), and relative sparing of distal deltoid muscle (*arrow 3*) along with the wasting of the trapezius (*arrowhead 1*), and atrophy of proximal deltoid muscles (*arrowhead 2*). Reversed anterior axillary fold (asterisk) is when the anterior axillary fold points medially, instead of laterally to the shoulder.

- ○ Patients with FSHD can exhibit a reversal of the anterior axillary folds, where the folds point toward the neck instead of the shoulder. This is termed the reversed anterior axillary fold (Fig. 18.10).
- Diamond on quadriceps sign is characterized by bulging of the mid-portion of the quadriceps muscle when a patient is in a semi-squatting position. This is due to atrophy of the proximal and distal portions of the quadriceps with relative sparing of the mid-portion. This sign is seen in the dysferlinopathies including limb-girdle muscular dystrophy type 2B (LGMD2B) and Miyoshi myopathy.

**QUESTION 29.** Which of the following statements is **CORRECT** regarding the extramuscular manifestations of facioscapulohumeral muscular dystrophy (FSHD)?
  A. These include cardiomyopathy, retinal vasculopathy, and hearing loss.
  B. Hearing loss is typically associated with late-onset FSHD.
  C. Retinal vasculopathy is typically associated with late-onset FSHD.
  D. Coats disease is associated with early-onset FSHD.
  E. Hearing loss and retinal vasculopathy are associated with high numbers of D4Z4 repeats.

**ANSWER:** D. Coats disease is associated with early-onset FSHD.

**COMMENTS AND DISCUSSION (see also comments and discussion from Question 26):**
- Important extramuscular manifestations of FSHD include:
  - ○ Retinal vasculopathy such as Coats disease, characterized by abnormal development of retinal vessels (e.g., retinal telangiectasia), and retinal microaneurysms
  - ○ High-frequency hearing loss
- Cardiomyopathy is not a feature of FSHD.
- Both retinal vasculopathy and hearing loss are associated with a very low number of D4Z4 repeats (1–3 repeats; normal 11–150; ≤10 in FSHD). Patients with a very low number of D4Z4 repeats typically have early-onset FSHD. Thus retinal vasculopathy and hearing loss are usually associated with early-onset FSHD.

**QUESTION 30.** Scapular winging is a common clinical feature in the following disorders **EXCEPT:**
  A. calpainopathy.
  B. dysferlinopathy.
  C. facioscapulohumeral muscular dystrophy.
  D. sarcoglycanopathy.
  E. valosin-containing protein (VCP)–related myopathy.

**ANSWER:** B. dysferlinopathy.

**COMMENTS AND DISCUSSION**
- Scapular winging is a common feature in various myopathies. The main differential diagnoses include:
  - ○ Facioscapulohumeral muscular dystrophy
  - ○ Calpainopathy (limb-girdle muscular dystrophy type 2A [LGMD2A])

- o Sarcoglycanopathies (LGMD2C–F)
- o Valosin containing protein (VCP)–related myopathy (aka inclusion body myopathy with Paget disease of bone and frontotemporal dementia [IBMPFD])
- Scapular winging is NOT a feature of dysferlinopathies.

## MNEMONICS

- FSHD is well known to have scapular winging
- For LGMDs, **SC**apular winging is a common feature in
  - **S**arcoglycanopathy and
  - **C**alpainopathy

**QUESTION 31.** A 45-year-old man reports difficulty using his hands including opening jars and buttoning in the past 2 years. His younger sister has early cataracts. His father died of sudden cardiac death in his 50s. When you shake the patient's hand, he has difficulty releasing his hand from yours. Motor strength is grade 4 for finger flexion bilaterally, while the other muscles are grade 5. What is the most likely genetic abnormality in this patient?

A. CTG repeat expansion in the *DMPK* gene
B. CCTG repeat expansion in the *CNBP* gene
C. Mutation in the *CLCN1* gene encoding for a chloride channel
D. Mutation in the *SCN4A* gene encoding for a sodium channel
E. Mutation in the *MYH7* gene encoding for myosin heavy chain

**ANSWER:** A. CTG repeat expansion in the *DMPK* gene

## COMMENTS AND DISCUSSION

- The diagnosis in this patient is *myotonic dystrophy* type 1. He has weakness involving the distal upper extremities. There is family history of sudden cardiac death and early cataracts. Difficulty releasing a hand after a hand grip is suggestive of myotonia. This can be confirmed clinically by testing for percussion myotonia and grip myotonia, and electrophysiologically, by demonstrating myotonic discharges on needle electromyography (EMG).
- There are two types of myotonic dystrophies: myotonic dystrophy type 1 (DM1) and type 2 (DM2). Table 18.5 demonstrates a comparison of these two types.
- Clinical features of DM1
  - o Variable age at onset
    - Age at onset has an inverse correlation with the number of CTG repeats: the higher number of CTG repeats, the earlier the age at onset.
    - "Anticipation" is a phenomenon that the number of CTG repeats expands in successive generations. This results in earlier ages at onset and increased severity of the disease in successive generations.
  - o Classic DM1
    - Classic onset occurs in adults when the number of CTG repeats is between 50 and 1000.
    - Weakness and atrophy mainly involve distal muscles. Long finger flexors are affected early. Ankle dorsiflexors may be affected.

**TABLE 18.5** Comparison between myotonic dystrophy type 1 and type 2.

| | Myotonic dystrophy type 1 | Myotonic dystrophy type 2 |
|---|---|---|
| Prevalence | Much more common | Less common |
| Distribution of weakness | Mainly distal | Mainly proximal |
| Myotonia | Prominent and distal | Subtle |
| Muscle pain | Rare | Can be prominent |
| Mutated gene | *DMPK* | *CNBP* (aka *ZNF9*) |
| Genetic abnormality | CTG repeat expansions | CCTG repeat expansion |
| Encoded protein | Myotonic dystrophy protein kinase | CCHC-type zinc finger nucleic acid–binding protein (aka zinc finger protein 9) |

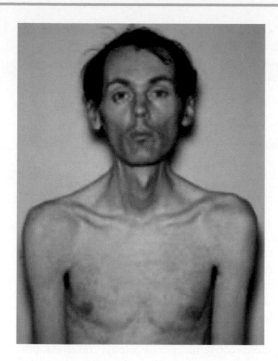

**Fig. 18.11** Facial features of a patient with myotonic dystrophy type 1. Note the characteristic facial diplegia, frontal balding, and temporal wasting, which give a "hatchet face" appearance. Herbert L Fred, Hendrik A. van Dik. Images of Memorable cases: 50 years at the bedside. 2009. Licensed under the Creative Commons Attributions License by 3.0

- Myotonia
  - Typically detected in the hands, tongue, and jaw.
  - Grip myotonia: impaired relaxation after handgrip
  - Percussion myotonia: impaired relaxation after percussion-induced contraction
  - Electrical myotonia is more sensitive than clinical myotonia. In some patients, myotonia may be detected only with needle EMG.
- Facial features (Fig. 18.11)
  - Facial diplegia: patients may have ptosis, and an inverted V-shaped upper lip (tent-shaped mouth).
  - Hatchet face (due to atrophy of facial muscles): narrow face, temporal wasting
  - Frontal balding (due to testosterone deficiency)
- Myotonic dystrophies are multisystem disorders (i.e., multiple organ systems are affected, in addition to the neuromuscular system). Multisystem involvement can be seen in both DM1 and DM2.
  - Cardiac involvement: cardiac conduction defects, supraventricular arrhythmias, and left ventricular dysfunction. Cardiac disease is the main cause of death in DM.
  - Endocrinologic involvement: hypogonadism, insulin resistance
  - Ophthalmologic involvement: early cataracts, classically "Christmas tree" cataracts
  - Sleep involvement: common in DM. Sleep abnormalities include excessive daytime sleepiness and sleep apnea.
  - Gastrointestinal involvement: dysphagia, gastroesophageal reflux disease
  - Cognitive involvement: impaired executive and visuospatial functions, behavioral symptoms
- Clinical features of DM2
  - Variable age at onset, typically ranging from early to late adulthood
  - Pain in muscles is a prominent feature. This can be mistaken for fibromyalgia or polymyalgia rheumatica.
  - Weakness affects mainly the proximal muscles. DM2 is formerly called proximal myotonic myopathy (PROMM).
  - The involvement of multiple systems in DM2 is similar to DM1, although it is often less severe.
- Laboratory features of myotonic dystrophies
  - Electrodiagnostic testing
    - Useful to demonstrate electrical myotonia, which is more sensitive than clinical myotonia
    - Myotonic discharges are spontaneous activities generated from muscle fibers. The key feature is waxing and waning of frequency and amplitude, producing a classic "revving engine" sound.
    - Myotonic discharges are more evident in DM1. In fact, occasional patients with DM2 lack electrical myotonia despite extensive muscle needle EMG.

- Serum creatine kinase (CK) levels can be modestly elevated.
- Muscle biopsy
  - DM1: increased internalized nuclei in type 1 muscle fibers
  - DM2: increased internalized nuclei in type 2 muscle fibers

---

**MNEMONICS**

Muscle pathology in myotonic dystrophies: increased internalized nuclei
In **DM1**, this is seen in **type 1** muscle fibers.
In **DM2**, this is seen in **type 2** muscle fibers.

---

- Genetic testing
  - DM1: CTG repeat expansion in the *DMPK* gene
  - DM2: CCTG repeat expansion in the *CNBP* gene
- Mutations in the *CLCN1* gene, which encodes a chloride channel, are associated with myotonia congenita. The disorders in this group are considered *chloride channelopathies*.
- Mutations in the *SCN4A* gene, which encodes a sodium channel, are associated with paramyotonia congenita, potassium-aggravated myotonia, and hyperkalemic periodic paralysis. These disorders are *sodium channelopathies*.
  - *Chloride and sodium channelopathies*, including myotonia congenita, paramyotonia congenita, potassium-aggravated myotonia, and hyperkalemic periodic paralysis, are non-dystrophic myotonias, in contrast to myotonic dystrophies, which are dystrophic myotonias. In non-dystrophic myotonia there is typically myotonia without fixed muscle weakness.
- Mutations in the *MYH7* gene are associated with Laing distal myopathy, in which the anterior leg compartment is preferentially affected. Patients may have weakness of the ankle dorsiflexors and the "hanging big toe" sign. The dropped finger sign due to weakness the of long finger extensors can also be seen in this disorder (see also comments and discussion from Questions 14 and 23).

**QUESTION 32.** Which of the following features is more prominent in myotonic dystrophy type 2, compared to type 1?
  A. Distal weakness
  B. Myotonia
  C. Pain
  D. Cataracts
  E. Cardiac conduction defect

**ANSWER:** C. Pain

**COMMENTS AND DISCUSSION (see also comments and discussion for Question 31):**
- Myotonic dystrophy type 2 (DM2) was formally called proximal myotonic myopathy (PROMM).
- In DM2, pain can be a prominent feature, whereas myotonia is more prominent in myotonic dystrophy type 1 (DM1).
- In DM2, weakness mainly involves proximal muscles. In contrast, in DM1, weakness involves the distal muscles predominantly, such as the long finger flexors and ankle dorsiflexors, as well as facial muscles (Table 18.5).
- Extramuscular manifestations such as cataracts, cardiac conduction abnormalities, and endocrine abnormalities can be seen in both DM1 and DM2. However, these features, as well as endocrinologic abnormalities (especially hypogonadism), sleep problems, and cognitive impairment, are usually more severe and prominent in DM1, compared to DM2.

**QUESTION 33.** Which of the following is the leading cause of death in patients with myotonic dystrophy?
  A. Aspiration from dysphagia
  B. Cardiac conduction abnormalities
  C. Diabetic ketoacidosis
  D. Neuromuscular respiratory failure
  E. Sleep apnea

**ANSWER:** B. Cardiac conduction abnormalities

**COMMENTS AND DISCUSSION (see also comments and discussion for Question 31):**

- Myotonic dystrophies, both type 1 (DM1) and type 2 (DM2), are multisystem disorders. In addition to the neuromuscular system, the cardiac, respiratory, gastrointestinal, endocrinologic, and ocular systems can be involved.
- The most common cause of death in myotonic dystrophies by far is cardiac conduction defects. This can be prevented by close and regular electrocardiography (ECG) monitoring.
- Dysphagia, insulin resistance, respiratory muscle weakness, sleep apnea, or sleep-disordered breathing can be seen in myotonic dystrophies. However, these manifestations are rarely the cause of death in patients with myotonic dystrophy.
- Cardiac surveillance is important in patients with myotonic dystrophies. Electrocardiography is recommended at diagnosis and at least once yearly. The most common cardiac conduction abnormality is a prolonged PR interval. Atrioventricular block can result in sudden cardiac death. Close monitoring with a cardiologist is required, and some patients may need a cardiac pacemaker or defibrillator implantation.

**QUESTION 34.** A newborn baby born from a mother with myotonic dystrophy type 1 has respiratory and feeding difficulties requiring admission to the neonatal intensive care unit. Examination reveals generalized hypotonia and bilateral talipes equinovarus. Which of the following statements is **CORRECT**?
   A. Oligohydramnios can be a finding during the prenatal period.
   B. This is due to placental transmission of autoantibodies from a mother to a baby.
   C. The baby most likely has a number of CTG repeats in the *DMPK* gene greater than 1000.
   D. The baby is more likely to have an affected father than an affected mother.
   E. This disorder does not affect intellectual skills.

**ANSWER:** C. The baby most likely has a number of CTG repeats in the *DMPK* gene greater than 1000.

**COMMENTS AND DISCUSSION**

- The baby in this vignette most likely has *congenital myotonic dystrophy*.
- Congenital myotonic dystrophy occurs in myotonic dystrophy type 1 when the number of CTG repeats in the *DMPK* gene is greater than 1000. The symptoms are present at birth.
- CTG repeats between 50 and 1000 can also result in "childhood-onset myotonic dystrophy type 1," in which the onset of symptoms is between the ages of 1 to 10 years.
- Congenital myotonic dystrophy and childhood-onset myotonic dystrophy represent a spectrum of myotonic dystrophy type 1.
- Due to anticipation, the parent of a patient with congenital myotonic dystrophy, usually the mother (more common than the father), may have classic myotonic dystrophy with fewer CTG repeats. Anticipation is a phenomenon where the number of multinucleotide repeats expands in successive generations, resulting in earlier onset and more severe symptoms.
- Clinical features of congenital myotonic dystrophy
  - Prenatal period: reduced fetal movements, polyhydramnios (due to poor swallowing of amniotic fluid)
  - Weakness and hypotonia
  - Facial features: marked facial diplegia, inverted V-shaped upper lip (tent-shaped mouth)
  - Skeletal abnormalities: talipes equinovarus and contractures
  - Patients can have intellectual disability, autistic spectrum disorders, attention- deficit/hyperactivity disorder.
  - It is also important to examine the parents, especially the mother, to look for signs of myotonic dystrophy, since they may remain undiagnosed.
- Unlike neonatal myasthenia gravis, congenital myotonic dystrophy is not due to placental transmission of autoantibodies from a mother to a baby.

**QUESTION 35.** Which of the following best describes the pathophysiology of myotonic dystrophy type 1?
   A. Impaired glycosylation
   B. Defects in muscle membrane repair
   C. Impaired alternative splicing of pre-mRNA
   D. Increased gene expression due to hypomethylation
   E. Premature stop codon resulting in truncation of protein

**ANSWER:** C. Impaired alternative splicing of pre-mRNA

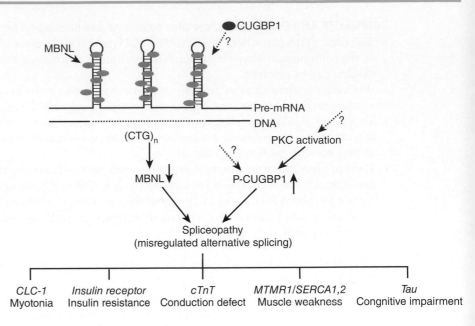

**Fig. 18.12 Pathophysiology of myotonic dystrophy type 1.** The expansion of CTG repeats in the DNA leads to the expansion of CUG repeats in pre-mRNA, resulting in the formation of hairpin loops that sequester RNA-binding proteins such as muscle blind-like protein (MBNL). As a consequence, alternative splicing of pre-mRNA is misregulated, leading to "spliceopathy" that affects various genes and causes multisystem involvement. Abbreviations: *MBNL*, muscleblind-like protein; *P-CUGBP1*, phosphorylated CUG-binding protein 1; *(CTG)ₙ*, CTG repeat expansion; *PKC*, protein kinase C. From Termsarasab P, Baajour W, Thammongkolchai T, Katirji B. The myotonic dystrophies. In: Katirji B., Kaminski H., Ruff R., eds. *Neuromuscular Disorders in Clinical Practice.* New York, NY: Springer; 2014:1221-1238

## COMMENTS AND DISCUSSION

- Pathophysiology of myotonic dystrophy type 1 (DM1) (Fig. 18.12)
  - CTG repeat expansion in the DNA → CUG repeat expansion in pre-mRNA → formation of hairpin loops → sequestration of RNA-binding proteins (e.g., muscle blind-like protein) to hairpin loops → impaired alternative splicing of pre-mRNA ("spliceopathy")
  - Impaired alternative splicing of pre-mRNA is thought to be key in the pathophysiology of DM1. Misregulated alternative splicing affects multiple genes, resulting in multisystem involvement in DM1. The affected genes include, for example:
    - *CLC1* gene, resulting in chloride channelopathy and myotonia
    - Insulin receptor gene, resulting in insulin resistance
    - Troponin T gene, resulting in cardiac conduction defects
    - *MTMR1* and *SERCA1,2* genes, resulting in muscle weakness
    - Tau gene, resulting in cognitive impairment
  - RNA-binding protein sequestration to hairpin loops has been supported by evidence of co-localization of RNA-binding proteins with CUG repeats within the nucleus. This is seen as RNA clumps by fluorescence in situ hybridization (FISH) technique, which support the RNA toxic gain-of-function mechanism in DM1.
- DM2 also has a similar mechanism. CCUG repeat expansion in the pre-mRNA forms hairpin loops, which then sequester RNA-binding proteins.
- Glycosylation is a posttranslational modification process in which sugar molecules are added to specific amino acid residues of a protein. Impaired glycosylation of α-dystroglycan is associated with dystroglycanopathies, which is a group of congenital muscular dystrophies.
- Defects in muscle membrane repair are the mechanism of dysferlinopathies.
- Hypomethylation of the D4Z4 region of the *FSHD1* gene resulting in increased expression of the *DUX4* gene is the key mechanism of facioscapulohumeral muscular dystrophy (FSHD). (see also comments and discussion from Question 26)
- Premature stop codon resulting in truncation of the dystrophin protein is the key mechanism in dystrophinopathies.

**QUESTION 36.** Which of the following statements is **CORRECT** regarding mexiletine?
  A. It reduces myotonia by blocking chloride channels.
  B. It can improve muscle strength.
  C. It is used in dystrophic myotonias but not non-dystrophic myotonias.
  D. It can be used in patients with coexisting cardiac conduction defects.
  E. Gastrointestinal discomfort is a common side effect.

**ANSWER:** E. Gastrointestinal discomfort is a common side effect.

## COMMENTS AND DISCUSSION

- *Mexiletine* is a sodium channel blocker that can reduce muscle hyperexcitability, especially in myotonia.
- It can be used to treat myotonia in both myotonic dystrophies (dystrophic myotonias) and non-dystrophic myotonias.
- It is contraindicated in patients with cardiac diseases, especially cardiac arrhythmias and coronary artery diseases, given due to potential cardiac side effects.
- Gastrointestinal discomfort or dyspepsia is a common side effects, which can be ameliorated by slow titration.
- Mexiletine has no effects on muscle strength improvement.

**QUESTION 37.** In addition to limb-girdle muscular dystrophy type 1C, mutations in the caveolin-3 (*CAV3*) gene are associated with which of the following disorders?
  A. Miyoshi myopathy
  B. Emery-Dreifuss muscular dystrophy
  C. Hypokalemic periodic paralysis
  D. Myotonia congenita
  E. Rippling muscle disease

**ANSWER:** E. Rippling muscle disease

## COMMENTS AND DISCUSSION

- In addition to limb-girdle muscular dystrophy type 1C (LGMD1C) in the old nomenclature, mutations in the *CAV3* gene, which encode the caveolin-3 protein, are associated with other phenotypes including rippling muscle disease, distal myopathy, and hyperCKemia. These disorders are considered to be allelic.
- *Rippling muscle disease*
  - Waves of contraction within muscles, typically triggered by stretching, percussion, or movements
  - Considered by some to be one of the muscle hyperexcitability syndromes
  - Can be hereditary (due to mutations in the *CAV3* gene) or acquired
  - On needle electromyography, rippling is electrically silent, except in occasional reports where active electrical activity has been found.

 **HIGH-YIELD FACT**

Mutations in the *CAV3* gene encoding caveolin-3 are associated with LGMD1C and rippling muscle disease.

- Other examples of allelic disorders that are caused by mutations in the same gene include:
  - *DYSF* (dysferlin) gene: LGMD2B and Miyoshi distal myopathy
  - *LMNA* (lamin A/C) gene: LGMD1A, Emery-Dreifuss muscular dystrophy, familial partial lipodystrophy, Hutchinson-Gilford progeria syndrome, and dilated cardiomyopathy, among others
  - *SCN4A* gene encoding for the sodium channel (Nav1.4): hyperkalemic periodic paralysis, potassium-aggravated myotonia, paramyotonia congenita, and hypokalemic periodic paralysis
- Hypokalemic periodic paralysis can be caused by mutations in the *CACNA1S* or *SCN4A* gene resulting in calcium or sodium channelopathy, respectively.
- Myotonia congenita is caused by mutations in the *CLCN1* gene, which encodes the skeletal muscle chloride channel (ClC-1).

**QUESTION 38.** Which of the following features is the most useful to differentiate between congenital muscular dystrophy and congenital myopathy?
  A. Cardiac involvement
  B. Central nervous system involvement
  C. Contracture
  D. Facial muscle weakness
  E. Respiratory involvement

**ANSWER:** B. Central nervous system involvement

**TABLE 18.6** Differentiating features between congenital muscular dystrophy and congenital myopathy.

|  | Congenital muscular dystrophy | Congenital myopathy |
|---|---|---|
| Progression of the disease | Variable; can be slowly or rapidly progressive | Usually stable or very slowly progressive |
| Central nervous system involvement | Can be seen; these include learning disability, seizures, white matter changes on MRI, lissencephaly | None |
| Serum creatine kinase | Elevated, typically greater than 3 times of UNL | Normal or mildly elevated |
| Muscle biopsy | Dystrophic features: muscle fiber necrosis and regeneration | Myopathic with specific findings and without dystrophic features |
| Location of abnormal protein | Mostly at the sarcolemmal membrane or extracellular matrix | Within the muscle; mostly involving muscle contraction (e.g., sarcomere, T-tubule, sarcoplasmic reticulum) |

Abbreviations: *MRI*, magnetic resonance imaging; *UNL*, upper normal limit.

**COMMENTS AND DISCUSSION**

- Several features are useful to differentiate between congenital muscular dystrophies and congenital myopathies, as shown in Table 18.6.
- Other features that are seen in both congenital muscular dystrophies and congenital myopathies include:
  - Onset of the disease: Patients often have onset of symptoms including hypotonia and weakness at birth or in the infantile period. However, the onset can be variable and patients may develop symptoms later.
  - Facial weakness, contracture, cardiac involvement, and respiratory involvement can be seen in some patients with congenital muscular dystrophies, as well as congenital myopathies.
- Involvement of extraocular muscles can be seen in some congenital myopathies.
- Long myopathic facies and a high-arched palate are seen in congenital myopathies.

**QUESTION 39.** A 1-week-old baby boy is referred for evaluation of generalized hypotonia and muscle weakness. He also has respiratory failure requiring endotracheal intubation and feeding difficulty requiring nasogastric tube placement. On examination, marked limitation of eye movements in multiple directions is noted. Serum creatine kinase is 40 U/L. Brain magnetic resonance imaging (MRI) is normal. Muscle biopsy shows internalized nuclei in most muscle fibers. This patient most likely has a mutation in which of the following genes?
A. *ACTA1* encoding α-actin 1
B. *DNM2* encoding dynamin 2
C. *MTM1* encoding myotubularin
D. *RYR1* encoding ryanodine receptor 1
E. *SEPN1* encoding selenoprotein N

**ANSWER:** C. *MTM1* encoding myotubularin

**COMMENTS AND DISCUSSION**

- The diagnosis in this baby is *centronuclear myopathy*, a type of congenital myopathy. This baby most likely has X-linked myotubular myopathy, which is the most severe form of centronuclear myopathy.
- *X-linked myotubular myopathy* is associated with mutations in the *MTM1* gene encoding myotubularin.
- Congenital myopathies can be categorized according to histopathological findings on muscle biopsy. Among many types of congenital myopathies, four main types include:
  - Centronuclear myopathy
  - Central core myopathy
  - Nemaline myopathy
  - Congenital fiber-type disproportion

- After discovery of the genes associated with these histopathological phenotypes, some overlaps have been found.
  - One gene may be associated with multiple phenotypes. For example,
    - *RYR1* mutations can be associated with central core myopathy and centronuclear myopathy.
    - *TTN* (encoding titin) mutations can be associated with central core myopathy and centronuclear myopathy.
  - One phenotype is associated with multiple genes.
    - There are several genes associated with each type of congenital myopathy.
- Centronuclear myopathy
  - Increased internalized or central nuclei are found on muscle biopsy. Normally internalized nuclei are present in less than 3% of all muscle fibers on biopsy.
    - On muscle biopsy, *DNM2* multiple can be associated with radiating sarcoplasmic strands around nuclei, giving a feature of spoke-like appearance (see also comments and discussion from Question 6 and Fig. 10.5A and B in Chapter 10).
  - Associated with mutations in multiple genes.
    - The most important ones include *MTM1*, *BIN1*, and *DNM2* genes (Table 18.7).
    - Other genes include *RYR1* (encoding ryanodine receptor 1), *TTN* (encoding titin), and *SPEG* (encoding striated muscle-enriched protein kinase).

**TABLE 18.7** Three most important genes associated with centronuclear myopathy.

| Gene | Inheritance | Encoded protein | Protein function | Typical onset | Phenotype |
|------|-------------|-----------------|------------------|---------------|-----------|
| *MTM1* | X-linked recessive | Myotubularin | Being PIP; important in membrane trafficking and endocytosis | Prenatal, neonatal to infantile periods | X-linked myotubular myopathy; most severe |
| *BIN1* | Mostly AR | Amphiphysin 2 (aka. bridging integrator 1) | Membrane remodeling | Late infancy to early childhood | Moderate (between those of *MTM1* and *DNM2* mutations) |
| *DNM2* | Mostly AD | Dynamin 2 | Membrane fission and T-tubule formation | Early adolescence to adulthood | Mild; spoke-like appearance on muscle biopsy |

Note: Other genes including *RYR1*, *TTN*, and *SPEG* are not shown in the table.
Abbreviations: *AD*, autosomal dominant; *AR*, autosomal recessive; *PIP*, phosphoinositide phosphatase.

## MNEMONICS

**Centronuclear myopathy**

Onset:    Infant  ————————————————————→  Adulthood
Severity: Severe  ←————————————————————  Mild
Gene:    *MTM1*                   *BIN1*                *DNM2*

- Onset has an inverse relationship with the severity. Earlier onset is associated with more severe phenotypes.
- *MTM1* encodes myotubularin. Think about **fetal** myotubes: very early onset; most severe
- The letter **B** is before the letter **D**. *BIN1* has the onset before *DNM2*.
- Most mutations in the *DNM2* gene are inherited in an autosomal **D**ominant manner.

  - Genes and encoded proteins associated with centronuclear myopathy share a common theme. Their functions are associated with the sarcolemmal membrane around T-tubules and triads (Fig. 18.13). The triad comprises a T-tubule and two terminal cisternae of the sarcoplasmic reticulum on both sides of the T-tubule (Fig. 18.14).
  - Clinical features of centronuclear myopathy
    - X-linked myotubular myopathy
      - Associated with *MTM1* mutations
      - The most severe phenotype: symptoms are present in the prenatal period (e.g., reduced fetal movements, polyhydramnios), neonatal, or early infantile period.

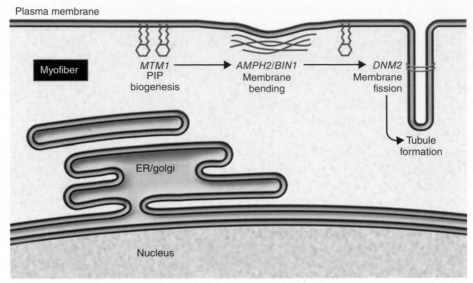

**Fig. 18.13** Function of three main proteins encoded from the genes associated with centronuclear myopathy. *MTM1* encodes myotubularin; *BIN1* encodes amphiphysin 2 (aka bridging integrator 1); *DNM2* encodes dynamin 2. These proteins are involved in various functions related to the sarcolemmal membrane, T-tubules, and triads. From Demonbreun AR, McNally EM. Dynamin 2 the rescue for centronuclear myopathy. *J Clin Invest.* 2014;124(3):976–978.

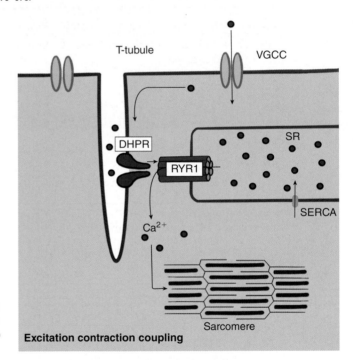

**Fig. 18.14** Physiology at the T-tubule. The triad consists of the T-tubule and two terminal cisternae of the sarcoplasmic reticulum (one on each side of the T-tubule; only one is shown in the figure). The dihydropyridine receptor *(DHPR)* couples with the ryanodine receptor 1 *(RYR1)* in skeletal muscle. RYR1 mediates calcium release from the sarcoplasmic reticulum. Sarco/endoplasmic reticulum calcium ATPase (SERCA) transports $Ca^{2+}$ from the cytosol back into the sarcoplasmic reticulum.

- Floppy infant, generalized weakness, feeding difficulty, respiratory weakness
- Ophthalmoparesis (weakness of the extraocular muscles), facial weakness including ptosis
- Milder phenotypes are associated with mutations in the other genes including *BIN1* and *DNM2*.
- Ophthalmoparesis or ptosis is a very important clue for the diagnosis of centronuclear myopathy. This feature is present in only a few congenital myopathies.
- *RYR1* mutations are associated with central core disease and centronuclear myopathy. However, this patient has a very severe phenotype with very early onset, so *RYR1* mutations are less likely.
- *ACTA1* mutations are associated with nemaline myopathy, not centronuclear myopathy.
- *SEPN1* mutations are associated with central core disease and rigid spine muscular dystrophy, not centronuclear myopathy.

◎ **HIGH-YIELD FACT**

**Ophthalmoparesis** and **ptosis** are very important clues for the diagnosis of centronuclear myopathy.

**QUESTION 40.** Mutations in which of the central core disease genes are associated with an increased risk of malignant hyperthermia?
A. *ACTA1* encoding α-actin 1
B. *MYH7* encoding myosin heavy chain 7
C. *RYR1* encoding ryanodine receptor
D. *SELENON* (*SEPN1*) encoding selenoprotein N
E. *TTN* encoding titin

**ANSWER:** C. *RYR1* encoding ryanodine receptor

**COMMENTS AND DISCUSSION**

- *Central core disease* is characterized by a central area that is devoid of enzymatic activity in the muscle fiber, most prominent on the NADH-TR stain. (see also comments and discussion from Question 6 and Fig. 10.5C in Chapter 10.)
- In central core disease, patients typically present with hypotonia and weakness since birth, but the onset can be variable.
- *Multiminicore myopathy*
  ◦ The cores are less prominent, smaller, and patchier.
  ◦ Clinical features are similar to those of central core disease.
  ◦ Of interest, some patients with multiminicore myopathy associated with the *RYR1* gene can have ophthalmoparesis and ptosis.

## ◎ HIGH-YIELD FACT

Ophthalmoparesis and ptosis are useful diagnostic clues in congenital myopathies, and can be seen in
- Centronuclear myopathy
- Multiminicore myopathy with *RYR1* mutations

- Central core disease is associated with various genes including:
  ◦ *RYR1* (encoding for ryanodine receptor)
  ◦ *SELENON* (aka *SEPN1*, encoding selenoprotein N)
  ◦ *MYH7* (encoding myosin heavy chain 7)
  ◦ *TTN* (encoding titin)
  ◦ *ACTA1* (encoding α-actin 1)
  ◦ *CCDC78* (encoding coiled-coiled domain-containing 78)
- The most important gene associated with central core disease is *RYR1*, which is responsible for the majority of cases.
- However, in multiminicore myopathy, the most common gene is *SELENON*, which can present as rigid spine syndrome.
- Malignant hyperthermia is also associated with mutations in the *RYR1* gene.
- Thus patients with central core disease due to *RYR1* mutations have an increased risk of malignant hyperthermia, especially when exposed to depolarizing muscle relaxants (e.g., succinylcholine) during anesthesia.
- Although the other genes in the options are also associated with central core disease, they do not increase the risk of malignant hyperthermia.

## ◎ HIGH-YIELD FACT

*RYR1* **mutations** are associated with **central core disease** and **malignant hyperthermia.**
Only central core disease associated with mutations in the *RYR1* gene (not the others) is at increased risk of malignant hyperthermia.

- *RYR1* gene encodes ryanodine receptor 1.
  ◦ Ryanodine receptor 1 is expressed in skeletal muscles.
  ◦ It mediates calcium ($Ca^{2+}$) release from the sarcoplasmic reticulum.
  ◦ This $Ca^{2+}$ release is important for excitation-contraction coupling.
- Physiology at the T-tubule (Fig. 18.14)
  ◦ T-tubule and two terminal cisternae of the sarcoplasmic reticulum (one on each side of the T-tubule) form the "triad."

- Action potential travels along the sarcolemmal membrane → opening of voltage-gated $Ca^{2+}$ channel → action potential travels along the T-tubule → activation of dihydropyridine receptor (L-type $Ca^{2+}$ channel) → activation of ryanodine receptor → $Ca^{2+}$ release from the sarcoplasmic reticulum → excitation-contraction coupling
  - Sarco/endoplasmic reticulum calcium ATPase (SERCA) transports $Ca^{2+}$ from the cytosol back into the sarcoplasmic reticulum.
- Genes responsible for calcium transport of sarcoplasmic reticulum and their disease associations
  - *RYR1* gene: associated with
    - Central core disease
    - Malignant hyperthermia: *RYR1* mutations cause excessive $Ca^{2+}$ release into the cytosol, resulting in sustained muscle contraction and excessive heat production.
  - *ATP2A1* gene affecting SERCA: associated with Brody myopathy
    - Impaired $Ca^{2+}$ transport from the cytosol back into the sarcoplasmic reticulum.
    - Clinical features: impaired muscle relaxation, muscle stiffness, and cramps that are exacerbated with cold temperature. The onset of symptoms typically occurs in childhood.

## ◎ HIGH-YIELD FACT

**Ryanodine receptor 1**
- $Ca^{2+}$ **release** from sarcoplasmic reticulum (SR)
- Impaired in **central core disease and malignant hyperthermia**

**SERCA1**
- $Ca^{2+}$ **transport back** into SR
- Impaired in **Brody myopathy**

**QUESTION 41.** Which of the following disorders is **NOT** associated with mutations in the *RYR1* gene?
  A. Centronuclear myopathy
  B. Central core myopathy
  C. Malignant hyperthermia
  D. Multiminicore myopathy
  E. Reducing body myopathy

**ANSWER:** E. Reducing body myopathy

**COMMENTS AND DISCUSSION (see also comments and discussion from Question 40)**
- *RYR1* mutations are associated with a variety of phenotypes including
  - Congenital myopathies
    - Central core disease
    - Multiminicore disease
    - Centronuclear myopathy
    - Congenital fiber-type disproportion
  - Other phenotypes
    - Malignant hyperthermia
    - Rhabdomyolysis-myalgia syndrome
- Reducing body myopathy is a subtype of congenital myopathy. It is associated with mutations in the *FHL1* gene (encoding four and a half LIM domains), and the *DES* gene (encoding desmin).
- Nemaline myopathy is generally not associated with *RYR1* mutations. However, rare case reports have suggested the presence of *RYR1* mutations in some patients with nemaline myopathy.

**QUESTION 42.** Which of the following statements is **CORRECT** regarding nemaline myopathy?
  A. The onset can vary from the neonatal period to late adulthood.
  B. Ophthalmoparesis is a frequent clinical feature.
  C. Cardiac involvement is absent.
  D. Mutations in the *ACTA1* gene are the most common.
  E. Nemaline rods are best demonstrated on NADH stain.

**ANSWER:** A. The onset can vary from the neonatal period to late adulthood.

## COMMENTS AND DISCUSSION

- *Nemaline myopathy* is a subtype of congenital myopathy.
- Clinical features of nemaline myopathy
  - Marked phenotypic variability with onset that can range from birth to late adulthood. The disease is usually more severe when the onset occurs earlier in life.
  - Several forms
    - Severe neonatal onset
    - Typical form: onset in early infancy, mild severity, non- or very slowly progressive
    - Childhood onset
    - Adult onset
      - Late-onset nemaline myopathy may present with neck extensor myopathy.
  - Common clinical features among these forms with variable severity
    - Hypotonia and muscle weakness
    - Weakness may affect the limbs, facial muscles, bulbar muscles (resulting in feeding difficulty or dysphagia), and respiratory muscles (resulting in hypoventilation).
    - Despite the presence of facial weakness in some patients, there is *no* ophthalmoparesis.
    - Cardiomyopathy may occur in some patients.
    - Dysmorphic features and skeletal deformities: long and narrow myopathic facies, high-arched palate, chest deformities, clinodactyly, foot deformities, kyphoscoliosis
    - No intellectual disability is typically associated with nemaline myopathy, as well as other congenital myopathies.
- Muscle biopsy in nemaline myopathy (see also commens and discussion from Question 6 and Fig. 10.14 in Chapter 10)
  - Nonspecific myopathic features: variation of muscle fiber size
  - Presence of nemaline rods
    - Best demonstrated on modified Gomori trichrome (mGT) stain, *not* NADH stain, which is best for demonstration of central cores
    - On electron microscopy, nemaline rods are seen as streaming of the Z discs.
- Genetics of nemaline myopathy
  - There is marked genetic heterogeneity with mutations in multiple genes.
  - Almost all genes in nemaline myopathy are associated with sarcomeric, thin-filament proteins important in excitation-contraction coupling (Fig. 18.15).

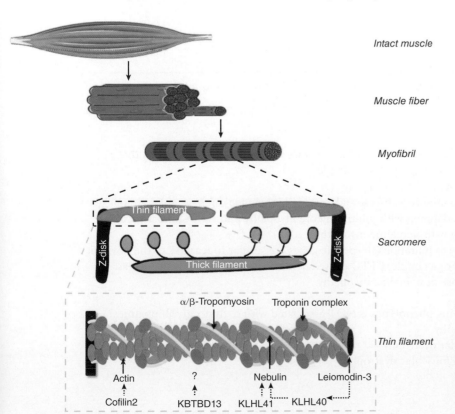

**Fig. 18.15** Genes associated with nemaline myopathy. Almost all genes responsible for nemaline myopathy and their encoded proteins are involved in the structure and functions of sarcomeric thin filaments. These genes include *NEB* encoding nebulin, *ACTA1* encoding α-actin 1, *TNNT1* encoding slow troponin T1, *KBTBD13*, *CFL2* encoding cofilin 2, *TPM2* and *TPM3* encoding tropomyosin 2 and tropomyosin 3, as well as *KLHL40* and *KLHL41* encoding kelch-like proteins 40 and 41. From de Winter JM, Ottenheijm CA. Sarcomere dysfunction in nemaline myopathy. *J Neuromusc Dis.* 2017;4:99–113. Creative Commons Attribution Non-Commercial License (CC BY-NC 4.0).

- ◦ Mutations occur in the following genes.
  - *NEB* encoding nebulin: the most common
  - *ACTA1* encoding α-actin 1: the second most common
  - *TNNT1* encoding slow troponin T1
  - *KBTBD13* encoding kelch repeat and BTB domain containing 13
  - *CFL2* encoding cofilin 2
  - *TPM2* and *TPM3* encoding tropomyosin 2 and tropomyosin 3
  - *KLHL40* and *KLHL41* encoding kelch-like protein 40 and kelch-like protein 41

 **HIGH-YIELD FACT**

> The most common genes associated with nemaline myopathy are ***NEB*** (encoding nebulin) followed by ***ACTA1*** (encoding α-actin 1).

**QUESTION 43.** Which of the following is a muscle biopsy feature typically seen in congenital fiber-type disproportion?
  A. Type 1 muscle fiber atrophy and predominance
  B. Type 2 muscle fiber atrophy and predominance
  C. Type 1 muscle fiber atrophy and type 2 muscle fiber predominance
  D. Type 2 muscle fiber atrophy and type 1 muscle fiber predominance
  E. Type 2 muscle fiber predominance without atrophy

**ANSWER:** A. Type 1 muscle fiber atrophy and predominance

**COMMENTS AND DISCUSSION**
- Type 1 muscle fiber atrophy and predominance are common features on muscle biopsy among all congenital myopathies.
- In *congenital fiber-type disproportion (CFTD)*, there are no other structural abnormalities (e.g., core structures, central nuclei or nemaline rods), in addition to type 1 muscle atrophy and predominance. The cutoff of 12%–15% size difference between type 1 and type 2 muscle fibers is typically used for diagnosis.

 **HIGH-YIELD FACT**

> Type 1 muscle fiber atrophy and predominance is a common feature among all congenital myopathies, not only congenital fiber-type disproportion (CFTD).

- CFTD is a controversial entity. Genes associated with CFTD have remarkable overlap with those associated with other congenital myopathies. For example:
  - ◦ *TPM3* gene: overlapping with nemaline myopathy
  - ◦ *RYR1* gene: overlapping with central core disease and others. This subtype can have ophthalmoplegia.
  - ◦ Other rarer genes: *SEPN1* overlapping with multiminicore myopathy and rigid spine muscular dystrophy; *TPM2* overlapping with nemaline myopathy
  - ◦ Clinical features of CFTD due to mutations in specific genes are similar to features of the disorder associated with those genes. For example, CFTD caused by mutations in the *TPM3* gene has clinical features similar to those of nemaline myopathy.

**QUESTION 44.** Which of the following phenotypes is **NOT** associated with α-dystroglycanopathies?
  A. Limb-girdle muscular dystrophy
  B. Fukuyama congenital muscular dystrophy
  C. Merosin-deficient congenital muscular dystrophy
  D. Muscle-eye-brain disease
  E. Walker-Warburg syndrome

**ANSWER:** C. Merosin-deficient congenital muscular dystrophy

## COMMENTS AND DISCUSSION

- α-*Dystroglycanopathies* are common causes of congenital muscular dystrophies.
- α-Dystroglycanopathies have marked phenotypic variability. The following phenotypes are in order of severity, from the most to least severe:
  - Walker-Warburg syndrome
    - The most severe form
    - Cobblestone lissencephaly (neuronal migration defect), intellectual impairment, seizures
  - Muscle-eye-brain disease
  - Fukuyama congenital muscular dystrophy
  - Limb-girdle muscular dystrophy phenotype
    - Mild form
- α-Dystroglycanopathies are associated with various genes such as *FKTN, POMT1, POMT2, FKRP, POMGnT1, POMGnT2,* and *LARGE,* among others. There is no need to remember these genes for the boards; however, their functions are worth knowing.
  - These genes are important in glycosylation of α-dystroglycan.
  - Glycosylation is a process of posttranslational modification of proteins by adding saccharides.
  - α-Dystroglycan has *O*-mannosyl-dependent glycosylation, where various sugar residues including mannose are added to form extensive chains.
  - α-Dystroglycan links β-dystroglycan to laminin α2 (aka merosin), which binds to the extracellular matrix (Fig. 18.16).
    - α-Dystroglycan and laminin α2 are important in the stabilization of the sarcolemmal membrane.
    - Impairment of these proteins results in congenital muscular dystrophies in which serum creatine kinase is typically elevated.
- Congenital muscular dystrophies include:
  - *LAMA2*-related muscular dystrophy (aka merosin-deficient muscular dystrophy)
  - α-Dystroglycanopathies
  - Collagen VI–related muscular dystrophies (see also comments and discussion from Question 21), specifically Ullrich congenital muscular dystrophy. In contrast, Bethlem myopathy is a milder from of collagen-VI related muscular dystrophies with a later onset.
  - *LMNA*-related congenital muscular dystrophy, which is one of the laminopathies (see also comments and discussion from Question 19)
  - Rigid spine muscular dystrophy due to *SEPN1* mutations
    - *SEPN1* mutations are also associated with multiminicore myopathy.
- Congenital muscular dystrophies are mostly autosomal recessive. They are associated with defects in proteins that link sarcolemma to the extracellular matrix (e.g., laminin α2 and α-dystroglycan), or proteins in the extracellular matrix (e.g., collagen VI). Impaired function of these proteins results in disruption of the sarcolemmal membrane and muscle fiber necrosis, which lead to elevated serum creatine kinase levels, a useful marker to distinguish congenital muscular dystrophies from congenital myopathies.

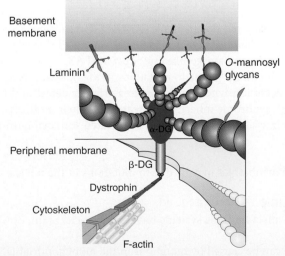

**Fig. 18.16** α-Dystroglycan. α-Dystroglycan links β-dystroglycan to laminin α2, which binds to extracellular matrix. α-Dystroglycan requires posttranslational modification by *O*-mannosyl–dependent glycosylation. Impaired glycosylation of α-dystroglycan is the key pathophysiological mechanism of α-dystroglycanopathies. From Taniguchi-Ikeda M, Morioka I, Iijima K, Toda T. Mechanistic aspects of the formation of α-dystroglycan and therapeutic research for the treatment of α-dystroglycanopathy: A review. *Mol Aspects Med.* 2016;51:115–124.

**QUESTION 45.**   A newborn has severe hypotonia, contractures of multiple joints and generalized muscle weakness at birth. A few days later, he develops feeding difficulty and respiratory failure. Brain magnetic resonance imaging (MRI) reveals hyperintense signals in the bilateral subcortical white matter on T2-weighted images. Serum creatine kinase is 1546 U/L. Muscle biopsy revealed absent merosin staining. This disorder is due to abnormalities in which of the following proteins?

A.  α-Dystroglycan
B.  Collagen VI
C.  Dystrophin
D.  Laminin α2
E.  Selenoprotein N

**ANSWER:** D. Laminin α2

**COMMENTS AND DISCUSSION**

- The diagnosis in this newborn is *LAMA2*-related congenital muscular dystrophy (aka merosin-deficient congenital muscular dystrophy).
- The elevated serum creatine kinase level indicates congenital muscular dystrophy rather than congenital myopathy. White matter changes can be seen on neuroimaging in this disorder. Absent merosin (laminin α2) confirms the diagnosis of *LAMA2*-related congenital muscular dystrophy.
- *LAMA2*-related congenital muscular dystrophy
   ○ The classic type typically has an onset at birth or in the early infantile period.
   ○ Floppy infant due to severe hypotonia and generalized muscle weakness
   ○ Joint contractures
   ○ Patients can have coexisting central nervous system (CNS) and peripheral nerve abnormalities.
      • CNS abnormalities
         • White matter changes on brain MRI
         • Seizures
         • Despite MRI changes, patients have normal intellectual function.
      • Peripheral nerve abnormalities
         • Hypomyelinating or demyelinating sensorimotor neuropathy
- *LAMA2*-related congenital muscular dystrophy is autosomal recessive, due to mutations in the *LAMA2* gene.
   ○ *LAMA2* gene encodes laminin α2.
   ○ Laminin α2 links α-dystroglycan to the basement membrane (extracellular matrix). This linking of proteins is essential for stabilizing the sarcolemmal membrane.
   ○ The most abundant isoform of laminin α2 in the skeletal muscle is laminin-211 (aka merosin; α2β1γ1 isoform of the α, β, and γ subunits).
   ○ Muscle biopsy in *LAMA2*-related congenital muscular dystrophy shows absent or markedly reduced merosin staining.

**QUESTION 46.**   Which of the following statements is **CORRECT** regarding mitochondrial myopathies?

A.  The ratio of mutated mitochondrial DNA is identical among all tissues in mitochondrial encephalomyopathy, lactic acidosis, and stroke-like episodes (MELAS).
B.  Mitochondrial myopathies may be due to mutations in the nuclear DNA.
C.  Mitochondrial DNA depletion syndrome is due to a primary defect in the mitochondrial DNA.
D.  All patients with Leigh syndrome inherit the disease from their mothers.
E.  Ragged-red fibers on muscle biopsy are best demonstrated with cytochrome oxidase (COX) staining.

**ANSWER:** B. Mitochondrial myopathies may be due to mutations in the nuclear DNA.

**COMMENTS AND DISCUSSION**

- Mitochondrial disorders affect multiple systems including muscle, brain, eye, heart, kidney, liver, and ear.
- Mitochondrial disorders can be caused by mutations in the mitochondrial DNA (mtDNA) or mutations in the nuclear DNA that affect the mitochondria.
- When mutations occur in the mtDNA, the principles of mitochondrial genetics are applied.
   ○ Maternal inheritance

- ○ Heteroplasmy: the number of mutated mtDNA varies among different cells or tissues. This phenomenon can explain why different tissues can be affected to varying degrees in different patients. In addition, testing in one tissue (e.g., blood) may yield a negative result due to low mutated mtDNA load, and testing in different tissues (e.g., muscle in mitochondrial myopathies) may be required.
- When the mutations occur in the nuclear DNA, the principles of Mendelian genetics (e.g., autosomal dominant, autosomal recessive) are applied.

## ◎ HIGH-YIELD FACT

Mitochondrial disorders can be due to mutations in either the mitochondrial or nuclear DNA.

- *Mitochondrial myopathies*
  - ○ Due to *mutations in the mitochondrial DNA (mtDNA)*
    - Mitochondria encephalomyopathy, lactic acidosis, and stroke-like episodes (MELAS) due to the A3243G mutation in the mtDNA tRNA$^{Leu}$ gene in the majority of cases
    - Myoclonic epilepsy with ragged-red fibers (MERRF) due to the A8344G mutation in the mtDNA tRNA$^{Lys}$ gene in the majority of cases
    - Kearns-Sayre syndrome, mostly due to large deletions in the mitochondrial DNA
      - Can have a milder phenotype of chronic progressive external ophthalmoplegia (CPEO) without cardiac involvement
    - Maternally-inherited Leigh syndrome (MILS)
      - Due to the same mutation as neuropathy ataxia retinitis pigmentosa (NARP), but there is no myopathy in NARP
  - ○ Due to *mutations in the nuclear DNA*
    - Leigh syndrome (other than MILS): associated with various mutations
    - *POLG*-related disorders (see also comments and discussion from Question 47)
    - Mitochondrial neurogastrointestinal encephalomyopathy (MNGIE) due to mutations in the *TYMP* (thymidine phosphorylase) gene
    - Mitochondrial myopathy due to thymidine kinase 2 (TK2) deficiency
- Leigh syndrome can be due to mtDNA mutations (maternally-inherited Leigh syndrome) or nuclear DNA mutations.
- Ragged-red fibers are due to accumulation of abnormal mitochondria. On muscle biopsy they are best demonstrated with modified Gomori trichrome (mGT) stain. (see also comments and discussion for Questions 6 in Chapter 10.)

**QUESTION 47.** Which of the following phenotypes is **NOT** associated with *POLG* mutations?
  A. Myocerebrohepatopathy in a toddler
  B. Myoclonic epilepsy, myopathy, and sensory ataxia
  C. Progressive external ophthalmoplegia
  D. Sideroblastic anemia with pancreatic dysfunction
  E. Sensory ataxia, neuropathy, dysarthria, and ophthalmoplegia

**ANSWER:** D. Sideroblastic anemia with pancreatic dysfunction

## COMMENTS AND DISCUSSION
- *POLG* encodes of a gamma subunit of mitochondrial DNA polymerase. It is a gene in the nuclear DNA.
- Mutations in the nuclear *POLG* gene result in mitochondrial disorders with a variety of phenotypes.
  - ○ Alpers-Huttenlocher syndrome (myocerebrohepatopathy)
    - Severe form with onset in early childhood, typically between 2–4 years of age
    - Myopathy, seizures, liver failure, intellectual impairment
  - ○ Myoclonic epilepsy, myopathy, sensory ataxia (MEMSA)
  - ○ Other phenotypes *without* myopathy
    - Sensory ataxia, neuropathy, dysarthria, ophthalmoplegia (SANDO)
    - Mitochondrial recessive ataxia syndrome (MIRAS)
    - Progressive external ophthalmoplegia
      - Autosomal dominant (adPEO)
      - Autosomal recessive (arPEO)
- Sideroblastic anemia and pancreatic dysfunction are seen in Pearson syndrome, which is due to mutations (mainly large deletions) in the mitochondrial DNA, not the *POLG* gene.

**QUESTION 48.** A 30-year-old man presents for further evaluation of weakness. He has had difficulty swallowing, chronic nausea, frequent vomiting after meals, abdominal pain, and diarrhea for more than 5 years. On examination, his weight is 70 lb (32 kg) and height is 168 cm (5 ft 6 in). He has bilateral ptosis, limitations of extraocular movements, and generalized and symmetrical muscle weakness, grade 3 proximally and grade 4 distally. Reflexes are diffusely reduced. This disorder is due to an abnormality in which of the following proteins?

A. Acid maltase
B. Docking protein 7 (DOK7)
C. Myophosphorylase
D. DNA polymerase-gamma
E. Thymidine phosphorylase

**ANSWER:** E. Thymidine phosphorylase

## COMMENTS AND DISCUSSION

- The diagnosis in this patient is *mitochondrial neurogastrointestinal encephalomyopathy (MNGIE)*.
- MNGIE is an autosomal recessive disorder caused by mutations in the *TYMP* gene that encodes thymidine phosphorylase. It is a mitochondrial disorder due to mutations in the nuclear DNA.
- Clinical features of MNGIE
  - Typical onset between the first and fifth decades
  - Neurological manifestations
    - Myopathy
    - Ptosis and external ophthalmoplegia
    - Neuropathy: often characterized by mixed demyelinating and axonal features, and may involve both sensory and motor nerves
    - Leukoencephalopathy: can be seen on brain MRI
  - Gastrointestinal and other systemic manifestations
    - Gastrointestinal dysmotility: nausea, postprandial emesis, dysphagia, episodic abdominal pain, diarrhea
    - Cachexia: this can be a very important clue, since most patients with MNGIE typically appear very emaciated.
- Acid maltase deficiency is associated with Pompe disease.
- Mutations in the *DOK7* gene are associated with congenital myasthenic syndromes that typically present with a limb-girdle weakness phenotype.
- Myophosphorylase deficiency is associated with McArdle disease.
- DNA polymerase-gamma is associated with *POLG*-related disorders. (see also comments and discussion from Question 47.)

**QUESTION 49.** A 52-year-old woman has long-standing ptosis, limited eye movements, and proximal muscle weakness for more than two decades. She has been diagnosed with myasthenia gravis and treated with pyridostigmine and immunosuppressive agents with no response. She denies diplopia. She has a medical history of second-degree atrioventricular block requiring pacemaker placement. On examination, there is prominent non-fatigable bilateral ptosis and moderately limited eye movements in both the horizontal and vertical directions. Muscle strength is grade 4 proximally and grade 5 distally in all extremities. What is the most likely genetic abnormality in this patient?

A. Mutation in the *DOK7* gene in the nuclear DNA
B. Mutation in the *POLG* gene in the nuclear DNA
C. Mutation in the mitochondrial tRNA$^{Leu}$ gene
D. Large deletion in the mitochondrial DNA
E. Mitochondria DNA depletion

**ANSWER:** D. Large deletion in the mitochondrial DNA

## COMMENTS AND DISCUSSION

- The diagnosis in this patient is *Kearns-Sayre syndrome (KSS)*.
- Some of these patients are misdiagnosed as myasthenia gravis and receive unnecessary treatment including immunotherapies.
- KSS is a mitochondrial disorder due to a large deletion in the mitochondrial DNA (mtDNA).

- Clinical features of KSS
  - Chronic progressive external ophthalmoplegia. Patients typically do not have diplopia.
  - Proximal myopathy
  - Cardiac conduction block
  - Other features: pigmentary retinopathy, ataxia, sensorineural hearing loss, elevated cerebrospinal fluid (CSF) protein
- Other disorders due to mtDNA deletions (aka mtDNA deletion syndromes) include Pearson syndrome, chronic progressive external ophthalmoplegia (CPEO), and Leigh syndrome.

## ◎ HIGH-YIELD FACT

Chronic progressive external ophthalmoplegia (CPEO) + Cardiac conduction block = Kearns-Sayre syndrome
CPEO can be due to
- Large mitochondrial DNA deletions as seen in KSS
- Mutations in the *POLG* gene in the nuclear DNA

- Mutations in the *DOK7* gene in the nuclear DNA are associated with a congenital myasthenic syndrome in which patients can present with a limb-girdle weakness phenotype.
- Mutations in the *POLG* gene in the nuclear DNA can be associated with autosomal dominant progressive external ophthalmoplegia (adPEO) and autosomal recessive progressive external ophthalmoplegia (arPEO). However, cardiac conduction defects are not a feature in these disorders.
- The A3243G mutation in the mitochondrial tRNA^Leu gene is associated with mitochondrial encephalomyopathy, lactic acidosis, and stroke-like episodes (MELAS). External ophthalmoplegia and cardiac conduction defects are not features in MELAS.
- Thymidine kinase 2 deficiency due to mutations in the *TK2* gene is an example of mitochondrial DNA depletion syndrome. In this disorder, affected infants have encephalopathy, myopathy, and seizure.

**QUESTION 50.** Which of the following is **CORRECT** regarding forearm exercise testing?
  A. The test is indicated in a patient with nocturnal muscle cramps.
  B. Blood pressure cuff insufflation above systolic blood pressure is the generally preferred method.
  C. The venous blood is drawn at baseline and 10 minutes after exercise.
  D. Each blood sample is tested for ammonia, lactate, and triglyceride.
  E. If a patient develops muscle contracture, the test should be terminated.

**ANSWER:** E. If a patient develops muscle contracture, the test should be terminated.

## COMMENTS AND DISCUSSION
- Forearm exercise test is useful when metabolic myopathies, especially glycogenoses, are suspected.
- Patients with metabolic myopathies have one of two main themes on clinical presentation.
  - Exercise intolerance, exercise-induced muscle pain/cramps, or myoglobinuria
  - Fixed weakness: weakness is persistent, and can be progressive over time.
  - Some patients can have mixed presentation between exercise intolerance and fixed weakness.
- Nocturnal muscle cramps, cramps unrelated to exercise, continuous muscle cramps/pain, and generalized fatigue are not compatible with metabolic myopathies, and forearm exercise test is not indicated.
- In the past, the forearm exercise test was performed under ischemic conditions (known as the "ischemic forearm exercise test") by using a blood pressure cuff to inflate above systolic blood pressure.
  - However, this blood pressure cuff insufflation is generally not recommended or preferred due to high risk of rhabdomyolysis and compartment syndrome in patients with metabolic myopathies.
  - Thus the forearm exercise test should be performed without blood pressure cuff insufflation.
- The forearm exercise procedure
  - The antecubital vein is typically used for venous access.
  - The patient performs isometric exercise. The protocol may be different among different laboratories. One method is to repetitively squeeze a dynamometer with the force of 80% of maximal voluntary contraction (MVC) and 1-Hz frequency for 1 minute.
  - During the forearm exercise, if the patient develops muscle cramps or contracture, the test should be terminated.
  - Venous blood is collected at 0, 1, 3, 6, and 10 minutes post-exercise (0, 1, 4, 6, and 10 minutes in some labs).
  - Each blood sample is analyzed for ammonia and lactate, not triglyceride.

- Interpretation
  - Normal pattern
    - Normal increase in lactate levels: at least 4 times of the baseline level
    - Normal increase in ammonia levels: at least 3–5 times of the baseline level
  - Abnormal patterns (Table 18.8 and Fig. 18.17)
- Potential complications of the forearm exercise test
  - Rhabdomyolysis: muscle pain, cramps, myoglobinuria
  - Compartment syndrome

**TABLE 18.8** Interpretation of the forearm exercise test.

| Lactate rise | Ammonia rise | Interpretation |
|---|---|---|
| Normal | Normal | Normal or CPT II deficiency (a disorder of lipid metabolism) |
| No | Normal | Disorders of carbohydrate metabolism: <br>• Myophosphorylase deficiency <br>• Phosphofructokinase deficiency <br>• Glycogen debranching enzyme deficiency |
| Normal | No | Myoadenylate deaminase deficiency |
| No | No | Inadequate exercise during test |

Abbreviation: *CPT II*, carnitine palmitoyltransferase II.

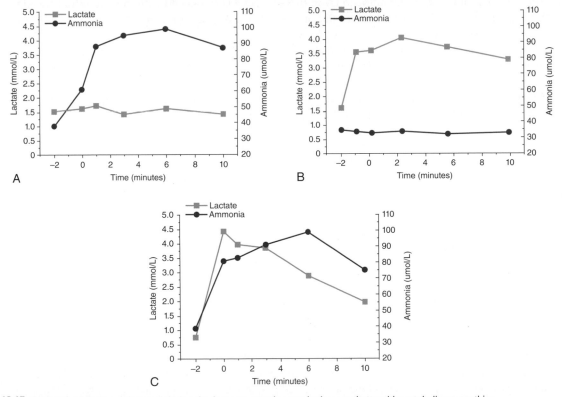

Fig. 18.17 Examples of patterns observed during the forearm exercise test in three patients with metabolic myopathies. (A) Myophosphorylase deficiency (McArdle disease). (B) Myoadenylate deaminase deficiency. (C) Carnitine palmitoyltransferase II deficiency. From Dulaney E, Katirji B. Forearm exercise testing. In: Katirji B, Kaminski H, Ruff R, eds. *Neuromusc Disord Clin Pract.* 2nd ed. New York, NY: Springer; 2014: 79–33.

**QUESTION 51.** A 22-year-old man comes for an evaluation of exercise-induced muscle cramps. Forearm exercise test shows no rise in venous lactate levels, but a six-fold rise in venous ammonia levels from baseline. Which of the following disorders is most compatible with this finding?
A. Acid maltase deficiency
B. Carnitine palmitoyltransferase II (CPT II) deficiency
C. Myoadenylate deaminase deficiency
D. Myophosphorylase deficiency
E. This result cannot be interpreted due to poor patient effort.

**ANSWER:** D. Myophosphorylase deficiency

**COMMENTS AND DISCUSSION (see also comments and discussion from Question 50, including Table 18.8 and Fig. 18.17):**

- No increase in lactate, but normal increase in ammonia levels on the forearm exercise test indicates disorders of carbohydrate metabolism or glycogen storage diseases (aka glycogenoses). However, it should be noted that not all glycogen storage diseases have necessarily exhibit this pattern.
    - Among the options, acid maltase deficiency (aka Pompe disease) and myophosphorylase deficiency (McArdle disease) are glycogenoses.
    - Myophosphorylase deficiency has this pattern, whereas acid maltase deficiency has a normal rise in lactate levels.
- Carnitine palmitoyltransferase II (CPT II) deficiency, a lipid storage disorder, results in a normal rise in lactate and ammonia levels.
- Myoadenylate deaminase deficiency results in a normal rise in lactate but no rise in ammonia levels.
- No increase in either lactate or ammonia indicates inadequate exercise and an uninterpretable result.

**QUESTION 52.** A 22-year-old man presents with recurrent episodes of muscle pain and cramps after intense running for about 5–10 minutes. He gets some relief of muscle pain and cramps after a few minutes of rest and then can continue his exercise. During some episodes his urine turns rusty in color. He feels normal at rest and denies weakness between these episodes. Serum creatine kinase level was 4552 U/L after one episode. What is the most likely diagnosis in this patient?
A. Acid maltase deficiency
B. Carnitine palmitoyltransferase II deficiency
C. Glycogen debranching enzyme deficiency
D. Myophosphorylase deficiency
E. Phosphofructokinase deficiency

**ANSWER:** D. Myophosphorylase deficiency

**COMMENTS AND DISCUSSION**
- The diagnosis in this patient is myophosphorylase deficiency (aka McArdle disease, glycogen storage disease type V [GSD V]).
- *Metabolic myopathies* can present with
    1. Exercise intolerance, exercise-induced muscle pain, or cramps. Examples include:
        - Myophosphorylase deficiency
        - Phosphofructokinase deficiency (aka Tarui disease, glycogen storage disease type VII [GSD VII])
        - Carnitine palmitoyltransferase II (CPT II) deficiency
    2. Fixed weakness. Weakness is persistent, and usually progressive over time. Examples include:
        - Acid maltase deficiency
        - Glycogen debranching enzyme deficiency (aka Cori-Forbes disease, glycogen storage disease type III [GSD III])
        - Glycogen branching enzyme deficiency (aka Andersen disease, glycogen storage disease type IV [GSD IV])
    - However, the presentation can be mixed in these disorders. For example, some patients with McArdle disease may have both exercise intolerance and fixed weakness, particularly in late adulthood.
    - Most of these disorders result from enzymatic defects and thus have autosomal recessive inheritance.
- *Myophosphorylase deficiency*
    - Clinical features
        - Typical onset in teenage to early adulthood
        - Exercise intolerance, exercised-induced muscle pain, or cramps
            - Symptoms mostly occur after brief intense exercise (anaerobic exercise), where glucose (converted from glycogen) is the main source of energy.
            - This is in contrast to disorders of lipid metabolism (e.g., CPT II deficiency) where exercise intolerance or exercise-induced muscle pain or cramps typically occur after prolonged low-intensity exercise, where blood-borne fatty acids are used as the main source of energy.

**HIGH-YIELD FACT**

Main source of energy during exercise
• Anaerobic glycolysis (the first few minutes) → aerobic glycolysis → fatty acid oxidation
Exercise intolerance, exercise-induced muscle pain or cramps after:
• **Brief intense** exercise – think about **glycogenoses** (e.g., myophosphorylase deficiency)
• **Prolonged low-intensity** exercise – think about **lipid storage myopathies** (e.g., CPT II deficiency)

- Second wind phenomenon is one of the key features of myophophorylase deficiency and not usually seen wth phosphofructokinase deficiency.
  - Characterized by improvement of symptoms (e.g., exercise intolerance, muscle pain or cramps) and improved exercise tolerance after:
    - Continuation of exercise at the same or reduced (moderate) intensity for ~10 minutes
    - A brief rest, which allows the patient to resume exercise
  - Second wind phenomenon can be evaluated by performing a cycle ergometry test or a walking test.
    - Decrease in heart rate and improvement of symptoms (muscle pain or cramps) after exercise at moderate constant workload for 10 minutes
  - Mechanism of second wind phenomenon: switching from muscle glycogen to alternative fuel sources such as free fatty acids, glucose, and amino acids.

**HIGH-YIELD FACT**

**Second wind phenomenon** is a key feature of **myophosphorylase deficiency**. It is characterized by improvement of symptoms (e.g., exercise intolerance and muscle pain) and a dramatic fall in heart rate after continuation of exercise for 10 minutes.

- Rhabdomyolysis and myoglobinuria can occur.
- Muscle contracture which is electrically silent on needle electromyography
- Fixed weakness: persistent progressive proximal muscle weakness in about one-fourth of patients
  - Laboratory features
    - Serum creatine kinase levels are usually high, greater than 1000 U/L after episodes.
    - Cycle ergometry or walking test: second wind phenomenon can be demonstrated as improvement of symptoms (e.g., exercise intolerance and muscle pain) and decreased heart rate after continuous exercise at a moderate constant workload for 10 minutes.
    - Forearm exercise test: no rise in lactate, but normal rise in ammonia levels
    - EMG: typically normal, except in muscle contracture, which is electrically silent
    - Muscle biopsy
      - Accumulation of glycogen vacuoles within muscle fibers seen on periodic acid–Schiff (PAS) stain. These glycogen vacuoles can be digested by diastase.
      - Absent or markedly reduced myophosphorylase staining
    - Genetic testing: mutations in the *PYGM* gene encoding myophosphorylase
  - Treatment and prevention
    - Avoid intense isometric and maximal aerobic exercise.
    - Promote second wind phenomenon by performing moderate-intensity exercise
    - Oral sucrose load before exercise. Oral sucrose can improve exercise tolerance by providing a consistent supply of glucose to the working muscles, despite the blockage in glycogen breakdown. Note that the myophosphorylase enzyme is upstream to the glucose breakdown in the metabolic pathway. However, the effects of sucrose load are short lasting.

**QUESTION 53.**    Which of the following features is **LEAST** likely to be seen in phosphofructokinase deficiency?
A. Exercise intolerance
B. Hemolytic anemia
C. Myoglobinuria
D. Second wind phenomenon
E. Worsening of symptoms after glucose administration

**ANSWER:** D. Second wind phenomenon

**TABLE 18.9** Comparison between myophosphorylase deficiency and phosphofructokinase deficiency.

|  | Myophosphorylase deficiency | Phosphofructokinase deficiency |
|---|---|---|
| Prevalence | More common | Rare |
| Involvement | Muscle only | Muscle and red blood cells (hemolytic anemia) |
| Myoglobinuria | More common | Less common |
| Second wind phenomenon | Yes | No |
| After glucose load | Improvement of symptoms (e.g., exercise intolerance and muscle pain) | Worsening of symptoms (out-of-wind phenomenon) |
| Diastase sensitivity of PAS-positive material | Sensitive | Resistant or partially sensitive, since they also contain polyglucosan body, in addition to glycogen |

Abbreviation: *PAS*, periodic acid–Schiff.

## COMMENTS AND DISCUSSION

- *Phosphofructokinase (PFK) deficiency* (aka Tarui disease, glycogen storage disease type VII [GSD VII])
  - Clinical features are similar to those of myophosphorylase deficiency: exercise intolerance, exercise-induced muscle pain or cramps; rhabdomyolysis is usually less than in myophosphorylase deficiency.
  - Features that are useful to distinguish PFK deficiency from myophosphorylase deficiency (Table 18.9)
    - Hemolytic anemia: increased reticulocyte count, hyperuricemia, and hyperbilirubinemia, since the PFK enzyme is also important for glycolysis within red blood cells
    - Worsening of symptoms after glucose loading is called "out-of-wind phenomenon." This is in contrast to the improvement of symptoms seen after glucose or sucrose loading in myophosphorylase deficiency.
      - The PFK enzyme is located downstream in the glycolytic pathway, compared to myophosphorylase. When this enzyme is deficient, glucose cannot be metabolized within muscle cells.
      - Increased blood glucose reduces other sources of energy including free fatty acids and ketones.
  - There are different forms of PFK deficiency:
    - Classic form has onset in childhood.
    - Late-onset form has milder symptoms.
    - Infantile form is typically severe and can also involve cardiomyopathy.
    - Hemolytic form has only predominantly hematologic involvement with no or minimal muscle involvement.
  - Laboratory features of PFK deficiency
    - Serum creatine kinase (CK): elevated
    - Forearm exercise test: no rise in lactate, but normal rise in ammonia levels
    - EMG: typically normal
    - Muscle biopsy
      - Vacuoles within muscle fibers, which are positive for periodic acid–Schiff (PAS) stain. These vacuoles are resistant or only partially sensitive to diastase, since they also contain polyglucosan bodies in addition to glycogen.
      - Absent or markedly reduced phosphofructokinase staining
    - Genetic testing: mutations in the *PFKM* gene encoding phosphofructokinase

**QUESTION 54.** Which of the following statements is **CORRECT** regarding lipid storage myopathies.
  A. Absence of lipid vacuoles on muscle biopsy excludes lipid storage myopathies
  B. Carnitine palmitoyltransferase II (CPT II) deficiency typically presents with fixed weakness.
  C. Primary carnitine deficiency rarely presents with encephalopathy.
  D. Multiple acyl-CoA dehydrogenase deficiency (MADD) has second wind phenomenon.
  E. MADD is a riboflavin-responsive disorder.

**ANSWER:** E. MADD is a riboflavin-responsive disorder.

### COMMENTS AND DISCUSSION

- *Lipid storage myopathies* include various disorders of lipid metabolism that affect muscles. Examples include
  - Carnitine palmitoyltransferase II (CPT II) deficiency
  - Primary carnitine deficiency
  - Multiple acyl-CoA dehydrogenase deficiency (MADD)
  - Neutral lipid storage disease
  - Very long-chain acyl-CoA dehydrogenase deficiency (VLCAD), long-chain acyl-CoA dehydrogenase deficiency (LCAD), medium-chain acyl-CoA dehydrogenase deficiency (MCAD)
- General principles
  - Many of these disorders present with exercise intolerance and recurrent myoglobinuria (e.g., CPT II deficiency), and some can present with fixed weakness (e.g., MADD).
  - Serum creatine kinase levels between exacerbations are usually normal (e.g., in CPT II deficiency, except in conditions of intense physical activity or fasting) or mildly elevated (e.g., in MADD).
  - Forearm exercise test: normal rise in lactate and ammonia levels
  - Plasma acylcarnitine profile is useful in the diagnosis of lipid storage myopathies. For example, in
    - MADD, there is elevation of various acylcarnitines from C4 to C18
    - VLCAD, there is elevation of C14, C12
  - Muscle biopsy
    - Lipid accumulation on Oil Red O stain. However, absence of accumulation of lipid droplets does not exclude lipid storage myopathies. For example, lipid accumulation on muscle biopsy may not be seen in several patients with CPT II, and other tests (e.g., genetic testing) are required.
  - Genetic testing

### ◎ HIGH-YIELD FACT

> Recurrent myoglobinuria especially after exercise is a common presentation of lipid storage myopathies.

- Important facts about selected lipid storage myopathies
  - Carnitine palmitoyltransferase II (CPT II) deficiency
    - CPT II is a part of the carnitine shuttle, and has a role in transport of long-chain fatty acids from the cytosol to the mitochondrial matrix for further fatty acid oxidation. CPT II is located at the inner mitochondrial membrane.
    - Patients typically present with recurrent myoglobinuria after prolonged or intense exercise. Fasting can be a precipitating factor. The onset varies from the first to the sixth decade.
    - In addition, there are severe infantile and late neonatal forms in which patients have hypoketotic hypoglycemia, cardiomyopathy, and seizures.
    - Serum creatine kinase levels are typically normal between attacks, but can be elevataed during intense physical activities or fasting.
  - Primary carnitine deficiency
    - Long-chain fatty acids cannot be transported from the cytosol to the mitochondrial matrix.
    - Patients often present with Reye-like syndrome: acute metabolic encephalopathy and hepatopathy. Cardiomyopathy can be present.
    - Treatment: oral L-carnitine
  - Multiple acyl-CoA dehydrogenase deficiency (MADD)
    - Due to mutations in the *EFTA*, *EFTB*, and *ETFDH* genes encoding electron transfer flavoprotein A, electron transfer flavoprotein B, and electron transfer flavoprotein dehydrogenase (aka ETF-ubiquinone [coenzyme Q] oxidoreductase)
    - These electron transfer flavoproteins accept electrons from all acyl-CoA dehydrogenases. Thus deficiency of these flavoproteins results in a secondary deficiency of multiple acyl-CoA dehydrogenases.
    - Plasma acylcarnitine profile shows elevation of all acylcarnitines including short-chain, medium-chain, long-chain, and very long-chain acylcarnitines.
    - Patients can present with recurrent myoglobinuria induced by exercise or fixed weakness.
    - This is a riboflavin-responsive lipid storage myopathy.
    - Second wind phenomenon is seen in myophosphorylase deficiency, not in MADD.

## ◎ HIGH-YIELD FACT

**Riboflavin-responsive neuromuscular disorders**
- Motor neuron diseases with bulbar and respiratory weakness
  - **Brown-Vialetto-Van Laere syndrome (BVVL)**: with sensorineural hearing loss
  - **Fazio-Londe syndrome**: no hearing loss
- Lipid storage myopathy
  - **Multiple acyl-CoA dehydrogenase deficiency (MADD)**

- ○ Neutral lipid storage diseases
  - Due to impaired degradation of cytoplasmic triglycerides (TGs) resulting in accumulation of TGs in various tissues
  - Two main forms
    - Neutral lipid storage disease with myopathy (NLSD-M)
    - Neutral lipid storage disease with ichthyosis (NLSD-I), also called Chanarin-Dorfman syndrome
  - Jordan anomaly, which is the accumulation of lipid vacuoles within the cytoplasm of granulocytes, can be seen in both forms of neutral lipid storage diseases (Fig. 18.18).

**QUESTION 55.** A 4-month-old infant presents with generalized hypotonia and weakness. He also has feeding difficulty, respiratory failure, and hypertrophic cardiomyopathy. An enlarged tongue is noted on physical examination. Serum creatine kinase is 1210 U/L. Muscle biopsy shows extensive large vacuoles within muscle fibers, which demonstrate positive periodic acid–Schiff staining with sensitivity to diastase and positive acid phosphatase staining. What is the most likely deficient enzyme in this patient?
A. Alpha-glucosidase
B. Alpha-galactosidase
C. Glycogen debranching enzyme
D. Myophosphorylase
E. Phosphofructokinase

**ANSWER:** A. Alpha-glucosidase

## COMMENTS AND DISCUSSION
- The most likely diagnosis in this patient is *infantile-onset Pompe disease*.
- Pompe disease (aka acid maltase deficiency, alpha-glucosidase deficiency, glycogen storage disease type II [GSD II])
- Pompe disease is a glycogen storage disease that is also a lysosomal storage disease.
- Pompe disease has variable age at onset and phenotypic variability. The phenotypes are typically more severe in the infantile-onset form.
  - ○ *Infantile-onset Pompe disease*
    - Onset before 12 months of age
    - Generalized hypotonia and muscle weakness
    - Feeding difficulty and respiratory distress

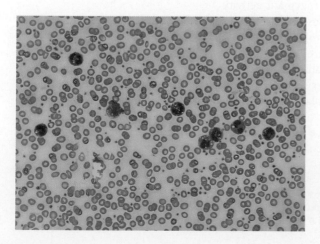

**Fig. 18.18** Jordan anomaly. This blood smear shows lipid vacuoles within the cytoplasm of granulocytes, known as Jordan anomaly. This finding can be seen in neutral lipid storage diseases, including neutral lipid storage disease with ichthyosis (Chanarin-Dorfman disease), which is the underlying diagnosis in this patient. From Paulo Henrique Orlandi Mourao (author). Wikipedia. Creative Commons License CC BY-SA 3.0.

- Cardiac involvement is an important feature in infantile-onset Pompe disease, which can include hypertrophic cardiomyopathy, cardiomegaly, left ventricular hypertrophy, short PR interval, and wide QRS complex on electrocardiography.
- Macroglossia (enlarged tongue)
- Hepatomegaly
- Hearing loss

## MNEMONICS

Glycogen storage disease (GSD) with muscle involvement
- **Pompe (GSD II)** – **Pumping** – Heart involvement (predominant feature)
- **McArdle (GSD V)** – **Muscle** – Muscle involvement (predominant feature)
- Other GSDs
  - o Cori-Forbes disease (GSD III)
  - o Andersen disease (GSD IV)
  - o Tarui disease (GSD VII)

- o *Late-onset Pompe disease*
  - Variable age at onset
  - No cardiomyopathy
  - Proximal muscle weakness: Gowers sign can be positive. Some patients have scapuloperoneal weakness and winged scapula.
  - Respiratory muscle weakness, dyspnea on exertion, orthopnea and respiratory failure. These symptoms may be dominant and overshadow the muscular weakness in limbs.
  - Macroglossia

## ◎ HIGH-YIELD FACT

Keep late-onset Pompe disease in the differential diagnosis in adults with respiratory failure and neuromuscular weakness.

- Laboratory features in Pompe disease
  - o Serum creatine kinase: elevated
  - o Cardiac involvement can be detected on electrocardiography and echocardiography.
  - o Muscle MRI: fatty replacement in the paraspinal muscles can be an early finding.
  - o Electromyography: myopathic findings (small short-duration polyphasic motor unit action potentials with early recruitment). Myotonic discharges in paraspinal muscles can be seen, especially in late-onset Pompe disease.
  - o Muscle biopsy
    - Glycogen vacuoles in muscle fibers: positive periodic acid–Schiff (PAS) stain, and sensitive to diastase. The vacuoles are prominent in the infantile-onset form.
    - In addition, these vacuoles are also positive for acid phosphatase staining, indicating accumulation of abnormal lysosomes. Pompe disease is also considered as a lysosomal storage disease.
  - o Biochemical testing of alpha-glucosidase (GAA) enzymatic activity
    - Enzymatic activity correlates with the age at onset and severity of the disease.
      - Complete deficiency (<1% of normal control): infantile-onset Pompe disease
      - Partial deficiency (2%–40% of normal control): late-onset Pompe disease
    - Dried blood spot (DBS) test. This is also available for newborn screening in the United States.
    - GAA activities can be tested in different tissues such as isolated lymphocytes, mixed leukocytes, and muscle. The testing of cultured skin fibroblasts is generally considered a gold standard.
  - o Genetic testing of the *GAA* gene
- It is important to diagnose Pompe disease early, since there are enzyme replacement therapies (ERTs) available for treatment. (see also comments and discussion from Question 57.)

## ◎ HIGH-YIELD FACT

**Paraspinal muscles** can be involved early in Pompe disease.
**Myotonic discharges in the paraspinal muscles** are a useful electrodiagnostic finding, especially in late-onset Pompe disease.

- Alpha-galactosidase deficiency is associated with Fabry disease. Fabry disease can present with small fiber neuropathy, renal involvement, skin involvement (angiokeratoma). and stroke in the young.
- In addition to Pompe disease, glycogen debranching enzyme deficiency, myophosphorylase deficiency, and phosphofructokinase deficiency are also glycogen storage diseases (types III, V, and VII, respectively). However, cardiomyopathy is highly suggestive of Pompe disease, rather than these disorders. While the accumulation of glycogen vacuoles with positive PAS staining can be seen in all of these disorders, only Pompe disease exhibits positive acid phosphatase staining.

### MNEMONICS

- **Pompe disease** – alpha-**gluco**sidase deficiency – glucose → think about glycogen storage disease
- **Fabry disease** – alpha-**galacto**sidase deficiency – not glucose; galactose is another simple sugar

**QUESTION 56.** A 51-year-old man has mild proximal muscle weakness for 3 years with shortness of breath, especially on exertion. He is admitted because of acute respiratory failure requiring endotracheal intubation. Electromyography shows small polyphasic motor unit action potentials with early recruitment in the proximal muscles. Myotonic discharges are detected in paraspinal muscles. Which of the following is most likely to be encountered in this patient?
A. CTG repeat expansion in the *DMPK* gene
B. Degeneration of anterior horn cells and corticospinal tracts
C. Deficiency of acid maltase enzyme
D. Mutation in the *DYSF* gene
E. Mutation in the *DOK7* gene

**ANSWER:** C. Deficiency of acid maltase enzyme

### COMMENTS AND DISCUSSION (see also comments and discussion from Question 55):
- This patient has late-onset Pompe disease (adult-onset acid maltase deficiency).
- Late-onset Pompe disease should be kept in the differential diagnosis of respiratory failure associated with neuromuscular weakness in adults.
- Myotonic discharges in paraspinal muscles are also suggestive of late-onset Pompe disease.
- Pompe disease is due to deficiency of the alpha-glucosidase (aka acid maltase) enzyme.
- CTG repeat expansion in the *DMPK* gene is associated with myotonic dystrophy type 1 (DM1). Myotonic discharges are a characteristic electrodiagnostic finding of DM1, but are typically seen in distal muscles rather than paraspinal muscles.
- Degeneration of anterior horn cells and corticospinal tracts is associated with amyotrophic lateral sclerosis. Myopathic findings and myotonic discharges in paraspinal muscles on needle electromyography are not expected in this disorder.
- Mutation in the *DYSF* gene is associated with dysferlinopathies, which can present with limb-girdle muscular dystrophy or Miyoshi distal myopathy. Mutation in the *DOK7* gene is associated with congenital myasthenic syndrome, which typically presents with a limb-girdle weakness phenotype. The clinical and electrodiagnostic features in this patient are not compatible with these two disorders.

**QUESTION 57.** Which of the following statements is **CORRECT** regarding alglucosidase alfa, an enzyme replacement therapy (ERT) in Pompe disease?
A. It has no benefit in the late-onset form.
B. It does not improve cardiac muscle function.
C. It provides symptomatic benefit without altering the natural history of the disease.
D. It has no impact on survival outcome.
E. It should be initiated as early as possible.

**ANSWER:** E. It should be initiated as early as possible.

### COMMENTS AND DISCUSSION
- The early diagnosis of Pompe disease is crucial, since it is treatable with enzyme replacement therapy (ERT).

- ERT for Pompe disease involves replacement of the deficient alpha-glucosidase (GAA) enzyme using two different main approaches:
  - Alglucosidase alfa
    - A recombinant human GAA (rhGAA) is a GAA analog. It is administered by intravenous infusion every 2 weeks.
    - Two different brands are available: Myozyme® and Lumizyme®.
    - Approval by the US Food and Drug Administration (FDA)
      - Myozyme® in 2006 for infantile-onset Pompe disease
      - Lumizyme® in 2010 for late-onset Pompe disease in patients aged 8 years and older. However, age restriction was removed in 2014.
    - Alglucosidase alfa should be started as early as possible, once the diagnosis is confirmed.

◎ **HIGH-YIELD FACT**

> Enzyme replacement therapy (ERT) for Pompe disease should be started as early as possible, once the diagnosis is confirmed.

- Studies have shown that alglucosidase alfa:
  - Improves ventilator-free survival in infantile-onset Pompe disease
  - Improves the mortality rate
  - Reduces decline in motor function
  - Reduces decline in respiratory function (measured as forced vital capacity [FVC] percent-predicted)
  - Reduces cardiac mass (in infantile-onset Pompe disease)
  - Changes the natural history of the disease
  - In late-onset Pompe disease, alglucosidase alfa stabilizes and reduces decline in motor and respiratory functions.
- Side effects
  - Infusion reactions
  - Development of antibodies: IgG more common than IgE
  - Avalglucosidase alfa
    - Increases glycogen clearance by targeting at the mannose-6-phosphate (M6P) receptor
    - Avalglucosidase alfa (Nexviazyme®) was approved by the US FDA in 2021 for late-onset Pompe disease in patients aged 1 year and older, based on a phase 3, randomized trial (COMET trial).
    - The COMET trial showed that avalglucosidase alfa led to greater improvements in FVC percent-predicted (the primary outcome), and 6-minute walk test (the secondary outcome), compared to the control group.

**QUESTION 58.** A 17-year-old woman presents with proximal muscle weakness. He has a hypertrophic cardiomyopathy and Wolff-Parkinson-White syndrome. Examination shows mild (grade 4) symmetrical weakness of the proximal muscles in the upper and lower extremities. Muscle biopsy demonstrates periodic acid–Schiff (PAS)-positive and acid phosphatase–positive vacuoles within muscle fibers. Biochemical testing shows normal alpha-glucosidase activity, and genetic testing shows no mutation in the *GAA* gene. Deficiency of which of the following proteins is most likely responsible for the disorder in this patient?
A. Alpha-galactosidase
B. Glycogen debranching enzyme
C. Lysosome-associated membrane protein 2
D. Myophosphorylase
E. Titin

**ANSWER:** C. Lysosome-associated membrane protein 2

**COMMENTS AND DISCUSSION**
- The diagnosis in this patient is *Danon disease*.
- Danon disease may present with similar clinical features to Pompe disease and should be considered in patients who have a Pompe-like clinical presentation but negative biochemical and genetic testing for Pompe disease.

**HIGH-YIELD FACT**

> Danon disease should be considered when a patient has a Pompe-like clinical presentation but negative testing for Pompe disease.

- Danon disease (aka X-linked vacuolar cardiomyopathy and myopathy, lysosomal glycogen storage disease without acid maltase deficiency)
  - Inherited as X-linked dominant: both males and females can be affected, but males have more severe phenotypes.
  - Caused by mutations in the *LAMP2* gene encoding lysosome-associated membrane protein 2, which plays an important role in autophagy, specifically fusion of lysosomes and autophagosomes
  - Clinical features
    - Cardiac involvement: prominent, including hypertrophic cardiomyopathy (rapidly progressive in affected males) and Wolff-Parkinson-White syndrome
    - Skeletal muscle involvement: progressive proximal muscle weakness, elevated serum creatine kinase levels
    - Retinal involvement: cone-rod dystrophy
    - Intellectual disability: this feature can be useful to distinguish Danon disease from Pompe disease. It is very rare in Pompe disease.
  - Muscle biopsy findings in Danon disease can resemble those seen Pompe disease:
    - Periodic acid–Schiff (PAS)–positive vacuoles within muscle fibers
    - These vacuoles are also positive for acid phosphatase stain, indicating abnormal accumulation of lysosomes.
- Alpha-galactosidase deficiency is associated with Fabry disease.
- Glycogen debranching enzyme deficiency is found in Cori-Forbes disease or glycogen storage disease type III.
- Myophosphorylase deficiency is associated with McArdle disease or glycogen storage disease type V.
- Titin mutations are associated with limb-girdle muscular dystrophy and cardiomyopathy. However, cardiac involvement in titinopathy is typically dilated cardiomyopathy.
- Fabry disease, Cori-Forbes disease, McArdle disease, and titinopathies are not lysosomal storage diseases; therefore, abnormal accumulation of lysosomes is not expected on muscle biopsy.

**QUESTION 59.** A 24-year-old man presents with slowly progressive weakness, affecting mainly his hands and feet, for over a decade. He also has a history of cardiomyopathy. Examination reveals hepatomegaly, as well as prominent atrophy and grade 3–4 weakness of muscles in the distal upper and lower extremities. The clinician suspects motor neuron disease. Needle electromyography (EMG) reveals small polyphasic short-duration motor unit action potentials with early recruitment. Muscle biopsy reveals periodic acid–Schiff (PAS)–positive, acid phosphatase–negative vacuoles within muscle fibers, which are sensitive to diastase. This patient most likely has a deficiency in which of the following enzymes?
A. Acid maltase
B. Carnitine palmitoyltransferase II
C. Glycogen debranching enzyme
D. Myophosphorylase
E. Phosphofructokinase

**ANSWER:** C. Glycogen debranching enzyme

**COMMENTS AND DISCUSSION**
- The diagnosis in this patient is *glycogen debranching enzyme deficiency* (aka Cori-Forbes disease, glycogen storage disease type III [GSD III])
- Needle EMG in this patient shows myopathic units. Muscle biopsy reveals evidence of glycogen vacuoles within muscle fibers. Among glycogen storage diseases, the one with distal muscle involvement, cardiomyopathy, and hepatomegaly is glycogen debranching enzyme deficiency.
- Glycogen in debranching enzyme deficiency can be digested by diastase. This is in contrast to branching enzyme deficiency, which is resistant to diastase.
- Glycogen debranching enzyme deficiency
  - Mutations in the *AGL* gene resulting in deficiency of the glycogen debranching (aka debrancher) enzyme

o  Clinical features
  • Skeletal muscle involvement
    • Fixed weakness: slowly progressive; distal muscle or generalized involvement
    • Prominent distal muscle weakness and atrophy can be mistaken for motor neuron disease or peripheral neuropathy.
    • Some patients can have exercise intolerance.
    • GSD IIIa has skeletal muscle and hepatic involvement. This type is more common than GSD IIIb, which has only hepatic involvement.

## MNEMONICS

Glycogen storage myopathy with **Distal** muscle involvement – think about **Debranching** enzyme deficiency (GSD III)

  • Hepatic involvement
    • Hepatomegaly, elevated transaminase enzymes, fasting ketotic hypoglycemia, cirrhosis
  • Cardiac involvement: hypertrophic obstructive cardiomyopathy, left ventricular hypertrophy
o  Laboratory features
  • Serum creatine kinase: elevated
  • Forearm exercise test: no increase in lactate, but normal increase in ammonia levels
  • Electromyography: myopathic findings
  • Muscle biopsy
    • Accumulation of glycogen vacuoles within muscle fibers, which is positive for periodic acid–Schiff stain
    • These vacuoles are sensitive to diastase, since they contain glycogen. This is in contrast to vacuoles in glycogen branching enzyme deficiency (Andersen disease or glycogen storage disease type IV [GSD IV]), which are resistant to diastase digestion, since they contain abnormally branched glycogen or polyglucosan body.
    • Of note, polyglucosan bodies that are diastase resistant are present in
      o  Glycogen branching enzyme deficiency (GSD IV)
      o  Phosphofructokinase deficiency (GSD VII)
      o  Adult polyglucosan body disease (which is also caused by glycogen branching enzyme deficiency)
  • Genetic testing for mutations in the *AGL* gene

## ◎ HIGH-YIELD FACT

PAS-positive materials that contain only glycogen are typically digestible with diastase (diastase sensitive). However, if they contain polyglucosan bodies, they are diastase resistant.
Diastase-**resistant** PAS-positive materials are seen in
  • Glycogen branching enzyme deficiency (GSD IV)
  • Phosphofructokinase deficiency (GSD VII)
Diastase-**sensitive** PAS-positive materials are seen in
  • Pompe disease (GSD II)
  • Glycogen debranching enzyme deficiency (GSD III)
  • McArdle disease (GSD V)

**QUESTION 60.** A 9-year-old boy presents with stiffness of his legs when walking for 2 years. After walking or running for a while, he feels better. Stiffness is worse with cold temperature. Examination reveals no muscle weakness. There is grip myotonia of both hands, which improves after repetitive hand opening and closing. Needle electromyography (EMG) shows myotonia in several proximal and distal muscles. The disorder in this patient is most likely caused by an abnormality in which of the following channels?
A. Sodium channel
B. Potassium channel
C. Calcium channel
D. Chloride channel
E. Either sodium or chloride channel

**ANSWER:** D. Chloride channel

## COMMENTS AND DISCUSSION

- The most likely diagnosis in this patient is *myotonia congenita*.
- This patient has myotonia without fixed weakness (non-dystrophic myotonia). Myotonia or muscle stiffness is aggravated by exercise or cold temperature. There is also a warm-up phenomenon. These features are compatible with myotonia congenita.
- Myotonic disorders are classified into two main groups:
  - *Dystrophic myotonia:* weakness is present. (see also comments and discussion from Question 31.)
    - Myotonic dystrophy type 1 (DM1)
    - Myotonic dystrophy type 2 (DM2), previously known as proximal myotonic myopathy (PROMM)
  - *Non-dystrophic myotonia:* generally there is no or rare fixed weakness but episodic weakness can be present. Patients present with muscle stiffness with or without pain. Disorders in this group are also channelopathies (Fig. 18.19 and Table 18.10).
    - Chloride channelopathies due to *CLCN1* mutations
      - Myotonia congenita (MC)
        - Autosomal dominant (AD) form: Thomsen disease
        - Autosomal recessive (AR) form: Becker disease

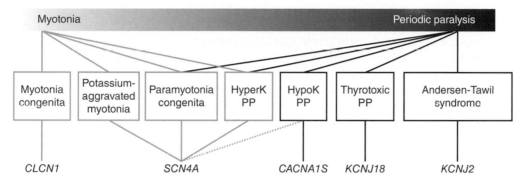

**Fig. 18.19** The spectrum of skeletal muscle channelopathies. Disorders with myotonia along with associated genes are shown on the left; those with periodic paralysis are on the right; those with mixed features between myotonia and periodic paralysis are in the middle. Hypokalemic periodic paralysis is caused by mutations in the *CACNA1S* gene in approximately 80% of patients, and the *SCN4A* gene in 20% (*dashed line*). Note that potassium-aggravated myotonia is also known as sodium channel myotonia. *HypoK PP*, Hypokalemic periodic paralysis; *HyperK PP*, Hyperkalemic periodic paralysis; *Thyrotoxic PP*, thyrotoxic periodic paralysis. Adapted from Cannon SC. Channelopathies of skeletal muscle excitability. *Compr Physiol.* 2015;5(2):761–790.

**TABLE 18.10** Summary of muscle channelopathies. Muscle channelopathies and their associated channels and clinical features, including myotonia and periodic paralysis, are shown in the table.

| Chloride channel | Sodium channel | Calcium channel | Potassium channel | Myotonia | Periodic paralysis |
|---|---|---|---|---|---|
| Myotonia congenita | | | | + | +/−* |
| | Paramyotonia congenita | | | + | + |
| | Potassium-aggravated myotonia | | | + | − |
| | Hyperkalemic periodic paralysis | | | + | + |
| | Hypokalemic periodic paralysis type 1 | | | − | + |
| | | Hypokalemic periodic paralysis type 2 | | − | + |
| | | | Andersen-Tawil syndrome | − | + |

*Present in some patients with Becker disease (an autosomal recessive form of myotonia congenita).

- Sodium channelopathies due to *SCN4A* mutations
  - Paramyotonia congenita (PMC)
  - Potassium-aggravated myotonia (PAM, aka sodium channel myotonia)
  - Hyperkalemic periodic paralysis (HyperPP)
  - Hypokalemic periodic paralysis type 2 (HypoPP2) is a sodium channelopathy due to *SCN4A* mutations, but there is *no associated myotonia*. Hence, it is *not* classified as non-dystrophic myotonia.

**MNEMONIC**

There is myotonia in hyperkalemic periodic paralysis.
However, there is **NO** myotonia in hy**PO**kalemic periodic paralysis.

- There is significant overlap between myotonic disorders, channelopathies, and periodic paralysis syndromes (Fig. 18.19 and Table 18.10).
  - Periodic paralysis syndromes *without* myotonia
    - Hypokalemic periodic paralysis (HypoPP)
      - Hypokalemic periodic paralysis type 1 (HypoPP1)
        - Constitutes about 80% of all HypoPP cases
        - Calcium channelopathy due to *CACNA1S* mutations
      - Hypokalemic periodic paralysis type 2 (HypoPP2)
        - Constitutes about 20% of all HypoPP cases
        - Sodium channelopathy due to *SCN4A* mutations
    - Andersen-Tawil syndrome
      - Potassium channelopathy due to *KCNJ2* mutations
- All non-dystrophic myotonia and periodic paralysis syndromes are autosomal dominant (AD) *except* Becker disease, which is autosomal recessive (AR).

**MNEMONICS**

Hy**PER**kalemic periodic paralysis – Sodium channel
Hy**PO**kalemic periodic paralysis – Calcium channel (in the majority)
**PO** has 2 letters. Calcium is in group 2 of the periodic table, and calcium ion has a 2+ charge: $Ca^{2+}$

- Myotonia congenita
  - Thomsen (AD form) and Becker (AR form) diseases may be differentiated by family history. In addition, Thomsen disease generally has an earlier onset, in infancy or early childhood, while Becker disease has a later onset in childhood.
  - Painless myotonia leading to muscle stiffness
    - Myotonia can involve limb muscles as well as facial muscles including the orbicularis oculi and tongue.
    - Legs are typically more affected than arms in Becker disease, and the opposite occurs in Thomsen disease.
  - Muscle hypertrophy ("Hercules-like" appearance) due to continuous muscle contraction
  - Myotonia is typically:
    - Worse after rest or with cold
    - Improves after exercise, known as the "warm-up phenomenon." This is in contrast to "paradoxical myotonia" in paramyotonia congenita. (see also comments and discussion for Question 61.)
  - Episodic weakness can occur in Becker disease. Although non-dystrophic myotonia typically does not cause fixed weakness, mild fixed proximal or distal weakness may occasionally be present in Becker disease. (n.b., Becker disease and Becker muscular dystrophy are completely separate disorders.)

**◎ HIGH-YIELD FACT**

In myotonia congenita, there is a warm-up phenomenon.
In **para**myotonia congenita, there is **para**doxical myotonia.

**QUESTION 61.** Which of the following features is seen in paramyotonia congenita, but **NOT** in myotonia congenita?
A. Episodic weakness
B. Eyelid myotonia
C. Myotonia provoked by cold
D. Myotonia provoked by exercise
E. Warm-up phenomenon

**ANSWER:** D. Myotonia provoked by exercise

**COMMENTS AND DISCUSSION (see also comments and discussion from Question 60)**
- Both myotonia congenita (MC) and paramyotonia congenita (PMC) are non-dystrophic myotonias.
- Several features distinguish MC from PMC (Table 18.11).
- One important clinical feature to distinguish between MC and PMC is whether myotonia and stiffness are improved or worse after repetitive contraction/exercise.
  - In MC, there is "*warm-up phenomenon*": *improvement* of myotonia and stiffness after repetitive contraction/exercise.
  - In PMC, there is "*paradoxical myotonia*": *worsening* of myotonia and stiffness after repetitive contraction/exercise.
- Eyelid myotonia can be seen in both PMC and MC, but may be more common in PMC. Myotonia in PMC involves predominantly the facial muscles, including the orbicularis oculi, and hands. MC often has generalized distribution of myotonia, and eyelids can also be involved.
  - In MC, after repeated contraction of the orbicularis oculi, there is improvement of myotonia (warm-up phenomenon).
  - In PMC, after repeated contraction of the orbicularis oculi, there is worsening of myotonia (paradoxical myotonia).

**TABLE 18.11** Comparison of myotonia congenita and paramyotonia congenita.

|  | **Myotonia congenita** | **Paramyotonia congenita** |
|---|---|---|
| Abnormal channel | Chloride | Sodium |
| Gene | *CLCN1* | *SCN4A* |
| Distribution of myotonia | Generalized, face (including orbicularis oculi), tongue | Face (including orbicularis oculi), tongue, hands |
| Myotonia after repetitive contraction | Improved (warm-up phenomenon) | Worse (paradoxical myotonia) |
| Trigger | Cold, rest | Cold, exercise |
| Relieving factor | Exercise | Warming |
| Episodic weakness | Can be present in AR form (Becker disease) | Present |
| Fixed (progressive weakness) | Rare in AR form (Becker disease) | No |

Abbreviation: *AR*, autosomal recessive.

**QUESTION 62.** Which of the following disorders is **NOT** associated with sodium channelopathies?
A. Episodic ataxia type 1
B. Familial erythromelalgia
C. Hypokalemic periodic paralysis
D. Hyperkalemic periodic paralysis
E. Potassium-aggravated myotonia

**ANSWER:** A. Episodic ataxia type 1

**COMMENTS AND DISCUSSION**
- *Sodium channelopathies* comprise a variety of neurological disorders. Examples include:
  - Disorders associated with *SCN4A* mutations
    - Paramyotonia congenita (PMC)

- Potassium-aggravated myotonia (PAM)
  - Myotonia fluctuans
  - Myotonia permanens
  - Acetazolamide-responsive myotonia
- Hyperkalemic periodic paralysis (HyperPP)
- Hypokalemic periodic paralysis type 2 (HypoPP2)
    ◦ Disorders associated with *SCN9A* mutations
      - Familial erythromelalgia
    ◦ Disorders associated with *SCN1A* mutations
      - Familial hemiplegic migraine type 3
      - Dravet syndrome (aka severe myoclonic epilepsy in infancy)
- PMC, PAM, and HyperPP are also disorders with non-dystrophic myotonia. HyperPP and HypoPP2 are also periodic paralysis syndromes (Fig. 18.19).
- There is *no* myotonia in HypoPP.
- To prevent attacks in HyperPP and HypoPP
  ◦ Diuretics
    - HyperPP: thiazide
    - HypoPP: potassium-sparing diuretics (e.g., spironolactone, triamterene)
  ◦ Carbonic anhydrase inhibitors
    - Can be used in both HyperPP and HypoPP
    - Acetazolamide or dichlorphenamide
- Episodic ataxia
  ◦ Episodic ataxia type 1 (EA1) is a potassium channelopathy due to mutations in the *KCNA1* gene.
  ◦ Episodic ataxia type 2 (EA2) is a calcium channelopathy due to mutations in the *CACNA1A* gene, which is allelic to spinocerebellar ataxia type 6 (SCA6).

## ◎ HIGH-YIELD FACT

Although potassium-aggravated myotonia, hyperkalemic periodic paralysis, and hypokalemic periodic paralysis type 2 have "potassium" or "-kalemic" in their names, they are actually *sodium* channelopathies, **NOT** potassium channelopathies.

Hypokalemic periodic paralysis type 1 is a *calcium* channelopathy.

- Muscle channelopathies are summarized in Table 18.10.

## MNEMONICS

Episodic ataxia type 1: Potassium channel. Potassium is in the 1st group of the periodic table, and the potassium ion has 1+ charge ($K^+$).
Episodic ataxia type 2: Calcium channel. Calcium is in the 2nd group of the periodic table, and the calcium ion has 2+ charge ($Ca^{2+}$).

**QUESTION 63.** A 12-year-old girl presents with multiple attacks of generalized muscle weakness, sometimes associated with pain. These attacks usually occur after prolonged rest. On examination, you note dysmorphic features including low set ears, broad nose, hypertelorism, and clinodactyly, in addition to short stature. Electrocardiography demonstrates a prolonged QT interval. This disorder is due to an abnormality in which of the following channels?
A. Sodium
B. Potassium
C. Chloride
D. Calcium
E. None of the above

**ANSWER:** B. Potassium

## COMMENTS AND DISCUSSION

- The diagnosis in this patient is *Andersen-Tawil syndrome*.
- Andersen-Tawil syndrome
  ○ A periodic paralysis syndrome due to mutations in the *KCNJ2* gene encoding the inward rectifier potassium channel 2 protein (Kir2.1). Therefore, this disorder is considered a potassium channelopathy.
  ○ Autosomal dominant, as all periodic paralysis syndromes
  ○ Typical onset is in the first to second decades.
  ○ Triad: periodic paralysis, cardiac arrhythmias, and dysmorphic features
    - Periodic paralysis
      - This may occur spontaneously, after prolonged rest, or following rest after exercise.
      - Patients can have mild fixed weakness such as neck flexor weakness.
    - Cardiac arrhythmias (Fig. 18.20)
      - Prolonged QT intervals, prominent U waves on electrocardiography
      - Ventricular arrhythmias: premature ventricular contraction, polymorphic ventricular tachycardia, bidirectional ventricular tachycardia
      - Patients can present with syncope or palpitation.
    - Dysmorphic features (Fig. 18.20)
      - Low-set ears
      - Hypertelorism (widely-spaced eyes), broad nose
      - Small mandible
      - Clinodactyly (abnormal curve) of the fifth digit
      - Syndactyly (fusion) of the 2nd and 3rd toes
      - Scoliosis, short stature
    - There is *no* myotonia.

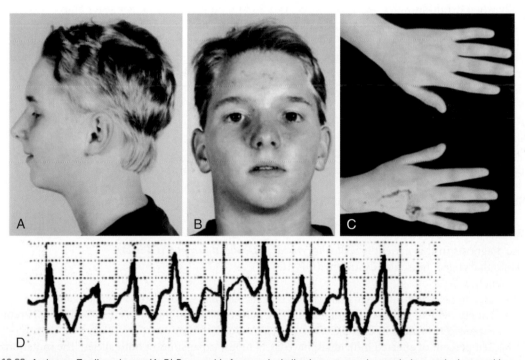

**Fig. 18.20** Andersen-Tawil syndrome. (A, B) Dysmorphic features including low set ears, hypertelorism, and micrognathia. (C) Bilateral fifth-digit clinodactyly. (D) A short run of polymorphic ventricular tachycardia on electrocardiography. From Plaster NM, Tawil R, Tristani-Firouzi M, et al. Mutations in Kir2.1 cause the developmental and episodic electrical phenotypes of Andersen's syndrome. *Cell.* 2001;105(4):511–519.

## ◎ HIGH-YIELD FACT

Periodic paralysis + Cardiac arrhythmia + Dysmorphic features = Andersen-Tawil syndrome
There is **NO** myotonia in this disorder.

**QUESTION 64.** Which of the following conditions is **NOT** electrically silent on needle electromyography?
  A. Contracture in McArdle disease
  B. Contracture after muscle cooling in paramyotonia congenita
  C. Cramps
  D. Severe paralytic attack of hypokalemic periodic paralysis
  E. Rippling muscle disease

**ANSWER:** C. Cramps

**COMMENTS AND DISCUSSION**
- Electrical silence on needle electromyography can be seen in the following conditions:
  o As a normal finding at rest in muscle outside the endplate zone (when there is no muscle contraction)
  o Contracture in metabolic myopathies such as myophosphorylase deficiency (McArdle disease)
  o During severe paralytic attacks of periodic paralysis syndromes such as hyperkalemic periodic paralysis and hypokalemic periodic paralysis
  o In most patients with rippling muscle disease, waves of contraction within muscles, typically triggered by stretching, percussion, or movements are electrically silent.
  o Muscle cooling in paramyotonia congenita. When the muscle is cooled below 20°C, myotonic discharges disappear, and the muscle has long-lasting electrically silent contracture.
- Cramps are not electrically silent. Cramp potentials are normal appearing motor unit action potentials firing at high frequencies repetitively and irregularly.

**QUESTION 65.** A 55-year-old man presents with slowly progressive proximal muscle weakness over 5 years. In addition, he reports difficulty swallowing for over a decade and has mild aspiration, especially when drinking water. He also complains of mild diplopia. His younger sister and mother have similar symptoms beginning in their late 40s. On examination, he has bilateral ptosis, which has remained unchanged since his early 40s according to his report. Extraocular movement examination shows mild limitation of upward gaze. There is grade 4 weakness of the proximal muscles in both arms and legs. Distal muscles are grade 5. What is the most likely underlying etiology of the disorder in this patient?
  A. Autoimmunity to the postsynaptic acetylcholine receptor
  B. CTG repeat expansion in the *DMPK* gene
  C. GCN repeat expansion in the *PABPN1* gene
  D. Large deletion in the mitochondrial DNA
  E. Mutation in the *POLG* gene encoding DNA polymerase-gamma

**ANSWER:** C. GCN repeat expansion in the *PABPN1* gene

**COMMENTS AND DISCUSSION**
- The diagnosis in this patient is *oculopharyngeal muscular dystrophy (OPMD)*.
- Oculopharyngeal muscular dystrophy (OPMD)
  o Genetics
    - Due to GCN repeat expansions (11-18 repeats; normal = 10) in the *PABPN1* gene
    - Ninety percent of affected individuals have autosomal dominant inheritance with GCN repeat expansions present in one allele.
    - Ten percent of affected individuals have GCN repeat expansions in both alleles. The mutations can be compound heterozygous (different number of repeats in both alleles) or homozygous (the same numbers of repeats in both alleles). These individuals tend to have more severe phenotypes.
    - No anticipation. The GCN repeat expansions are stable during mitosis and meiosis.
  o Clinical features
    - Patients may have French-Canadian or Bukhara Jewish background. This disorder has a high prevalence in these populations but can also be seen in others.
    - Ptosis and dysphagia. These are typically initial symptoms beginning around the fifth to sixth decade. The onset can be earlier in individuals with a higher number of GCN repeat expansions or with expansions in both alleles.
    - Extraocular movements can be affected, and patients may have diplopia. However, complete external ophthalmoplegia is rare.

- In contrast, chronic progressive external ophthalmoplegia (CPEO) and Kearns-Sayre syndrome (KSS) are characterized by prominent external ophthalmoplegia, which is typically more severe than in OPMD, and more predominant than dysphagia. Patients with CPEO or KSS usually do not complain of diplopia, since ophthalmoplegia develops chronically.
- Proximal muscle weakness usually occurs 10 years after the onset of dysphagia and ptosis.
- There is no cardiac involvement.

## ◎ HIGH-YIELD FACT

- In OPMD, dysphagia and ptosis are early and predominant features. External ophthalmoplegia can occur later but should not be severe or complete. Diplopia can be present.
- In CPEO, external ophthalmoplegia is a predominant feature, along with ptosis. Dysphagia occurs later. Ophthalmoplegia is typically severe or complete, and **NOT** associated with diplopia due to its chronicity.

- ○ Laboratory features
  - Muscle biopsy (see also comments and discussion from Question 7 and Fig. 10.9 in Chapter 10)
    - Electron microscopy: intranuclear tubulofilamentous inclusions, 8.5 nm in external diameter
  - Genetic testing to detect GCN repeat expansions in the *PABPN1* gene
- CPEO and KSS are associated with large deletions in the mitochondrial DNA. KSS has cardiac conduction abnormalities, in addition to ophthalmoplegia.
- Mutations in the *POLG* gene encoding the gamma subunit of DNA polymerase are also associated with CPEO, among other phenotypes. (see also comments and discussion for Question 47.)
- In CPEO, external ophthalmoplegia is a predominant feature. Patients with CPEO typically also have ptosis. Dysphagia is not an early feature in CPEO.
  - ○ This is in contrast to OPMD in which dysphagia and ptosis are early and predominant features, and external ophthalmoplegia can occur later, but is not severe or complete as in CPEO.
  - ○ External ophthalmoplegia in OPMD can result in diplopia, whereas patients with CPEO do not typically have diplopia.
- CTG repeat expansions in the *DMPK* gene are associated with myotonic dystrophy type 1 (DM1). DM1 can have ptosis early, but dysphagia typically comes later in the course of the disease. Weakness and myotonia in DM1 affect predominantly distal muscles. In addition, there are also systemic features such as cardiac abnormalities. Ophthalmoplegia is not a typical feature in myotonic dystrophies. (see also comments and discussion from Question 31.)
- Autoimmunity to the postsynaptic acetylcholine receptor of the skeletal muscle is associated with myasthenia gravis (MG). Fluctuation is a feature in MG, but not in OPMD.

## SUGGESTED READINGS

Bonne G, Leturcq F, Ben Yaou R. Emery-Dreifuss muscular dystrophy. In: Adam MP, Ardinger HH, Pagon RA, et al., eds. *GeneReviews* (R). Seattle, WA. September 29, 2004 [Updated August 15, 2019].

Bonnemann CG, Wang CH, Quijano-Roy S, et al. Diagnostic approach to the congenital muscular dystrophies. *Neuromuscul Disord*. 2014;24:289-311.

Brais B, Chrestian N, Dupré N, Bouchard JP, Rouleau G. Oculopharyngeal muscular dystrophy. In: Katirji B, Kaminski HJ, Rff RL, eds. *Neuromuscular Disorders in Clinical Practice*. New York, NY: Springer New York; 2014:1239–1245. 2nd ed.

Cenacchi G, Papa V, Pegoraro V, et al. Review: Danon disease: review of natural history and recent advances. *Neuropathol Appl Neurobiol*. 2020;46:303-322.

Di Mauro S. Muscle glycogenoses: an overview. *Acta Myol*. 2007;26:35-41.

Diaz-Manera J, Kishnani PS, Kushlaf H, et al. Safety and efficacy of avalglucosidase alfa versus alglucosidase alfa in patients with late-onset Pompe disease (COMET): a phase 3, randomised, multicentre trial. *Lancet Neurol*. 2021;20:1012-1026.

Dimachkie MM, Barohn RJ. Distal myopathies. *Neurol Clin*. 2014;32:817-842.

Dimauro S, Akman HO, Paradas C. Metabolic myopathies. In: Katirji B, Kaminski HJ, Ruff RL, eds. *Neuromuscular Disorders in Clinical Practice*. New York, NY: Springer New York; 2014a.

Dimauro S, Nishino I, Hirano M. Mitochondrial myopathies. In: Katirji B, Kaminski HJ, Ruff RL, eds. *Neuromuscular Disorders in Clinical Practice*. New York, NY: Springer New York; 2014b:1273-1296.

Duan D, Goemans N, Takeda S, et al. Duchenne muscular dystrophy. *Nat Rev Dis Primers*. 2021;7(1):13.

Dulaney E, Katirji B. Forearm exercise testing. In: Katirji B, Kaminski HJ, Ruff RL, eds. *Neuromuscular Disorders in Clinical Practice*. New York, NY: Springer New York; 2014:79-88. 2nd ed.

Fichna JP, Maruszak A, Zekanowski C. Myofibrillar myopathy in the genomic context. *J Appl Genet*. 2018;59:431-439.

Hamel J, Tawil R. Facioscapulohumeral muscular dystrophy: update on pathogenesis and future treatments. *Neurotherapeutics*. 2018;15:863-871.

Jungbluth H, Treves S, Zorzato F, et al. Congenital myopathies: disorders of excitation-contraction coupling and muscle contraction. *Nat Rev Neurol*. 2018;14:151-167.

Kishnani PS, Corzo D, Nicolino M, et al. Recombinant human acid [alpha]-glucosidase: Major clinical benefits in infantile-onset Pompe disease. *Neurology*. 2007;68:99-109.

Lampe AK, Bushby KM. Collagen VI related muscle disorders. *J Med Genet*. 2005;42:673-685.

Lilleker JB, Keh YS, Roncaroli F, Sharma R, Roberts M. Metabolic myopathies: a practical approach. *Pract Neurol*. 2018;18:14-26.

Mahjneh I, Marconi G, Bushby K, et al. Dysferlinopathy (LGMD2B): a 23-year follow-up study of 10 patients homozygous for the same frameshifting dysferlin mutations. *Neuromuscul Disord*. 2001;11:20-26.

Mendell JR, Goemans N, Lowes LP, et al. Longitudinal effect of eteplirsen versus historical control on ambulation in Duchenne muscular dystrophy. *Ann Neurol*. 2016;79:257-271.

Meola G, Cardani R. Myotonic dystrophies: an update on clinical aspects, genetic, pathology, and molecular pathomechanisms. *Biochim Biophys Acta*. 2015;1852:594-606.

Mercuri E, Muntoni F. Congenital muscular dystrophies. In: Darras BT, Jones HR, Ryan MM, De Vivo DC, eds. *Neuromuscular Disorders of Infancy, Childhood, and Adolescence*. 2nd ed. San Diego: Academic Press; 2015: 538–550.

Miller TM. Differential diagnosis of myotonic disorders. *Muscle Nerve*. 2008;37:293-299.

Mohassel P, Bönnemann CG Limb-girdle muscular dystrophies. In: Darras BT, Jones HR, Ryan MM, De Vivo DC, eds. *Neuromuscular Disorders of Infancy, Childhood, and Adolescence*. 2nd ed. San Diego: Academic Press; 2015:635-666.

North KN, Wang CH, Clarke N, et al. Approach to the diagnosis of congenital myopathies. *Neuromuscul Disord*. 2014;24:97-116.

Pradhan S. Clinical and magnetic resonance imaging features of 'diamond on quadriceps' sign in dysferlinopathy. *Neurol India*. 2009;57:172-175.

Preston DC, Shapiro BE. Myotonic muscle disorders and periodic paralysis syndromes. In: *Electromyography and Neuromuscular Disorders*. 4th ed. Philadelphia: Elsevier; 2021:693-712.

Ruff RL, Shapiro BE. Disorders of skeletal muscle membrane excitability: myotonia congenita, paramyotonia congenita, periodic paralysis, and related syndromes. In: Katirji B, Kaminski HJ, Ruff RL, eds. *Neuromuscular Disorders in Clinical Practice*. 2nd ed. New York, NY: Springer New York; 2014:1111-1147.

Selcen D. Myofibrillar myopathies. *Neuromuscul Disord*. 2011;21:161-171.

Statland JM, Fontaine B, Hanna MG, et al. Review of the diagnosis and treatment of periodic paralysis. *Muscle Nerve*. 2018;57:522-530.

Statland JM, Tawil R. Facioscapulohumeral muscular dystrophy. *Continuum (Minneap Minn)*. 2016;22:1916-1931.

Stunnenberg BC, Lorusso S, Arnold WD, et al. Guidelines on clinical presentation and management of nondystrophic myotonias. *Muscle Nerve*. 2020;62:430-444.

Suetterlin KJ, Raja Rayan D, Matthews E, Hanna MG. Mexiletine (NaMuscla) for the treatment of myotonia in non-dystrophic myotonic disorders. *Expert Opin Orphan Drugs*. 2020;8:43-49.

Termsarasab P, Baajour W, Thammongkolchai T, Katirji B. The myotonic dystrophies. In: Katirji B, Kaminski HJ, Ruff RL, eds. *Neuromuscular Disorders in Clinical Practice*. 2nd ed. New York, NY: Springer New York; 2014:1221-1238.

Trollet C, Boulinguiez A, Roth F, et al. Oculopharyngeal muscular dystrophy. In: Adam MP, Ardinger HH, Pagon RA, et al., eds. *GeneReviews((R))*. Seattle, WA. March 8, 2001 [Updated October 22, 2020].

Van Der Ploeg AT, Clemens PR, Corzo D, et al. A randomized study of alglucosidase alfa in late-onset Pompe's disease. *N Engl J Med*. 2010;362:1396-1406.

Watts GD, Wymer J, Kovach MJ, et al. Inclusion body myopathy associated with Paget disease of bone and frontotemporal dementia is caused by mutant valosin-containing protein. *Nat Genet*. 2004;36:377-381.

Wicklund MP. The limb-girdle muscular dystrophies. *Continuum (Minneap Minn)*. 2019;25:1599-1618.

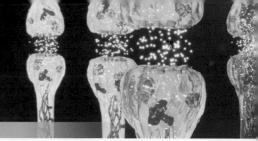

# Peripheral Nerve Hyperexcitability (PNH) Syndromes

## PART 1 | PRACTICE TEST

**Q1.** Which of the following is **NOT** associated with peripheral nerve hyperexcitability?
- A. Isaacs syndrome
- B. Morvan syndrome
- C. Cramp-fasciculation syndrome
- D. Stiff-person syndrome
- E. Neuromyotonia

**Q2.** Which of the following is **FALSE** about Morvan syndrome?
- A. Hyperhidrosis is a common manifestation.
- B. Hallucinations, agitation, and delirium are often seen.
- C. Neuromyotonia is common, while myokymia is not typically present.
- D. It is associated with elevated potassium channel-complex antibodies.
- E. It may be associated with thymoma.

**Q3.** Which of the following can eliminate neuromyotonic discharges in Isaacs syndrome?
- A. Curare
- B. Baclofen
- C. Sleep
- D. General anesthesia
- E. Diazepam

**Q4.** Which of the following is **NOT** associated with high-titer voltage-gated potassium channel-complex antibodies?
- A. Cerebellar syndrome
- B. Isaacs syndrome
- C. Rippling muscle disease
- D. Intractable epilepsy
- E. Limbic encephalitis

**Q5.** Which of the following is **CORRECT** about cramp-fasciculation syndrome?
- A. Needle electromyography (EMG) shows large motor unit action potentials.
- B. It is characterized by myalgia and cramps with muscle weakness.
- C. Needle EMG shows fasciculation and fibrillation potentials.
- D. Voltage-gated potassium channel-complex antibodies are seen in all patients.
- E. Slow-rate repetitive nerve stimulation may show afterdischarges.

**Q6.** Which of the following is **CORRECT** about abnormal discharges in peripheral nerve hyperexcitability syndromes?
- A. Myokymic and neuromyotonic discharges are similar discharges.
- B. Myokymic discharge is a burst of a single motor unit action potential firing at 150 to 250 Hz.
- C. Neuromyotonic discharge is grouped discharge of motor unit action potentials occurring spontaneously at rates of 2 to 60 Hz.
- D. Neuromyotonic discharges are fairly specific for peripheral nerve hyperexcitability syndromes.
- E. Neuromyotonic discharges are seen only in Isaacs syndrome, whereas myokymic discharges are detected only in Morvan syndrome.

**Q7.** Which of the following statements regarding Isaacs syndrome is **FALSE**?
- A. Muscle stiffness and abnormal discharges are not eliminated by curare.
- B. Associated with antibodies against LGI-1 (leucine-rich glioma-inactivated protein 1) or CASPR2 (contactin-associated protein-like 2).
- C. It is sometimes referred to as acquired neuromyotonia.
- D. It is responsive to carbamazepine and immunomodulation.
- E. Abnormal posture is common is severe cases.

**Q8.** Which of the following statements is **CORRECT** regarding voltage-gated potassium channel (VGKC)-complex antibodies?
A. Leucine-rich glioma-inactivated 1 (LGI1) is more common in Isaacs syndrome.
B. Contactin-associated protein-like 2 (CASPR2) is more common in limbic encephalitis.
C. LGI1 and CASPR2 antibodies are never elevated in epilepsy and cerebellar syndrome.
D. LGI1 and CASPR2 antibodies are directed against intracellular antigens.
E. LGI1 and CASPR2 antibodies are directed against cell-surface antigens.

**Q9.** Which of the following disorders is **LEAST** likely to be clinically confused with Isaacs syndrome is?
A. Rippling muscle disease
B. Stiff-person syndrome
C. Charcot-Marie-Tooth disease
D. Myotonia congenita
E. Morvan syndrome

## PART 2 | QUESTIONS WITH ANSWERS AND DISCUSSION

**QUESTION 1.** Which of the following is **NOT** associated with peripheral nerve hyperexcitability?
A. Isaacs syndrome
B. Morvan syndrome
C. Cramp-fasciculation syndrome
D. Stiff-person syndrome
E. Neuromyotonia

**ANSWER:** D. Stiff-person syndrome

### COMMENTS AND DISCUSSION

- Peripheral nerve hyperexcitability (PNH) syndromes are a group of disorders characterized by muscle stiffness, cramps, and muscle twitches with involuntary abnormal electrical activity on needle electromyography (EMG). Dysautonomia and encephalopathy may also accompany these syndromes.
- Despite the presence of several distinguishing clinical and electrophysiological features of PNH syndromes, a significant overlap exists among the main PNH syndromes: Isaacs syndrome (neuromyotonia), Morvan syndrome, and cramp-fasciculation syndrome.
- PNH syndromes are distinct from the disorders of muscle stiffness originating in the central nervous system, such as spasticity from brain or spine disorders and stiff-person syndrome. In addition, PNH syndromes differ significantly from muscle disorders associated with stiffness such as the dystrophic and non-dystrophic myotonias and rippling muscle disease.
- The terminology, clinical phenomenology, and neurophysiological findings used in the past in PNH syndromes are often confusing.
  - The medical literature has used multiple terms to describe PNH syndromes, including idiopathic generalized myokymia, acquired neuromyotonia, Armadillo syndrome, syndrome of continuous muscle fiber activity, and quantal squander, among others.
  - PNH syndromes include Isaacs syndrome (neuromyotonia), Morvan syndrome, and cramp-fasciculation syndrome, which are the preferred terms.
  - The electrophysiological terms, including myokymia, neuromyotonia, continuous muscle fiber activity, continuous motor neuron discharges, and neuromyotonia, are used interchangeably and inconsistently.
  - Myokymic and neuromyotonic discharges are the preferred electrophysiological terms.
- *Stiff-person syndrome* is a central nervous system disorder characterized by progressive and fluctuating muscle stiffness, lumbar hyperlordosis, and gait stiffness, with painful muscle spasms in the limbs, trunk, and neck.
- *Stiff-person* syndrome is associated with type 1 diabetes, epilepsy, and other organ-specific autoimmunity.
- In more than 70% of patients with stiff-person syndrome, antibodies are detected in serum directed against glutamic acid decarboxylase (GAD), the enzyme responsible for the biosynthesis of γ-aminobutyric acid (GABA). In about 5 % of patients, anti-amphiphysin antibodies are seen in serum and cerebrospinal fluid (CSF), and their presence in women can be associated with breast cancer.

- The needle EMG in stiff-person syndrome reveals nonspecific continuous normal motor unit activity at rest. These manifestations are abolished by sleep, anesthesia, peripheral nerve blockade, and curare.

**QUESTION 2.** Which of the following is **FALSE** about Morvan syndrome?
   A. Hyperhidrosis is a common manifestation.
   B. Hallucinations, agitation, and delirium are often seen.
   C. Neuromyotonia is common, while myokymia is not typically present.
   D. It is associated with elevated potassium channel-complex antibodies.
   E. It may be associated with thymoma.

**ANSWER:** C. Neuromyotonia is common, while myokymia is not typically present.

## COMMENTS AND DISCUSSION

- *Morvan syndrome* is a disorder with features of peripheral nerve hyperexcitability (PNH), dysautonomia, and encephalopathy.
- Morvan syndrome affects males more than females, with symptoms of muscle stiffness, cramps, and PNH that are often the presenting features. Neuropathic pain in the limbs may be a feature.
- Hyperhidrosis is a common dysautonomic symptom. Other signs of autonomic dysfunction reported in patients with Morvan syndrome include tachycardia, arrhythmias, and urinary dysfunction.
- Central nervous system (CNS) features include hallucinations, agitation, delirium, amnesia, and confusion. Sleep disturbances are common, especially insomnia.
- As with other PNH syndromes, needle electromyography (EMG) shows evidence of motor unit hyperexcitability in the form of fasciculations, multiplets, as well as myokymic and neuromyotonic discharges. Also, after-discharges or repetitive muscle action potentials are often noted following motor nerve stimulation with a single stimulus. These are best seen with the F wave montage (0.2 mV sensitivity and 10 msec/division).
- Voltage-gated potassium channel (VGKC)-complex antibodies can be detected in serum, typically in a high titer, in a majority of patients with Morvan syndrome. As with Isaacs syndrome, VGKC-complex antibodies are actually directed against proteins associated with the potassium channel, including CASPR2 (contactin-associated protein-like 2) and LGI1 (leucine-rich glioma-inactivated 1). In patients with Morvan syndrome, antibodies to CASPR2, LGI1, or both, can be detected.
- Thymoma may be present in up to one-third of patients with Morvan syndrome, with CASPR2 antibody–positive patients having thymoma more often than LGI1-positive patients.
- Morvan syndrome shares some features with limbic encephalitis, a CNS disorder associated with LGI1 antibodies (Table 19.1). PNH may be associated with limbic encephalitis, but is much less common or prominent than the major PNH syndromes including Isaacs syndrome, Morvan syndrome and cramp-fasciculation syndrome. In contrast to limbic enceaphlitis, Morvan syndrome is characterized by prominent PNH, neuropathic pain, and dysautonomia. Magnetic resonance imaging (MRI)

**TABLE 19.1** Characteristic clinical findings in patients with peripheral nerve hyperexcitability syndromes and voltage-gated potassium channel (VGKC)-complex antibodies

| | Cramp-fasciculation syndrome | Isaacs syndrome | Morvan syndrome | Limbic encephalitis |
|---|---|---|---|---|
| Muscle twitching | ++ | ++ | ++ | + / - |
| Muscle cramps | ++ | ++ | ++ | + / - |
| Myokymic discharges | - | ++ | ++ | + / - |
| Neuromyotonic discharges | - | ++ | +++ | + / - |
| Autonomic features | - | ++ | ++ | - |
| Agitation | - | - | ++ | +++ |
| Seizures | - | - | - | +++ |
| Memory loss | - | - | + | +++ |
| VGKC-complex antibodies | + / - | + | + | + |
| • LGI1 antibodies | - | ± | ± | +++ |
| • CASPR2 antibodies | + / - | ++ | ++ | ++ |
| Brain MRI changes | - | - | +/- | + |

*CASPR2*, contactin-associated protein-like 2; *LGI1*, leucine-rich glioma-inactivated 1; *MRI*, magnetic resonance imaging. -, not present; +/-, may/may not present; +, can present; ++, moderately present; +++, obviously present.

abnormalities in limbic encephalitis include unilateral or bilateral medial temporal hyperintensities, rarely seen in Morvan syndrome. Morvan syndrome may be associated with thymoma, unlike limbic encephalitis.

**QUESTION 3.** Which of the following can eliminate neuromyotonic discharges in Isaacs syndrome?
A. Curare
B. Baclofen
C. Sleep
D. General anesthesia
E. Diazepam

**ANSWER:** A. Curare

### COMMENTS AND DISCUSSION
- The needle electromyography (EMG) examination in Isaacs syndrome reveals a variety of spontaneous motor unit activities that include fasciculation potentials, myokymic discharges, and neuromyotonic discharges. These originate from one or more segments of the peripheral motor axon and persist during sleep or general anesthesia. However, they can be eliminated by neuromuscular junction blockade.
- Symptomatic treatment in peripheral nerve hyperexcitability (PNH) syndromes including Isaacs syndrome, includes phenytoin or carbamazepine, which are often effective in reducing muscle stiffness, twitching, and cramps.
- Muscle stiffness and spasms in stiff-person syndrome, but not Isaacs syndrome, respond to γ-aminobutyric acid (GABA) agonists including baclofen and diazepam.

**QUESTION 4.** Which of the following is **NOT** associated with high-titer voltage-gated potassium channel-complex antibodies?
A. Cerebellar syndrome
B. Isaacs syndrome
C. Rippling muscle disease
D. Intractable epilepsy
E. Limbic encephalitis

**ANSWER:** C. Rippling muscle disease

### COMMENTS AND DISCUSSION
- The classical syndromes associated with high-level voltage-gated potassium channel (VGKC)-complex antibodies include Isaacs syndrome, Morvan syndrome, limbic encephalitis, and possibly cramp-fasciculation syndrome.
- High-level VGKC-complex antibodies are occasionally seen in patients with other possible autoimmune disorders such as cerebellar syndrome, intractable epilepsy, and pain syndromes.
- Low-level VGKC-complex antibodies are less specific and present in a variety of non-autoimmune disorders.
- Rippling muscle disease is *not* associated with elevated VGKC-complex antibodies.

**QUESTION 5.** Which of the following is **CORRECT** about cramp-fasciculation syndrome?
A. Needle electromyography (EMG) shows large motor unit action potentials.
B. It is characterized by myalgia and cramps with muscle weakness.
C. Needle EMG shows fasciculation and fibrillation potentials.
D. Voltage-gated potassium channel-complex antibodies are seen in all patients.
E. Slow-rate repetitive nerve stimulation may show afterdischarges.

**ANSWER:** E. Slow-rate repetitive nerve stimulation may show afterdischarges.

### COMMENTS AND DISCUSSION
- *Cramp-fasciculation syndrome* is a benign peripheral nerve hyperexcitability syndrome.
- Patients present with myalgia and cramps without weakness. Examination may show fasciculations, myokymia, or both, in muscles with an otherwise normal neuromuscular examination. Patients often respond to treatment with carbamazepine.

- The pathophysiology involves instability of the distal motor axon.
- Needle EMG demonstrates fasciculation potentials without fibrillation potentials, and normal motor unit action potential morphology and recruitment.
- Supramaximal stimulation of motor nerves at 0.5, 1, 3, and 5 Hz may show afterdischarges following the initial motor response.
- Voltage-gated potassium channel-complex antibodies may be detected in some patients, suggesting an autoimmune pathogenesis.

**QUESTION 6.** Which of the following is **CORRECT** about abnormal discharges in peripheral nerve hyperexcitability syndromes?
  A. Myokymic and neuromyotonic discharges are similar discharges.
  B. Myokymic discharge is a burst of a single motor unit action potential firing at 150 to 250 Hz.
  C. Neuromyotonic discharge is grouped discharge of motor unit action potentials occurring spontaneously at rates of 2 to 60 Hz.
  D. Neuromyotonic discharges are fairly specific for peripheral nerve hyperexcitability syndromes.
  E. Neuromyotonic discharges are seen only in Isaacs syndrome, whereas myokymic discharges are detected only in Morvan syndrome.

**ANSWER:** D. Neuromyotonic discharges are fairly specific for peripheral nerve hyperexcitability syndromes.

### COMMENTS AND DISCUSSION
- Both myokymic and neuromyotonic discharges are generated in the motor neuron/axon and have a motor unit action potential morphology. The difference between them appears largely related to firing rate and pattern (Table 19.2).
- A myokymic discharge is a repetitive grouped discharge of a single motor unit action potential occurring spontaneously with a slow frequency between bursts (typically 1–5 Hz) and a much higher frequency inside the burst (typically 5–60 Hz). Neuromyotonic discharge includes bursts of a single

**TABLE 19.2** Needle EMG abnormal spontaneous discharges

| EMG discharge | Generator/ source | Firing frequency | Stability | Sound on loudspeaker | Clinical setting |
|---|---|---|---|---|---|
| **Myokymic discharge** | Motor axon | 1–5 Hz (interburst) 5–60 Hz (intraburst) | Fairly stable | Marching band | • Radiation plexopathy<br>• Peripheral nerve hyperexcitability syndromes |
| **Neuromyotonic discharge** | Motor axon | 150–250 Hz | Wax and wane in frequency and amplitude | Pinging sound | • Peripheral nerve hyperexcitability syndromes<br>• Limbic encephalitis<br>• Extremely chronic motor neuron disorders<br>• Familial cases |
| **Myotonic discharge** | Muscle membrane | 20–50 Hz | Wax and wane in frequency and amplitude | Revving engine or dive-bomber | • Myotonic dystrophies<br>• Non-dystrophic myotonias<br>• Pompe disease, Scwhartz-Jampel syndrome<br>• Myotubular myopathy<br>• Statin- or colchicine-induced myopathy |
| **Complex repetitive discharge** | Muscle fiber | 5–100 Hz | Stable | Machine | • Chronic myopathies and chronic neurogenic disorders (radiculopathy, polyneuropathy) |

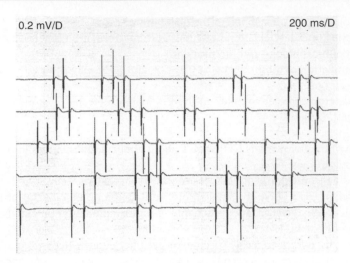

0.2 mV/D 200 ms/D

**Fig. 19.1** Myokymic discharge. Myokymic discharges are shown in a raster mode with a long sweep speed of 200 ms/division. Note that the number of potentials often changes from one burst to another, varying in this example from one to four potentials. In addition, note the relatively slow interburst frequency of ~2 Hz, whereas the intraburst frequency is ~18–20 Hz. Adapted from Katirji B. Electromyography in Clinical Practice. 2nd ed. Philadelphia: Mosby/Elsevier; 2007: 31.

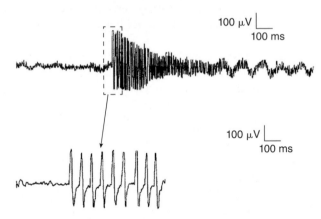

100 μV ⌐
     100 ms

100 μV ⌐
     100 ms

**Fig. 19.2** Neuromyotonic discharges. Neuromyotonic discharges are recorded in the top tracing with a long sweep speed of 100 ms per division, and in the inset below with a regular sweep speed of 10 ms per division. Very high-frequency (150-250 Hz), decrementing, repetitive discharges of a single motor unit are demonstrated. The inset identifies each potential as the same motor unit action potential. Adapted from Preston DC, Shapiro BE. *Electromyography and Neuromuscular Disorders.* 3rd ed. London: Elsevier/Saunders; 2013.

motor unit action potential initially firing at 150 to 250 Hz, often starting and stopping abruptly, and waning in amplitude and frequency (Figs. 19.1 and 19.2). Neuromyotonic discharges have the fastest frequency of any discharge.

- Both neuromyotonic and myokymic discharges may be detected in patients with Isaacs and Morvan syndromes, and less commonly in limbic encephalitis and cramp-fasciculation syndrome.
- Neuromyotonic discharges are more common and specific for peripheral nerve hyperexcitability syndromes, although rarely they are seen in extremely chronic motor neuron disorders (e.g., adult-onset spinal muscular atrophy) and in inherited forms of neuromyotonia (e.g., those due to mutations in the *KCNA1* gene).
- Myokymic discharges occur either focally or in a more generalized fashion in many other peripheral nerve disorders. This includes, in addition to peripheral nerve hyperexcitability syndromes, radiation plexopathy, carpal tunnel syndrome, Guillain–Barré syndrome, gold toxicity, pontine glioma, and multiple sclerosis.
- Myokymic and neuromyotonic discharges should also be distinguished from myotonic discharges and complex repetitive discharges. The latter are discharges of single muscle fiber action potential, whereas the former are motor unit action potentials.

**QUESTION 7.** Which of the following statements regarding Isaacs syndrome is **FALSE**?
- A. Muscle stiffness and abnormal discharges are not eliminated by curare.
- B. Associated with antibodies against LGI-1 (leucine-rich glioma-inactivated protein 1) or CASPR2 (contactin-associated protein-like 2).
- C. It is sometimes referred to as acquired neuromyotonia.
- D. It is responsive to carbamazepine and immunomodulation.
- E. Abnormal posture is common is severe cases.

**ANSWER:** A. Muscle stiffness and abnormal discharges are not eliminated by curare.

**COMMENTS AND DISCUSSION**
- Isaacs described the clinical syndrome in 1961 and suspected that the origin of the spontaneous motor activity was the distal segments of peripheral nerves, since it was not eliminated by blockade of the peripheral nerve but could be eliminated by curare, a non-depolarizing acetylcholine receptor blocker at the postsynaptic neuromuscular junction.
- The disorder is sometimes referred to as acquired neuromyotonia, or idiopathic generalized myokymia. Isaacs syndrome is the preferred term, since both myokymia and neuromyotonia are seen and these discharges may be encountered in other disorders.
- Isaacs syndrome may affect patients at any age and varies significantly in severity. In most cases it manifests with generalized muscle stiffness, which persists during sleep. On examination, there is muscle hypertrophy, continuous muscle twitching, undulation (myokymia), and slowness of movement. Signs of dysautonomia including hyperhidrosis, sialorrhea, and piloerection may be present. The symptoms of Isaacs syndrome may fluctuate, but are usually slowly progressive over years.
- Anti-voltage-gated potassium channel (VGKC) antibodies are directed mainly at proteins surrounding the potassium channel, rather than the channel itself, and are thus now known as anti-VGKC-complex antibodies. These autoantibodies are directed against LGI1 (leucine-rich glioma-inactivated protein 1) and CASPR2 (contact-associated protein-like 2), which are cell-surface proteins.
- The majority of patients with Isaacs syndrome respond to carbamazepine or phenytoin.
- Immunomodulation and immunotherapy is also indicated in patients with confirmed autoimmune origin who remain symptomatic. Plasmapheresis or intravenous immunoglobulin (IVIG) treatment can be used, often in combination with prednisone, azathioprine, cyclosporine, rituximab, or cyclophosphamide.

**QUESTION 8.** Which of the following statements is **CORRECT** regarding voltage-gated potassium channel (VGKC)-complex antibodies?
- A. Leucine-rich glioma-inactivated 1 (LGI1) is more common in Isaacs syndrome.
- B. Contactin-associated protein-like 2 (CASPR2) is more common in limbic encephalitis.
- C. LGI1 and CASPR2 antibodies are never elevated in epilepsy and cerebellar syndrome.
- D. LGI1 and CASPR2 antibodies are directed against intracellular antigens.
- E. LGI1 and CASPR2 antibodies are directed against cell-surface antigens.

**ANSWER:** E. LGI1 and CASPR2 antibodies are directed against cell-surface antigens.

**COMMENTS AND DISCUSSION**
- Identification of antibodies against voltage-gated potassium channel (VGKC) has been recently developed, significantly changing our understanding of the peripheral nerve hyperexcitability (PNH) syndromes. It is now understood that VGKC antibodies identified earlier are not directed against the VGKC subunits, but actually against associated cell-surface proteins surrounding the potassium channel (Fig. 19.3), primarily leucine-rich glioma-inactivated 1 (LGI1) and contactin-associated protein-like 2 (CASPR2).
- Most patients with PNH syndromes including Isaacs syndrome have autoantibodies against CASPR2, whereas patients with limbic encephalitis have autoantibodies against LGI1. However, this is not exclusive, and there is significant overlap.
- Neuropathic pain, cerebellar ataxia, and intractable epilepsy may be associated with antibodies against CASPR2.

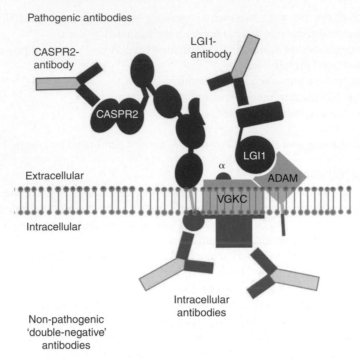

**Fig. 19.3** Antibodies against the voltage-gated potassium channel (VGKC)-complex. Pathogenic antibodies (*in purple*) including anti-LGI and anti-CASPR2 antibodies are directed against the extracellular domains of the LGI1 and CASPR2 which are the proteins surrounding the voltage-gated potassium channel (VGKC). In contrast, non-pathogenic antibodies (*in red*) found in double-negative patients (i.e., those with seronegativity of both anti-LGI1 and anti-CASPR2 antibodies) bind to the intracellular domain of the VGKCs, and likely other intraceullar antigenic epitopes. *CASPR2*, contactin-associated protein-like 2; *LGI1*, leucine-rich glioma-inactivated 1. Adapted from Michael S, Waters P, Irani SR. Stop testing for autoantibodies to the VGKC-complex: only request LGI1 and CASPR2. Practical Neurology 2020;20:377-384.

**QUESTION 9.** Which of the following disorders is **LEAST** likely to be clinically confused with Isaacs syndrome?
  A. Rippling muscle disease
  B. Stiff-person syndrome
  C. Charcot-Marie-Tooth disease
  D. Myotonia congenita
  E. Morvan syndrome

**ANSWER:** C. Charcot-Marie-Tooth disease

### COMMENTS AND DISCUSSION
- Rippling muscle disease, stiff-person syndrome, myotonia congenita, and Morvan syndrome are associated with muscle stiffness and enter into the differential diagnosis of Isaacs syndrome. Charcot-Marie-Tooth disease is an inherited polyneuropathy manifesting with pes cavus, distal weakness and sensory loss, and areflexia with occasional muscle cramps.
- Rippling muscle disease is a benign myopathy with symptoms and signs of muscle stiffness, cramps, and muscular hyperexcitability. The typical finding is a rolling, wavelike mounding of the muscle provoked by mechanical stimuli and stretch. On electromyography (EMG), the muscle is electrically silent. Rippling muscle disease is associated with mutations in the *CAV3* gene encoding caveolin-3, a membrane-associated protein localized to skeletal muscle fibers. The disorder has immunologic associations, including acetylcholine receptor antibody–positive myasthenia gravis and thymoma. In addition to the genetic form, there is also an immune-mediated form of rippling muscle disease.
- The non-dystrophic myotonias, specifically myotonia congenita, often present with muscle stiffness that manifests when attempting to initiate movements after a period of rest, and diminishes with repeated activity and muscle contractions. Needle EMG in these patients shows prominent myotonic discharges without myopathic changes of motor unit action potentials.

## SUGGESTED READINGS

Ahmed A, Simmons Z. Isaacs syndrome. A review. *Muscle Nerve.* 2015;52:5-12.

Gutmann L, Gutmann L. Myokymia and neuromyotonia. *J Neurol.* 2004;251:138-142.

Irani SR, Alexander S, Waters P. Antibodies to Kv1 potassium channel-complex proteins leucine-rich, glioma inactivated 1 protein and contactin-associated protein-2 in limbic encephalitis, Morvan's syndrome and acquired myotonia. *Brain.* 2010;133(9):2734-2748.

Irani SR, Pettingill P, Kleopa KA, et al. Morvan syndrome: Clinical and serological observations in 29 cases. *Ann Neurol.* 2012;72(2):241-255.

Jamieson PW, Katirji MB. Idiopathic generalized myokymia. *Muscle Nerve.* 1994;17:42-51.

Jammoul A, Shayya L, Mente K, et al. Clinical utility of seropositive voltage-gated potassium channel-complex antibody. *Neurol Clin Pract.* 2016;6:409-418.

Josephs KA, Silber MH, Fealey RD, Nippoldt TB, Auger RG, Vernino S. Neurophysiologic studies in Morvan syndrome. *J Clin Neurophysiol.* 2004;21:440-445.

Katirji B. Peripheral nerve hyperexcitability. *Handb Clin Neurol.* 2019;161:281-290.

Liewluck T, Klein CJ, Jones Jr LK. Cramp-fasciculation syndrome in patients with and without neural autoantibodies. *Muscle Nerve.* 2014;49(3):351-356.

Lo HP, Bertini E, Mirabella M, et al. Mosaic caveolin-3 expression in acquired rippling muscle disease without evidence of myasthenia gravis or acetylcholine receptor autoantibodies. *Neuromuscul Disord.* 2011;21:194-203.

Paterson RW, Zandi MS, Armstrong R, et al. Clinical relevance of positive voltage-gated potassium channel (VGKC)-complex antibodies: experience from a tertiary referral centre. *J Neurol Neurosurg Psychiatry.* 2014;85:625-630.

Sawlani K, Katirji B. Peripheral nerve hyperexcitability syndromes. *Continuum (Minneap Minn).* 2017;23(5): 1437-1450.

Tahmoush AJ, Alonso RJ, Thamoush GP, et al. Cramp-fasciculation syndrome: a treatable hyperexcitable peripheral nerve disorder. *Neurology.* 1991;41(7):1021-1024.

Tan KM, Lennon VA, Klein CJ, et al. Clinical spectrum of voltage-gated potassium channel autoimmunity. *Neurology.* 2008;70:1883-1890.

Termsarasab T, Thammongkolchai T, Katirji B. *Stiff-Person Syndrome and Related Disorders.* New York: Springer; 2020.

Torbergsen T. Rippling muscle disease: a review. *Muscle Nerve.* 2002;11(suppl):S103-S107.

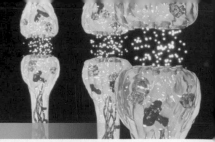

# CHAPTER 20

# Small Fiber Neuropathy

## PART 1 | PRACTICE TEST

**Q1.** A 62-year-old woman with type 2 diabetes mellitus is referred for evaluation of burning feet for 3 months. Examination shows normal muscle bulk, tone, and strength. Sensory exam shows hyperesthesia in both soles, and normal pinprick, vibration, and proprioception. Reflexes are all normal. Which types of nerve fibers are most likely involved in this patient?
A. Aα and Aβ nerve fibers
B. Aα and C nerve fibers
C. Aβ and Aδ nerve fibers
D. Aβ and C nerve fibers
E. Aδ and C nerve fibers

**Q2.** Which of the following symptoms or signs are the **LEAST** likely seen in a patient with a small fiber neuropathy?
A. Hyperesthesia in the soles
B. Allodynia in the dorsum of the feet
C. Decreased vibratory sense in the toes
D. Hair loss over the toes
E. Skin flushing in the feet

**Q3.** Which of the following statements is **CORRECT** regarding small fiber neuropathy (SFN)?
A. Clinical presentation is exclusively a length-dependent pattern.
B. Positive symptoms (e.g., pain, burning, or pricking sensation) are uncommon.
C. Intolerance to the bedsheets is one common complaint.
D. Sensory ataxia can be seen in severe cases.
E. Autonomic function is normal in SFN.

**Q4.** A 30-year-old woman presents with hyperesthesia and numbness in both feet up to the ankles. The neurological examination is normal except for hyperesthesia in both soles. Nerve conduction study and needle electromyography (EMG) are completely normal. Which is the most appropriate next step in the evaluation of this patient?
A. Low-frequency repetitive nerve stimulation
B. Repetitive nerve stimulation after 10-second exercise
C. Single-fiber EMG
D. Quantitative sudomotor axon reflex test (QSART)
E. Muscle biopsy

**Q5.** A 50-year-old woman presents with hyperesthesia in both feet for 5 months. She reports no weakness, but cannot walk barefoot due to pain. At night she cannot sleep well due to pain when the bedsheets touched her feet. She has no known underlying diseases. Neurological examination in the office is completely normal, except for hyperesthesia of both feet. What is the MOST LIKELY etiology of this condition?
A. Diabetes mellitus
B. Obesity
C. Obstructive sleep apnea
D. Vitamin B12 toxicity
E. Menopause

**Q6.** Which of the following medications is most effective for treating neuropathic pain in small fiber neuropathy?
A. Naproxen
B. Diclofenac gel
C. Pregabalin
D. Carbamazepine
E. Mirtazapine

**Q7.** A 50-year-old woman presents with tingling and numbness in hands and feet for 6 months. She has a history of multiple syncopal episodes in the past 2 years and bilateral carpal tunnel syndrome treated with surgical release 5 years ago. On examination, macroglossia and periorbital petechiae are noted. Nerve conduction study (NCS) and electromyography (EMG) are normal. Hemoglobin A1c, fasting glucose, complete blood count (CBC), and thyroid function tests are normal. What is the most appropriate next step of investigation for this patient?
A. Serum iron level
B. Serum protein electrophoresis with immunofixation
C. Computerized tomography (CT) of the chest with contrast
D. Magnetic resonance imaging (MRI) of the cervical spine
E. Clinical observation without further investigation

**Q8.** A 68-year-old man has tingling and numbness in his hands and feet for the past 6 months. He reports dyspnea on exertion and has been diagnosed with cardiomyopathy. Cardiac magnetic resonance imaging (MRI) is pending. The patient also has a history of bilateral carpal tunnel syndromes, which were surgically released 3 years ago. Which of the following laboratory findings can confirm the diagnosis in this patient?
A. Spared sensory action potentials on nerve conduction study
B. IgE kappa monoclonal protein on serum immunofixation electrophoresis
C. Myeloid hyperplasia from bone marrow biopsy
D. Extracellular deposition of amorphous eosinophilic material on nerve biopsy
E. Restrictive cardiomyopathy on echocardiography

**Q9.** A 38-year-old man is referred to you for evaluation of neuropathy. He has numbness in both hands and neuropathic pain in both feet for 10 months. He wakes up during the night due to pain and tingling in both hands. He recently developed dyspnea on exertion and near-syncope when changing position from sitting to standing. His father had similar symptoms when he was in his 40s and passed away from a cardiac condition at 50 years of age. Fasting blood sugar (FBS), hemoglobin A1c (HbA1c), complete blood count (CBC), lipid profile, renal and liver function tests, and serum protein electrophoresis and immunofixation are all within normal limits. What is the most appropriate diagnostic test in this patient?
A. Electromyography
B. Echocardiography
C. Nerve biopsy
D. Transthyretin gene testing
E. Acid α-glucosidase activity

**Q10.** Which of the following treatments is a small-interfering RNA?
A. Nusinersen
B. Onasemnogene
C. Tafamidis
D. Patisiran
E. Casimersen

**Q11.** A 20-year-old woman presents with episodic burning pain in both feet and hands since childhood. The pain is accompanied by redness and warmth, worsened by physical activity, and more severe at night. The pain is relieved by limb elevation and applying cold packs. Examination in the office is unremarkable. What is the underlying pathophysiology of this condition?
A. Misfolded protein causing amyloid deposition in multiple organs
B. Mutation in the gene encoding α-subunit of $Na_V1.7$
C. Reduced alpha-galactosidase A enzyme
D. Inflammation of the vasa vasorum resulting in nerve infarction
E. *PMP22* duplication

**Q12.** A 20-year-old woman is referred for evaluation of intermittent burning sensation of her hands and feet for 3 years. Symptoms are triggered by exertion, especially in the summer, and include pain, burning sensation, and tightness in both hands and feet. Episodes last for 30 minutes followed by a slow spontaneous recovery. Elevating the limbs and applying cold packs can relieve the symptoms. Neurological examination in the office between episodes of pain is normal. Her mother has end-stage renal disease on hemodialysis and a history of chest pain of unknown etiology. Which of the following clinical features can be seen in this condition?
A. Angiokeratoma
B. Sicca syndrome
C. Self-mutilation
D. Neuropathic arthropathy
E. Dark reddish urine

**Q13.** A 45-year-old woman presents with absence of sweat over the right chest wall and right arm for 5 years. However, there is excessive sweating over the left side. She also reports heat intolerance for the past 2 years. Examination reveals anisocoria with the right pupil being dilated and showing a sluggish pupillary response to light. However, the pupil is strongly responsive to near vision. Motor power is grade 5 in all muscle groups, but reflexes are diffusely diminished. What is the MOST LIKELY diagnosis?
A. Neurosyphilis
B. Ross syndrome
C. Harlequin syndrome
D. Frey syndrome
E. Leprosy

## PART 2 | QUESTIONS WITH ANSWERS AND DISCUSSION

**QUESTION 1.** A 62-year-old woman with type 2 diabetes mellitus is referred for evaluation of burning feet for 3 months. Examination shows normal muscle bulk, tone, and strength. Sensory exam shows hyperesthesia in both soles, and normal pinprick, vibration, and proprioception. Reflexes are all normal. Which types of nerve fibers are most likely involved in this patient?

A. Aα and Aβ nerve fibers
B. Aα and C nerve fibers
C. Aβ and Aδ nerve fibers
D. Aβ and C nerve fibers
E. Aδ and C nerve fibers

**ANSWER:** E. Aδ and C nerve fibers

### COMMENTS AND DISCUSSION

- Nerve fibers are classified based on their size, conduction velocity and function (Fig. 20.1). There are two commonly used classifications systems:
  - The Erlanger-Gasser classification divides nerve fibers into three categories based on their diameter: A, B, and C fibers. The A fibers are further subdivided into Aα, Aβ, Aγ, and Aδ fibers. This classification applies to motor, sensory, and autonomic nerves.
  - The Lloyd classification only applies to sensory fibers. This system categorizes them into four groups based on diameter: I, II, III, and IV fibers.
  - Faster conduction velocities are observed in fibers with larger diameters, and myelinated fibers conduct faster than unmyelinated fibers.
  - C fibers are the only fiber type that is unmyelinated, and these fibers have the smallest diameters, and accordingly the slowest conduction velocities.
  - C fibers mediate slow or dull pain, warm and cold temperatures, and crude touch, as well as post-ganglionic sympathetic fibers.
  - "Small" sensory fibers include A**δ** and C fibers, which mediate pain and temperature.
  - "Large" sensory fibers include Aα and Aβ, which carry vibration and proprioception.
    - Deep pressure is received by Pacinian corpuscles. The signals generated by these receptros are then conducted through Aα and Aβ fibers, which are myelinated and have large diameters.

 **HIGH-YIELD FACT**

Aδ and C fibers convey pain sensation. Impairment of Aδ and C fibers results in small fiber neuropathies.

- Small fiber neuropathy
  - Dysfunction is limited to the small nerve fibers.
  - Small fibers = thin myelinated (Aδ) fibers + unmyelinated (C) fibers
- Thinly myelinated (Aδ) fibers
  - Moderately slow velocity (3–13 m/s)
  - Terminate as free nerve endings
  - Conduct high threshold mechanical and mechanothermal nociceptors (pressure, pricking pain, and cold)
  - Stimulation causes sharp, well-localized pain sensation.
- Unmyelinated (C) fibers
  - Very slow conduction velocity (0.6–1.2 m/s)
  - Terminates as free nerve endings
  - Conduct polymodal nociceptors (crude touch, pressure, aching pain, cold, and warmth)
  - Also serve as efferents for the autonomic system
  - Stimulation causes dull, burning or aching, and poorly localized pain.

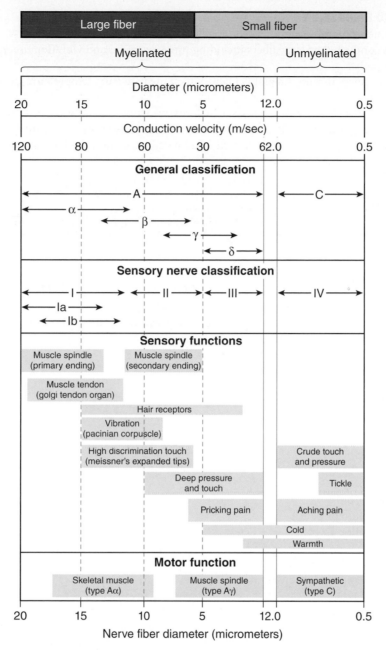

**Fig. 20.1** Nerve fiber classification based primarily on diameter. Note that types I to IV of the Llyod classification are only applicable to sensory nerves fibers. (Adapted from Hall JE, Hall ME. Sensory receptor, neuronal circuits for processing information. In: *Guyton and Hall textbook of medical physiology.* 14th ed., 2021:587–598.)

**QUESTION 2.** Which of the following symptoms or signs is the **LEAST** likely seen in a patient with a small fiber neuropathy?
A. Hyperesthesia in the soles
B. Allodynia in the dorsum of the feet
C. Decreased vibratory sense in the toes
D. Hair loss over the toes
E. Skin flushing in the feet

**ANSWER:** C. Decreased vibratory sense in the toes

## COMMENTS AND DISCUSSION

- In small fiber neuropathy, the lesion is confined to small fibers.
  - Sensations conducted by large fibers including proprioception and vibration *are spared* in small fiber neuropathy.
- "Small" sensory fibers include Aδ and C fibers, which mediate pain, temperature, and autonomic functions.
- "Large" sensory fibers include Aα and Aβ, which receive vibration and proprioception.
  - Deep pressure is received by Pacinian corpuscles. The signals generated by these receptros are then conducted through Aα and Aβ fibers, which are myelinated and have large diameters.

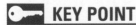 **KEY POINT**

Loss in proprioception and vibration senses is **NOT** a clinical feature of small fiber neuropathy.

**QUESTION 3.** Which of the following statements is **CORRECT** regarding small fiber neuropathy (SFN)?
  A. Clinical presentation is exclusviely a length-dependent pattern.
  B. Positive symptoms (e.g., pain, burning, or pricking sensation) are uncommon.
  C. Intolerance to the bedsheets is one common complaint.
  D. Sensory ataxia can be seen in severe cases.
  E. Autonomic function is normal in SFN.

**ANSWER:** C. Intolerance to the bedsheets is one common complaint.

## COMMENTS AND DISCUSSION

- Clinical presentation of SFN include somatic sensory and autonomic symptoms, since only sensation and autonomic fibers are supplied by small nerve fibers.
- Sensory symptoms
  - Pricking sensation
  - Burning sensation or pain
  - Shooting sensation or pain
  - Aching pain
  - Intolerance to bedsheets/socks
  - Alteration of temperature sensation
  - Pruritus
  - Cramps
  - Restless legs syndrome

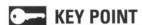 **KEY POINT**

In small fiber neuropathy (SFN), large fiber functions (e.g., vibration, proprioception senses) are COMPLETELY normal.

- Sensory deficits can present in two patterns:
  - Length-dependent (LD-SFN): symptoms begin in the toes and then ascend up, affecting at least the mid-calves before the fingertips are involved.
  - Non–length-dependent (NLD-SFN)
- Autonomic symptoms
  - Dry eyes
  - Dry mouth
  - Abnormal sweating
  - Hair loss

- ○ Altered gastrointestinal motility
- ○ Altered bladder control
- ○ Abnormal heart-rate variability
- ○ Orthostatic hypotension or tachycardia
- ○ Erectile dysfunction

**QUESTION 4.** A 30-year-old woman presents with hyperesthesia and numbness in both feet up to the ankles. The neurological examination is normal except for hyperesthesia in both soles. Nerve conduction study and needle electromyography (EMG) are completely normal. Which is the most appropriate next step in the evaluation of this patient?
A. Slow-frequency repetitive nerve stimulation
B. Repetitive nerve stimulation after 10-second exercise
C. Single-fiber EMG
D. Quantitative sudomotor axon reflex test (QSART)
E. Muscle biopsy

**ANSWER:** D. Quantitative sudomotor axon reflex test (QSART)

**COMMENTS AND DISCUSSION**
- Patients presenting with pure small-fiber sensory symptoms may have an isolated small fiber neuropathy or a classical polyneuropathy (with involvement of both small and large fibers).
- To accurately diagnose small fiber neuropathy (SFN), it is important to perform nerve conduction study to exclude any involvement of large fibers (Fig. 20.2).
- While there are no universal criteria for diagnosing small fiber neuropathy, most neurologists or neuromuscular neurologists typical rely on a combination of clinical signs and diagnostic tests as shown below. The available criteria that have been proposed are outlined in Table 20.1.

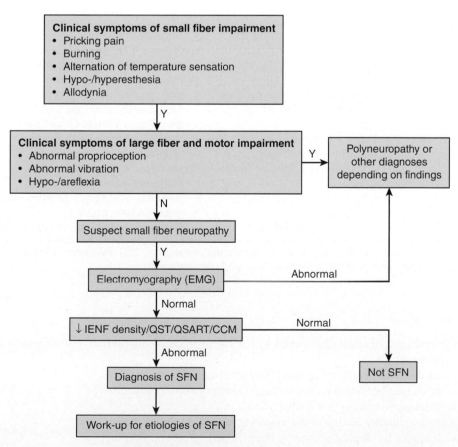

**Fig. 20.2** Making a diagnosis of SFN.

**TABLE 20.1** Available criteria of SFN used in clinical practice

|  | **NEURODIAB** |  | **Besta Criteria** |
|---|---|---|---|
| **Definite** | • Length-dependent symptoms and/or signs of small fiber damage<br>• Normal sural nerve conduction study<br>• **AND** reduced IENF density at ankle<br>• **AND/OR** abnormal QST (temperature thresholds) at foot | At least two of<br><br><br><br>**AND**<br><br>**AND** | • Clinical signs of small fiber neuropathy<br>• Abnormal QST (temperature thresholds) at foot*<br>• Reduced IENF density at distal leg<br>Absence of large fiber neuropathy signs<br>Normal NCS |
| **Probable** | • Length-dependent symptoms and/or signs of small fiber damage<br>• Normal sural nerve conduction study | N/A | N/A |
| **Possible** | Length-dependent symptoms and/ or signs of small fiber damage | N/A | N/A |

*IENF*, intraepidermal nerve fiber; *NCS*, nerve conduction study; *NEURODIAB*, Diabetic Neuropathy Study Group of the European Association of the Study of Diabetes; *QST*, quantitative sensory test.
*Several authorities substitute QST with QSART (quantitative sudomotor axon reflex test).

**TABLE 20.2** Investigations for small fiber neuropathy

| Tests | Pros | Cons |
|---|---|---|
| IENF density | • Objective measurement | • Slightly invasive<br>• Normal IENF density have been reported in some SFNs (e.g., erythromelalgia). |
| QST | • Noninvasive<br>• Evaluate both loss and gain of sensory functions | • Psychophysical test; may contain bias<br>• Time-consuming<br>• Nonspecific and cannot localize a lesion; can be peripheral or central sensory lesion |
| QSART | • Objective measurement<br>• Autonomic testing<br>• Localize to peripheral lesion | • Requires special equipment; not widely available<br>• Moderately time-consuming<br>• Requires good preparation |
| CCM | • Objective measurement<br>• Noninvasive<br>• Not time-consuming | • Available data mostly from patients with diabetic neuropathy.<br>• Requires more data in other SFNs |

*CCM*, corneal confocal microscopy; *IENF*, intraepidermal nerve fiber; *QST*, quantitative sensory test; *QSART*, quantitative sudomotor axon reflex test; *SFN*, small fiber neuropathy.

- ○ Clinical signs of small fiber deficit with a polyneuropathy distribution (either length-dependent or non–length-dependent)
  - • Examination confirming small fiber involvement
  - • No large fiber involvement on clinical history and examination
- ○ Normal nerve conduction study (NCS)
- ○ Any abnormality on one of the following tests (Table 20.2):
  - • Reduced intraepidermal nerve fiber (IENF) density on skin biopsy
  - • Quantitative sensory testing (QST)
  - • Quantitative sudomotor axon reflex test (QSART)
  - • Corneal confocal microscopy (CCM)

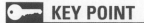 **KEY POINT**

Before making a diagnosis of SFN:
- Exclude large fiber impairment (light touch/vibration/proprioception/deep tendon reflexes should all be intact)
- Exclude motor fiber impairment
- Exclude abnormality on nerve conduction study (NCS)

**QUESTION 5.** A 50-year-old woman presents with hyperesthesia in both feet for 5 months. She reports no weakness, but cannot walk barefoot due to pain. At night she cannot sleep well due to pain when the bedsheets touched her feet. She has no known underlying diseases. Neurological examination in the office is completely normal, except for hyperesthesia of both feet. What is the **MOST LIKELY** etiology of this condition?

A. Diabetes mellitus
B. Obesity
C. Obstructive sleep apnea
D. Vitamin B12 toxicity
E. Menopause

**ANSWER:** A. Diabetes mellitus

**COMMENTS AND DISCUSSION**
- Etiology of Small Fiber Neuropathy (SFN).
  - SFN can have various etiologies, and although some have been identified (Table 20.3), a significant proportion of cases remain idiopathic.
  - The cause remains unknown in 30%–50% of all SFN cases.
  - The most common cause of SFN is diabetes (~30% of cases).

**TABLE 20.3** Etiology of small fiber neuropathy

| Primary | Secondary | Idiopathic |
|---|---|---|
| **Hereditary** | **Metabolic causes** | • Idiopathic small fiber neuropathy |
| • Na$_v$1.7 (due to *SCN9A* mutations) | • DM, IGT, rapid glycemic control | • Burning mouth syndrome |
| • Na$_v$1.8 (due to *SCN10A* mutations) | • Hypothyroidism | |
| • Fabry disease | • Hypertriglyceridemia | |
| • Familial amyloid polyneuropathy (FAP) | • Uremia | |
| • Tangier disease | • Vitamin B12 deficiency | |
| | **Infection** | |
| | • HIV | |
| | • Hepatitis C | |
| | • Influenza | |
| | • Lyme | |
| | **Toxic/drugs** | |
| | • Alcohol | |
| | • Antiretroviral drugs | |
| | • Antibiotics (metronidazole, nitrofurantoin, linezolid) | |
| | • Chemotherapy (e.g., bortezomib) | |
| | • Vitamin B6 toxicity | |
| | **Immune mediated** | |
| | • Vasculitis | |
| | • SLE | |
| | • Celiac | |
| | • Sarcoidosis | |
| | • Sjögren syndrome | |
| | • Rheumatoid arthritis | |
| | • Monoclonal gammopathy | |
| | • Primary systemic amyloidosis | |

*DM,* diabetes mellitus; *HIV,* human immunodeficiency syndrome; *IGT,* impaired glucose tolerance; *QST,* quantitative sensory test; SLE, systemic lupus erythematosus.

**QUESTION 6.** Which of the following medications is most effective for treating neuropathic pain in small fiber neuropathy?
A. Naproxen
B. Diclofenac gel
C. Pregabalin
D. Carbamazepine
E. Mirtazapine

**ANSWER:** C. Pregabalin

**COMMENTS AND DISCUSSION**
- Treatment of small fiber neuropathy (SFN) includes specific and symptomatic therapies.
- In cases with a known etiology, treatment is based on the underlying cause such as:
  - Diabetic control in cases of diabetic-related SFN
  - Removal of toxic agents in cases of toxic SFN
  - Liver transplant in cases of SFN associated with AL amyloidosis
  - Intravenous immunoglobulin (IVIG) in cases of SFN associated with Sjögren syndrome
- Symptomatic treatment
  - Aims to control pain, as well as sensory and autonomic symptoms (Table 20.4)

**TABLE 20.4** Recommendations for treatment in painful neuropathy

| Recommended Level | Medication Classes | Medication |
| --- | --- | --- |
| A | Anticonvulsants | Pregabalin |
| B | Anticonvulsants | Gabapentin |
| | | Sodium valproate |
| | Selective serotonin and norepinephrine reuptake inhibitors (SNRIs) | Venlafaxine |
| | | Duloxetine |
| | Tricyclic antidepressants | Amitriptyline |
| | Antitussives | Dextromethrophan |
| | Narcotics | Morphine sulphate |
| | | Tramadol |
| | | Oxycodone |
| | Tropical analgesics | Capsaicin cream |
| | | Lidoderm patch |
| | Tropical nitrates | Isosorbide dinitrate spray |
| | Neuromodulation therapy | Percutaneous electrical nerve stimulation |

**QUESTION 7.** A 50-year-old woman presents with tingling and numbness in hands and feet for 6 months. She has a history of multiple syncopal episodes in the past 2 years and bilateral carpal tunnel syndrome treated with surgical release 5 years ago. On examination, macroglossia and periorbital petechiae are noted. Nerve conduction study (NCS) and electromyography (EMG) are normal. Hemoglobin A1c, fasting glucose, complete blood count (CBC), and thyroid function tests are normal. What is the most appropriate next step of investigation for this patient?
A. Serum iron level
B. Serum protein electrophoresis with immunofixation
C. Computerized tomography (CT) of the chest with contrast
D. Magnetic resonance imaging (MRI) of the cervical spine
E. Clinical observation without further investigation

**ANSWER:** B. Serum protein electrophoresis with immunofixation

## COMMENTS AND DISCUSSION

- This patient presents with symptoms consistent with possible acquired amyloidosis including small fiber neuropathy and bilateral carpal tunnel syndromes.
- Amyloidosis is a heterogeneous group of disorders with a wide spectrum of clinical manifestations.
- Amyoloidosis is caused by misfolding of proteins, which become insoluble and deposit in tissues.
- Amyloidosis can involve multiple organs.
- There are inherited and acquired forms of amyloidosis.
  - Acquired forms of amyloid neuropathy include:
    - Primary systemic AL amyloidosis:
      - Extensive misfolded free light chains produced in plasma cell dyscrasias or B-cell lymphoproliferative disorders
      - Light chain fibrils deposit in tissues.
      - Seventeen percent of patients with AL amyloidosis have peripheral neuropathy.
      - Initial symptoms include small fiber neuropathy and/or carpal tunnel syndrome.
      - Small fiber neuropathy can then progresses to sensorimotor axonal polyneuropathy
      - Secondary demyelination can be seen.
      - Autonomic involvement is also commonly seen.
    - Primary systemic AL amyloidosis can also involve other major organs including heart (cardiomyopathy), liver (hepatomegaly), kidney (proteinuria), and soft tissue (macroglossia).
    - Diagnosis
      - Monoclonal gammopathy is an important diagnostic clue.
      - Both serum protein electrophoresis (quantitative) with immunofixation (to identify an immunoglobulin subtype) are required.
      - Definite diagnosis is based on a finding from biopsy.
        - Evidence of amyloid deposition in tissue **OR**
        - Presence of lambda or kappa light chains on immunohistochemical staining

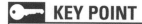 **KEY POINT**

> *AL amyloidosis* = Small fiber neuropathy (including autonomic failure) + Carpal tunnel syndrome + Cardiomyopathy

- Other causes of acquired amyloidosis
  - Reactive AA amyloidosis: rarely involved in the neurological system
  - β2-Microglobulin amyloidosis: associated with autonomic neuropathy
  - Senile systemic amyloidosis: commonly associated with carpal tunnel syndrome

**QUESTION 8.** A 68-year-old man has tingling and numbness in his hands and feet for 6 months. He reports dyspnea on exertion and has been diagnosed with cardiomyopathy. Cardiac magnetic resonance imaging (MRI) is pending. The patient also has a history of bilateral carpal tunnel syndromes, which was surgically released 3 years ago. Which of the following laboratory findings can confirm the diagnosis in this patient?

A. Spared sensory action potentials on nerve conduction study
B. IgE kappa monoclonal protein on serum immunofixation electrophoresis
C. Myeloid hyperplasia from bone marrow biopsy
D. Extracellular deposition of amorphous eosinophilic material on nerve biopsy
E. Restrictive cardiomyopathy on echocardiography

**ANSWER:** D. Extracellular deposition of amorphous eosinophilic material on nerve biopsy

## COMMENTS AND DISCUSSION

- Diagnosis of *primary AL amyloidosis*
  - Monoclonal gammopathy is an important diagnostic clue.
  - Both serum protein electrophoresis (quantitative) with immunofixation (to identify an immunoglobulin [Ig] subtype) are required.

- IgG lambda (λ) or IgA λ paraprotein is more common than IgG kappa (κ) or IgA κ.
- Sensorimotor axonal polyneuropathy is the most common polyneuropathy in primary AL amyloidosis.
  - Can have secondary demyelination mimicking chronic inflammatory demyelinating polyneuropathy (CIDP)
  - Pure small fiber involvement can be an early presentation.
- Confirmation of cardiac involvement on:
  - Electrocardiography
    - Diffusely low voltages
  - Echocardiography
    - Restrictive cardiomyopathy
    - Left ventricular thickening
    - Presence of the above abnormalities in the absence of aortic valve diseases or significant systemic hypertension
  - Cardiovascular magnetic resonance imaging
    - Subendocardial and/or transmural late gadolinium enhancement
- Definite diagnosis is based on histopathologic findings in various tissues such as abdominal fat pad, nerve, muscle, rectum and bone marrow
  - Extracellular deposition of amyloid in tissue, which is characterized by an amorphous eosinophilic material with a salmon-pink color on Congo red staining and apple-green birefringence under polarized light) OR
  - Presence of λ or κ light chains on immunohistochemical staining

**QUESTION 9.** A 38-year-old man is referred to you for evaluation of neuropathy. He has numbness in both hands and neuropathic pain in both feet for 10 months. He wakes up during the night due to pain and tingling in both hands. He recently developed dyspnea on exertion and near-syncope when changing position from sitting to standing. His father had similar symptoms when he was in his 40s and passed away from a cardiac condition at 50 years of age. Fasting blood sugar (FBS), hemoglobin A1c (HbA1c), complete blood count (CBC), lipid profile, renal and liver function tests, and serum protein electrophoresis and immunofixation are all within normal limits. What is the most appropriate diagnostic test in this patient?

A. Electromyography
B. Echocardiography
C. Nerve biopsy
D. Transthyretin gene testing
E. Acid α-glucosidase activity

**ANSWER:** D. Transthyretin gene testing

## COMMENTS AND DISCUSSION

- This patient most likely has a hereditary form of amyloid neuropathy (aka familial amyloid polyneuropathy [FAP]), which is most commonly caused by transthyretin amyloidosis (TTR amyloidosis or ATTR).
- *Transthyretin amyloidosis*
  - The most common cause of FAP
  - Autosomal dominant
  - Transthyretin gene (*TTR*) is located on chromosome 18.
  - The most common *TTR* mutation worldwide is Val30Met (substitution of methionine for valine at position 30).
  - In the United States, Val122Ile mutation (substitution of isoleucin for valine at position 122) is the most common.
  - Neurological features
    - Carpal tunnel syndrome is a common and early presentation
    - Small fiber neuropathy usually precedes sensorimotor axonal polyneuropathy. The symptoms of small fiber neuropathy include pins-and-needles sensation, burning pain or sensation, and allodynia.

- When large fibers are affected, severe sensory loss and distal muscle weakness commonly occur.
  - Autonomic dysfunction is common, affecting:
    - Cardiovascular system: orthostatic hypotension
    - Genitourinary system: urinary retention or incontinence, sexual dysfunction
    - Gastrointestinal system: postprandial diarrhea, constipation, gastroparesis
- Apolipoprotein A1-related FAP
  - Relatively rare
  - Can manifest as a length-dependent polyneuropathy
- Gelsolin-related FAP
  - Rare
  - Clinical presentation includes:
    - Corneal lattice dystrophy
    - Progressive cranial neuropathies, commonly facial and trigeminal neuropathies
    - Cutis laxa

**QUESTION 10.** Which of the following treatments is a small-interfering RNA?
  A. Nusinersen
  B. Onasemnogene
  C. Tafamidis
  D. Patisiran
  E. Casimersen

**ANSWER:** D. Patisiran

**COMMENTS AND DISCUSSION**
- Treatment in transthyretin amyloidosis includes disease-modifying therapies (Fig. 20.3), liver transplantation, and symptomatic treatment.

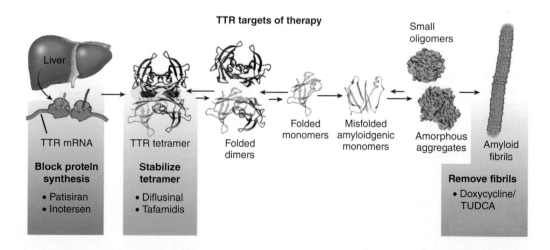

**Fig. 20.3** Targets of disease-modifying therapies in transthyretin amyloidosis (ATTR). The aims are to reduce circulating transthyretin (TTR) protein and to slow down the organ damage or progression of the disease. TTR silencers inhibit TTR synthesis by silencing the *TTR* gene, such as by promoting degradation of *TTR* mRNA. Inortersen is an anti-sense oligonucleotide (ASO), while patisiran is a small interfering RNA (siRNA). TTR stabilizers stabilize TTR tetramers. Medications in this group include diflunisal and tafamidis. Patisiran, inotersen, and tafamidis have been approved by the US Food and Drug Administration (FDA). A combination of doxycycline and tauroursodeoxycholic acid can disrupt existing TTR amyloid fibrils, but has not been approved by the US FDA. *TTR*, Transthyretin; *TUDCA*, tauroursodeoxycholic acid. Adapted from Ruberg FL, Grogan M, Hanna M, Kelly JW, Maurer MS. Transthyretin amyloid cardiomyopathy: JACC State-of-the-Art Review. *J Am Coll Cardiol.* 2019;73(22):2872–2891.

- Disease-modifying therapies include transthyretin (TTR) stabilizers and TTR silencers.
  - TTR stabilizers prevents misfolding of mutant TTR proteins and include:
    - Diflunisal
      - Non-steroidal anti-inflammatory drug (NSAID) that binds to thyroxine (T4) binding sites of tetrameric TTR
      - Stabilizes TTR and decreases fibril formation
    - Tafamidis
      - Thyroxine-like small ligand inhibitor
      - Stabilizes mutant TTR tetramers
  - TTR silencers inhibits the production of TTR proteins in the liver. TTR silencers include:
    - Inotersen
      - Anti-sense oligonucleotide (ASO) that prevents translation of the TTR protein
    - Patisiran
      - Small interfering RNA (siRNA) that inhibits TTR synthesis in the liver
- Liver transplantation
  - Liver is a major site of amyloid production.
  - Liver transplantation is a treatment that removes the main source of TTR production.
- Symptomatic treatment include the management of symptoms related to peripheral and autonomic neuropathies.
- Nusinersen is an ASO that facilitates the integration of exon 7 into the mRNA and thereby enhances full-length SMN protein levels in patients with genetically confirmed spinal muscular atrophy.
- Onasemnogene is an adeno-associated virus (AAV) vector-based gene therapy that delivers a fully functional copy of the human *SMN* gene into the target motor neuron cells. It is indicated in children younger than 2 years of age with genetically confirmed spinal muscular atrophy.
- Casimersen is an ASO that is indicated for the treatment of patients with Duchenne muscular dystrophy (DMD) who have a mutation in the *DMD* gene that is amenable to exon 45 skipping.

**QUESTION 11.**  A 20-year-old woman presents with episodic burning pain in both feet and hands since childhood. The pain is accompanied by redness and warmth, worsened by physical activity, and more severe at night. The pain is relieved by limb elevation and applying cold packs. Examination in the office is unremarkable. What is the underlying pathophysiology of this condition?

A. Misfolded protein causing amyloid deposition in multiple organs
B. Mutation in the gene encoding $\alpha$-subunit of $Na_V1.7$
C. Reduced alpha-galactosidase A enzyme
D. Inflammation of the vasa vasorum resulting in nerve infarction
E. *PMP22* duplication

**ANSWER:** B. Mutation in the gene encoding $\alpha$-subunit of $Na_V1.7$

**COMMENTS AND DISCUSSION**
- This patient most likely has *primary erythromelalgia*, an inherited pain disorder.
- Inherited pain disorders include primary erythromelalgia and other less-common episodic pain syndromes.
- Primary erythromelalgia
  - Genetic form of erythromelalgia
  - Episodic symptoms of the clinical triad of:
    - Redness
    - Warmth
    - Burning pain
  - Most commonly affects the feet and less commonly the hands
  - Usually bilateral
  - Onset in the first two decades of life
  - Aggravating factors
    - Exercise
    - Warm climates
    - Standing
    - Wearing tight shoes or garment
    - Nighttime

- ○ Relieving factors
  - Cooling (fans, ice pack)
  - Elevating the affected limb
- ○ Diagnosis
  - Genetic testing to identify mutations in the *SCN9A* gene which encodes the voltage-gated sodium channel $Na_V1.7$
  - Mutations responsible for primary erythromelalgia lower the activation threshold of $Na_V1.7$, leading to increased neuronal excitability and pain.
  - Secondary erythromelalgia (e.g., myeloproliferative disorders, systemic lupus erythematosus [SLE]) should be excluded.
- Other inherited pain disorders include:
  - ○ Paroxysmal extreme pain disorder (PEPD)
    - Characterized by paroxysmal attacks of pain in the lower body (e.g., rectum), eye, and jaw
    - Mutations in the *SCN9A* gene that impair inactivation of the sodium channel $Na_V1.7$, resulting prolonged action potentials
  - ○ Familial episodic pain syndrome types 1, 2 and 3
    - Episodes of severe upper body pain (type 1), distal lower limb pain (type 2), and lower and sometimes upper body pain (type 3)
    - Onset in infancy (type 1), adulthood (type 2), or childhood (type 3)
    - Triggered by fasting, fatigue, exercise, or cold temperatures
    - Autosomal dominant inheritance
    - Caused by mutations in the *TRPA1* gene (type 1), *SCN10A* gene (type 2), and *SCN11A* gene (type 3)
- Misfolded protein causing amyloid deposition in multiple organs is the pathophysiology of amyloidosis.
- Reduction in alpha-galactosidase A enzyme occurs in Fabry disease.
- Inflammation of the vasa vasorum resulting in nerve infarction is the pathophysiology of vasculitic neuropathy.
- *PMP22* duplication is the cause of Charcot-Marie-Tooth disease type 1A.

**QUESTION 12.** A 20-year-old man is referred for evaluation of intermittent burning sensation of his hands and feet for 3 years. Symptoms are triggered by exertion, especially in the summer, and include pain, burning sensation, and tightness in both hands and feet. Episodes last for 30 minutes followed by a slow spontaneous recovery. Elevating the limbs and applying cold packs can relieve the symptoms. Neruological examination in the office between episodes of pain is normal. His mother has end-stage renal disease on hemodialysis and a history of chest pain of unknown etiology. Which of the following clinical features can be seen in this condition?
A. Angiokeratoma
B. Sicca syndrome
C. Self-mutilation
D. Neuropathic arthropathy
E. Dark reddish urine

**ANSWER:** A. Angiokeratoma

**COMMENTS AND DISCUSSION**
- The most likely diagnosis in this patient most is *Fabry disease.*
- Fabry disease is an X-linked recessive lysosomal storage disorder
- Despite being an X-linked recessive disorder, heterozygous females can also be affected.
- Fabry disease is caused by mutations in the *GLA* gene, which encodes the α-galactosidase A enzyme.
- Mutations result in the accumulation of glycolipids, particularly globotriaosylceramide (GL-3 or Gb3), leading to cellular dysfunction and tissue damage.
- Clinical presentation
  - ○ Acroparesthesia: chronic pain and episodic severe pain (or Fabry's cries)
  - ○ Hypohidrosis
  - ○ Angiokeratomas (Fig. 20.4).

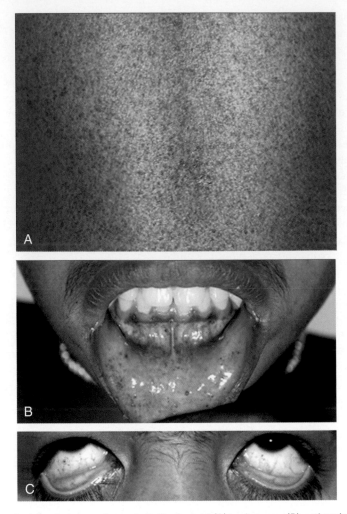

**Fig. 20.4** Angiokeratoma. Angiokeratomas are demonstrated in the back (A), oral mucosa (B), and conjunctivae (C) in a patient with Fabry's disease. From Sethuraman G, Chouhan K, Kaushal S, Sharma VK. Fabry's disease. *Lancet.* 2011;378(9798):1254.

- ○ Gastrointestinal disturbances
  - ○ Early-onset end-stage renal disease (ESRD)
  - ○ Cardiomyopathy and strokes at an early age
  - ○ Hearing loss
  - ○ Cornea verticillata (corneal opacity)
- Laboratory investigations
  - ○ Activity of enzyme α-galactosidase A in plasma, isolated leukocytes or cultured cells
  - ○ Genetic testing for mutations in the *GLA* gene
- Treatment
  - ○ Enzyme replacement therapy (ERT), either agalsidase alfa or agalsidase beta
  - ○ Supportive treatment
- Sicca syndrome is a manifestation of Sjögren syndrome.
- Self-mutilation can occur in children with congenital sensory neuropathy and psychological disorders.
- Neuropathic arthropathy, aka Charcot joint, occurs in severe chronic ganglionopathy, large fiber sensory polyneuropathy, and tabes dorsalis.
- Dark reddish urine follows rhabdomyolysis and metabolic myopathy.

**QUESTION 13.** A 45-year-old woman presents with absence of sweat over the right chest wall and right arm for 5 years. However, there is excessive sweating over the left side. She also reports heat intolerance for the past 2 years. Examination reveals anisocoria with the right pupil being dilated and showing a sluggish pupillary response to light. However, the pupil is strongly responsive to near vision. Motor power is grade 5 in all muscle groups, but reflexes are diffusely diminished. What is the **MOST LIKELY** diagnosis?

A. Neurosyphilis
B. Ross syndrome
C. Harlequin syndrome
D. Frey syndrome
E. Leprosy

**ANSWER:** B. Ross syndrome

**COMMENTS AND DISCUSSION**

- Ross syndrome is a rare entity characterized by segmental or patchy anhidrosis, tonic pupils, and areflexia.
- Etiology remains unknown.
- Triad of Ross syndrome includes:
  - Tonic pupils. This is due to parasympathetic denervation. There is light near dissociation: pupillary constriction to light is impaired, while pupillary constriction to accommodation is relatively preserved.
  - Hyporeflexia and areflexia
  - Segmental anhidrosis
- Due to segmental anhidrosis
  - Excessive sweating can be seen on the contralateral side.
  - Patients often have heat intolerance.
- Disorders that may be in the same spectrum as Ross syndrome include:
  - Holmes-Adie syndrome (tonic pupils and hyporeflexia without anhidrosis)
  - Harlequin syndrome (segmental hypohidrosis without pupillary abnormalities)
- Frey syndrome is a rare neurological disorder that causes excessive sweating (hyperhidrosis) on the cheek, temple, or behind the ear, while eating or thinking about food (gustatory sweating). It most often occurs as a complication of surgeries involving the parotid gland, but may follow neck dissection, facelift procedures, or trauma to the area near the parotid gland.
- Leprosy causes segmental sensory loss with hypohidrosis, whereas neurosyphilis does not cause hyperhidrosis or hypohidrosis.

## SUGGESTED READINGS

Bril V, England J, Franklin GM, et al. Evidence-based guideline: treatment of painful diabetic neuropathy: report of the American Academy of Neurology, the American Association of Neuromuscular and Electrodiagnostic Medicine, and the American Academy of Physical Medicine and Rehabilitation. *Neurology*. 2011;76(20):1758-1765. Erratum in: *Neurology*. 2011;77(6):603. Dosage error in article text. PMID: 21482920; PMCID: PMC3100130.

Chan AC, Wilder-Smith EP. Small fiber neuropathy: getting bigger! *Muscle Nerve*. 2016;53(5):671-682.

Devigili G, Tugnoli V, Penza P, et al. The diagnostic criteria for small fibre neuropathy: From symptoms to neuropathology. *Brain*. 2008;131(Pt 7):1912-1925.

Farhad K. Current diagnosis and treatment of painful small fiber neuropathy. *Curr Neurol Neurosci Rep*. 2019;19(12):103.

Hoy SM. Patisiran: first global approval. *Drugs*. 2018;78(15):1625-1631.

Jha SK, Karna B, Goodman MB. Erythromelalgia. [Updated 2022 Jan 17]. In: *StatPearls* [Internet]. Treasure Island (FL): StatPearls Publishing; 2022 Jan.

Kaku M, Berk JL. Neuropathy associated with systemic amyloidosis. *Semin Neurol*. 2019;39(5):578-588.

Katirji B. Disorders of peripheral nerves. In: Jankovic J, Mazziotta JC, Pomeroy SL, Newman NJ, eds. *Bradley and Daroff's Neurology in Clinical Practice*. 8th ed. Philadelphia: Elsevier; 2022, Chap 106.

McArthur JC. Painful small fiber neuropathies. *Continuum (Minneap Minn)*. 2012;18(1):106-125.

Müller ML, Butler J, Heidecker B. Emerging therapies in transthyretin amyloidosis—A new wave of hope after years of stagnancy? *Eur J Heart Fail.* 2020;22:39-53.

Nolano M, Provitera V, Perretti A, et al. Ross syndrome: a rare or a misknown disorder of thermoregulation? A skin innervation study on 12 subjects. *Brain.* 2006;129(Pt 8):2119-2131.

Ranieri M, Bedini G, Parati EA, Bersano A. Fabry disease: recognition, diagnosis, and treatment of neurological features. *Curr Treat Options Neurol.* 2016;18(7):33.

Shin SC, Robinson-Papp J. Amyloid neuropathies. *Mt Sinai J Med.* 2012;79(6):733-748.

Terkelsen AJ, Karlsson P, Lauria G, et al. The diagnostic challenge of small fibre neuropathy: clinical presentations, evaluations, and causes. *Lancet Neurol.* 2017;16(11):934-944. doi:10.1016/S1474-4422(17)30329-0. Erratum in: *Lancet Neurol.* 2017 Dec;16(12):954. PMID: 29029847.

Tesfaye S, Boulton AJ, Dyck PJ, et al. Diabetic neuropathies: Update on definitions, diagnostic criteria, estimation of severity, and treatments. *Diabetes Care.* 2010;33(12):2285-2293.

Themistocleous AC, Ramirez JD, Serra J, Bennett DL. The clinical approach to small fibre neuropathy and painful channelopathy. *Pract Neurol.* 2014;14(6):368-379.

Zhou Lan Small Fiber Neuropathy. Semin Neurol. 2019;39(5):570–577.

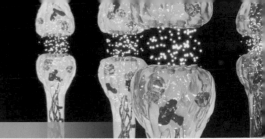

# CHAPTER 21

# Miscellaneous Topics in Neuromuscular Diseases

## REHABILITATION IN NEUROMUSCULAR DISEASES

**Q1.** Which type of exercises is most appropriate for patients with neuromuscular disease?
A. Bicycling at a slow rate
B. Vigorous aerobic dancing
C. Moderate-intensity eccentric strengthening
D. High-intensity concentric strengthening
E. None, since exercise is harmful and increases muscle damage

**Q2.** Which of the following statements is **CORRECT** regarding exercise in McArdle disease?
A. Exercise is contraindicated due to the risk of post-exercise rhabdomyolysis.
B. A patient should start with moderate-intensity aerobic exercise and increase as tolerated.
C. When a patient develops a second wind phenomenon, exercise should be stopped.
D. A patient should start with high-intensity exercise to avoid painful cramps and weakness.
E. There are no exercise limitations.

**Q3.** Which of the following statements is **CORRECT** regarding rehabilitation in amyotrophic lateral sclerosis (ALS)?
A. High-intensity exercise can improve motor power in end-stage ALS.
B. Eccentric exercise is recommended in weakened muscles.
C. Ankle-foot orthoses (AFOs) can improve gait in ALS patients with foot drop.
D. Pain does not occur in ALS because it is a pure motor syndrome.
E. No rehabilitation options are useful in ALS.

**Q4.** A 60-year-old man with amyotrophic lateral sclerosis (ALS) presented to the emergency department (ED) after a fall. His symptoms started in the right lower extremity 8 months ago. He has had right foot drop, and recently weakness of the right hand. Today, he fell after tripping over the office floor with his right foot. Which of the following are two factors that increase the risk of falls in patients with ALS?
A. Spasticity and weakness of ankle dorsiflexion
B. Fatigue and dysarthria
C. Pseudobulbar affect and disinhibition
D. Ankle-foot orthoses and cane
E. Fasciculations and cramps

**Q5.** A 62-year-old woman presents with a 6-month history of spasticity in both legs, and is diagnosed with primary lateral sclerosis. She has recently experienced multiple falls, and reports discomfort while using the walker due to backward falls. Which of the following statements is **CORRECT**?
A. While functional falls and weakness are concerns, spasticity without weakness does not cause falls.
B. Maintaining the patient on their feet using a cane or walker can prolong ambulation.
C. At least 10 falls per month is needed to be eligible for a power wheelchair.
D. Medicare eligibility for a power wheelchair requires its use to complete basic activities of daily living (ADLs) inside the house.
E. Without weakness, the patient is not Medicare eligible for a power wheelchair.

**Q6.** Which of the following factors is associated with an increased risk of complicatoins after percutaneous endoscopic gastrostomy (PEG) placement in patients with amyotrophic lateral sclerosis (ALS)?
- A. Neck flexor weakness
- B. Anarthria
- C. Tongue atrophy
- D. Forced vital capacity (FVC) <50%
- E. None of the above

**Q7.** A 55-year-old man presents to the neuromuscular clinic with a 3-year history of lower extremity weakness. He reports difficulty moving the left thigh while walking, resulting in near falls. He has also weakness of his grip in the past year. Examination demonstrates atrophy and severe weakness of the quadriceps and forearm flexors, worse on the left. What is the recommended treatment for this patient at this time?
- A. Prednisolone
- B. IVIG (intravenous immunoglobulin)
- C. Rituximab
- D. Power scooter
- E. Left knee-ankle-foot orthoses

**Q8.** A 55-year-old man with inclusion body myositis presents with foot drop and knee buckling. Which of the following equipment is the most beneficial in this case?
- A. Plastic posterior leaf spring (PLS) ankle-foot orthoses
- B. Floor reaction orthoses
- C. Non-ambulatory ankle-foot-orthoses
- D. Axillary crutch
- E. Ankle brace

**Q9.** Your patient with neck extensor myopathy is experiencing worsening head drop, and asks for a recommendation to improve this symptom. What is the **BEST** course of action?
- A. Refer him to orthopedics for cervical posterior fusion
- B. Recommend a baseball cap orthosis to keep the head up
- C. Recommend a thoracic-lumbar-sacral orthosis (TLSO) to support the neck
- D. Inject botulinum toxin to the neck flexors to improve balance of the neck muscles
- E. Reassure that there is no evidence-based treatment for head drop syndrome

## ETHICS IN NEUROMUSCULAR DISEASES

**Q10.** Your colleague asks you for the electromyography (EMG) result of his neighbor because his wife wants to know the diagnosis. Your colleague is not involved professionally in this patient's care. Which of the following statements is **CORRECT**?
- A. Because your colleague is also a medical staff, the EMG result can be shared.
- B. Without the patient's permission, all personal medical information is confidential.
- C. You can discuss the case in the physician lounge, so your colleague can hear the result.
- D. You can only share information with the patient's wife, since she is the person who wants to know the result.
- E. You cannot share data verbally, but you can fax the report to your colleague.

**Q11.** A 75-year-old woman with end-stage amyotrophic lateral sclerosis (ALS) appears fatigued and is using her accessory muscles for breathing. Her vital signs show a blood pressure (BP) of 100/70 mm Hg, a pulse of 105 bpm, and a respiratory rate of 26 per minute. During a previous clinic visit, you discussed with her issues related to advanced life support, and she expressed her lack of interest in any assisted mechanical ventilation. What is the most appropriate next step?
- A. Respect her previous discussion and consult palliative care
- B. Wait until she becomes confused and ask permission from her relatives to initiate assisted ventilation
- C. Start a morphine intravenous (IV) drip
- D. Refer her to the emergency department for intubation as she is at risk for respiratory collapse
- E. Send her home without any new management

**Q12.** While you are busy performing needle electromyography (EMG) on a patient in the lab, your technologist informs you that another patient, who arrived later and is waiting for needle EMG in the other room, is complaining and wants to have the test done now. What is the most appropriate next step?
- A. Have a neurology resident perform the needle EMG instead of you
- B. Have the patient leave without the needle EMG
- C. Stop the needle EMG of the current patient even though there are three more muscles to be tested
- D. Inform the patient that you are performing the test on another patient who arrived earlier, and that you will be with him for the needle EMG as soon as possible
- E. Call the referring physician to discuss cancelling the test due to patient's inability to wait

**Q13.** A primary care physician refers a 35-year-old woman with right arm weakness to the electromyography (EMG) lab to rule out cervical radiculopathy. Upon pretest evaluation, the patient reports that weakness has recently progressed to the left arm. Examination reveals atrophy of the right arm and a "split hand" pattern of weakness and atrophy on the left. She has hyperreflexia throughout. She states that her grandfather passed away from Lou Gehrig's disease and hopes that she does not have the same. The EMG shows widespread denervation and reinnervation in both upper extremities and the thoracic paraspinal muscles. What is the best next step?

A. Make an appointment for her in your amyotrophic lateral sclerosis (ALS) clinic

B. Contact the referring physician about the result and recommend patient referral to the neuromuscular clinic

C. Refer the patient to another neuromuscular colleague

D. Send blood for genetic ALS testing

E. Suggest the patient to change her primary care physician, since the diagnosis of ALS is missed.

**Q14.** A 25-year-old woman is referred to the electromyography (EMG) lab to confirm a diagnosis of myasthenia gravis. Before starting the test, you notice that the patient is dysarthric and short of breath. She states that 5 days prior she developed a urinary tract infection, and has been taking antibiotics. Two days prior, she developed weakness of the neck, head drop, and difficulty breathing, especially when lying flat, and difficulty swallowing with food getting stuck in her throat. You are concerned that she is developing a myasthenic crisis. You try to contact her referring and primary care physician, but are unable to reach them. What is the best next step?

A. Send the patient home and recommend her to contact the referring/primary physician

B. Continue the test and then send the result to the referring physician

C. Discontinue the test and start the patient on pyridostigmine and prednisone

D. Complete the test and start the patient on pyridostigmine and prednisone

E. Send the patient to the emergency department

---

# PART 2 | QUESTIONS WITH ANSWERS AND DISCUSSION

## REHABILITATION IN NEUROMUSCULAR DISEASES

**QUESTION 1.** Which type of exercises is most appropriate for patients with neuromuscular disease?

A. Bicycling at a slow rate

B. Vigorous aerobic dancing

C. Moderate-intensity eccentric strengthening

D. High-intensity concentric strengthening

E. None, since exercise is harmful and increases muscle damage

**ANSWER:** A. Bicycling at a slow rate

## COMMENTS AND DISCUSSION

- Goals of rehabilitation of neuromuscular disorders (NMDs) are to:
  - Assist patients in maximizing function and quality of life
  - Help patients reach their full potential despite disability
- *Eight general aspects of rehabilitation in NMDs.* In every NMD, there are eight main aspects of rehabilitation that depend on the level of deficits and stage of the disease:
  1. Exercise
  2. Fall assessment and lower extremity orthoses
  3. Adaptive equipment for activities of daily living and upper extremity orthoses
  4. Musculoskeletal symptoms
  5. Transfers
  6. Assistive devices for ambulation
  7. Articulation, swallowing, and nutrition
  8. Environmental modification and safety
- Exercise
  - To maintain and improve strength, increase endurance, and improve function
  - Strength training
    - Progressive resistance exercise
    - To maintain existing strength or reduce progression of weakness

- Mild-and-moderate-intensity exercises show benefits in NMDs.
- Avoid high resistance or high-intensity excercises as they can cause muscle overload and damage
- Avoid eccentric contractions (muscles contractions in a lengthened state) due to possibility of muscle damage
- Avoid exercises that trigger cramping or fatigue
  o Aerobic exercise
   - Improve endurance and reduce fatigue
   - **Submaximal** workloads (e.g., brisk walking, water aerobics, slow bicycling) are recommended.
   - Targeted heart rate is 50%–70% of maximum heart rate (moderate-intensity exercise).
   - **Avoid** aerobic exercises that cause significant dyspnea.

## 🔑 KEY POINT

> In patients with neuromuscular diseases:
> - Moderate-intensity aerobic exercise → increases endurance
> - Moderate-intensity concentric strengthening exercise → maintains strength
> - AVOID vigorous or high-intensity exercise
> - AVOID eccentric strengthening exercises

**QUESTION 2.** Which of the following statements is **CORRECT** regarding exercise in McArdle disease?
  A. Exercise is contraindicated due to the risk of post-exercise rhabdomyolysis.
  B. A patient should start with moderate-intensity aerobic exercise and increase as tolerated.
  C. When a patient develops a second wind phenomenon, exercise should be stopped.
  D. A patient should start with high-intensity exercise to avoid painful cramps and weakness.
  E. There are no exercise limitations.

**ANSWER:** B. A patient should start with moderate-intensity aerobic exercise and increase as tolerated.

### COMMENTS AND DISCUSSION
- McArdle disease (glycogen storage disease type V) is a metabolic disease caused by the absence of muscle glycogen phosphorylase (see also comments and discussion Question 52 in Chapter 18)
- The muscle glycogen phosphorylase is necessary for the breakdown of glucogen into glucose, which is then used to produce energy during exercise. Without this enzyme, the muscle cannot break down glycogen, leading to an accumulation of glycogen in the muscle and a decreased ability to produce energy during exercise.
- Clinical presentation of McArdle disease
  o Physical activity or exercise intolerance
  o Painful muscle cramps
  o Weakness
  o Fatigue
  o High-intensity exercise can cause severe muscle damage and can result in rhabdomyolysis.
  o Second wind phenomenon is a unique characteristic of McArdle disease, in which symptoms improve after 10 minutes of gentle aerobic activity.
- Moderate-intensity aerobic exercise in McArdle disease can improve exercise capacity.
- Gentle exercise should be preceded by a warm-up period of 5-10 minutes. This is to:
  o Promote second-wind phenomenon
  o Increase exercise capacity

## 🔑 KEY POINT

> Although exercise can worsen symptoms or trigger rhabdomyolysis in metabolic myopathies, moderate-intensity exercise can improve motor function.

**QUESTION 3.** Which of the following statements is **CORRECT** regarding rehabilitation in amyotrophic lateral sclerosis (ALS)?
  A. High-intensity exercise can improve motor power in end-stage ALS.
  B. Eccentric exercise is recommended in weakened muscles.
  C. Ankle-foot orthoses (AFOs) can improve gait in ALS patients with foot drop.

    D. Pain does not occur in ALS because it is a pure motor syndrome.

    E. No rehabilitation options are useful in ALS.

**ANSWER:** C. Ankle-foot orthoses (AFOs) can improve gait in ALS patients with foot drop.

## COMMENTS AND DISCUSSION

- Rehabilitation in amyotrophic lateral sclerosis (ALS)
  - Multidisciplinary care including rehabilitation can improve quality of life in patients with ALS.
  - Rehabilitation strategies in ALS should take into account the stage of the disease.
- The general aspects of rehabilitation in neuromuscular diseases apply to ALS.
  1. Exercise
  2. Fall assessment and lower extremity orthoses
  3. Adaptive equipment for activities of daily living and upper extremity orthoses
  4. Management of musculoskeletal symptoms
  5. Transfers
  6. Assistive devices for ambulation
  7. Management of dysphagia and dysarthria
  8. Palliative care
- However, these rehabilitation aspects differ in various stages of ALS.
  - **Aspects in early-stage ALS**
    - Exercise
    - Fall assessment and lower extremity orthoses (if disease starts in the lower extremity)
    - Adaptive equipment for activities of daily living and upper extremity orthoses (if disease starts in the upper extremity)
    - Management of musculoskeletal symptoms
  - **Aspects in middle- and end-stage ALS**
    - Transfers
    - Assistive devices for ambulation
    - Management of dysphagia and dysarthria
- *Exercise*
  - To maintain and improve strength, increase endurance, and improve function
  - Strength training
    - Progressive resistance exercise
    - To maintain existing strength or reduce progression of weakness
    - Mild-and-moderate intensity exercises show benefits in neuromuscular diseases.
    - Avoid high-resistance or high-intensity exercises because they cause muscle overload and damage
    - Avoid eccentric contractions (contractions in a lengthened state) due to the possibility of muscle damage
    - Avoid exercise that trigger cramping or fatigue
  - Aerobic exercise
    - Increase endurance and reduce fatigue
    - Submaximal workload (e.g., brisk walking, water aerobics, slow bicycling) is recommended.
    - Targeted heart rate is 50% to 70% of maximum heart rate (moderate-intensity exercise).
    - Avoid aerobic exercises that cause significant dyspnea
- *Fall assessment and lower extremity orthoses*
  - In patients with lower limb involvement, foot drop is very common.
  - Foot-drop patients compensate with circumduction and hip-hiking gait (elevation of an ipsilateral hip or pelvis during the swing phase to achieve foot clearance), which can increase the risk of falls.
    - Ankle-foot orthoses (AFOs) can help keep the ankle dorsiflexed and improve gait.
  - Proximal leg weakness results in difficulty with tasks such as getting up, transferring, or climb stairs.
    - Knee-ankle-foot orthoses (KAFOs) can stabilize the knee, but the weight of the orthoses can be a downside.
  - Leg spasticity results in difficulty moving the leg.
    - Anti-spastic medications or botulinum toxin injections can be used to mange severe spasticity.

**HIGH-YIELD FACT**

Foot drop is one of the most common causes of falls in neuromuscular diseases. AFOs often help.

- *Adaptive equipment for activities of daily living and upper extremity orthoses*
  - Hand weakness and intrinsic hand atrophy are common in ALS.
    - Hand weakness interferes with daily activities (e.g., grasping, pinching).
    - Special utensils (e.g., large-handled utensils, rocker knives, straw holders, plate guard, button-hook, zipper pull) can aid daily functions.
    - Speech-recognition applications on a smart phone, tablet or computer can be useful.
    - Guidance from an occupational therapist is crucial in selecting appropriate equipment and adaptations.
    - Hand orthoses such as a resting hand splint can help prevent flexion contractures in patients with intrinsic hand atrophy.
- *Management of musculoskeletal symptoms*
  - Patients can develop secondary pain and discomfort from disability, weakness, spasticity, malposition, and contractures.
  - Musculoskeletal pain, especially in the low back and neck regions are common.
  - Pharmacologic treatment
    - Pain: nonsteroidal anti-inflammatory drugs (NSAIDs) or neuropathic pain medications (e.g., gabapentin, pregabalin)
    - Spasticity: baclofen, tizanidine, or botulinum toxin injections
  - Non-pharmacologic treatment
    - Stretching exercises
    - Bracing for support
    - Application of heat or cold packs
    - Transcutaneous electrical nerve stimulation (TENS) therapy
- *Transfers*
  - When weakness has progressed, equipment for assisting with transfers is required to ensure patient safety and reduce the risk of musculoskeletal strain or injury.
    - Cushions, which allow the hips to be higher than the knees while sitting. Patients can stand up easier.
    - Power lift recliners or power lift chairs, which can assist patients in standing up and sitting down
    - Sliding boards, which help transfer patients from one surface to another
    - Transfer belts, which provide support and assistance during transfers
  - Proper caregiver education and training are essential for:
    - Proper technique
    - Patient safety
    - Caregiver safety
    - Avoiding musculoskeletal strain or injury from inappropriate transfers
    - Preventing caregiver burden
- *Assistive devices for ambulation*
  - The choice of assistive devices depend on the degree of lower-extremity weakness, as well as upper body and grip strength.
  - Cane or walkers (standard or wheeled)
    - Can be used if upper body and handgrip strength is preserved or relatively good
    - For four-wheeled walkers, a break system is essential. Push-down brakes may be easier to use compared to squeeze brakes for patients with handgrip weakness.
  - Wheelchair
    - Ultimately, most ALS patients will require a power wheelchair due to progression of leg weakness.
    - Coordination with a physical therapist is crucial in determining the appropriate assistive device.
    - A wheelchair can significantly improve a patient's quality of life.
    - To be eligible for a power wheelchair through Medicare, patients need to be certified that a power wheelchair is necessary to complete basic activities of daily living (ADLs) inside the house.
    - House and transportation adjustments such as ramps or lifts are needed, when patients become wheelchair dependent.
    - Home evaluation is recommended to ensure safety and accessibility.

- *Management of dysphagia and dysarthria*
  - Management of dysphagia
    - Evaluate swallowing function in collaboration with speech and language pathologists (SLPs).
    - Dieticians can also help with managing caloric intake and recommending nutritional supplements.
    - Early consideration of alternative routes (e.g., percutaneous endoscopic gastrostomy [PEG]) is recommended.
    - Higher rate of procedure-related and anesthesia-related complications of gastrostomy tube placement when the forced vital capacity (FVC) is <50% predicted. Thus the procedure is preferable when the FVC is >50% predicted.
    - Even though gastrostomy tube is placed, oral feeding for pleasure is still allowed.
  - Management of dysarthria
    - Speech therapists can help developing compensatory speech techniques.
    - Communication boards
    - Portable voice amplifiers
    - Text-to-speech applications on smart phones, tablets or computers
    - Message banking: recommended before patients become anarthric.
    - Augmentative and alternative communication (AAC) devices such as eye tracking technology

**QUESTION 4.** A 60-year-old man with amyotrophic lateral sclerosis (ALS) presented to the emergency department (ED) after a fall. His symptoms started in the right lower extremity 8 months ago. He had right foot drop, and recently weakness of the right hand. Today, he fell after tripping over the office floor with his right foot. Which of the following are two factors that increase the risk of falls in patients with ALS?

A. Spasticity and weakness of ankle dorsiflexion
B. Fatigue and dysarthria
C. Pseudobulbar affect and disinhibition
D. Ankle-foot orthoses and cane
E. Fasciculations and cramps

**ANSWER:** A. Spasticity and weakness of ankle dorsiflexion

**COMMENTS AND DISCUSSION (see also comments and discussion from Question 3)**
- Fall assessment and lower extremity orthoses are essential in patients with ALS and leg weakness.
- In patients with lower limb involvement, foot drop is very common.
- Patients with foot drop compensate with circumduction and hip hiking gait, which increases the risk of falls.
  - Ankle-foot orthoses (AFOs) keep the weak ankle dorsiflexed and improve gait.
- Proximal leg weakness results in difficulty with tasks such as getting up, transferring, or climbing stairs.
  - Knee-ankle-foot orthoses (KAFOs) can stabilize the knee, but the weight of the orthoses can be a downside.
- Leg spasticity results in difficulty moving the leg.
  - Anti-spastic medications or botulinum toxin injections can be considered.
- Cane can be considered when upper body and handgrip strength is preserved or relatively good.
- Fatigue, dysarthria, pseudobulbar affect, fasciculations, and cramps have no effects on falls.

**QUESTION 5.** A 62-year-old woman presents with a 6-month history of spasticity in both legs, and is diagnosed with primary lateral sclerosis. She has recently experienced multiple falls, and reports discomfort while using the walker due to backward falls. Which of the following statements is **CORRECT**?

A. While functional falls and weakness are concerns, spasticity without weakness does not cause falls.
B. Maintaining the patient on their feet using a cane or walker can prolong ambulation.
C. At least 10 falls per month is needed to be eligible for a power wheelchair.
D. Medicare eligibility for a power wheelchair requires its use to complete basic activities of daily living (ADLs) inside the house.
E. Without weakness, the patient is not Medicare eligible for a power wheelchair.

**ANSWER:** D. Medicare eligibility for a power wheelchair requires its use to complete basic activities of daily living (ADLs) inside the house.

### COMMENTS AND DISCUSSION (see also comments and discussion from Question 3)

- Assistive devices for ambulation should be selected based on the degree of lower extremity weakness and upper body/grip strength of the patient.
- Cane or walker (standard or wheeled)
  - Can be used when upper body and handgrip strength is preserved or relatively good
  - For four-wheeled walkers, a brake system is essential. In patients with handgrip weakness, push-down brakes may be easier to use compared to squeeze brakes.
- Wheelchair
  - Ultimately, most patients with ALS will require a power wheelchair due to progression of weakness.
  - Coordination with a physical therapist is crucial in determining the appropriate assistive device
  - A wheelchair can significantly improve a patient's quality of life.
  - To be eligible for a power wheelchair through Medicare, patients need to be certified that a power wheelchair is neccessary to complete basic activities of daily living (ADLs) inside the house.
  - House and transportation adjustments such as ramps or lifts are needed, when patients become wheelchair dependent.
  - Home evaluation is recommended to ensure safety and accessibility.

 **HIGH-YIELD FACT**

To be eligible for a power wheelchair through Medicare, an ALS patient needs to be certified that a power wheelchair is needed in order to complete basic activities of daily living (ADLs) **inside** the house.

**QUESTION 6.** Which of the following factors is associated with an increased risk of complications after percutaneous endoscopic gastrostomy (PEG) placement in patients with amyotrophic lateral sclerosis (ALS)?

A. Neck flexor weakness
B. Anarthria
C. Tongue atrophy
D. Forced vital capacity (FVC) <50%
E. None of the above

**ANSWER:** D. Forced vital capacity (FVC) <50%

### COMMENTS AND DISCUSSION

- Evaluation of swallowing function is done in collaboration with speech and language pathologists (SLPs).
- Dieticians can also help with managing caloric intake and recommending nutritional supplements.
- Early consideration of alternative routes (e.g., percutaneous endoscopic gastrostomy [PEG]) is recommended.
- There is a higher rate of procedural-related or anesthesia-related complications of gastrostomy tube placement when the FVC is <50% predicted. Thus the procedure is preferrable when the FVC is >50% predicted.
- Although gastrostomy tube is placed, oral feeding for pleasure is still allowed.

 **HIGH-YIELD FACT**

Consideration of alternative dietary routes (e.g., PEG) is recommended early, since complication rates tend to be higher when FVC is < 50% predicted.

**QUESTION 7.** A 55-year-old man presents to the neuromuscular clinic with a 3-year history of lower extremity weakness. He reports difficulty moving the left thigh while walking, resulting in near falls. He has also developed weakness of his grip in the past year. Examination demonstrates atrophy and severe weakness of the quadriceps and forearm flexors, worse on the left. What is the recommended treatment for this patient at this time?

A. Prednisolone
B. IVIG (intravenous immunoglobulin)
C. Rituximab
D. Power scooter
E. Left knee-ankle-foot orthoses

**ANSWER:** E. Left knee-ankle-foot orthoses

**COMMENTS AND DISCUSSION**

- The patient's clinical manifestations and profile are most consistent with inclusion body myositis (IBM).
- Clinical features of IBM include:
  o Typical onset after 45 years of age
  o Gradually progressive course over years
  o Muscle atrophy and weakness
    • Asymmetric involvement is common.
    • Pattern of weakness: predilection to the long finger flexors, quadriceps, and tibialis anterior
    • Atrophy of the ventral forearm and anterior thigh muscles
    • Dysphagia is often present.
- Due to quadriceps weakness, patients with IBM usually complain of knee buckling and instability when standing or walking.
- Knee-ankle-foot orthoses (KAFOs) can help stabilize the knee and prevent falls.
- A power scooter may be useful when patients experience falls.
- Treatment
  o Immunotherapies have failed to show improvement in several studies.
  o Once a diagnosis of IBM is made, immunotherapies are often discontinued.

**QUESTION 8.** A 55-year-old man with inclusion body myositis presents with foot drop and knee buckling. Which of the following equipment is the most beneficial in this case?

A. Plastic posterior leaf spring (PLS) ankle-foot orthoses
B. Floor-reaction orthoses
C. Non-ambulatory ankle-foot orthoses
D. Axillary crutch
E. Ankle brace

**ANSWER:** B. Floor-reaction orthoses

**COMMENTS AND DISCUSSION**

- In this case, the patient would benefit most from floor-reaction orthoses (FROs) as he has weakness in ankle dorsiflexion and knee extension (Table 21.1).

**TABLE 21.1** Comparison of different types of lower extremitiy orthoses.

| Lower extremity orthoses | Pros | Appropriate for | Cons |
|---|---|---|---|
| Posterior leaf spring (PLS) | • Lightweight<br>• Flexible<br>• Allows some plantar flexion during heel strike | Mild ankle dorsiflexion weakness | • Not good with spasticity<br>• Does not stabilize ankle in the medio-lateral direction |

*Continued*

**TABLE 21.1**  Comparison of different types of lower extremitiy orthoses—cont'd

| Lower extremity orthoses | Pros | Appropriate for | Cons |
|---|---|---|---|
| Hinged AFOs | • Easier for transferring from sitting to standing and climbing stairs<br>• With additional plantar flexion stop → prevent plantar flexion beyond the setting angle, → which can be useful in spasticity<br>• Helps stabilize the mediolateral movement of the ankle | Moderate ankle dorsiflexion weakness | • Requires good quadriceps strength |
| Solid AFOs | • Fixed position<br>• Help stabilize the mediolateral movement of the ankle<br>• Set at 5-degree plantar flexion angle → enhance knee stability<br>• Can be used with quadriceps weakness (in plantar flexion setting) | Severe ankle dorsiflexion weakness | • Due to fixed position, transferring from sitting to standing, climbing stairs and inclines are difficult<br>• Also requires good quadriceps strength |
| Floor-reaction orthoses (FROs) | • Utilize the ground spring reaction force to assist with propulsion by pushing off at toe-off<br>• Create knee extension → good with quadriceps weakness | Ankle dorsiflexion weakness with mild quadriceps weakness<br>Quadriceps and gastrocnemius weakness | Contraindicated in<br>• Severe hamstring spasticity<br>• Knee flexion contracture >20 degrees |
| KAFOs | • Control stability of the knee and ankle<br>• Good for quadriceps weakness<br>• Can be used in paraplegia (Craig-Scott KAFO) | Significant quadriceps and ankle dorsiflexion weakness | Heavy |

*AFO*, ankle-foot orthoses; *FROs*, floor-reaction orthoses; *KAFOs*, knee-ankle-foot orthoses.

- Ankle-foot orthoses (AFOs) are the most commonly prescribed orthoses by neuromuscular specialists.
  - AFOs are used in patients with foot drop or weakness of ankle dorsiflexion to improve gait function and safety, and prevent ankle plantar flexion contractures.
  - AFOs need to be customized by physical therapists and orthotists
  - Sessions of gait training can optimize gait with orthoses.
  - The use of hinged and solid AFOs requires good quadriceps strength.
- There are several differences between FROs and AFOs. FROs are designed to provide support for both the ankle and the knee, while AFOs primarily provide support for the ankle. In addition, FROs are typically used in patients with both ankle dorsiflexion and knee extension weakness, while AFOs are more commonly used for patients with isolated ankle dorsiflexion weakness.

## ◎ HIGH-YIELD POINT

Fixed ankle dorsiflexion → Helps stabilize the ankle but needs a strong quadriceps
Slight ankle plantar flexion → Enhances knee stability and can be used in mild quadriceps weakness

**QUESTION 9.** Your patient with neck extensor myopathy is experiencing worsening head drop, and asks for a recommendation to improve this symptom. What is the **BEST** course of action?

A. Refer him to orthopedics for cervical posterior fusion
B. Recommend baseball cap orthosis to keep the head up
C. Recommend a thoracic-lumbar-sacral orthosis (TLSO) to support the neck
D. Inject Botulinum toxin to the neck flexors to improve balance of the neck muscles
E. Reassure that there is no evidence-based treatment for head drop syndrome

**ANSWER:** B. Recommend a baseball cap orthosis to keep the head up

**COMMENTS AND DISCUSSION**

- Dropped head syndrome is characterized by marked flexion of the neck, which can be due to neuromuscular, orthopedic (e.g. severe cervical spondylosis) etiologies, or dystonic (i.e., overactivation of the neck flexors) etiologies. Neuromuscular dropped head syndrome is due to weakness of the neck extensor muscles, which can result from various causes, including:
  - Neck extensor myopathy
  - Myopathies affecting axial muscles such as sporadic late-onset nemaline myopathy
  - Amyotrophic lateral sclerosis (ALS)
  - Myasthenia gravis
  - Congenital myasthenic syndrome
- Head drop can cause difficulty with activities such as walking, reading, and swallowing
- The main treatment for dropped head syndrome is addressing the underlying cause of the weakness.
- Supportive measures can improve a patient's quality of life:
  - Orthoses (e.g., neck collars, head-up collar, baseball cap orthoses [Fig. 21.1]) can be helpful.
  - Thoracic-lumbar-sacral orthoses (TLSOs) can support the spine in cases of camptocormia or increased lordosis seen in congenial myopathy or chronic muscular dystrophy, but they are not indicated for head drop.
  - Botulinum toxin injections to the neck flexors are not recommended in dropped head syndrome due to weakness of the neck extensor muscles.

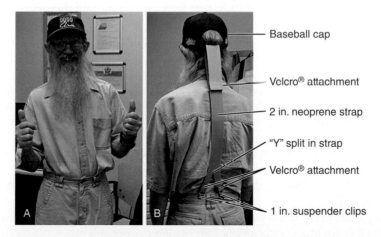

**Fig. 21.1** Baseball cap orthoses. Elastic head support system connecting the pants to the back of baseball cap, known as ("baseball cap orthosis") can help support head drop. From Hansen A, Bedore B, Nickel E, Hanowski K, Tangen S, Goldish G. Elastic head support for persons with amyotrophic lateral sclerosis. *J Rehabil Res Dev.* 2014;51(2):297–303.

## ETHICS IN NEUROMUSCULAR DISEASES

**QUESTION 10.** Your colleague asks you for the electromyography (EMG) result of his neighbor because his wife wants to know the diagnosis. Your colleague is not involved professionally in this patient's care. Which of the following statements is **CORRECT**?

A. Because your colleague is also a medical staff, the EMG result can be shared.
B. Without the patient's permission, all personal medical information is confidential.
C. You can discuss the case in the physician lounge, so your colleague can hear the result.

D. You can only share information with the patient's wife, since she is the person who wants to know the result.

E. You cannot share data verbally, but you can fax the report to your colleague.

**ANSWER:** B. Without the patient's permission, all personal medical information is confidential.

### COMMENTS AND DISCUSSION
- Patient privacy and confidentiality is of utmost importance.
- Personal medical information cannot be shared without permission from a patient or his/her medical power of attorney.
- Patient information can only be shared among medical professionals who are directly involved in the patient's care.

**QUESTION 11.** A 75-year-old woman with end-stage amyotrophic lateral sclerosis (ALS) appears fatigued and is using her accessory muscles for breathing. Her vital signs show a blood pressure (BP) of 100/70 mm Hg, a pulse of 105 bpm, and a respiratory rate of 26 per minute. During a previous clinic visit, you discussed with her issues about advanced life support, and she expressed her lack of interest in any assisted mechanical ventilation. What is the most appropriate step?

A. Respect her previous discussion and consult palliative care

B. Wait until she becomes confused and ask permission from her relatives to initiate assisted ventilation

C. Start a morphine intravenous (IV) drip

D. Refer her to the emergency department for intubation as she is at risk for respiratory collapse

E. Send her home without any new management.

**ANSWER:** A. Respect her previous discussion and consult palliative care

### COMMENTS AND DISCUSSION
- Autonomy is a one of the key ethical principles.
- Respecting patient autonomy while ensuring patient safety and promoting their best interests is essential.
- Patients have the right to make decisions affecting their health care, and they may change their decisions when their circumstances change.
- When a patient is competent to make a decision, it is unethical to ask relatives or intentionally wait until the patient becomes incompetent.

**QUESTION 12.** While you are busy performing needle electromyography (EMG) on a patient in the lab, your technologist informs you that another patient, who arrived later and is waiting for needle EMG in the other room, is complaining and wants to have the test done now. What is the most appropriate next step?

A. Have a neurology resident perform the needle EMG instead of you

B. Have the patient leave without the needle EMG

C. Stop the needle EMG of the current patient even though there are three more muscles to be tested.

D. Inform the patient that you are performing the test on another patient who arrived earlier, and that you will be with him for the needle EMG as soon as possible

E. Call the referring physician to discuss cancelling the test due to patient's inability to wait

**ANSWER:** D. Inform the patient that you are performing the test on another patient who arrived earlier, and that you will be with him for the needle EMG as soon as possible

### COMMENTS AND DISCUSSION
- Professional competence
  - Should perform the test within the scope of expertise
  - Perform the test under standard, well-established, evidence-based techniques and accepted interpretation
- Appropriate services
  - The physician is responsible for nerve conduction study examination even if it is performed by technicians.

- ○ All needle EMG examinations should be performed by a trained physician or trainee physician under supervision.
- ○ Needle EMG should *not* be performed by trainees without supervision.

**QUESTION 13.** A primary care physician refers a 35-year-old woman with right arm weakness to the electromyography (EMG) lab to rule out cervical radiculopathy. Upon pretest evaluation, the patient reports that weakness has recently progressed to the left arm. Examination reveals atrophy of the right arm and a "split hand" pattern of weakness and atrophy on the left. She has hyperreflexia throughout. She states that her grandfather passed away from Lou Gehrig's disease and hopes that she does not have the same. The EMG shows widespread denervation and reinnervation in both upper extremities and the thoracic paraspinal muscles. What is the best next step?
A. Make an appointment for her in your amyotrophic lateral sclerosis (ALS) clinic
B. Contact the referring physician about the result and recommend patient referral to the neuromuscular clinic
C. Refer the patient to another neuromuscular colleague
D. Send blood for genetic ALS testing
E. Suggest the patient to change her primary care physician, since the diagnosis of ALS is missed

**ANSWER:** B. Contact the referring physician about the result and recommend patient referral to the neuromuscular clinic.

## COMMENTS AND DISCUSSION

- The patient-physician relationship in electrodiagnostic medicine
  - ○ It is essential for an electrodiagnostic (EDX) physician to conduct a pretest clinical evaluation.
  - ○ If the pretest evaluation reveals that EMG is not necessary for patient care, the EDX physician could discuss with the referring physician directly before performing the test.
  - ○ After completion of the test, the EDX physician should relinquish the patient to the care of the referring physician unless the referring physician, patient, and EDX physician all agree that the EDX physician should take over the care of the patient.
  - ○ In the case of a potentially serious condition, direct communication to the referring physician is the appropriate behavior.
  - ○ Referring a patient to yourself or to others without permission from the primary care and/or referring physician is an unacceptable behavior.

**QUESTION 14.** A 25-year-old woman is referred to the electromyography (EMG) lab to confirm a diagnosis of myasthenia gravis. Before starting the test, you notice that the patient is dysarthric and short of breath. She states that 5 days prior she developed a urinary tract infection and has been taking antibiotics. Two days prior, she developed weakness of the neck, head drop, and difficulty breathing, especially when lying flat, and difficulty swallowing with food getting stuck in her throat. You are concerned that she is developing a myasthenic crisis. You try to contact her referring and primary care physician, but are unable to reach them. What is the best next step?
A. Send the patient home and recommend her to contact the referring/primary physician
B. Continue the test and then send the result to the referring physician
C. Discontinue the test and start the patient on pyridostigmine and prednisone
D. Complete the test and start the patient on pyridostigmine and prednisone
E. Send the patient to the emergency department

**ANSWER:** E. Send the patient to the emergency department

## COMMENTS AND DISCUSSION

- In an emergency or urgent situation, the needs of the patient must come first.
- The referring or primary care physician should be contacted if possible.
- If they are not accessible, it is the responsibility of the electrodiagnostic (EDX) physician to take appropriate measures to ensure that the patient receives proper care and remains safe.

## SUGGESTED READINGS

Abel NA, De Sousa EA, Govindarajan R, Mayer MP, Simpson DA. Guidelines for ethical behavior relating to clinical practice issues in neuromuscular and electrodiagnostic medicine. *Muscle Nerve*. 2015;52(6):1122-1129.

Abresch RT, Han JJ, Carter GT. Rehabilitation management of neuromuscular disease: the role of exercise training. *J Clin Neuromuscul Dis*. 2009;11(1):7-21.

American Association of Neuromuscular & Electrodiagnostic Medicine Ethics Committee. Guidelines for ethical behavior relating to clinical practice issues in neuromuscular and electrodiagnostic medicine. *Muscle Nerve*. 2022;65(4):391-399.

Fox JR, Lovegreen W. Lower limb orthoses. In: Webster JB, Murphy DP, eds. *Atlas of Orthoses and Assistive Devices*. 5th ed. Philadelphia: Saunders/Elsevier; 2019, Chap 22.

Hansen A, Bedore B, Nickel E, et al. Elastic head support for persons with amyotrophic lateral sclerosis. *J Rehabil Res Dev*. 2014;51(2):297-303.

Jorgensen S, Lau M, Arnold WD. Motor neuron disease. In: Cifu D, ed. *Branddom's Physical Medicine and Rehabilitation*. 6th ed. Philadelphia, PA: Saunders/Elsevier; 2021.

Khattak ZE, Ashraf M. McArdle disease. [Updated 2022 Jan 9]. In: *StatPearls* [Internet]. Treasure Island, FL: StatPearls Publishing; 2022 Jan.

Majmudar S, Wu J, Paganoni S. Rehabilitation in amyotrophic lateral sclerosis: why it matters. *Muscle Nerve*. 2014;50(1):4-13.

Novacheck TF, Kroll G, Rasmussen A. Orthoses for cerebral palsy. In: Webster JB, Murphy DP, eds. *Atlas of Orthoses and Assistive Devices*. 5th ed. Philadelphia, PA: Saunders/Elsevier; 2019.

Paganoni S, Ensrud E. The rehabilitation of neuromuscular diseases. In: Amato AA, Russell JA, eds. *Neuromuscular Disorders*. 2nd ed. New York, NY: McGraw Hill; 2016. Accessed March 27, 2022.

Voet NBM. Exercise in neuromuscular disorders: a promising intervention. *Acta Myol*. 2019;38(4):207-214.

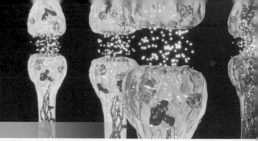

# INDEX

## A

Aα fiber, 38t

Aβ fiber, 38t

A-band, of sarcomere, during muscle contraction, 34, 45b, 48

*ABCA1* mutations, associated with Tangier disease, 411

Abductor digiti minimi (ADM), 8t, 9–11t
  forearm recording from, 349, 367

Abductor pollicis brevis, 8, 8t, 9–11t, 11

Abductor pollicis longus, lesion of posterior cord of brachial plexus, 310–314, 316

Abnormal jitter, in ocular myasthenia gravis, 146

Abnormal spontaneous activity, 78, 83, 84–85t

Accessory peroneal nerve, 72f, 161–162, 161f, 162b

Acetylcholine (ACh)
  iontophoresis of, 175
  in parasympathetic nervous system, 170, 172, 174b
  in quantitative sudomotor axon reflex test (QSART), 170, 175, 175f

Acetylcholine receptor antibody, for ocular myasthenia, 138

ACh vesicles, steps in exocytosis of, 421

AChR Abb, in myasthenia gravis, 424–425

Acid maltase deficiency, 224, 482, 535

Acid phosphatase, 190–191, 190f, 216, 216f, 222b

Acquired demyelinating peripheral polyneuropathy, 122, 380t

Acquired myopathies, 448–476

Acquired neuropathies, 347–352

Acquired peripheral polyneuropathies, 351, 379

*ACTA1* gene mutation, 189, 189f, 212, 212f

Actinin, 43

Action hand tremor, 396

Activation, in MUAPs, 98, 99b

Active (peripheral) denervation
  evidence of, 79, 89
  signs of, 102b

Acute cervical radiculopathy, 138

Acute flaccid myelitis, 303

Acute inflammatory demyelinating polyneuropathy (AIDP), 350, 373

Acute motor axonal neuropathy (AMAN), 124, 375, 378

Aδ fibers, 37b, 38t, 556, 558, 558b

Adductor brevis, 21–22t

Adductor gracilis, 21–22t

Adductor longus, 2, 19t, 21–22t, 23, 23t
  needle electromyography and, 313, 337, 337b

Adductor magnus, 3, 21–22t, 25

Adenosine triphosphatase (ATPase) stain, 222, 222b, 222f

ADM *see* Abductor digiti minimi

Adrenoreceptors, 172

Adult polyglucosan body disease (APBD), 240, 241f, 306f

Aerobic exercise
  for amyotrophic lateral sclerosis, 577
  for neuromuscular disease, 576

AFOs *see* Ankle-foot orthoses

Aγ fiber, 38t

Age
  conduction velocity and, 54, 76, 76b, 76f
  in nerve conduction study (NCS), 153

Agrin, in postsynaptic membrane, 415, 423

AIDP *see* Acute inflammatory demyelinating polyneuropathy

AIN *see* Anterior interosseous nerve

Aliasing, in electromyography, 51, 59, 60b, 60f

Alkaline phosphatase (ALP), 222, 222b
  elevation of, 464

All-ulnar hand, 54, 74

Allodynia, 354

Alpha-glucosidase, 482, 533

ALS *see* Amyotrophic lateral sclerosis

AMAN *see* Acute motor axonal neuropathy

Ambulation, assistive devices for, in amyotrophic lateral sclerosis, 578

Amiodarone, as amphiphilic drugs, 466

A-mode ultrasound (U/S), 251–252, 251f

Amorphous eosinophilic extracellular deposition, on nerve biopsy, 557, 565

Amphiphilic drugs, amphiphilic drug myopathy and, 466

Amplification, 55

Amplitude
  high-frequency filter and, 162
  morphology of, 97, 98b
  reduced, in axonal degeneration, 118, 118t, 124, 124t, 125f
  waning of, neuromyotonia, 80, 94

Amyloid neuropathy
  acquired forms of, 565, 565b
  causes of, 565
  diagnosis of, 240, 240b, 240f, 565
  hereditary form of, 566–567

Amyloidosis
  diagnosis of, 557
  transthyretin, treatment in, 567, 567f

Amyotrophic lateral sclerosis (ALS), 286f, 286t
  adaptive equipment for activities for, 578
  assistive devices for ambulation in, 578
  cervical spinal stenosis *versus*, 281, 287
  early-stage, aspects in, 577
  end-stage, 574
  exercise for, 577
  fall assessment and lower extremity orthoses in, 577
  familial percentage of, 283, 293
  forced vital capacity (FVC) in, 283, 297
  gastrostomy in, 283, 297, 297b
  genetics of, 294f
  middle- and end-stage, aspects in, 577
  multifocal motor neuropathy from, 282, 290
  muscle biopsy in, 191–192, 191f, 225, 225f
  musculoskeletal symptoms of, 578
  in nerve conduction studies, 287
  neuropathology of, 296f
  orthostatic hypotension and, 186

Amyotrophic lateral sclerosis *(Continued)*
  pathophysiology of, 296f
  patterns of weakness, 281, 287, 287b
  percutaneous endoscopic gastrostomy in, 574, 580, 580b
  rehabilitation in, 573, 577–579
  revised El Escorial criteria for, 289t
  risk of falls in, 573, 579
  transfers in, 578

Anconeus
  in differentiating lesion locations, 18t
  innervation of, 30t

Andersen-Tawil syndrome, 543, 543b, 543f

Angiokeratoma, 570f

Anisotropy, 246, 262, 262b, 263f, 265

Ankle dorsiflexion, spasticity and weakness of, 573, 579

Ankle-foot orthoses (AFOs), 576–577, 581–582t

Ankle inversion, 27
  common peroneal neuropathy and, 349, 369
  L5 radiculopathy and, 314, 314b, 343, 343b

Ankle reflex, 396

Anoctaminopathy, 478, 497, 498b

Anterior axillary line, 248, 277

Anterior interosseous nerve (AIN), 8t, 13, 13b
  lesion of, 348, 364
  "OK" sign in, 13, 14f

Anterior interosseous neuropathy, 364f

Anti-3-hydroxy-3-methylglutaryl coenzyme A reductase (anti-HMGCR), 460–461

Anti-cytosolic 5'-nucleotidase 1A (anti-cN1a), 448, 451, 454
  in inclusion body myositis, 448, 456, 460

Anti-HMG-CoA reductase (anti-HMGCR) antibody syndrome, 449, 462

Anti-HU (ANNA-I) antibodies, elevated, 351, 386

Anti-Jo-1, 449, 459

Anti-MDA-5, 459

Anti-Mi-2, 192–193, 192f, 228, 228f
  in classic dermatomyositis, 459, 460

Anti-microtubular myopathy, medications causing, 466

Anti-myelin-associated glycoprotein (MAG) neuropathy, electron microscopic finding in, 242–243, 243f

Anti-myostatin antibody, 488

Anti-NXP-2
  associated with calcinosis cutis, 459
  in dermatomyositis, 460

Anti-signal recognition particle (anti-SRP), 461

Anti-synthetase syndrome, 452, 460
  clinical features of, 460
  diagnosis in, 449f, 459, 459f

Anti-TIF1γ, 448, 459

Antibiotics, for trigger myasthenic crisis, 429

Anticholinergic agents, QSART and, 177

Antidromic sensory recording, 167, 167t

Antidromic technique, for sensory studies, 52, 59t, 63

Antisense oligonucleotide (ASO), 488, 488t